Practical 3D Echocardiography

Joseph F. Maalouf
Francesco F. Faletra
Samuel J. Asirvatham
Krishnaswamy Chandrasekaran
Editors

Practical 3D Echocardiography

Springer

Editors
Joseph F. Maalouf
Rochester, MN, USA

Francesco F. Faletra
Lugano, Switzerland

Samuel J. Asirvatham
Rochester, MN, USA

Krishnaswamy Chandrasekaran
Rochester, MN, USA

ISBN 978-3-030-72940-0 ISBN 978-3-030-72941-7 (eBook)
https://doi.org/10.1007/978-3-030-72941-7

This Springer imprint is published by the registered company Springer Nature Switzerland AG
The registered company address is: Gewerbestrasse 11, 6330 Cham, Switzerland

Preface

The ultimate goal of any imaging modality is to present cardiac anatomy and pathology in a three-dimensional (3D) format that faithfully depicts the dynamic in vivo morphology fundamental to accurate diagnosis for optimal therapy. Over the past two decades, giant strides were made in the field of 3D echocardiography (3DE) due in large part to the tremendous advances in computer technology coupled to the miniaturization of electronic circuitry. This enabled the development of the fully sampled matrix array transducer, a milestone in the history of 3DE and currently the basis for all 3DE imaging platforms.

With 3DE, it is possible to obtain en face views of an entire region of interest from a single acoustic window with little probe manipulation. The images obtained can be viewed in multiple perspectives and are readily appreciated by non-imaging cardiologists and cardiac surgeons. As a result, 3DE has become essential for the diagnosis of a host of cardiac diseases including the entire spectrum of native and prosthetic mitral valve pathologies, aortic valve perforations, and atrial septal defects. Moreover, because catheters, devices, and wires are better seen in the 3D space than in the 2D space, 3DE, and mainly three-dimensional transesophageal echocardiography (3D TEE), has emerged as an indispensable tool to guide many catheter-based interventions with a particular emphasis on mitral interventions. A thorough appreciation of cardiac anatomy and pathology is a major prerequisite for 3D imaging. We, therefore, used a correlative approach to 3D imaging that incorporates anatomically correct spatial orientation of images in normal and disease states.

3DE is also increasingly assuming a quantitative role. By eliminating the need for speculative geometric assumptions, a major limitation of 2D echocardiography, three-dimensional transthoracic echocardiography (3D TTE) is currently being routinely used for the quantitation of left ventricular chamber volumes and function. Moreover, quantitative analysis of the 3D volumetric data set is assuming a greater role in the morphologic and physiologic assessments of stenotic and regurgitant lesions to guide surgical or catheter-based therapies; these include transcatheter mitral or tricuspid valve repair, and aortic and mitral valve-in-native or prosthetic valve implantation. Additionally, 3D TEE is used to guide percutaneous left atrial appendage occlusion in patients with atrial fibrillation. These added quantitative values of 3D are amplified by recent developments in fully automatic quantification algorithms and "artificial intelligence," which make 3D quantification easy, fast, and reproducible.

This book, which draws on the extensive experience in 3DE at Mayo Clinic and Cardiocentro Ticino, is written in a practical user-friendly format to guide 3D imaging in daily practice and addresses the needs and concerns of both novice and experienced 3D echocardiographers by providing a best practice methodology to 3D imaging (what to look for, how to look for, optimal views, etc.) including caveats, pitfalls, and limitations. It is written in a highly instructive practical disease and problem-oriented approach that is supported by illustrative high-quality images (and supplemental video clips where applicable) and includes cases that demonstrate the incremental value of 3DE over 2D echocardiography. Additionally, a step-by-step approach to image acquisition and optimization is utilized and includes clinical pearls, pointers, and the navigation of complicated vendor-specific 3D "knobology" that has made even the most experienced echocardiographers weary of embracing this technology. For beginners in 3D echocardiography, we strongly urge you to start exploring the imaging capabilities of the matrix array transducer, and in the process to appreciate its immense value as a diagnostic tool. For all others, we hope that the information provided in this book will be useful in your daily practice.

Rochester, MN	Joseph F. Maalouf
Lugano, Switzerland	Francesco F. Faletra
Rochester, MN	Samuel J. Asirvatham
Rochester, MN	Krishnaswamy Chandrasekaran

Contents

Editors and Contributors

Editors

Joseph F. Maalouf, MD, FAHA, FACC, FASE, maalouf.joseph@mayo.edu Professor of Medicine, Mayo Clinic College of Medicine; Director, Interventional Echocardiography; Consultant, Department of Cardiovascular Medicine, Mayo Clinic, Rochester, MN, USA

Francesco F. Faletra, MD, Francesco.Faletra@cardiocentro.org Director of Cardiac Imaging Lab, Cardiocentro Ticino Institute, Lugano, Switzerland

Samuel J. Asirvatham, MD, Asirvatham.Samuel@mayo.edu James M. and Lee S. Vann Professorship in Cardiovascular Diseases; Consultant, Department of Cardiovascular Medicine; Division of Pediatric Cardiology, Department of Anatomy & Department of Physiology and Biomedical Engineering; Professor of Medicine and Pediatrics; Mayo Clinic College of Medicine; Vice Chair, Innovation in the Midwest; Program Director, EP Fellowship Program; Medical Director, Electrophysiology Laboratory, Mayo Clinic, Rochester, MN, USA

Krishnaswamy Chandrasekaran, MD, FACC, FASE, KChandra@mayo.edu Professor of Medicine, Mayo Clinic College of Medicine; Consultant, Department of Cardiovascular Medicine, Mayo Clinic, Rochester, MN, USA

Contributors

Nandan S. Anavekar, MB, BCh, Anavekar.Nandan@mayo.edu Professor of Medicine, Mayo Clinic College of Medicine; Consultant, Department of Cardiovascular Medicine, Mayo Clinic, Rochester, MN, USA

Htin Aung, aung.htin@mayo.edu Cardiovascular Disease, Mayo Clinic, Rochester, MN, USA

Jared G. Bird, MD, bird.jared@mayo.edu Instructor of Medicine, Mayo Clinic College of Medicine, Senior Associate Consultant, Department of Cardiovascular Medicine, Mayo Clinic, Rochester, MN, USA

Thomas A. Foley, MD, Foley.Thomas@mayo.edu Assistant Professor of Radiology, Mayo Clinic College of Medicine; Consultant, Division of Cardiovascular Radiology, Department of Radiology, Mayo Clinic, Rochester, MN, USA

Elisa Gherbesi, MD, elisa.gherbesi@cardiocentro.org Cardiac Imaging Lab, Cardiocentro Ticino Institute, Lugano, Switzerland

Pedrazzini Giovanni, MD, pedrazzini.giovanni@cardiocentro.org Professor, Division of Cardiology, Cardiocentro Ticino Institute, Lugano, Switzerland

S. Yen Ho, yen.ho@imperial.ac.uk Professor, Cardiac Morphology Unit, Royal Brompton Hospital and Imperial College, London, UK

Tae-Yop Kim, MD, Ph.D., Professor, Research institute of Medical Science, Konkuk University School of Medicine, Department of Cardiovascular Medicine, Konkuk University Medical Center, Neungdong-ro, Gwangjin-gu, Seoul, Korea

Laura A. Leo, MD, lauraanna.leo@cardiocentro.org Cardiac Imaging Lab, Cardiocentro Ticino Institute, Lugano, Switzerland

Sushil Allen Luis, MBBS, FRACP, FACC, FASE, Luis.S@mayo.edu Associate Professor of Medicine, Mayo Clinic College of Medicine; Consultant, Rochester, MN, USA

Joseph J. Maleszewski, MD, FCAP, FACC, Maleszewski.Joseph@mayo.edu Professor of Laboratory Medicine & Pathology, College of Medicine & Science; Professor of Medicine, College of Medicine & Science; Section Head, Cardiovascular Pathology; Consultant, Departments of Laboratory Medicine & Pathology, Cardiovascular Medicine, and Medical Genomics, Mayo Clinic, Rochester, MN, USA

Vera L. Paiocchi, MD, vera.paiocchi@cardiocentro.org Cardiac Imaging Lab, Cardiocentro Ticino Institute, Lugano, Switzerland

Francois Regoli, MD PhD, francois.regoli@cardiocentro.org Division of Arrhythmology and Electrophysiology, Cardiocentro Ticino Institute, Lugano, Switzerland

Prajwal Reddy, reddy.prajwal@mayo.edu Cardiovascular Disease, Mayo Clinic, Rochester, MN, USA

Susanne A. Schlossbauer, MD, Susanne.schlossbauer@cardiocentro.org Cardiac Imaging Lab, Cardiocentro Ticino Institute, Lugano, Switzerland

Korosh Sharain, MD, Sharain.Korosh@mayo.edu Assistant Professor in Medicine, Mayo Clinic College of Medicine; Resident, Department of Cardiovascular Medicine, Mayo Clinic, Rochester, MN, USA

Jeremy J. Thaden, MD, FASE, Thaden.Jeremy@mayo.edu Assistant Professor of Medicine, Mayo Clinic College of Medicine; Co-Chair for Clinical Practice and Quality, Division of Cardiovascular Ultrasound; Consultant, Department of Cardiovascular Medicine, Mayo Clinic, Rochester, MN, USA

Marco Valgimigli, Prof, MD, PhD, marco.valgimigli@cardiocentro.org Professor, Division of Cardiology, Cardiocentro Ticino Institute, Lugano, Switzerland

Hyun Suk Yang, MD, Ph.D., yang.hyun@kuh.ac.kr Professor, Research institute of Medical Science, Konkuk University School of Medicine, Department of Cardiovascular Medicine, Konkuk University Medical Center, Neungdong-ro, Gwangjin-gu, Seoul, Korea

Kathleen A. Young, MD, Young.Kathleen1@mayo.edu Instructor in Medicine, Mayo Clinic College of Medicine; Resident, Department of Cardiovascular Medicine, Mayo Clinic, Rochester, MN, USA

Part I

Basic, Practical Principles of 3D Echocardiography

Imaging Principles and Acquisition Modes

1

Joseph F. Maalouf and Francesco F. Faletra

The concept of visualizing the heart by using ultrasound imaging evolved in the fifth decade of the twentieth century, when the engineer Helmut Hertz and the cardiologist Inge Edler obtained the first echo images of the heart with an ultrasonic machine used in the industry setting to detect flaws in metals.

The first ultrasound image of the heart was displayed in ***A-mode*** (A = amplitude). The returning echoes were represented as sharp deflections of the main signal appearing as spikes of different heights. The intensity of echoes determined the height of the spikes and the time necessary for the ultrasound wave to reach the structure of interest and to return to the probe determined the interval between spikes. These spikes were displayed on an oscilloscope and documented by a Polaroid instant camera. The main limitation of A-mode consisted in the fact that, while the operator could see the spikes moving within the oscilloscope, the photograph failed to capture this motion. A mode was shortly superseded by another modality: ***B-mode*** (B = Brightness) where the returning ultrasound echoes were represented by dots rather than spikes and the intensity of the signal was proportional to the brightness of the dots. This modality would have undergone the same ignominious destiny of A-mode, had it not been for an ingenious and unknown engineer who had the idea to record the dot's motion on a strip-chart recorder. This modality, called M-*mode* (M for Motion), became for many years the "state-of-the-art" of echocardiography. The classic "M" shape of the anterior leaflet of the mitral valve with its E and A waves, the "box" of the aortic valve opening, the flat slope characteristic of mitral stenosis, the thickening of the posterior wall of the left ventricle and several other "classic" M-mode features were significant contributions to the history of echocardiography. Several books have been written on acquired and congenital cardiac diseases using this modality. Feigenbaum coined the name "echocardiography" to reflect ultrasound imaging of the heart as opposed to other organs such as the brain (echoencephalography).

Two Dimensional Echocardiography

Two-dimensional transthoracic echocardiography (2D-TTE) was introduced in the 1970s and represented a major step in the evolution of echocardiography. In fact, for the first time in its history, two-dimensional (2D) imaging showed cross-sectional images that approximated sections of pathological specimens, thus replacing the undulating waves of M-mode echocardiography.

As illustrated in Fig. 1.1, a 2D image sector is built up pulse line by line, by emitting an ultrasound pulse, waiting for the reflected echoes to return to the transducer, before tilting the beam and emitting the next ultrasound pulse. The time to generate the image therefore, is contingent on the **number of pulse lines** emitted, the **depth of the image sector** and the **image sector width**. The **frame rate** is the number of 2D images per second and determines the **temporal resolution**. Pulse line density is an important determinant of the image detail or **spatial resolution** which is highest in the near field where the ultrasound beam is narrow and pulse line density is maximal, and is lowest in the far field because of dispersion of the ultrasound beam. With 2D imaging, the ultrasound beam can be steered in two dimensions (vertical also referred to as axial or y-axis, and lateral also referred to as azimuthal or x-axis). Resolution in the elevation

Supplementary Information The online version of this chapter (https://doi.org/10.1007/978-3-030-72941-7_1) contains supplementary material, which is available to authorized users.

J. F. Maalouf (✉)
Professor of Medicine, Mayo Clinic College of Medicine; Director, Interventional Echocardiography; Consultant, Department of Cardiovascular Medicine, Mayo Clinic, Rochester, MN, USA
e-mail: maalouf.joseph@mayo.edu

F. F. Faletra
Director of Cardiac Imaging Lab, Cardiocentro Ticino Institute, Lugano, Switzerland
e-mail: Francesco.Faletra@cardiocentro.org

J. F. Maalouf et al. (eds.), *Practical 3D Echocardiography*, https://doi.org/10.1007/978-3-030-72941-7_1

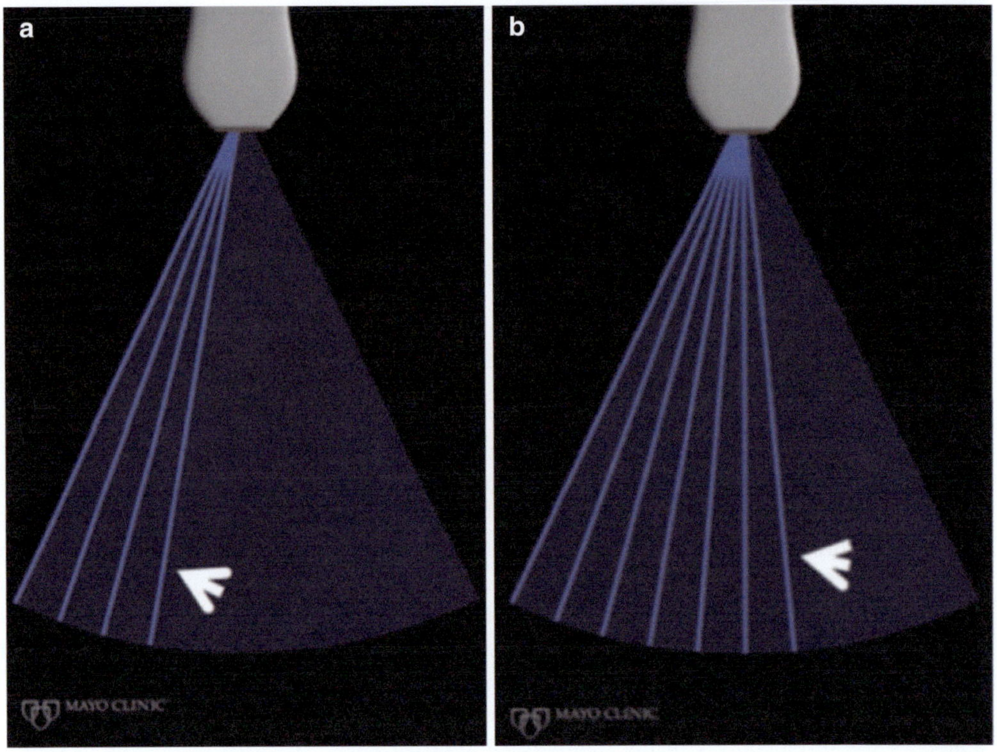

Fig. 1.1 (**a**, **b**) 2D image generation. Arrows point to leading ultrasound pulse line. Used with permission of Mayo Foundation for Medical Education and Research. All rights reserved

(antero-posterior) dimension also referred to as z-axis is fixed by the thickness of the tomographic slice.

An explosion of other evolutionary steps followed. Within few years, mechanical scanners were replaced by more flexible electronic scanners and the early 1980s witnessed the introduction of ***second harmonic imaging***, with a tremendous improvement in the quality of 2D imaging.

Two-dimensional transesophageal echocardiography (2D-TEE) represented further improvement. The dramatic success of such a modality was mainly due to the fact that 2D TEE images had a quality that was superior to that of 2D TTE, due to lack of interference with image acquisition by the interposition of the lungs and chest wall tissues, and use of high-frequency transducers. The first 2D-TEE probe was monoplane (i.e. a single transducer scanning through one single transverse plane), but a bi-plane 2D-TEE probe (with two transducers scanning through two orthogonal planes) soon became available. Multiplane 2D-TEE was a logical advancement that allowed continuous visualization of cardiac structures initially through manual and eventually through electronic steering of the ultrasound beam through 180°. 2D-TEE allowed the visualization of anatomic structures such as the left atrial appendage (LAA) and pulmonary veins that otherwise could not be seen or did not lend themselves to adequate visualization using 2D-TTE. Of note that currently one of the most frequent indications for 2D-TEE is the exclusion of thrombus within the LAA prior to cardioversion or atrial fibrillation ablation. Moreover, the ability of multiplane 2D-TEE to view cardiac structures in multiple sequential adjacent planes provided a better understanding of the spatial relationship of normal cardiac structures and a deeper insight into the complex morphology of cardiac diseases. Because the TEE probe is inserted into the esophagus and hence does not invade the sterile operative field, intraoperative TEE during cardiac surgery emerged as an invaluable imaging tool to plan the surgical strategy, assess the operative results and guide anesthetic management. It was soon evident that the routine use of TEE during cardiac surgery was beneficial, reduced patient morbidity, and was cost-effective in the mid-term.

Doppler echocardiography was a concomitant amazing evolutionary development. The capability of the Doppler phenomenon to register differences in ultrasound wave frequency (the so-called "Doppler shift") of a moving target opened the door to an impressively wide array of clinical applications. Furthermore, with its different modalities [i.e. continuous (CW), pulsed (PW) waves and eventually color Doppler] Doppler echocardiography allowed, for the first time, the assessment and quantification of valve gradients and the "visualization" of valve regurgitation. By providing reliable data on most hemodynamic parameters, such as cardiac output, diastolic filling pressure, vascular resistances and pulmonary arterial pressures, Doppler echocardiography became the main non-invasive modality to determine the hemodynamic profile of patients with any type of coronary, myocardial or valve pathology.

Contrast echocardiography using sonicated gases became clinically available in the late 1980s. The venous injection of microbubbles which were able to cross the pulmonary circulation and to reach the left heart chambers, were used for better delineation of the endocardial contour, thus allowing both a more precise quantitative assessment of left ventricular (LV) volumes, especially in obese patients, and better discrimination of intraventricular masses and thrombi and, to some extent, myocardial perfusion. At the same time, *Stress echocardiography* emerged as the most cost-effective method to evaluate patients with suspected coronary artery disease and to assess the ischemic burden of intermediate coronary stenosis and the hemodynamic significance of moderate valvular heart disease.

Doppler tissue imaging (DTI) and speckle tracking emerged into the clinical arena in the late 1990s. DTI conceptually derived from Doppler technology, measures myocardial rather than blood velocity. A few years later this technique, despite several limitations, became integral to the routine echocardiographic examination providing relevant data on systolic and diastolic function. *Speckle tracking* was a completely new technology. By tracking speckles (i.e. the agglomerate of echocardiographic dots which form the 2D texture of the myocardium), this new technique could detect subtle changes in myocardial deformation. Longitudinal, radial and circumferential deformations and their changes in the setting of several pathological states were extensively studied providing new insights into myocardial mechanics.

Three Dimensional Echocardiography (3DE)

The ultimate goal of any imaging modality is to image in a three dimensional (3D) format because the image generated closely reflects true anatomy or pathology (Fig. 1.2).

Therefore, whereas a 2D image represents a tomographic slice of a region of interest through one of the three primary planes of the heart (frontal or coronal, transverse, vertical or sagittal), a 3D image encompasses the entire region of interest (Fig. 1.3).

The first attempts to produce ultrasound images in a 3D format date back to the 1970s. The first 3D images required an extensive off-line reconstruction from consecutive serial cross-sectional images. A short-lived attempt in the application of 3D imaging in clinical practice involved *transthoracic free-hand scanning*. A series of adjacent 2D tomographic slices were obtained by manually tilting the transducer in one direction. A magnetic field transmitter was positioned near the patient's bed. The transmitter generated a spherical electromagnetic field that exceeded the earth magnetic field by five times. An electromagnetic receiver was attached directly to a standard ultrasound transthoracic transducer. The transducer could therefore, move freely in the hemisphere generated by the transmitter and its position was recorded into a 3D coordinate Cartesian system. This provided information as to exactly where the image plane was being acquired. The images were thus assembled (according to the transducer position) to form a 3D image. Free-hand 3D echocardiography was able to provide diagnostic 3D images of both acquired and congenital heart diseases (Fig. 1.4) as well as to determine the volumes of the left cardiac chambers.

An alternative to the free-hand method was the application of a *mechanical driven rotating transducer*, which captured sequential 2D slices by pivoting around a fixed axis in a rotational fanlike manner. Because the intervals between slices and volumetric data set were more uniformly sampled than with the free-hand scanning, diagnostic 3D images were more consistently obtained. However, both systems provided an average quality of imaging which was by far inferior to

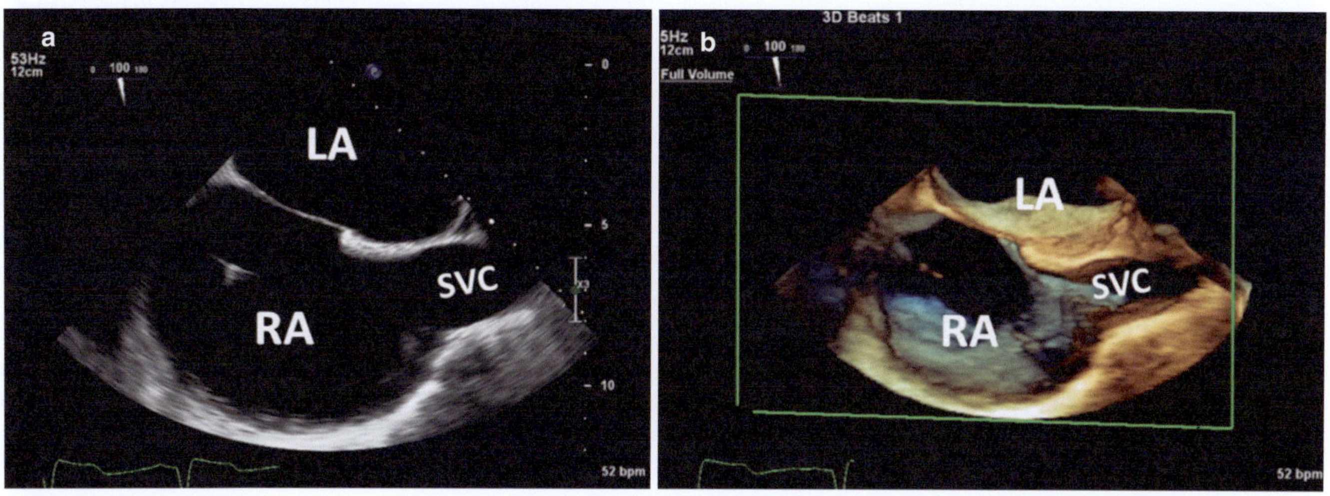

Fig. 1.2 (**a**) 2D TEE bicaval view. (**b**) 3D TEE of same 2D view. Note the added depth to all structures in the image. LA, left atrium; RA, right atrium; SVC, superior vena cava. Used with permission of Mayo Foundation for Medical Education and Research. All rights reserved

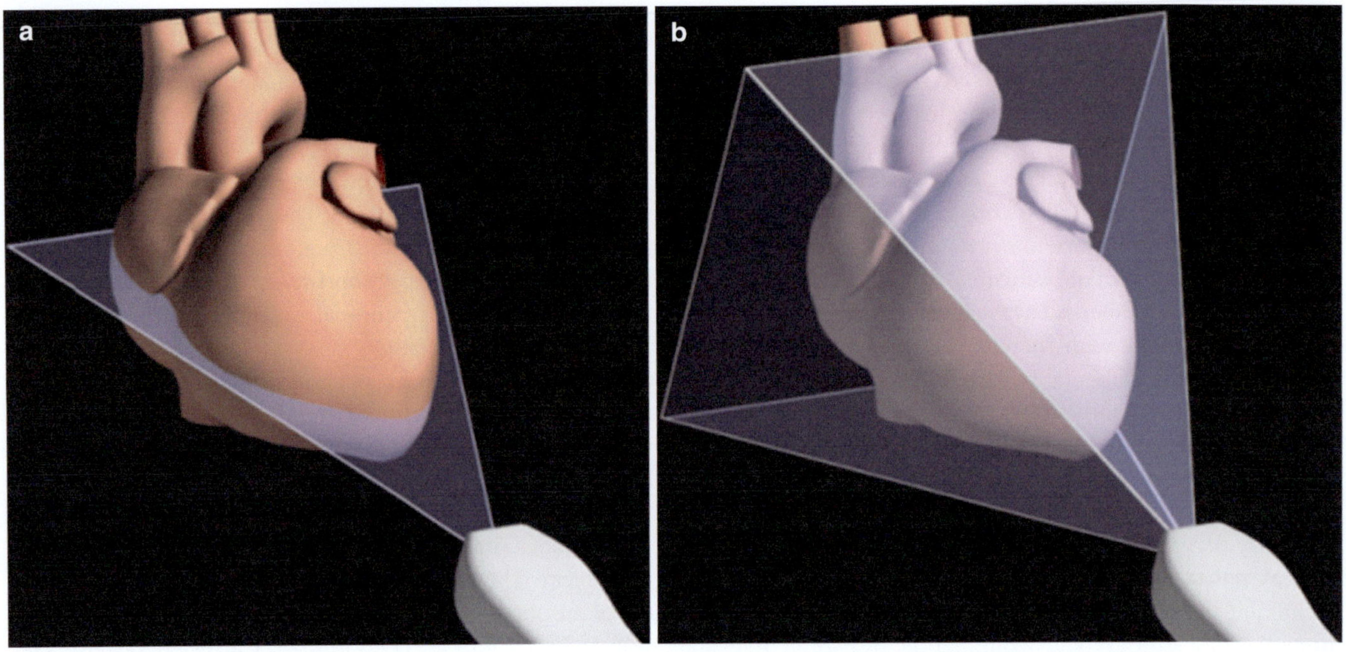

Fig. 1.3 Schematic diagrams of 2D (**a**) versus 3D (**b**) acquisition. Used with permission of Mayo Foundation for Medical Education and Research. All rights reserved

that of 2D-TTE and therefore, they were seldom used in clinical practice. Both free hand and rotational 3D-TTE were shortly removed from the echocardiographic armamentarium. *The transesophageal rotational system* was the only one that provided 3D reconstruction of valuable and "diagnostic" images due to the high quality of the original 2D slices. Respiratory and ECG gating were used to capture only those slices coinciding with a specific phase of the respiratory cycle and within the preset limits of the R-R interval, thus minimizing spatial and temporal malalignment of the 2D tomographic slices due to respiration and heart rate variability (stitching artifacts) (Fig. 1.5).

The Matrix Revolution

The aforementioned technique would certainly have remained the "state of art" of 3D echocardiography for many years had it not been for the unexpected "evolutionary leap" in 3D transducer technology that occurred shortly afterwards. An innovative new transducer architecture, the matrix array probe emerged whereby piezoelectric crystals are arranged in rows and columns, instead of in a single row (as is the case in two-dimensional transducers) thus forming a "pyramidal-shaped" beam. This matrix array architecture allowed electronical scanning of a 3D volume in multiple planes thus embracing a volumetric 3D space.

The Sparse Array Matrix Transducer

The "sparse" array matrix transducer was the first product of this new generation of transducers. This first transthoracic transducer had a number of limitations and was ultimately short-lived. Although the number of crystals that was technically feasible to assemble in one matrix was relatively low (289 crystals), the transducer had a large footprint which did not fit in the intercostal spaces. Moreover, if each crystal were to have its own electrical connection, the transducer cable would have been extremely large and commercially unrealistic. To overcome this limitation, engineers devised a method whereby only a percentage of crystals in the "sparse" array matrix transducer are electrically connected and acoustically active, thus allowing the connecting cable to have a more "realistic" size. However, this technical solution implied an unacceptable degradation in image quality due to reduced number of crystals transmitting and receiving ultrasound data, which eventually resulted in a loss of signal-to-noise ratio (the ratio of the strength of the desired signal carrying information to that of noise interference hence image quality). Moreover, this transducer, with only a fraction of transmitted crystals, was not able to generate waveforms of sufficient pressures to create harmonic echoes. In summary, the quality of 2D images was worse as compared to traditional 2D probes. Last but not least, while the transducer was able to simultaneously generate different tomo-

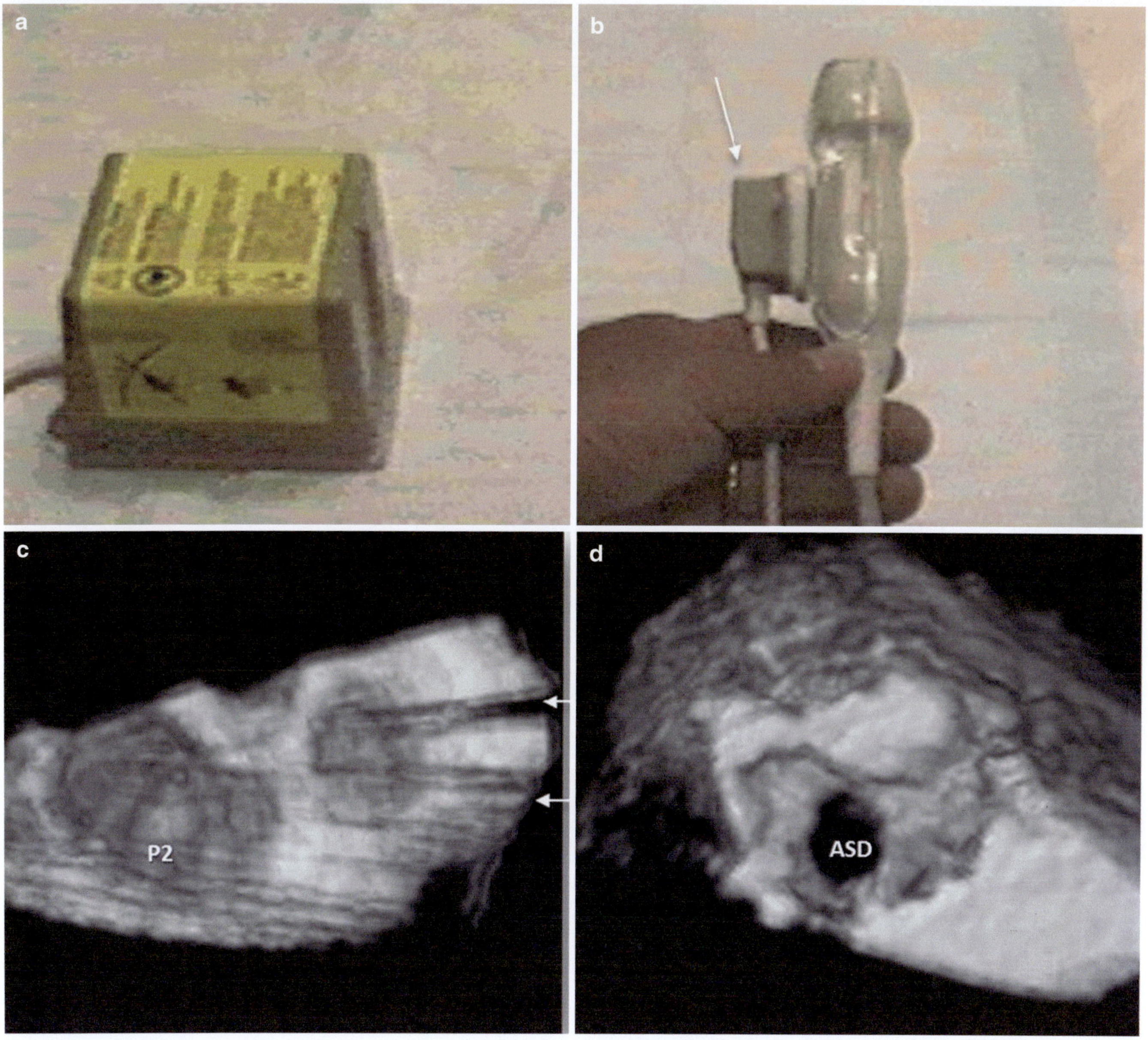

Fig. 1.4 Transthoracic "free-hand" 3D echocardiography (TTE). (**a**) Magnetic field generator. (**b**) A spatial magnetic locator attached to the transducer (arrow), recorded the transducer position into the 3D coordinate Cartesian system. (**c**) 3D TTE image of a P2 flail. Please note the gaps between slices (arrows) due to different time intervals between slices. (**d**) 3D TTE image of an atrial septal defect (ASD) recorded from a subcostal window

graphic cutting planes, it was not capable of displaying real-time surface rendered 3D images. For all these reasons, the "sparse" phased-array matrix transducer was very soon rejected by clinicians and, consequently, abandoned by manufacturers. Nevertheless, the probe had the theoretical advantage of being the first of a new class of transducers, in which a single ultrasound scanner could operate in two imaging planes simultaneously. In other words, for the first time, the word "scan", referred to the transducer location with respect to the patient, as opposed to "view" (i.e. which slice within the pyramidal data set is displayed).

Current Matrix Array Transducers

The ensuing decade witnessed the development of a new generation of piezoelectric crystals, and further advances in the crystals' manufacturing process. The ultimate miniatur-

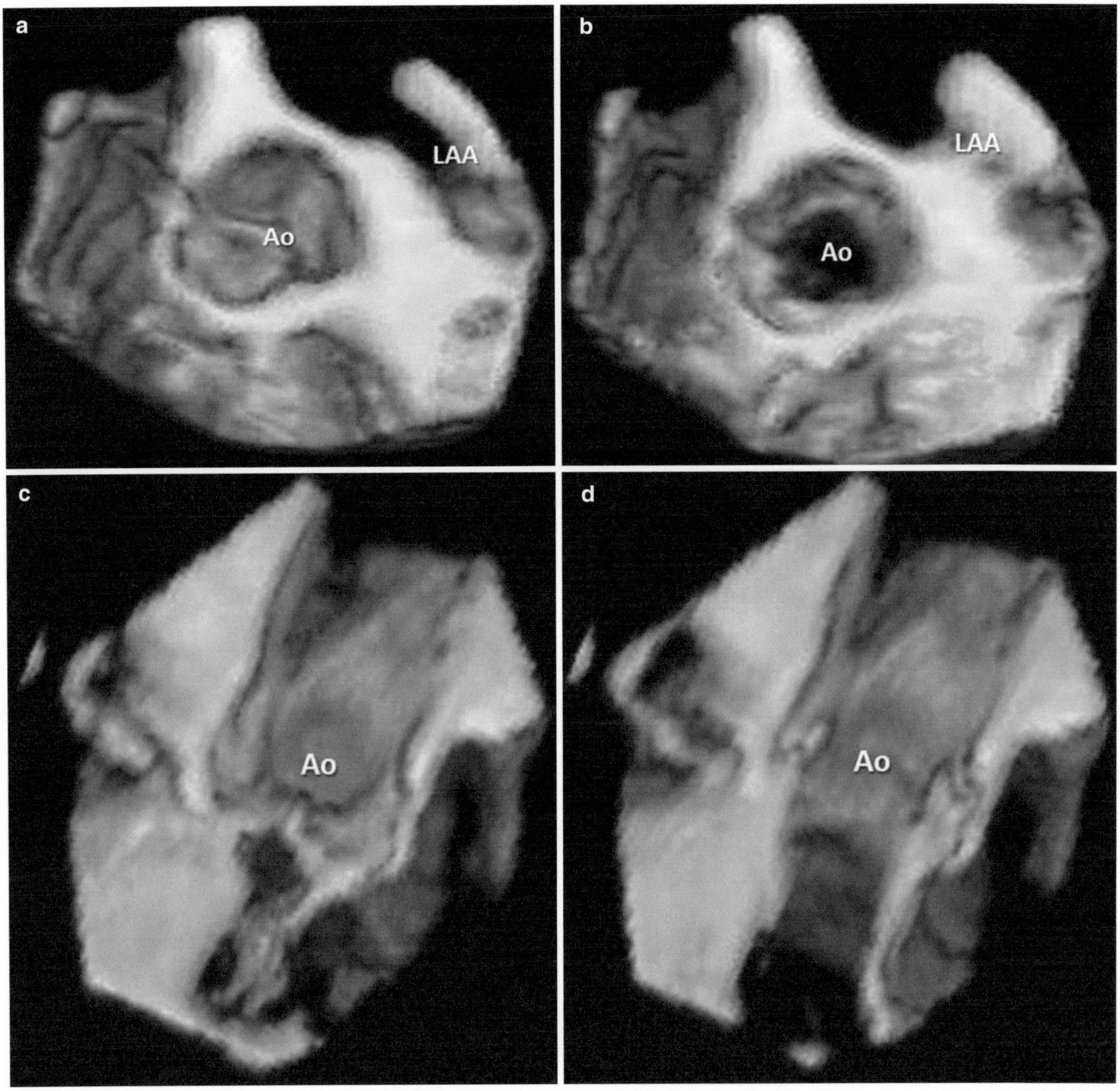

Fig. 1.5 (**a**, **b**) 3D transesophageal rotational echocardiography showing a normal aortic valve (Ao) in short axis view in (**a**) diastole and (**b**) systole. (**c**, **d**) Same patient in long axis view in (**c**) diastole and (**d**) systole. LAA, left atrial appendage

ization of electronic circuitry and tremendous advances in computer technology led to the real time 3DE we have today.

The New Generation of Piezoelectric Crystals

Some material have a "piezoelectric" capability, which means that they change their volume and shape when appropriately placed in an alternating electrical field. The mechanical deformation depends upon the disposition of highly polarized particles (dipole) in the material. Such particles have a polar axis (i.e. the imaginary line in the center of the dipole). In a monocrystalline material all the particles (and hence, the polar axis) lie in one direction. This crystalline material is believed to be symmetric. The polycrystalline compounds are, on the contrary, asymmetric since particles lie in different directions in different regions within the material. When this material is subjected to a strong electrical field, particles tend to be oriented perpendicularly to the surface of the material (polarization) causing an expansion of the polycrystalline material. A rapid on-off of the electrical field produces rapid changes both in volume and shape. These mechanical vibrations generate compression and rarefaction of the same frequency in the surrounding medium, creating sound waves. The same material also has the opposite propriety: when mechanical stress is applied, it generates an electrical charge proportional to the strength of the mechanical stress. When all the electrical energy is converted to mechanical energy, the electro-mechanical coupling is 100%. It is well known that electro-mechanical coupling is of paramount relevance for the quality of an image. These groups of piezoelectric crystals are made from ceramic. These crystals contain natural impurities and boundaries between different areas of the same element. Consequently, under an electrical field the dipoles are not perfectly oriented, thus preventing an optimal electro-mechanical coupling. The new generation of piezoelectric crystals has a more uniform atomic structure with few impurities and boundaries. The alignment of dipoles under an electrical field is more homogeneous, producing changes in terms of volume and shape of the crystals (strain) that is ten times greater than the traditional ceramic with a greater efficacy in converting electrical energy into mechanical energy and vice versa. Such an increase in efficacy during transduction results in a reduction in the production of heat (Fig. 1.6).

Last but not least, such new crystals have a larger band width. When vibrating, they produce a larger spectrum of frequencies than the traditional ceramics allowing better flexibility between resolution and penetration. Moreover, with a large spectrum of frequencies, multiple harmonic frequencies can be utilized providing images which combine optimal spatial resolution and good penetration.

Miniaturization of Piezoelectric Crystals and Electronic Circuitries

An advanced crystal manufacturing process generates piezoelectric crystals as small as 200 µm. This sub-millimetrical size allows the assembling of nearly 3000 active elements in a traditional transthoracic transducer or nearly 2500 active elements in a normal-sized transesophageal transducer. Furthermore, the miniaturization of electronic circuitries allows the insertion of nearly eight million of electronic devices and thousands of microchannels inside a transthoracic and transesophageal probe while maintaining the same probe size. The huge amount of electronic circuitries inevitably produces heat during imaging. An active cooling system whereby the heat is transported actively through the cable into the ultrasound machine minimizes heat generation without reducing transmit power.

The "Full" Sampled Matrix Array Transducer [1]

The introduction of the full sample matrix array transducer, in which all its thousands of elements are capable of <u>**both**</u> *transmitting* <u>**and**</u> *receiving* a signal, represented a major step forward in 3D technology. This was made possible by the introduction of *micro-beamforming circuitry* (Fig. 1.7)

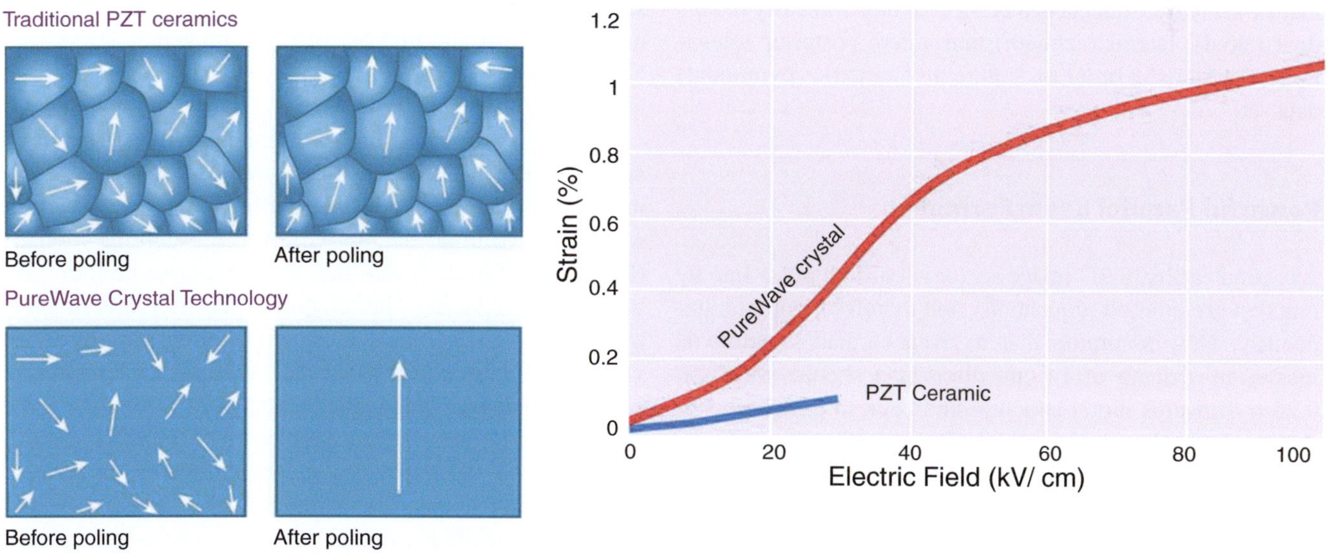

Fig. 1.6 Dipole orientation under an electrical field in traditional PZT ceramics (upper row) and in new pure wave crystals. The deformation (strain) of the new crystals is greater than that of PZT ceramic (courtesy of Philips)

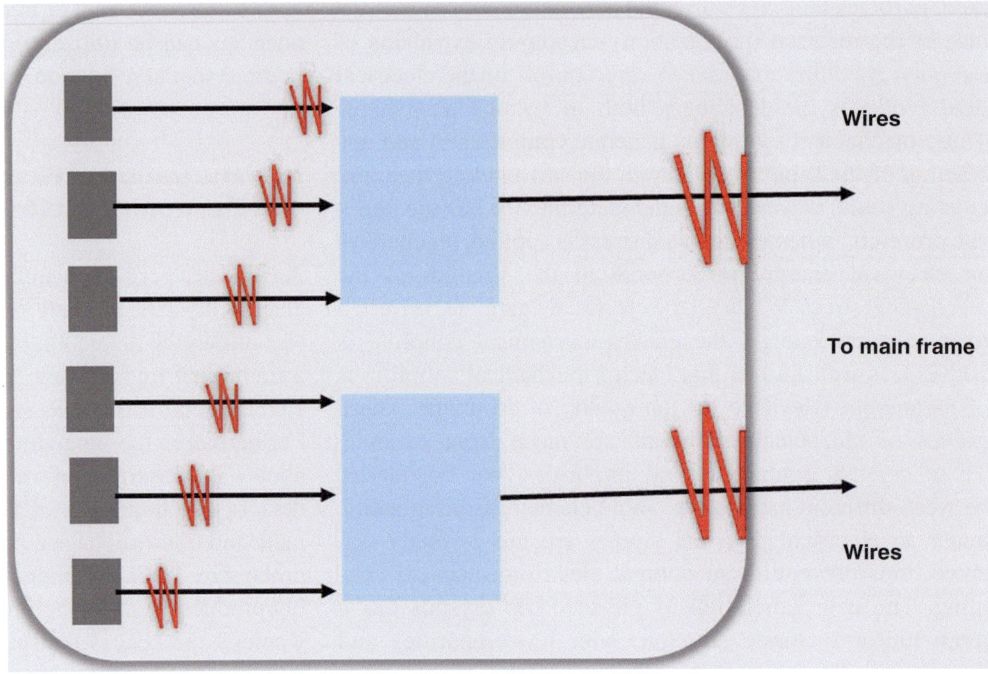

Fig. 1.7 Beamforming circuitry

whereby a small group of elements (i.e. patches of 25 crystals) combine their output to a single connecting wire. In fact, only 128 wires connect 3000 crystals to the mainframe. This eliminates the need for large connecting cables and provides a fully sampled array of 3000 elements. Maintaining the electric interconnection for every element so that each element remains independent with respect to transmission and reception provides the same uncompromised performance as a fully sampled array having 3000 wires and 3000 converters. The ultrasound scan lines that are generated by matrix-array transducers can be steered electronically in vertical (axial), lateral (azimuth) and antero-posterior (elevation) directions in order to acquire a volumetric (pyramidal) data set.

Powerful Parallel Beam Forming

As stated earlier, a 2D image sector is built up pulse line by line that are emitted sequentially and therefore, not simultaneously. Now assuming that a given cardiac structure is located at a depth of 14 cm, ultrasound should travel for 0.28 m (towards target structure and back to transducer) at the standard velocity of 1540 m/s. Because distance (d) is the product of velocity (v) and time (t), at this distance the number of pulses or beams per second (frame rate; 1/t or v/d) that can be transmitted without interferences is 5500 (1540/0.28). Assuming a pyramidal data set is formed by 60 × 60 beams with a space between beams of 1° and therefore non uniform distances traveled by the ultrasound beam in both lateral (x-axis) and elevation (z-axis) dimensions, we would need 3600 beams to resolve a 60 × 60 degrees volume which means a frame rate of 1.52 per second (5500/3600) that is clinically useless (Fig. 1.8).

In more simple terms, when a 3D volume of interest is obtained in one single beat (see 3D acquisition modes later), 3D frame rate (also referred to as volume rate), analogous to 2D imaging, is a function of the total number of transmitted ultrasound pulses needed to generate the 3D image which in turn is a function of the 3D volume size and scanning density (i.e. the number of 2D sectors in the volume of interest and number of pulse lines in a 2D sector). Scanning density also determines 3D spatial or detail resolution (Fig. 1.9).

Therefore, the 3D frame rate can be increased by either reducing the volume of the pyramidal data-set while maintaining same spatial resolution or by keeping the same 3D volume but reducing the scanning density (Fig. 1.9). The 3D frame rate can of course be increased by simply reducing the distance between the imaging transducer and region of interest (axial or vertical depth; y-axis) without altering the 3D volume dimensions or scanning density (Fig. 1.10).

The development of parallel beam forming or parallel processing i.e. the ability to receive multiple beams for each transmit thus reducing the number of transmit beams needed to generate the 3D pyramidal data set has been instrumental in increasing the 3D frame rate. This means that rather than a 1:1 pattern of one receiving line for every transmit line, a new ratio of 1:8, 1:16 or even 1:64 is possible. In other

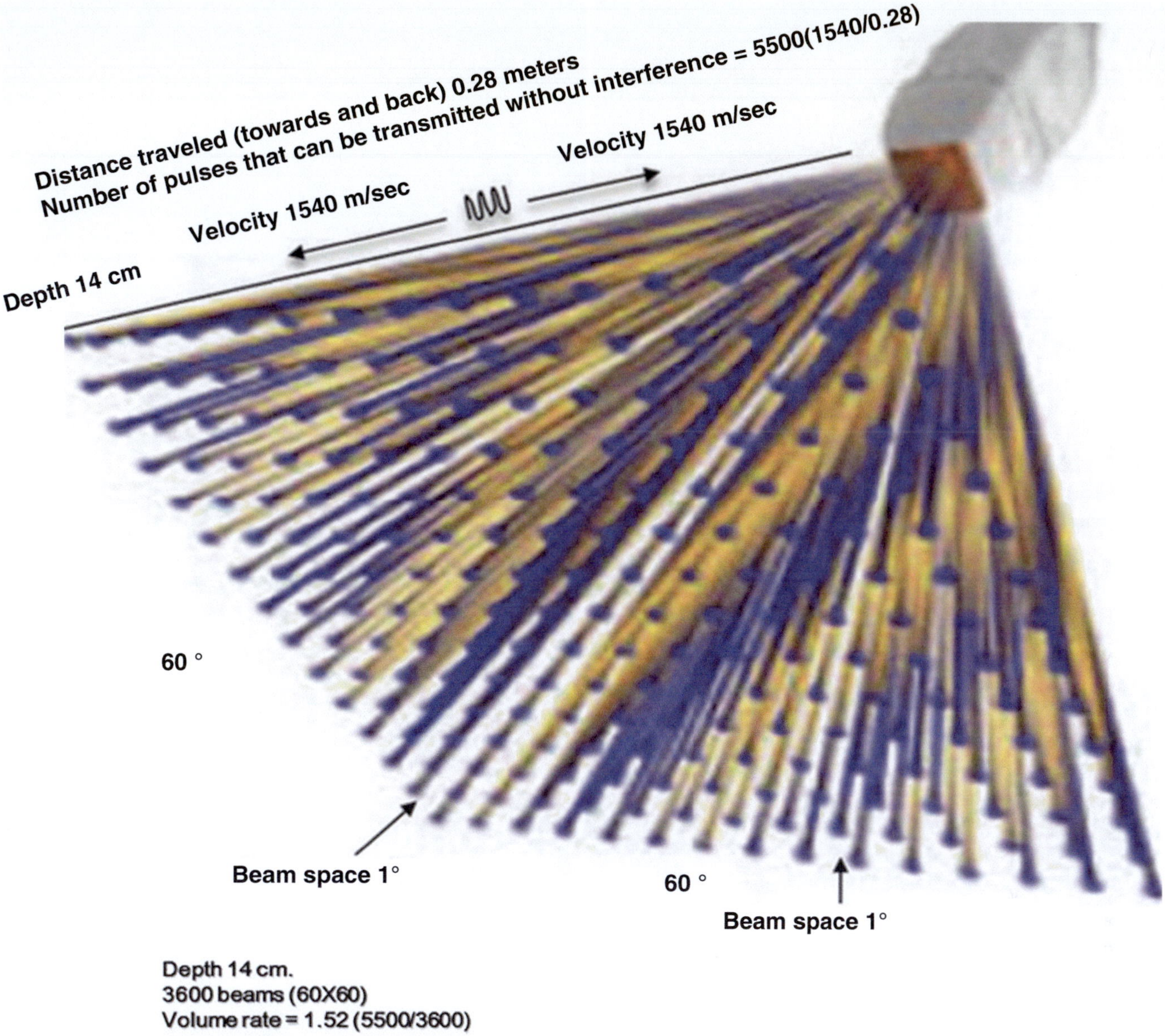

Fig. 1.8 Full sample matrix array transducer

words, this multi-line acquisition enables analysis of multiple scan lines in parallel for each transmitted pulse. In this manner, the reconstruction of a 3D image is accelerated by a factor equal to the number of the received beams thus increasing the volume or frame rate. The tradeoff for increasing the number of received beams is an increase in the width of the transmitted beam. And, because the transmit beam is not perfectly flat the outer lines would have lower signal strength than the inner lines. This in turn results in decrease in the signal to noise ratio and objectionable receive line to line gain artifacts hence reduced image quality. Moreover, the larger the transmitted beam, the lower the sound wave pressures of the propagating pulses which, in turn, affect the formation of second harmonic signals that are necessary for generating 3D images. Color Doppler is a phased based detection technique that is not sensitive to small line-to-line

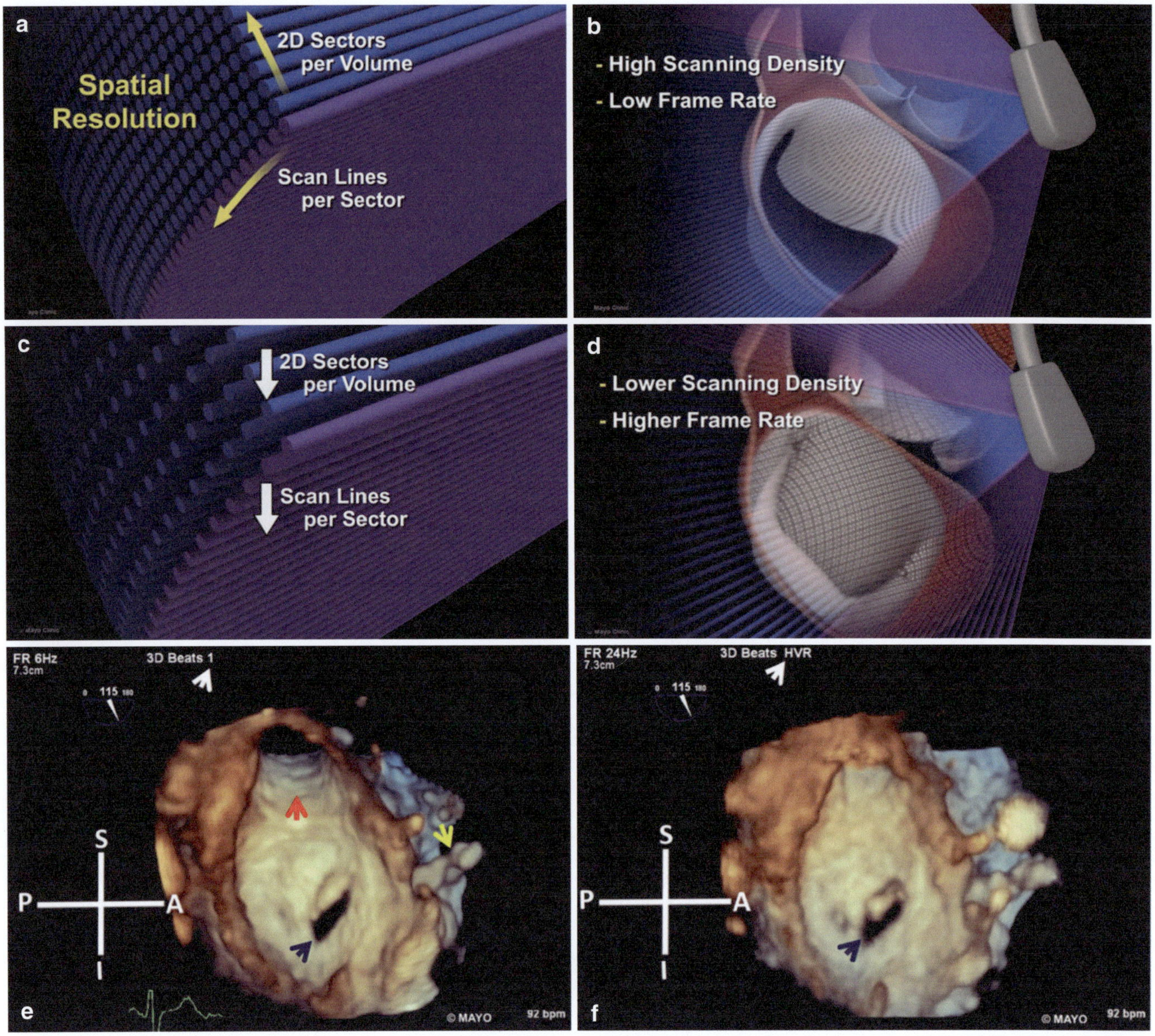

Fig. 1.9 Tradeoff between spatial and temporal resolution**: Top Panel**: (**a**) 3DE spatial or detail resolution is a function of both the number of 2D sectors that make up the 3D volume and number of scan lines within each 2D sector. (**b**) A high scanning density results in low frame rates (FR). **Middle panel**: Reducing scanning density reduces spatial resolution (**c**) but increases the frame rate (**d**). **Bottom panel**: (**e**) Single beat 3D TEE of ASD (dark blue arrow) as viewed from the RA. Yellow arrow points to aortic valve cusp, and red arrow points to SVC. Compared with this image, the image in **f** is blurred because of reduced scanning density but the FR is 4 times higher (24 versus 6). Used with permission of Mayo Foundation for Medical Education and Research. All rights reserved. A, anterior; HVR, high volume rate; I, inferior; P, posterior; RA, right atrium; S, superior; SVC, superior vena cava

gain variations, however, and multiline parallel processing provides for higher frame rates without loss of spatial resolution. Recently introduced overlapping transmit beam capability allows for increase in 3D image frame rate with good image quality without gain artifacts.

3D temporal resolution can also be increased while maintaining the ***same*** 3D volume dimensions ***and*** scanning density hence spatial resolution, by dividing the 3D volume of interest into sub-volumes, that are electrocardiographically triggered, and acquiring each sub-volume separately (Fig. 1.11).

By doing so, the 3D volume or frame rate will be a function of the time needed to acquire the sub-volume and not the entire volume. With two beat acquisitions (that is two sub-

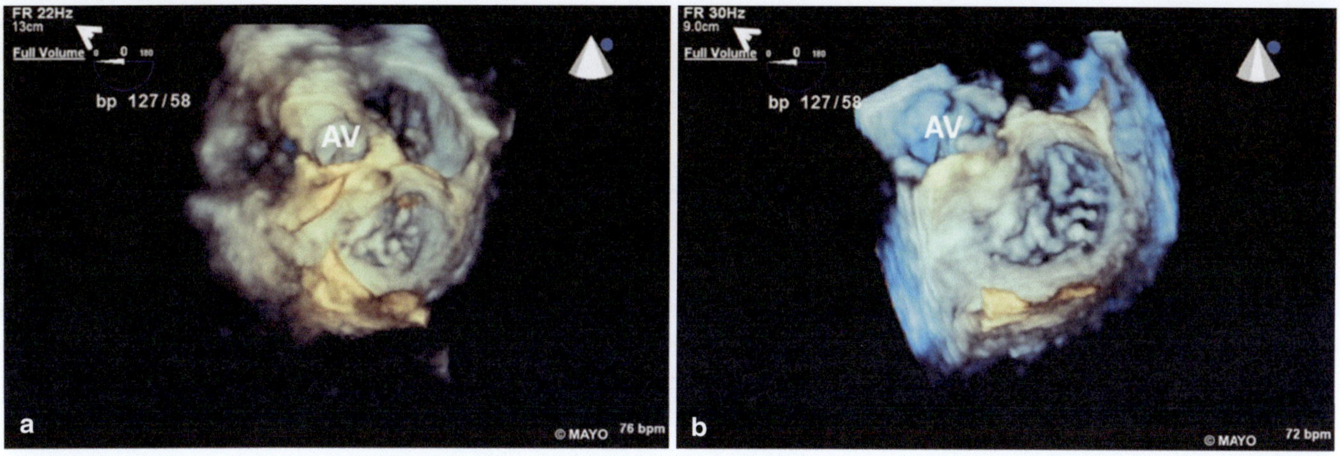

Fig. 1.10 (**a**) 3D image FR is 22 Hz at a depth of 13 cm. (**b**) By reducing the image depth to 9 cm, the FR increases to 30 Hz. Used with permission of Mayo Foundation for Medical Education and Research. All rights reserved. AV, aortic valve, FR, frame rate

volumes) the volume rate will double and with a six beat acquisition, the frame rate is increased sixfold. The subvolumes are electronically "stitched" together to form a complete volume. This process is referred to as multi-beat acquisition. Patient motion, patient breathing or arrhythmias can disturb this acquisition process resulting in stitch artifacts (Fig. 1.12).

Rarely, fine stich-like line artifacts can be seen during single beat acquisition with a very high frame rate and consequently very low line density that results in wide ultrasound line spacing (Fig. 1.13).

Simultaneous Multiplane and 3D Imaging Acquisition Modes

Simultaneous multiplane mode also referred to as x-Plane (Philips Healthcare), and Bi-Plane (GE Healthcare) mimics the 3D multiplanar reconstruction (see Chap. 2) with in contrast to 3D imaging only a minimal impact on spatial resolution that is comparable to standard 2D imaging with a 2D transducer. Two independent 2D scanning planes are obtained simultaneously (Fig. 1.14). Images are displayed using a split-screen format, with the primary image plane as the reference plane, displayed on the left side of the screen. By default, the initial two planes are at a 90° angle to each other. The image on the right panel display can be changed by moving the cursor line to alter the angulation in the reference plane. In the x-Plane mode, color Doppler can be displayed in both images although with lower temporal resolution (Fig. 1.14).

There are three 3D acquisition modes available. The smallest in size is referred to as 3D or Live 3D (Philips Healthcare) or Bird's View (GE Healthcare), and the largest is referred to as a Full Volume (Philips Healthcare); 4D Large size option (GE Healthcare) or simply 4D mode (Siemens Healthineers). 3D zoom (Philips; 4D Zoom on GE) is a truncated 3D pyramid of a region of interest within a larger 3D volume (Fig. 1.15) with adjustable size and position. Maintaining spatial orientation is key regardless of mode of 3D/4D acquisition. This entails including fixed anatomic landmarks in the acquired 3D/4D dataset. Note that the fourth dimension in 4D refers to time.

The size of any of these three 3D acquisition modes can be made smaller or larger using the Lateral Size/Width (azimuthal or x-axis) and Elevation Width (antero-posterior or z-axis) (Philips Healthcare) or 4D Zoom prepare (GE Healthcare) function controls (Fig. 1.16).

When the entire volume of interest is acquired in a single heart beat (referred to as 3D Beats 1 on Philips 3D platforms) regardless of mode of acquisition, it is effectively live or in real time (see Figs. 1.9e and 1.15e, f). The HVR mode on Philips 3D platforms (see Fig. 1.9f) refers to high volume rate and is a real time mode. As such, there are no stitch artifacts associated with the HVR mode, but spatial resolution is inferior to single beat acquisition as illustrated in Fig. 1.9. With multi-beat acquisition (Phillips and GE platforms), the image obtained is <u>*not*</u> in real time.

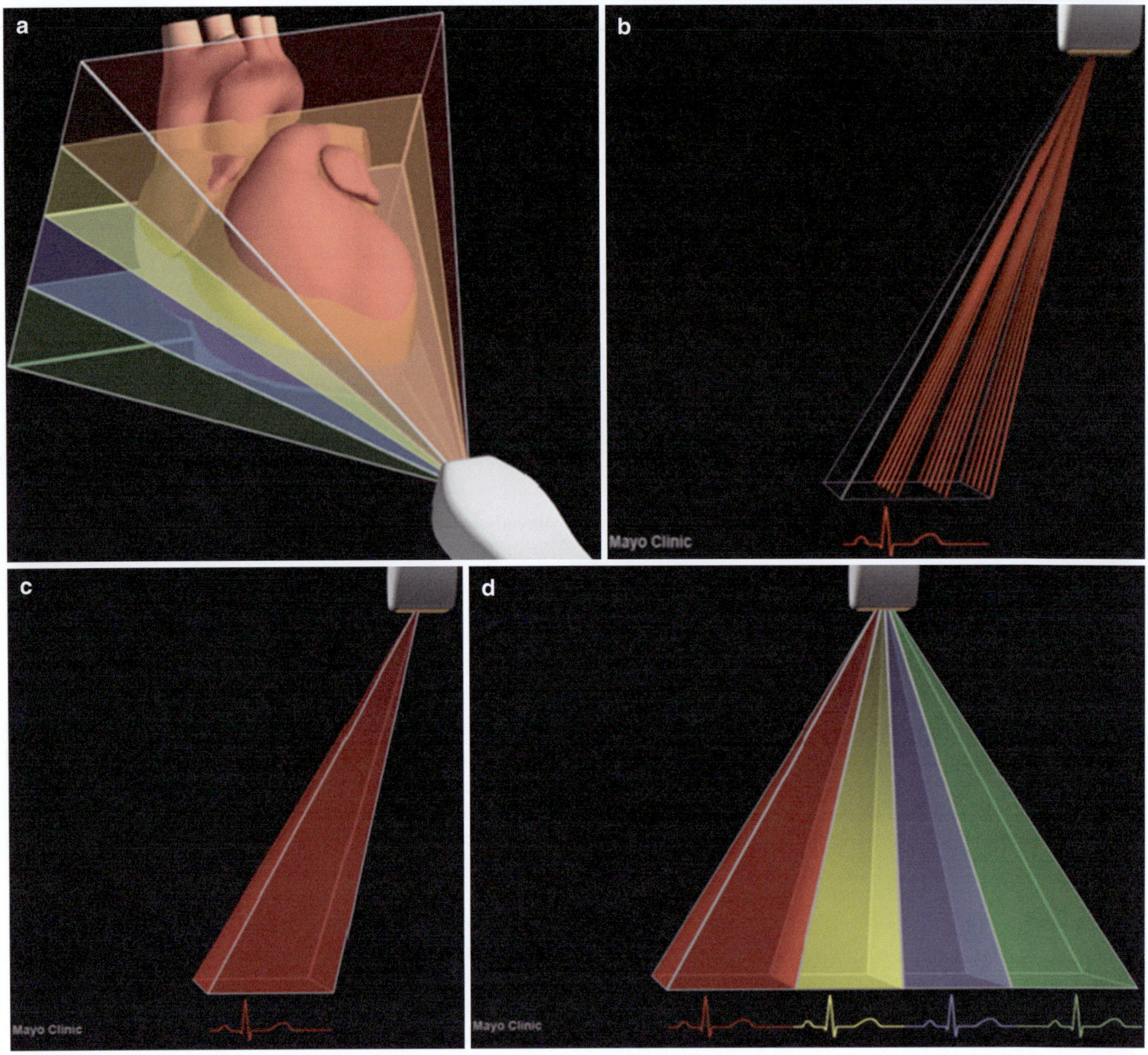

Fig. 1.11 Schematic illustration of method of multibeat acquisition. From top left to bottom right. The 3D volume of interest is divided into four subvolumes that are color coded (**a**). Each subvolume is ECG gated and acquired separately (**b**, **c**). The resulting four subvolumes are then electronically "stitched" together to produce the entire 3D volume (**d**). Note that the scanning density for each subvolume is not altered, but the FR is determined by the time needed to acquire the subvolume, and not the entire 3D volume. The FR, in this illustration, would be four times higher than if the entire 3D volume were to be obtained in a single beat. FR, frame rate. Used with permission of Mayo Foundation for Medical Education and Research.

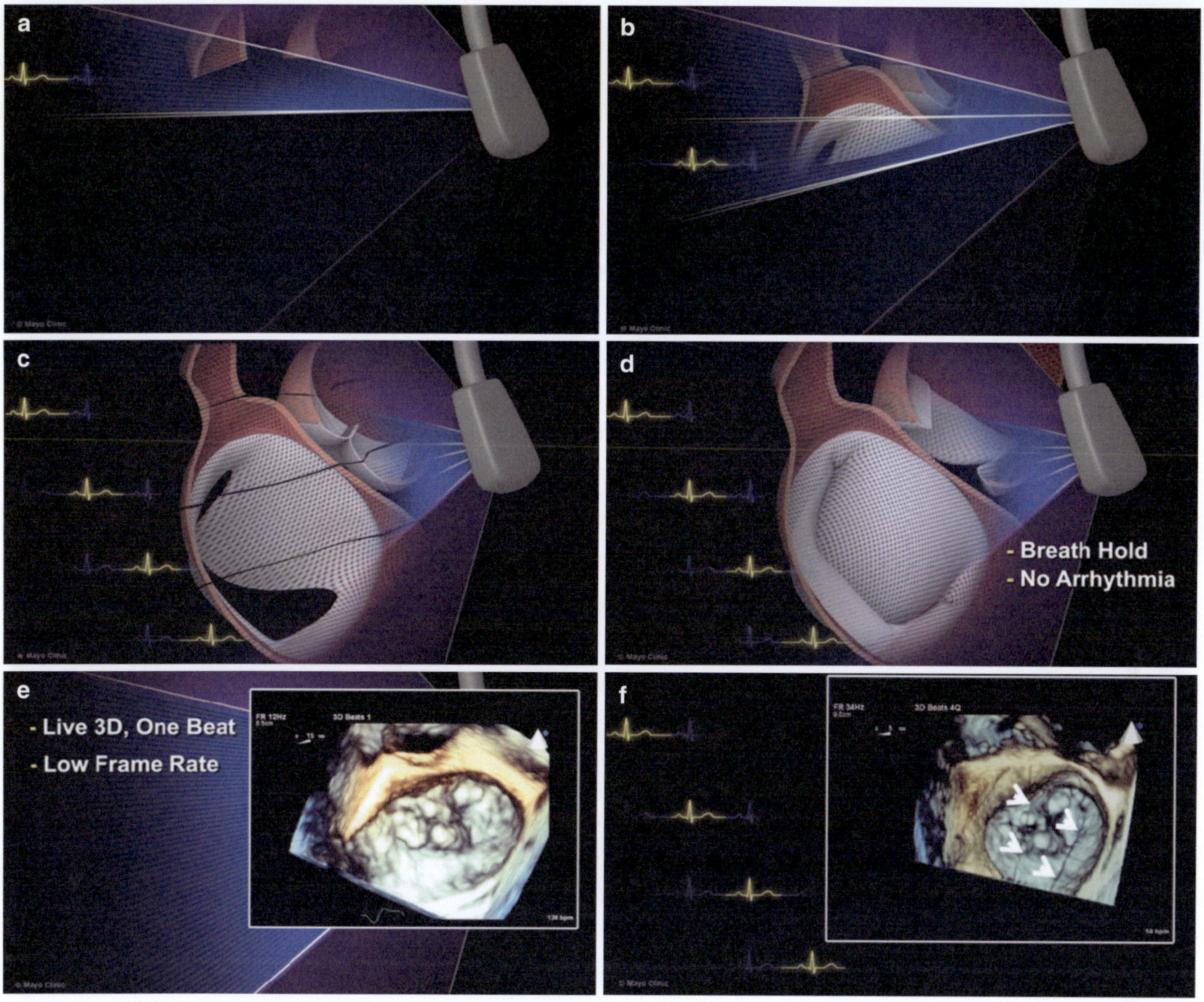

Fig. 1.12 Multibeat acquisition of MV: (**a–d**) Sequential schematic diagrams of a 4 ECG gated beat acquisition. Note that the acquired subvolumes are electronically stitched together to form the completed image (right, middle panel). (**e**) Single beat image acquisition with low frame rate. (**f**) Multibeat acquisition of same view. Note the stich artifacts (arrows). Used with permission of Mayo Foundation for Medical Education and Research. All rights reserved

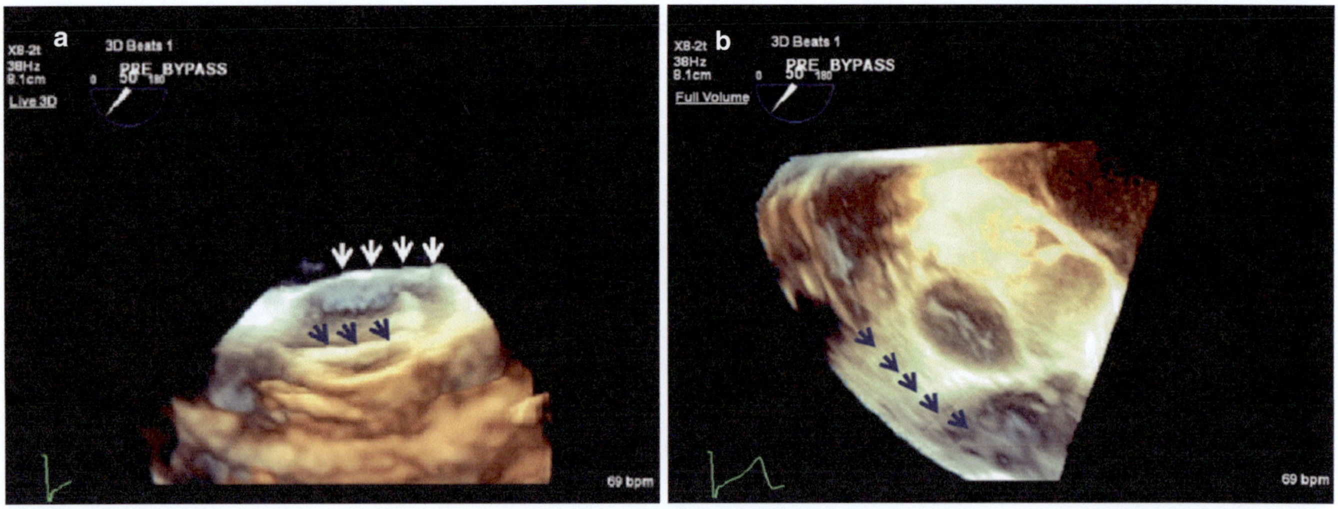

Fig. 1.13 (**a**, **b**) Fine stitch-like line to line artifact (arrows) in a patient with single beat (3D Beats 1), high frame rate (38) acquisition of the aortic valve. Used with permission of Mayo Foundation for Medical Education and Research. All rights reserved

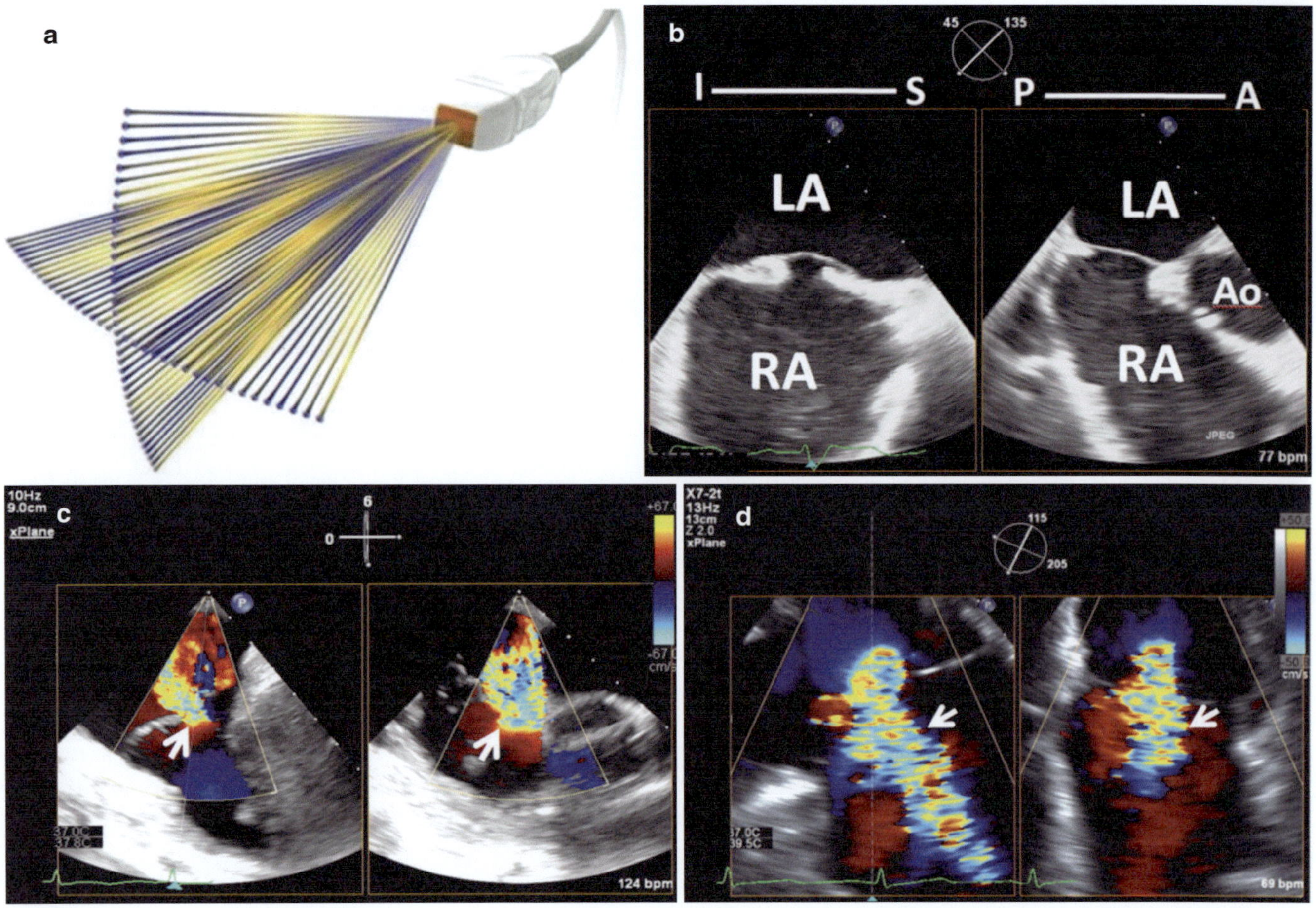

Fig. 1.14 Multiplane mode (x-Plane) examples**. Top panel**: (**a**) schematic diagram of two orthogonal two-dimensional tomographic planes (adapted from https://echoracle.wordpress.com). (**b**) x-Plane of atrial septum showing the superior, inferior, anterior and posterior spatial coordinates. **Bottom panel**: (**c**, **d**) CFD x-Planes of TR (arrows). Figures **b**, **c** and **d** are used with permission of Mayo Foundation for Medical Education and Research. All rights reserved. A, anterior; Ao, aorta; I, inferior; LA, left atrium; P, posterior; RA, right atrium; S, superior; TR, tricuspid regurgitation

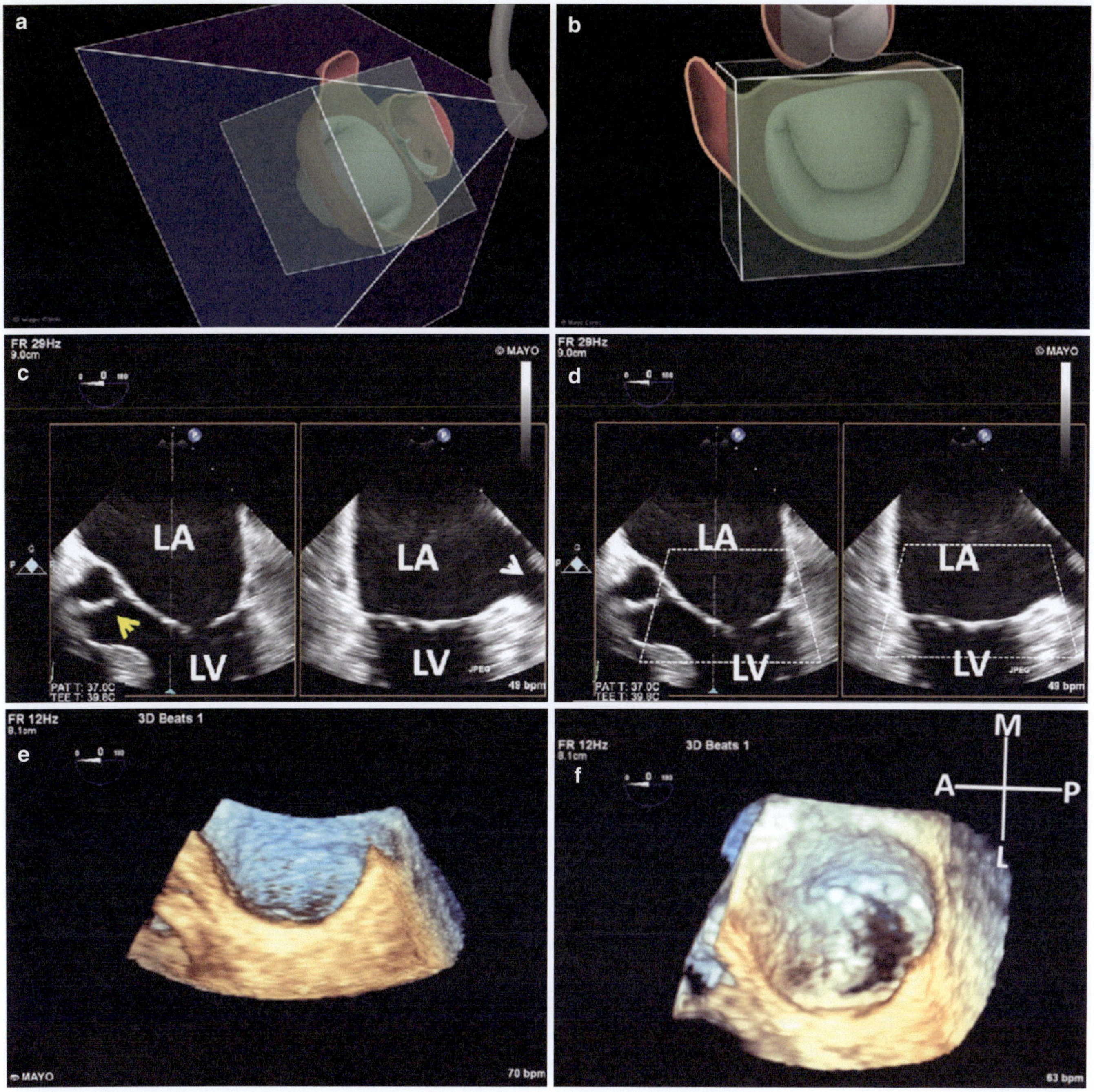

Fig. 1.15 **Top panel**: (**a**, **b**) Schematic illustration of 3D zoom acquisition. **Middle panel**: (**c**) orthogonal 2D views of the MV with left side of the image being the primary or reference plane (Philips Healthcare). (**d**) Preparing 3D zoom. Two trapezoid shaped boxes appear together with a Box Position and Box Size function buttons that can be used to reposition the reference plane box, and determine its lateral width (see Fig. 1.16). The dimension of the other box is adjusted using the elevation width button (see Fig. 1.16). It is always recommended to include in any 3D image fixed reference spatial coordinates such as the AV (yellow arrow) and LAA (white arrow). **Bottom panel**: (**e**) Acquired 3D zoom. (**f**) Same 3D zoom after tilting the image to better view the MV. Used with permission of Mayo Foundation for Medical Education and Research. A, anterior; AV, aortic valve; L, lateral; LA, left atrium; LAA, left atrial appendage; LV, left ventricle; M, medial; MV, mitral valve; P, posterior

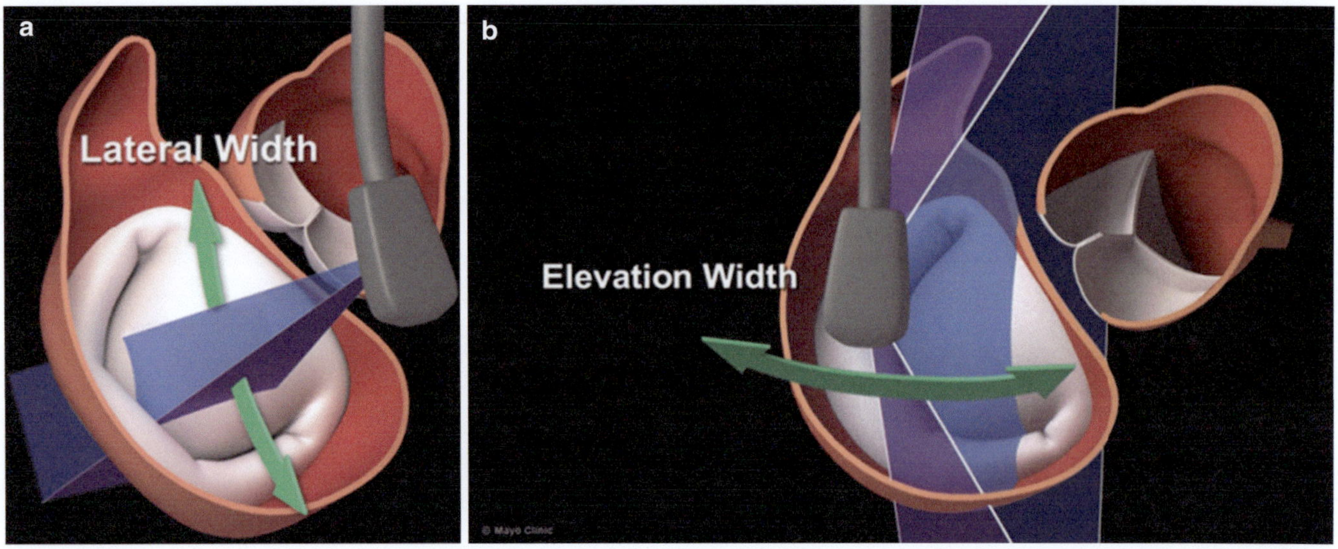

Fig. 1.16 Schematic illustrations of lateral (**a**) and elevation (**b**) width adjustments. Used with permission of Mayo Foundation for Medical Education and Research. All rights reserved

Reference

1. Lang RM, et al. EAE/ASE recommendations for image acquisition and display using three dimensional echocardiography. Eur Heart J Cardiovasc Imaging. 2012;13:1–46.

Image Optimization Tools and Image Display

2

Joseph F. Maalouf and Francesco F. Faletra

3D Image Optimization [1, 2]

The first step regardless of mode of 3D acquisition is to obtain the highest quality 2D image possible of the region of interest (ROI; Fig. 2.1). Next the 3D counterpart of the 2D image is obtained by pressing the desired 3D mode button (Fig. 2.1).

Regardless of mode of acquisition, 3D image size can be optimized using the Lateral Size/Width and Elevation Width (Philips Healthcare) or Volume Size/Volume Shape (GE Healthcare) function controls (Figs. 2.2, 2.3, and 2.4).

As expected, there is a progressive decrease in the 3D volume rate or frame rate as the 3D volumetric data set gets larger. On the Philips 3D platforms, the initial 3D Full Volume image obtained represents only the posterior half of the entire 3D volume because the anatomic crop plane used to obtain the image is a coronal plane that bisects the heart into two equal anterior and posterior halves. The missing anterior half is restored by pressing a Reset Crop button (Fig. 2.5).

After appropriate image display (discussed later), the 3D image/video clip is initially optimized by using the lowest compression settings possible (Fig. 2.6). Lower compression produces a high contrast image with better fine image details.

Persistent noise and other echo artifacts can be removed through a process known as tissue cropping. Tissue cropping is also very useful to highlight or view the ROI within the 3D volumetric data set and therefore, is crucial for image optimization. The different vendors offer several methods to achieve adequate tissue cropping. These include use of tomographic crop planes that can be advanced into the 3D volumetric data set in parallel to the primary planes of the heart [coronal, sagittal, or transverse which are perpendicular to the elevation or z-axis, azimuthal or x-axis, and axial depth or y-axis respectively [Crop Adjust Box (Philips Healthcare); Crop Tool (GE Healthcare), Box Edit (Siemens Healthineers) Fig. 2.7] or from any angle [Translate (GE Healthcare; Fig. 2.8), Crop Adjust Plane or Plane Crop (Philips Healthcare) a freely adjustable arbitrary cropping plane that has a purple color when in front the 3D volumetric data set (Fig. 2.9)], or alternatively, crop lines or boxes [iCrop , Face Crop, or Quick Vue (Philips Healthcare), 2 Click Crop (GE Healthcare); D'art (Siemens Healthineers)] that determine the ROI within the 3D volumetric data set to be viewed (Figs. 2.10 and 2.11).

Care should be taken to avoid over cropping and thus creation of artefactual defects. The effects of excessive gain or too low a gain setting are illustrated in Fig. 2.12.

Smoothing is the process by which the texture of a rough surface is evened out. Too much smoothing masks fine image details (Fig. 2.13).

3D Image Display

Appropriate image display is important. For the enface left atrial view of the mitral valve, the 3D image is rotated so that the anterior aortic valve is at the top of the image with the medial atrial septum to the right and the anterolateral left atrial appendage to the left of the image (Figs. 2.6 and 2.14).

This view is referred to as the surgeon's view because it closely resembles how the cardiac surgeon sees the mitral valve upon opening up the left atrium. *Current 3D imaging platforms offer the option of automatic display of the mitral valve in a surgeon's view format.* By simply rotating the 3D

Supplementary Information The online version of this chapter (https://doi.org/10.1007/978-3-030-72941-7_2) contains supplementary material, which is available to authorized users.

J. F. Maalouf (✉)
Professor of Medicine, Mayo Clinic College of Medicine; Director, Interventional Echocardiography; Consultant, Department of Cardiovascular Medicine, Mayo Clinic, Rochester, MN, USA
e-mail: maalouf.joseph@mayo.edu

F. F. Faletra
Director of Cardiac Imaging Lab, Cardiocentro Ticino Institute, Lugano, Switzerland
e-mail: Francesco.Faletra@cardiocentro.org

J. F. Maalouf et al. (eds.), *Practical 3D Echocardiography*, https://doi.org/10.1007/978-3-030-72941-7_2

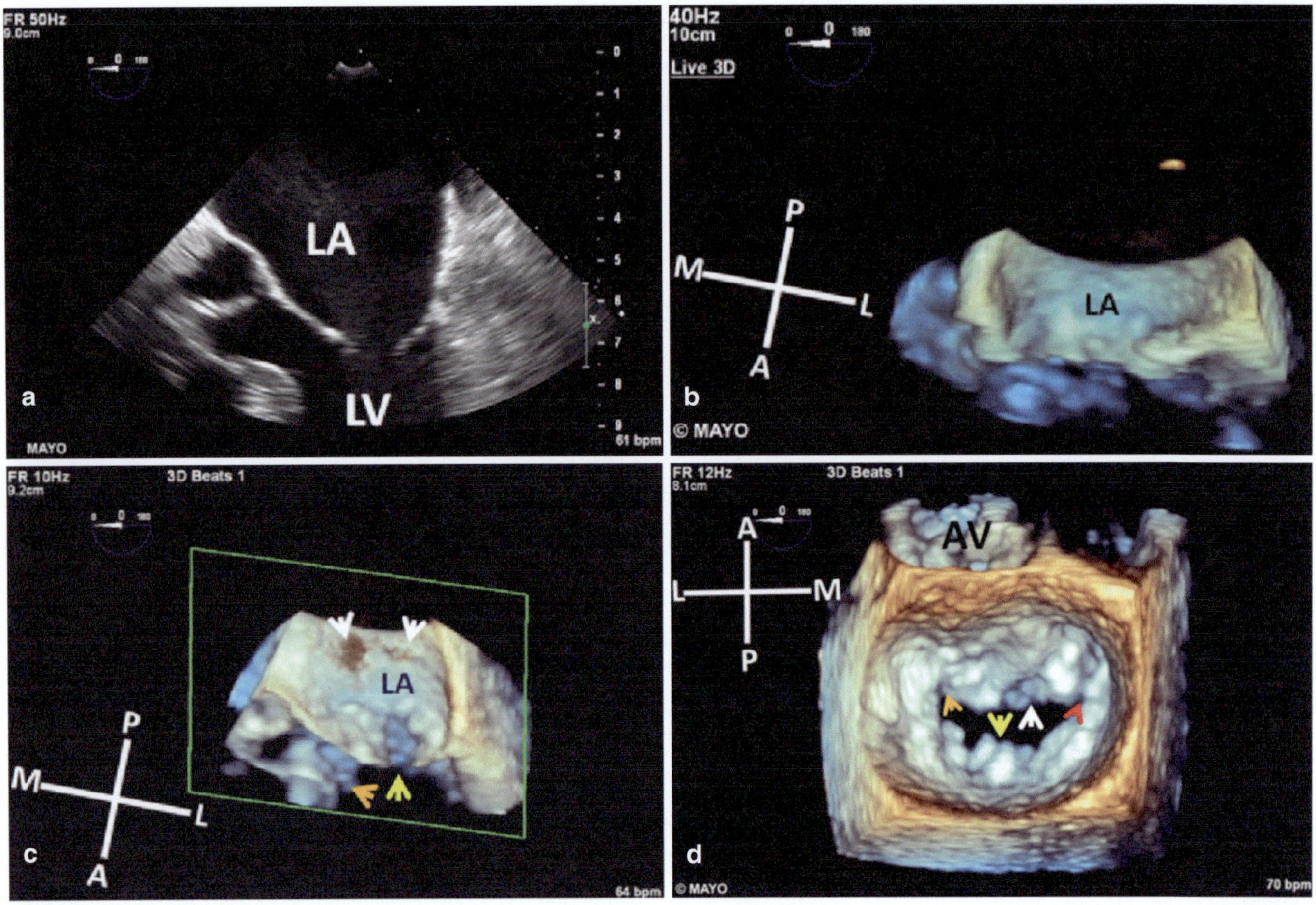

Fig. 2.1 **Top panel**: 2D TEE (**a**) and corresponding live 3D (**b**). Note the small 3D volume acquisition and high FR (40) also referred to as VR. **Bottom panel**: Live single beat FV and 3D zoom of the same 2D TEE. (**c**) FV acquisition . Note the larger 3D image data set compared with live 3D and consequently marked drop in FR to 10 despite the slightly lower image depth. White arrows point to posterior mitral annulus, yellow arrow points to MV and orange arrow points to LVOT. Green box indicates that the FV is autocropped with only the posterior half of the image being displayed. (**d**) 3D zoom acquisition at an even shallower depth . The entire MV including AML (white arrow), PML (yellow arrow), medial and lateral commissures (red and orange arrows respectively) is seen at an adequate FR. Used with permission of Mayo Foundation for Medical Education and Research. All rights reserved. A, anterior; AML, anterior mitral leaflet; AV, aortic valve; FR, frame rate; FV, full volume; L, lateral; LA, left atrium; LV, left ventricle; LVOT, left ventricular outflow tract; M, medial; MV, mitral valve; P, posterior; PML, posterior mitral leaflet; VR, volume rate

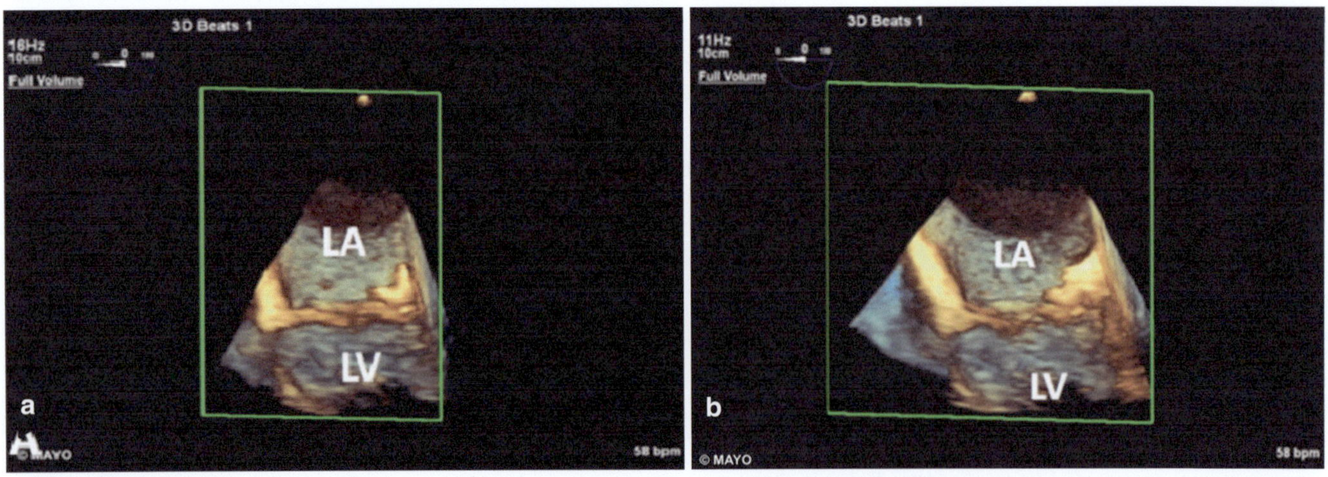

Fig. 2.2 Optimizing live single beat FV size using Lateral Size function. As expected, the FR decreases from **a** to **b** with increase in lateral width. Used with permission of Mayo Foundation for Medical Education and Research. All rights reserved. FR, frame rate; FV, Full Volume; LA, left atrium; LV, left ventricle

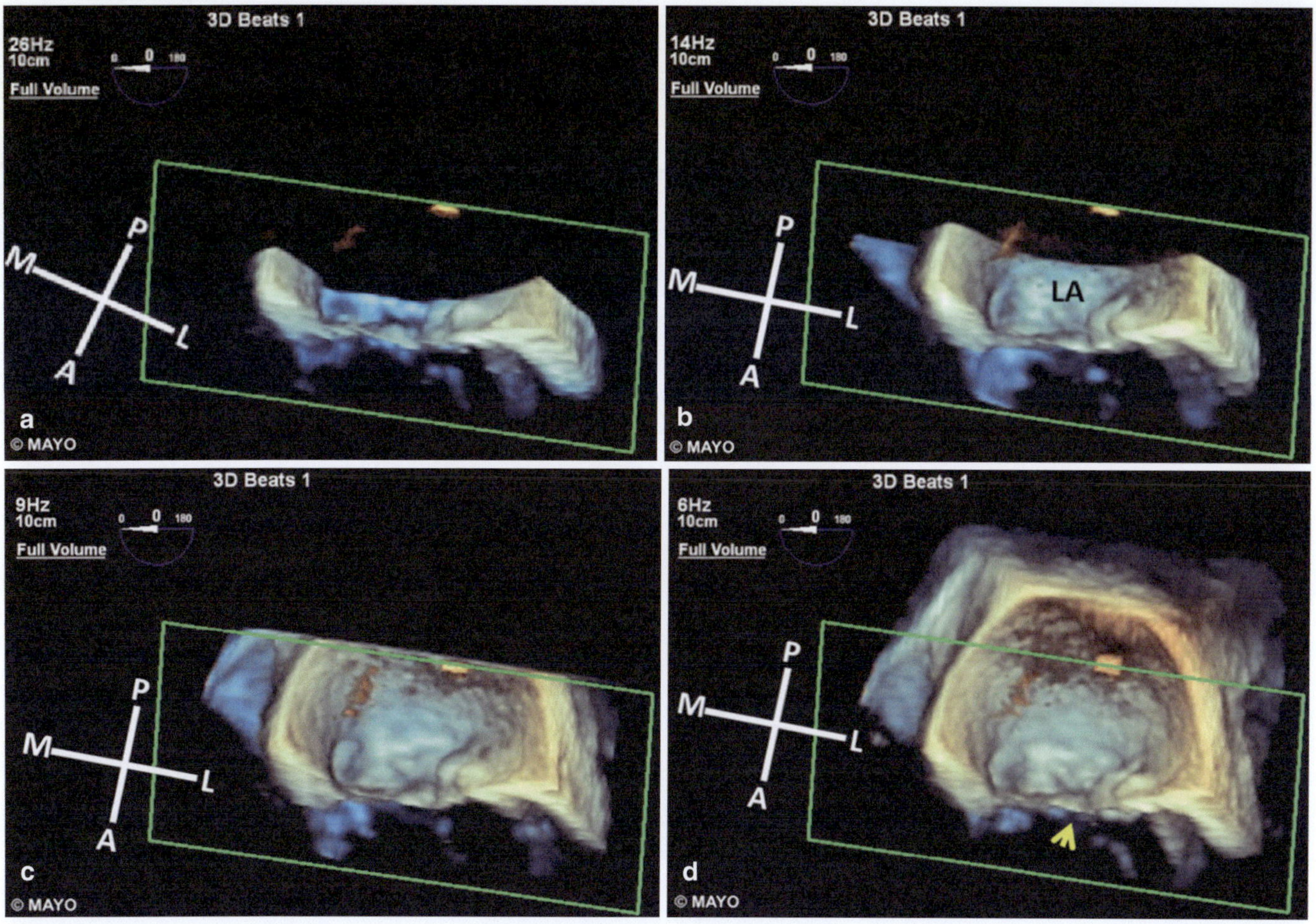

Fig. 2.3 (**a–d**) Adjusting elevation in a live FV acquisition while keeping the lateral width the same. Note the progressive increase in posterior image depth and corresponding decrease in FR with increase in size of 3D data set. Because the FV is autocropped, the progressive increase in anterior image dimensions can only be appreciated after crop reset (see Fig. 2.5). Arrow points to MV. Used with permission of Mayo Foundation for Medical Education and Research. All rights reserved. A, anterior; FR, frame rate; FV, Full Volume; L, lateral; LA, left atrium; M, medial; MV, mitral valve; P, posterior

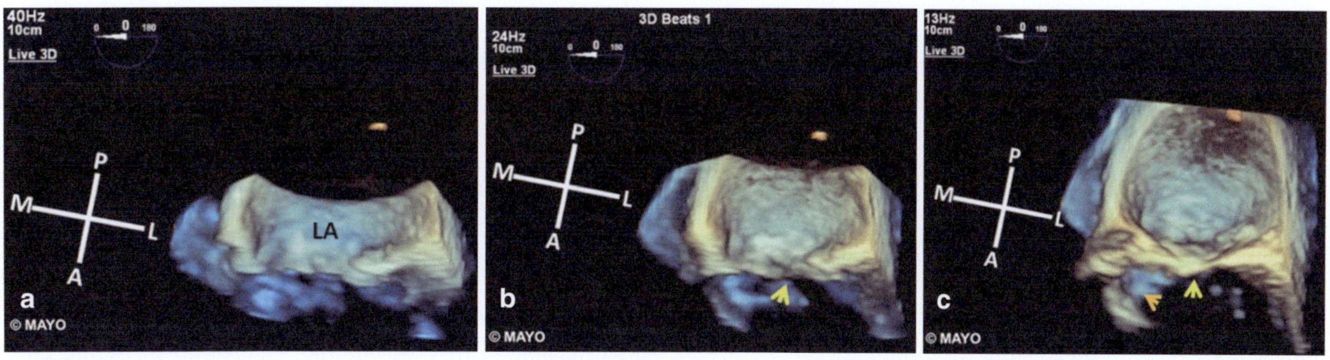

Fig. 2.4 (**a–c**) Adjusting elevation in a Live 3D acquisition of the MV. Note the progressive increase in posterior dimensions of the 3D data set accompanied by progressive decrease in the FR. Yellow arrow points to MV and orange arrow points to LVOT. Used with permission of Mayo Foundation for Medical Education and Research. All rights reserved. A, anterior; FR, frame rate; L, lateral; LA, left atrium; LVOT, left ventricular outflow tract; M, medial; MV, mitral valve; P, posterior

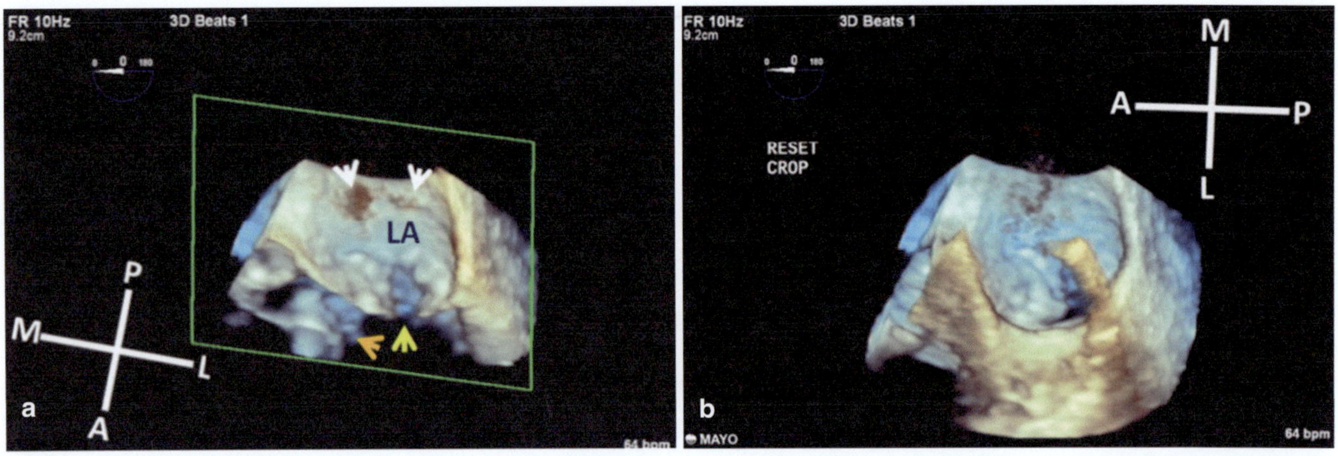

Fig. 2.5 (**a**) Auto cropped live FV image of MV. Only the posterior half of the 3D data set can be seen. White arrows point to posterior MV annulus. (**b**) FV after restoring the anterior half of the 3D data set (Reset Crop). Note that the FR remains the same. Yellow arrow points to MV and orange arrow points to LVOT. Used with permission of Mayo Foundation for Medical Education and Research. All rights reserved. A, anterior; FR, frame rate; FV, Full Volume; L, lateral; LA, left atrium; LVOT, left ventricular outflow tract; M, medial; MV, mitral valve; P, posterior

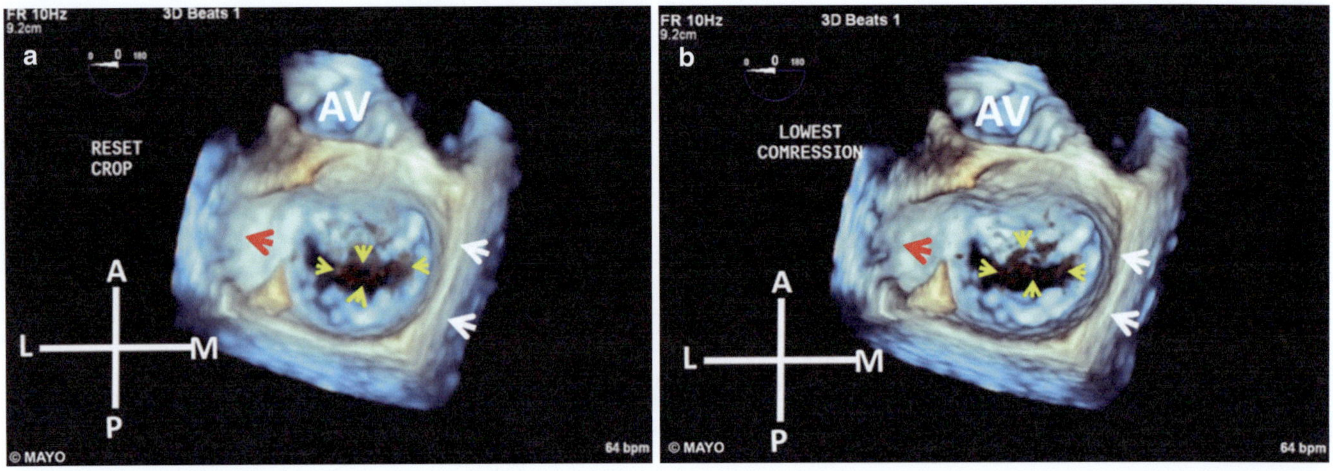

Fig. 2.6 (**a**) Fully restored FV image in Fig. 2.5 rotated such that the AV is at top of the image (surgeon's view). (**b**) Same view after dialing down the compression to the lowest possible without creating artifactual defects. White arrows point to atrial septum and red arrows point to LAA. Note the noise artifacts in both images (yellow arrows). Used with permission of Mayo Foundation for Medical Education and Research. All rights reserved. A, anterior; AV, aortic valve; FV, Full Volume; L, lateral; LAA, left atrial appendage; M, medial; P, posterior

"surgeon's view" of the mitral valve, enface views from the left ventricular apex can be obtained, and provide an excellent perspective of the left ventricular outflow tract after appropriate image optimization (Fig. 2.15). The enface left ventricular view of the mitral valve closely resembles the interventional cardiologist's fluoroscopic view.

3D/4D Zoom Dual layout (Philips and GE platforms) and 4D Dual view (Siemens) provide simultaneous enface views of *both* surfaces of the structure of interest (e.g. left atrial and left ventricular views of the mitral valve and left and right atrial views of the atrial septum) (Fig. 2.16). Dual Layout is also feasible with Full Volume acquisition including CFD

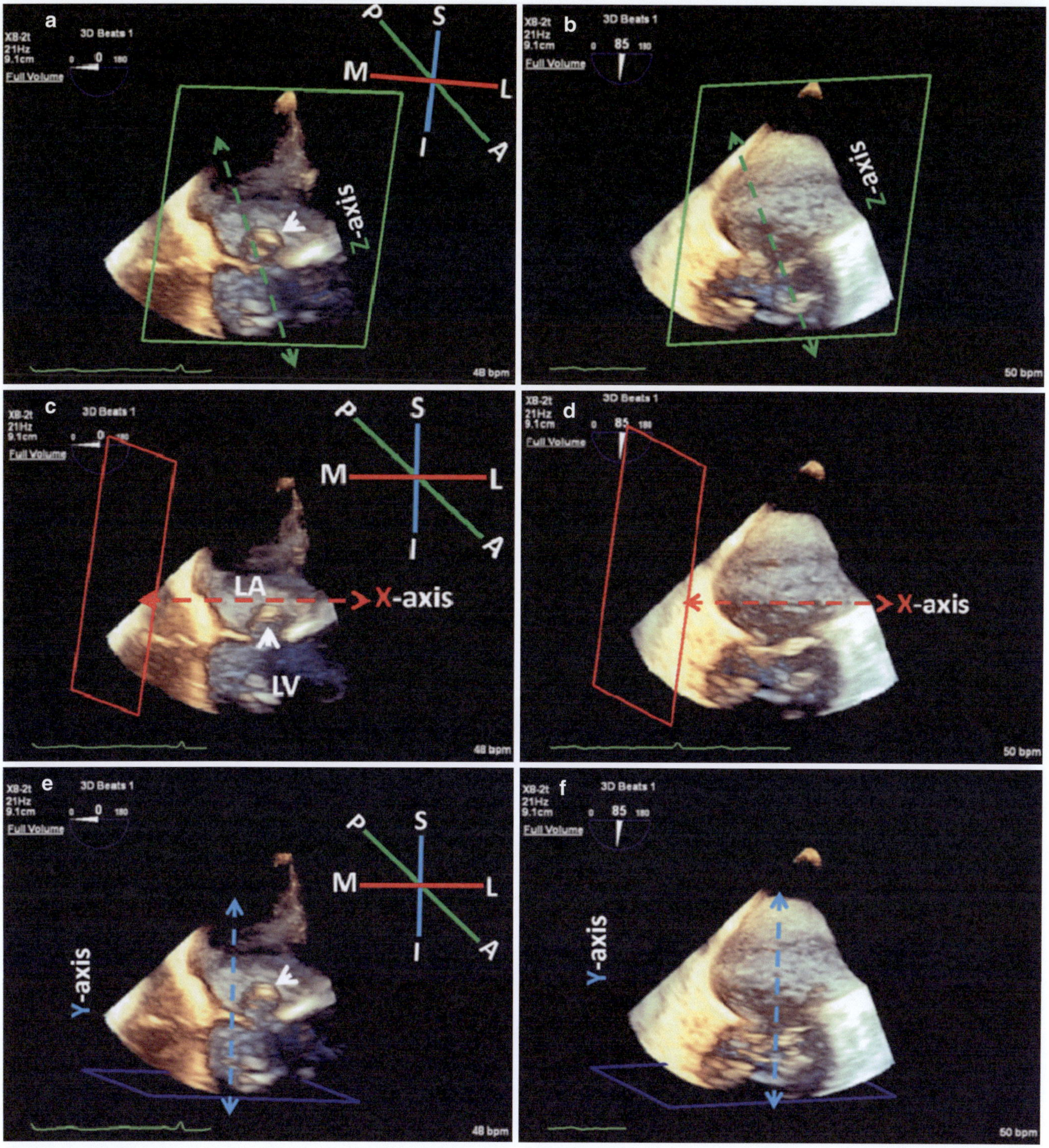

Fig. 2.7 Crop Adjust Box (Philips Healthcare) using color coded planes. Cropping of 3D TEE volumetric data set using the three primary planes of the heart. **Top panel**: (**a**, **b**) Green for coronal or frontal plane divides the heart into anterior and posterior portions and is perpendicular to the elevation or z-axis. **Middle panel**: (**c**, **d**) Red for sagittal or vertical plane divides the heart into right and left portions and is perpendicular to the azimuthal or x-axis. **Bottom panel**: (**e**, **f**) Blue for transverse short-axis plane divides the heart into superior and inferior portions and is perpendicular to the axial or *y*-axis. Note that although the 3D data sets were obtained from 2D images that are nearly orthogonal to each other (0 and 85° left and right column respectively), cropping direction remains the same. Used with permission of Mayo Foundation for Medical Education and Research. All rights reserved. A, anterior; I, inferior; L, lateral; LA, left atrium; LV, left ventricle; M, medial; P, posterior; S, superior. Arrows point to P2 prolapse

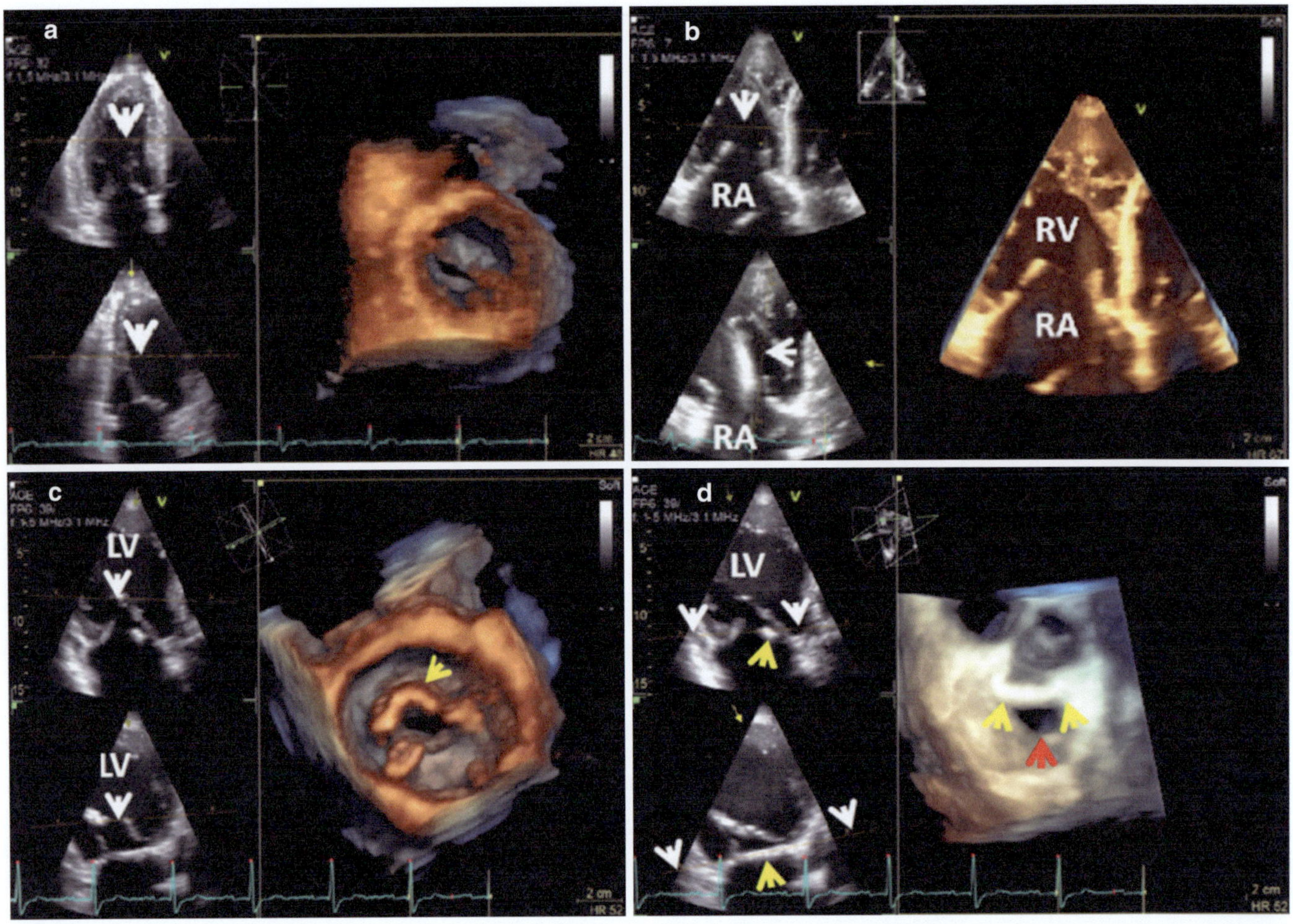

Fig. 2.8 3D TTE cropping using Translate function (moves crop plane within the 3D volume). **Top panel**: (**a**) cropping of MV from LV side (white arrows). (**b**) Cropping of TV from RV side. Note that the Translate crop plane can be repositioned in any direction by the track ball (white arrow bottom of image). **Bottom panel**: Use of Translate crop plane to view posterior annuloplasty ring dehiscence post MV repair. (**c**) Translate crop plane at tips of MV leaflets viewed from LV perspective (white arrows). Yellow arrow points to AML. (**d**) Translate crop plane moved towards the LA (white arrows) to be at level of annuloplasty ring (yellow arrows). Red arrow points to defect caused by the annuloplasty ring dehiscence. Used with permission of Mayo Foundation for Medical Education and Research. All rights reserved. AML, anterior mitral leaflet; LA, left atrium; LV, left ventricle; MV, mitral valve; RA, right atrium; RV, right ventricle; TV, tricuspid valve

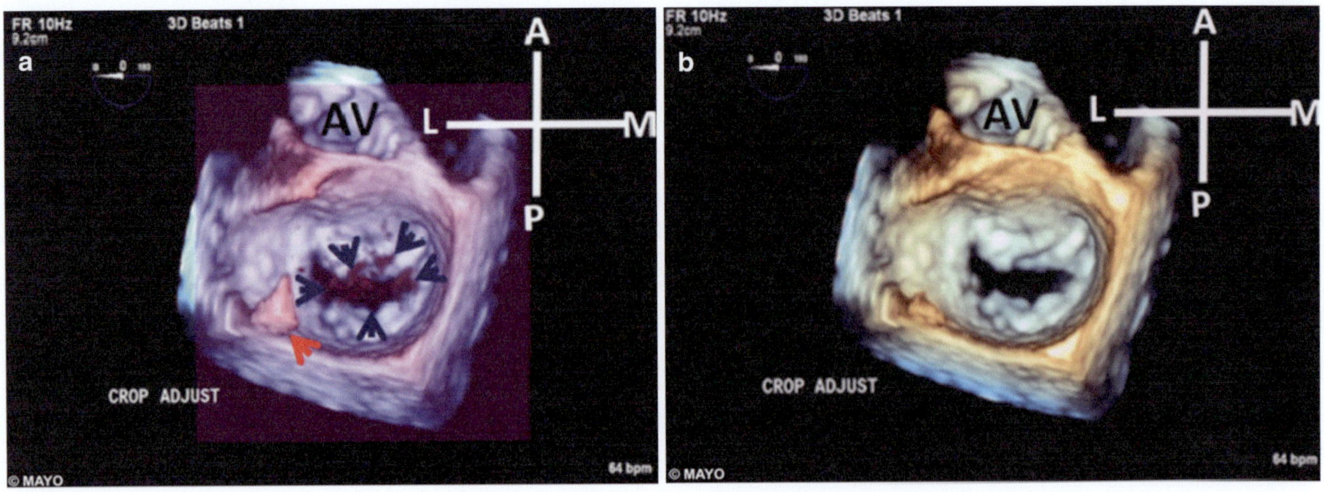

Fig. 2.9 Use of freely adjustable arbitrary "purple" plane to crop out artifacts. (**a**) Crop plane above plane of MV aligned parallel to transverse plane of the heart. Note the noise (dark blue arrows) and tissue (red arrow) artifacts that need to be cropped out. (**b**) Same image after tissue cropping. Used with permission of Mayo Foundation for Medical Education and Research. All rights reserved. A, anterior; AV, aortic valve; L, lateral; M, medial; MV, mitral valve; P, posterior

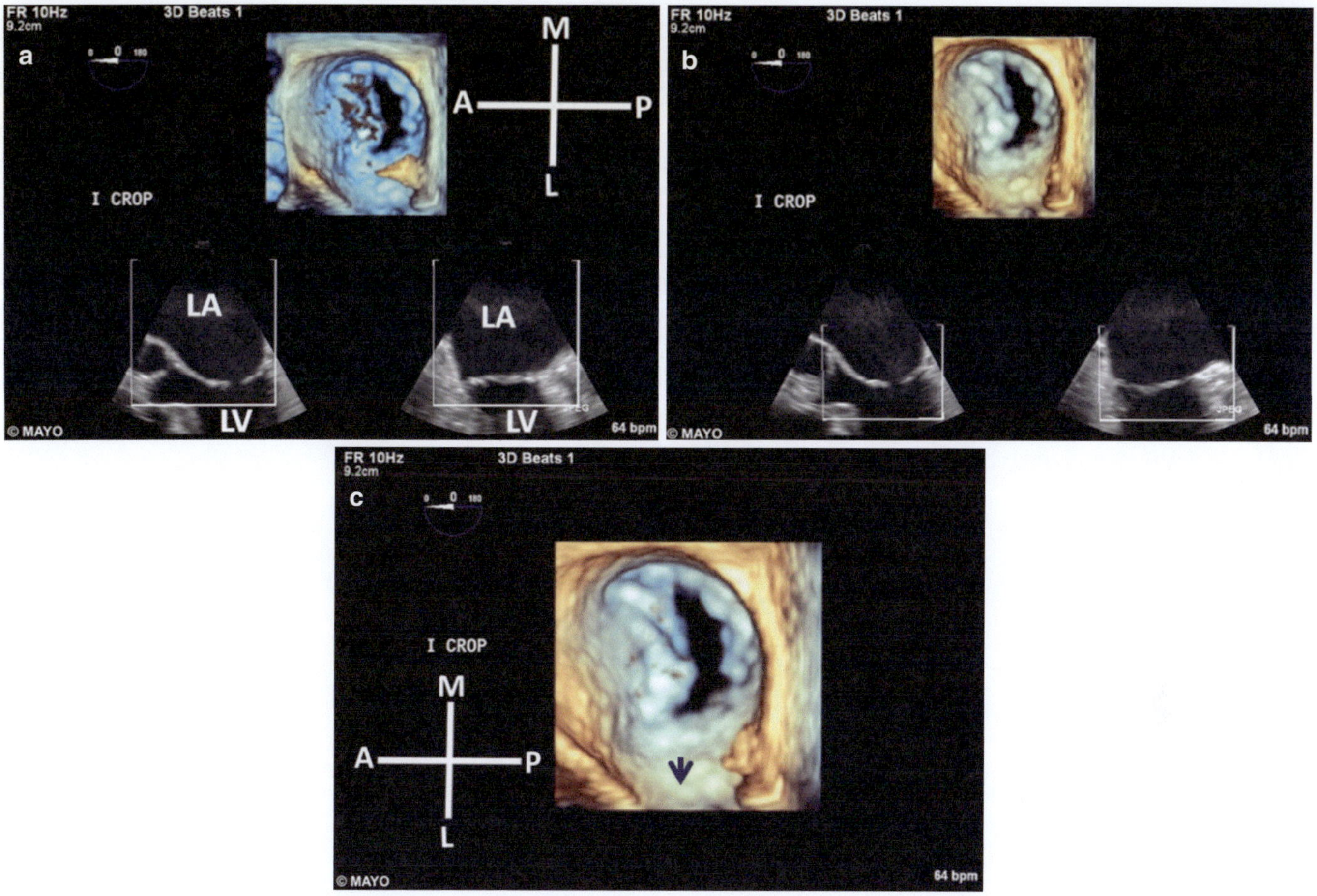

Fig. 2.10 iCrop of MV 3D data set. Selection of the ROI on two orthogonal MPR reference images within the 3D data set (**a**) and image optimization (**b**). The 3D image of the MV can then be viewed from either the LA or LV perspective. (**c**) Final iCrop 3D image as viewed sideways from LA perspective. Arrow points to ostium of LAA. Used with permission of Mayo Foundation for Medical Education and Research. All rights reserved. A, anterior; L, lateral; LA, left atrium; LAA, left atrial appendage; LV, left ventricle; M, medial; MPR, multiplanar reconstruction; MV, mitral valve; P, posterior; ROI, region of interest

(Fig. 2.16) on the Epic Philips 3D platforms. TrueVue (Philips Healthcare) provides a different perspective of the 3D image tissue characteristics by adjusting the position of a light source within the 3D volumetric data set (Figs. 2.17 and 2.18b). GlassVue (Philips Healthcare) with its internal light source provides more transparent 3D visualization of anatomy of interest thus allowing shapes and boundaries of intracardiac structures including soft tissues to be more easily seen (Fig. 2.18).

3DE Multiplanar Reconstruction

Multiplanar reconstruction (MPR) of 3D volume rendered data sets, analogous to its use in other imaging modalities such as CT and MRI, allows for viewing cardiac structures from any perspective, assessing cardiac pathology simultaneously in multiple planes, quantifying complex geometric lesions and flow, and obtaining measurements needed prior to structural heart interventions. Three crop planes color coded blue, red, and green (Philips Healthcare and Siemens Healthineers) and green, white, and yellow (GE Healthcare) form the basis for MPR. They can be orthogonal to each other in the default setting (3DQ Philips Healthcare) aligned parallel to one of the three primary planes of the heart (Fig. 2.7) analogous to Crop Box, and therefore, perpendicular to one of the three axes [elevation (z-axis), azimuthal (x-axis) or axial (y-axis)] in which the matrix transducer transmits and receives acoustic data. Accordingly, in 3DQ MPR, the coronal or frontal plane divides the heart into anterior and posterior portions and is color coded green, the sagittal or vertical plane divides the heart into right and left portions and is color coded red, and the transverse short-axis or depth plane divides the heart into superior and inferior portions and is color coded blue. The green, red and blue planes are perpendicular to the elevation or z-axis, the azimuthal or x-axis, and axial or y-axis respectively (Figs. 2.19, 2.20, and 2.21).

MPR crop planes and lines may be arbitrary however, with the crop direction of a color coded line/plane depending

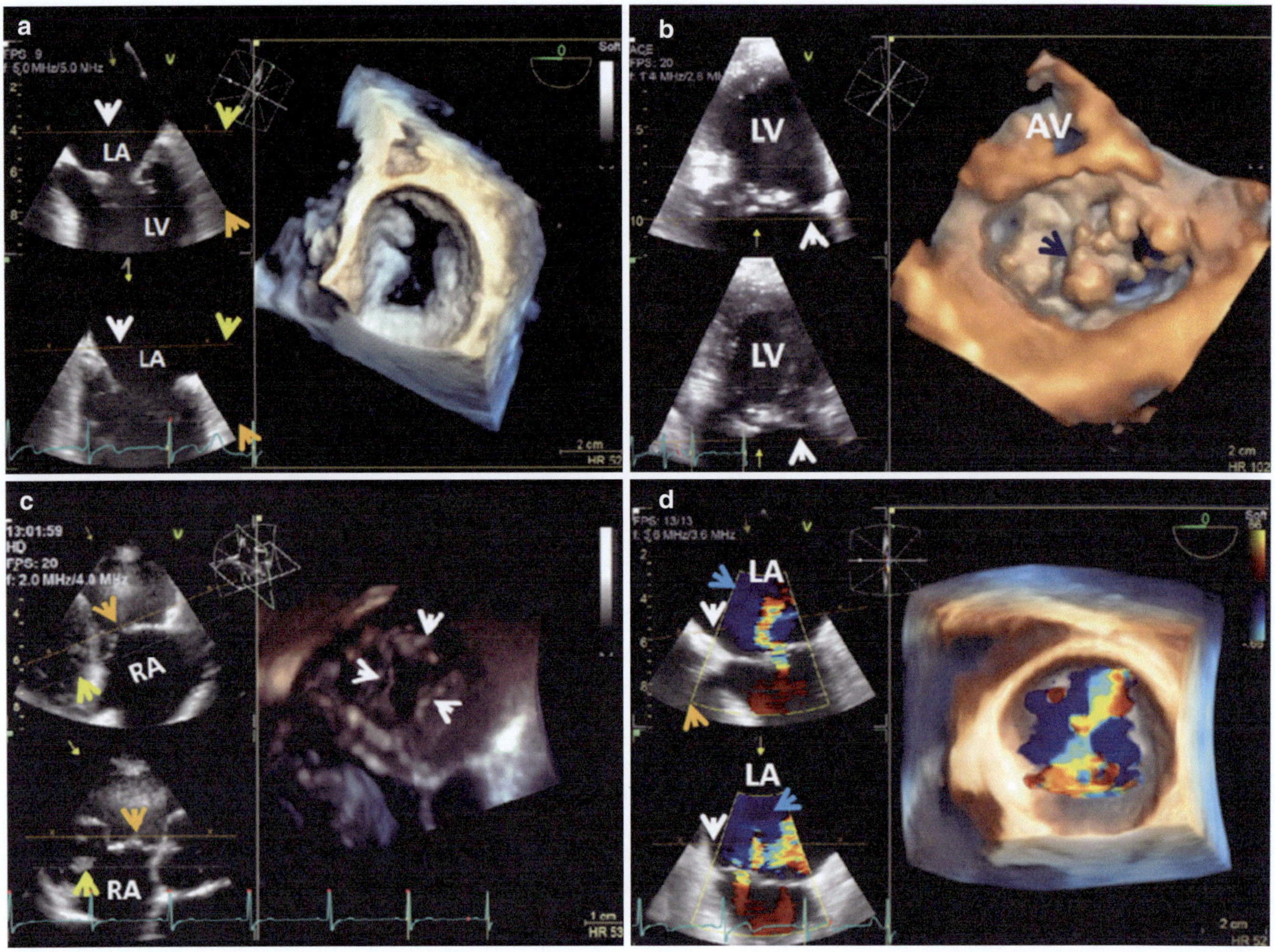

Fig. 2.11 2 Click Crop **Top panel**: MV 3D TEE (**a**) and 3D TTE (**b**) viewed from LA (white arrows). Yellow and orange arrows point to position of the LA and LV crop planes respectively. Dark blue arrow points to flail P2 segment. **Bottom panel**: (**c**) 3D TTE of TV leaflets in late diastole viewed from RV perspective (white arrows). Yellow and orange arrows point to position of RA and RV crop planes respectively. (**d**) 3DTEE MR viewed from LA side (white arrows). Orange arrow points to LV side of the cropped image. Note low velocity flow (blue arrows) that can be cropped out. Used with permission of Mayo Foundation for Medical Education and Research. All rights reserved. AV, aortic valve; LA, left atrium; LV, left ventricle; MR, mitral regurgitation; MV, mitral valve; RA, right atrium; RV, right ventricle; TV, tricuspid valve

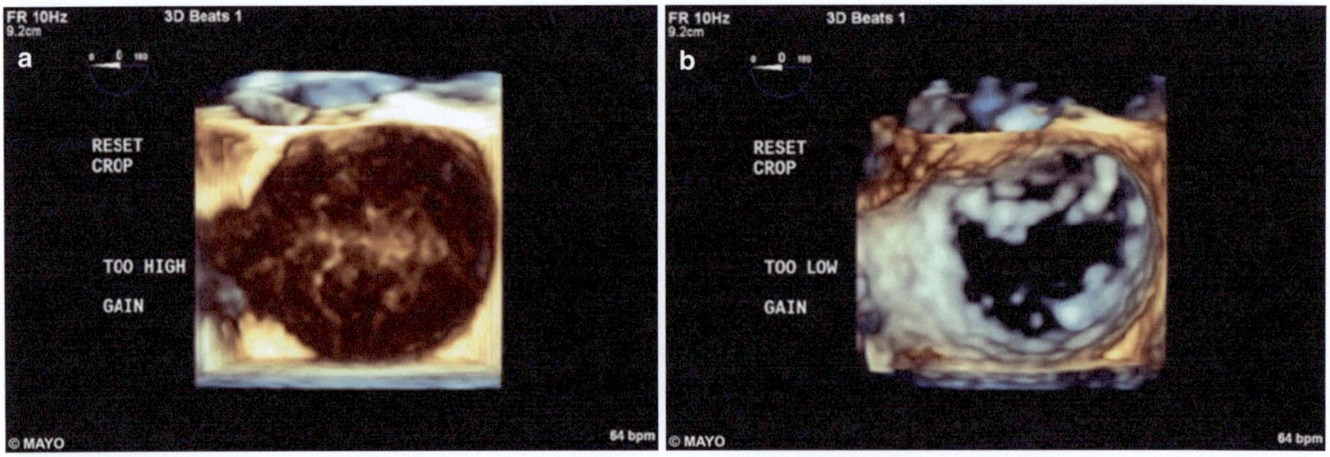

Fig. 2.12 (**a**) Too high a gain setting shows marked noise that resembles dense SEC. (**b**) Too low a gain setting creates drop out MV leaflet artifacts. Used with permission of Mayo Foundation for Medical Education and Research. All rights reserved. MV, mitral valve; SEC, spontaneous echo contrast

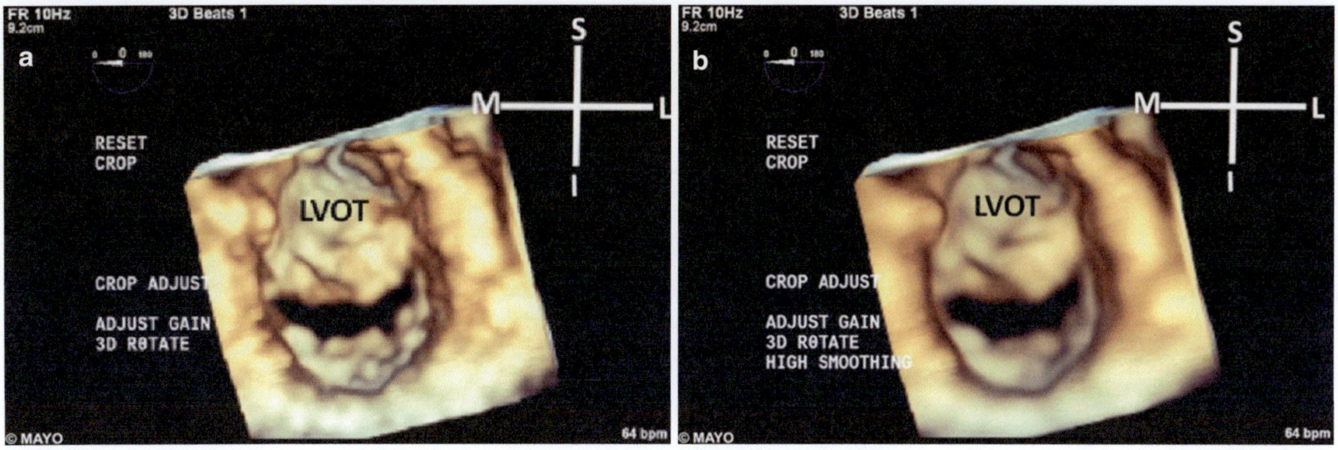

Fig. 2.13 3D TEE enface LV view of MV. (**a**) Optimal image view. (**b**) Too much smoothing. Note the loss of fine image details. Used with permission of Mayo Foundation for Medical Education and Research. I, inferior; L, lateral; LVOT, left ventricular outflow tract; LV, left ventricle; M, medial; MV, mitral valve; S, superior

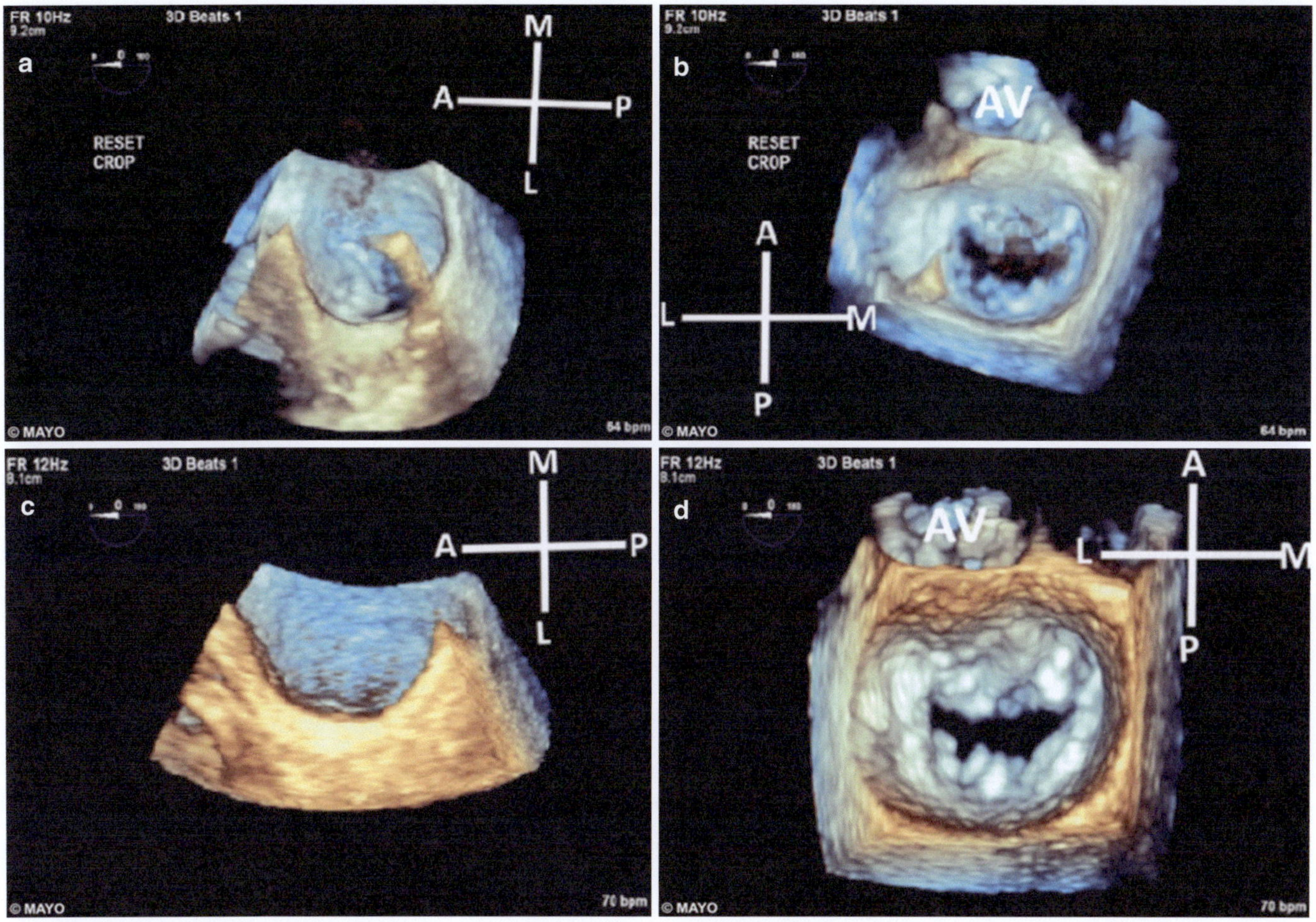

Fig. 2.14 3D TEE enface LA views of the MV. Appropriate image display for a FV (top panel-**b**) and 3D Zoom clip (bottom panel-**d**). Note that the acquired 3D data set for either FV (**a**) or 3D Zoom (**c**) needs to be rotated such that the AV is displayed on top of the image (surgeon's view). Used with permission of Mayo Foundation for Medical Education and Research. A, anterior; AV, aortic valve; FV, Full Volume; L, lateral; LA, left atrium; LV, left ventricle; M, medial; MV, mitral valve; P, posterior

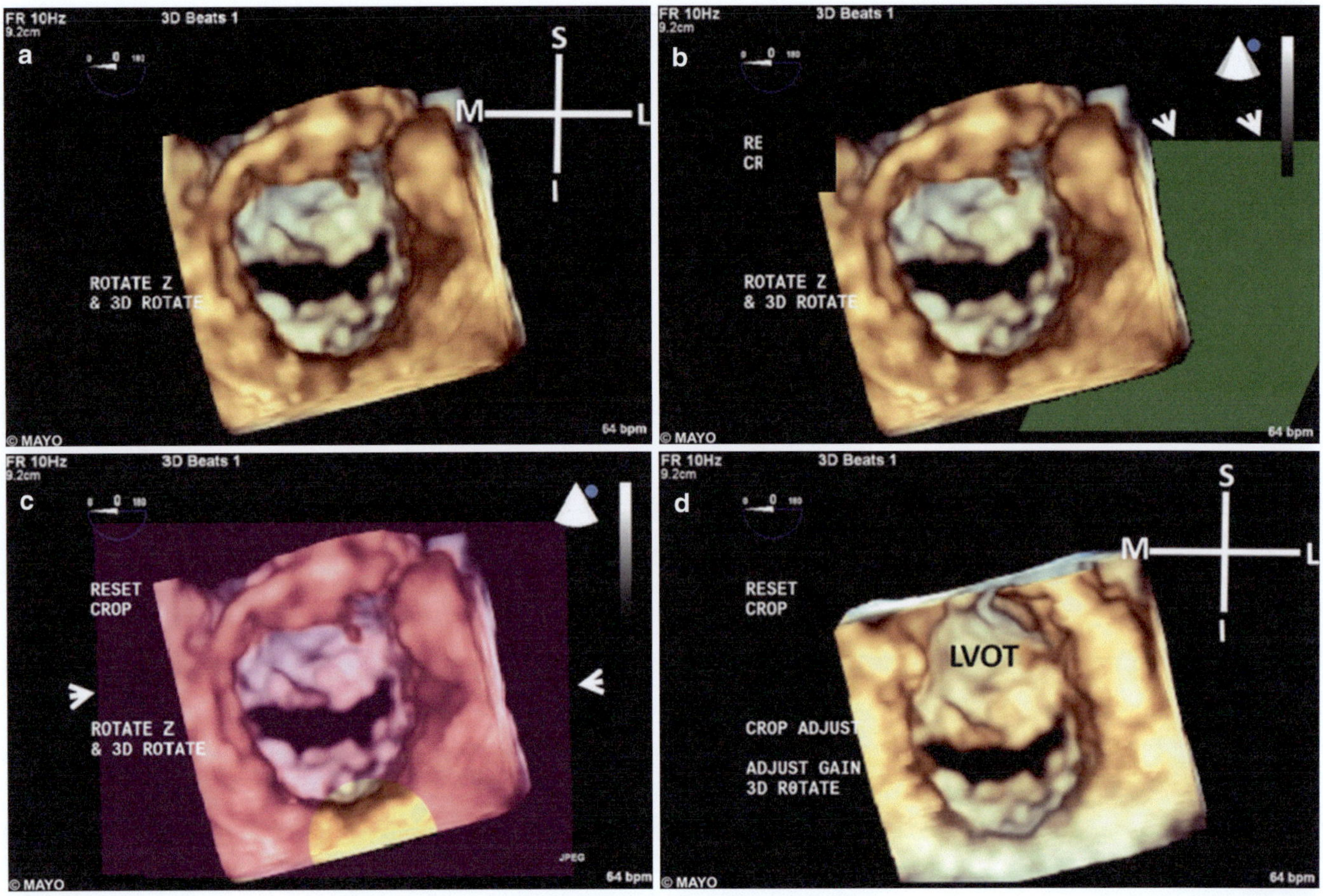

Fig. 2.15 (**a**–**d**) 3D TEE enface LV views of the MV: Image optimization is achieved using the freely adjustable "purple" plane (white arrows) and by adjusting both gain and compression settings to obtain the final image **d** at bottom right. Note that cropping using the freely adjustable plane is only possible when the plane is purple. This is achieved by simply rotating this crop plane from green (**b**) to enface purple (**c**). Used with permission of Mayo Foundation for Medical Education and Research. All rights reserved. I, inferior; L, lateral; LVOT, left ventricular outflow tract; LV, left ventricle; M, medial; MV, mitral valve; S, superior

on the 2D image view from which the 3D volumetric data set is generated [MultiVue (Philips Healthcare) and FlexiSlice (GE Healthcare)] (Figs. 2.22, 2.23, and 2.24). MPR can be used in any 3D acquisition mode.

The availability of the MPR software on the machine allows for timely analysis of the 3D data set either in real time [MultiVue (Philips Healthcare) and Flexi-Slice (GE Health Care)] or after 3D data acquisition [post processing (Figs. 2.25 and 2.26)]. Real time Flexi-Slice or MultiVue can be very helpful during transcatheter interventions (see Chap. 33). iSlice (Philips Healthcare) or Multi-Slice (GE Healthcare and Philips Healthcare) enable simultaneous display of equidistant short axis views generated from a 3D volume acquisition, and are very useful for quantitation of left ventricular ejection fraction and regional wall motion analysis (Fig. 2.26).

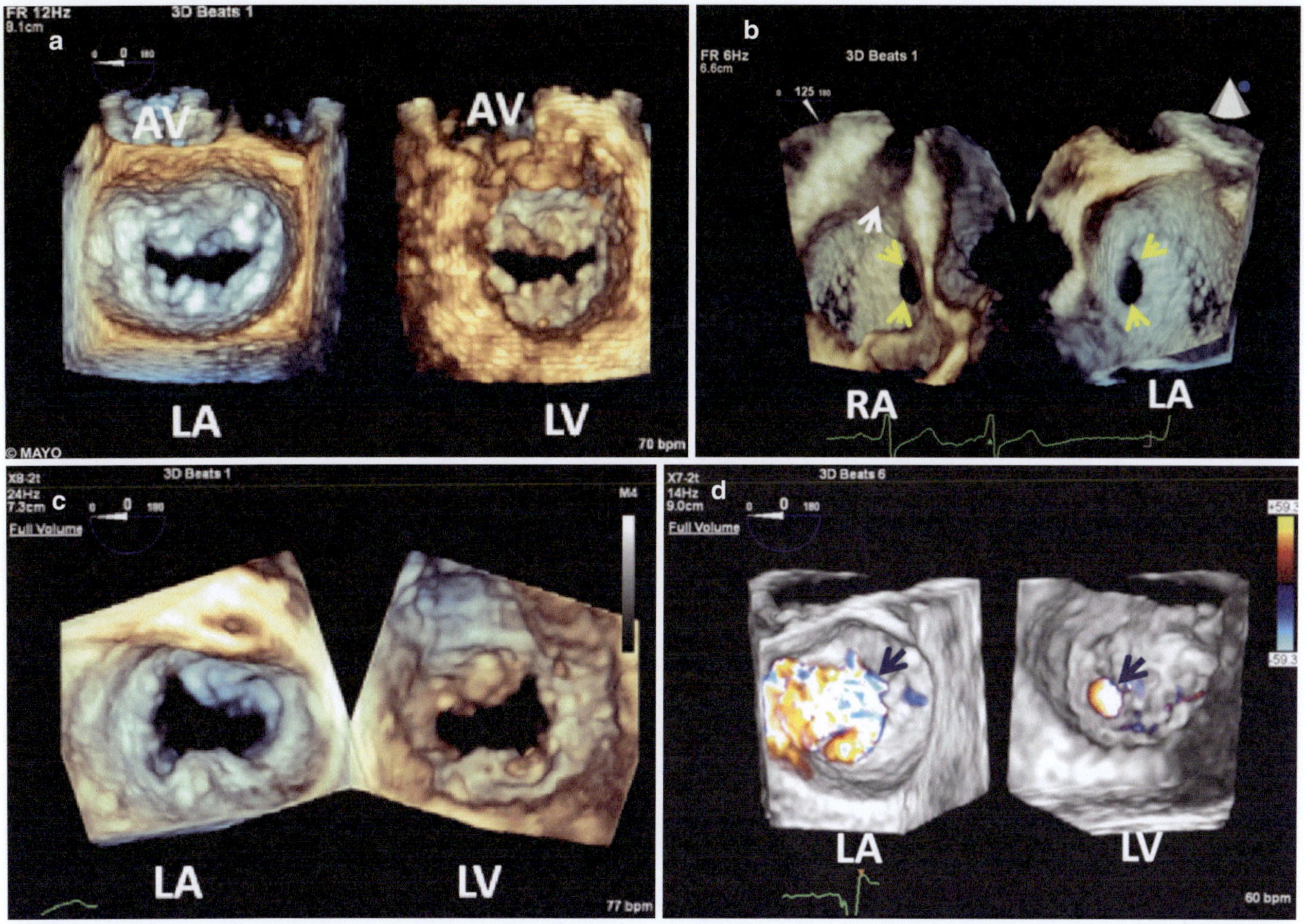

Fig. 2.16 **Top panel**: 3D zoom dual layout of MV (**a**) and ASD (yellow arrows, **b**). White arrow points to SVC. **Bottom panel**: (**c**) Dual layout FV acquisition of MV. (**d**) Dual layout FV MR CFD (arrows). Used with permission of Mayo Foundation for Medical Education and Research. All rights reserved. ASD, atrial septal defect; AV, aortic valve; CFD, color flow Doppler; FV, Full Volume; LA, left atrium; LV, left ventricle; MR, mitral regurgitation; MV, mitral valve; RA, right atrium; SVC, superior vena cava

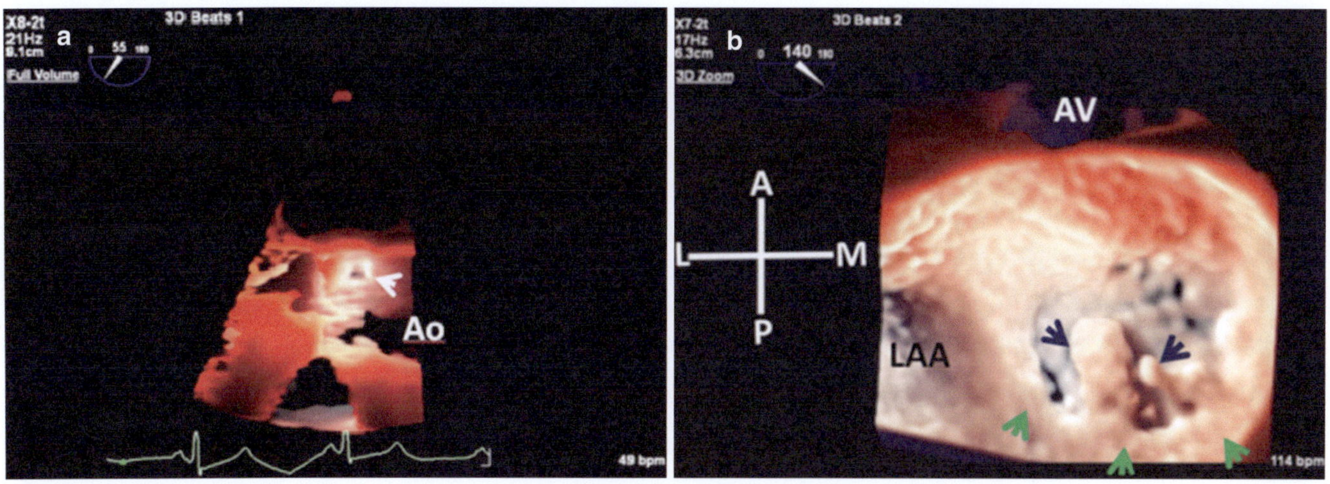

Fig. 2.17 TrueVue (Philips Healthcare) 3D TEE. (**a**) Coronary artery ostium (arrow). (**b**) Thrombus (dark blue arrows) on SR (green arrows). Used with permission of Mayo Foundation for Medical Education and Research. All rights reserved. A, anterior; Ao, ascending aorta; AV, aortic valve; L, lateral; LAA, left atrial appendage; M, medial; P, posterior; SR, sewing ring

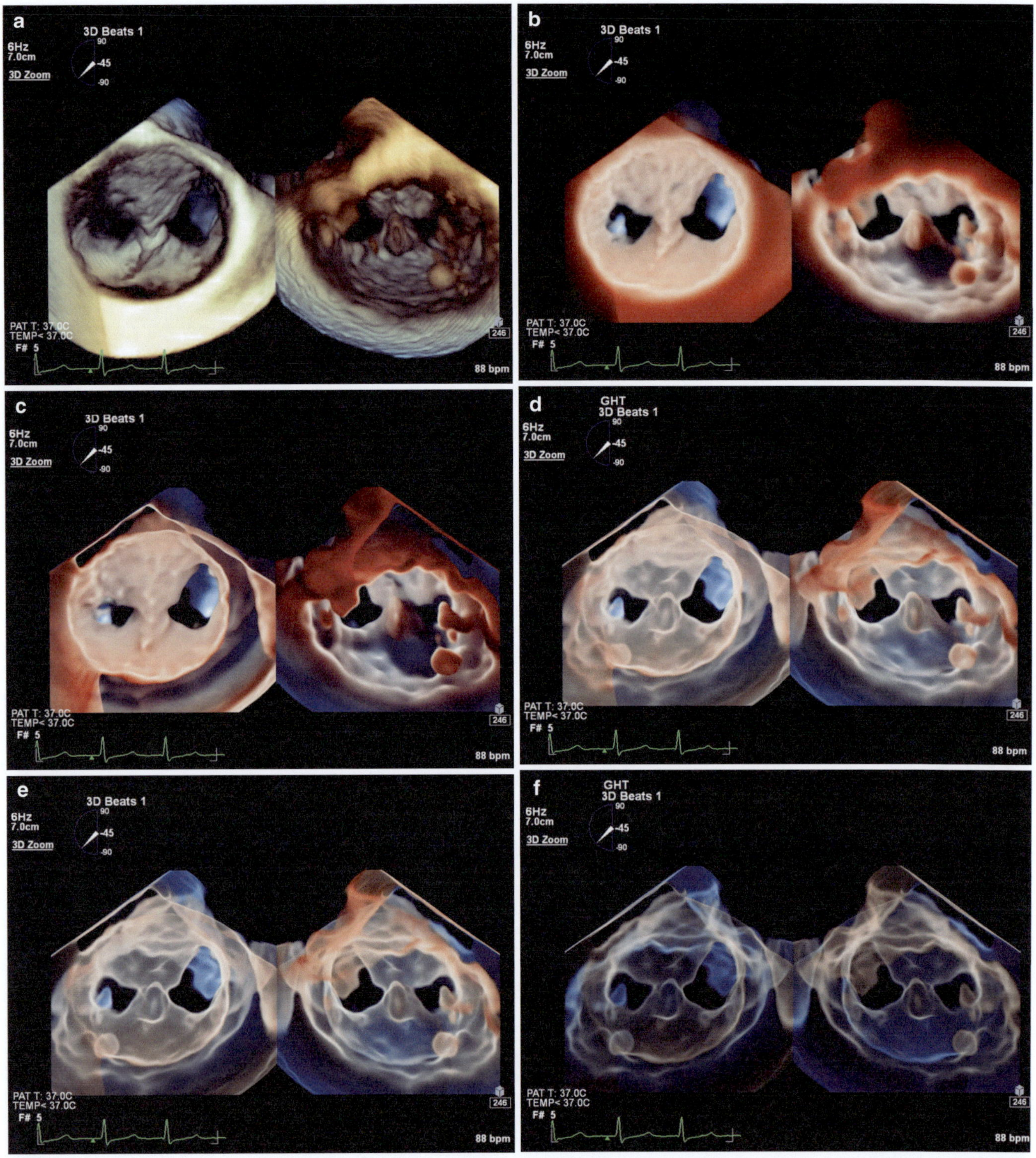

Fig. 2.18 3D Zoom Dual layout collage of double orifice MV post MitraClip deployment with focus on GlassVue (Philips Healthcare). **Panels a and b:** Default 3D Zoom (**a**) and same image in TrueVue format (**b**) after optimizing compression and smoothing options. **Panels c–f:** GlassVue of same TrueVue image in panel b using progressively higher transparency settings [0(**c**),10(**d**),15(**e**), and 20(**f**)]. Images courtesy of Dr. Sari Padang. Used with permission of Mayo Foundation for Medical Education and Research. All rights reserved

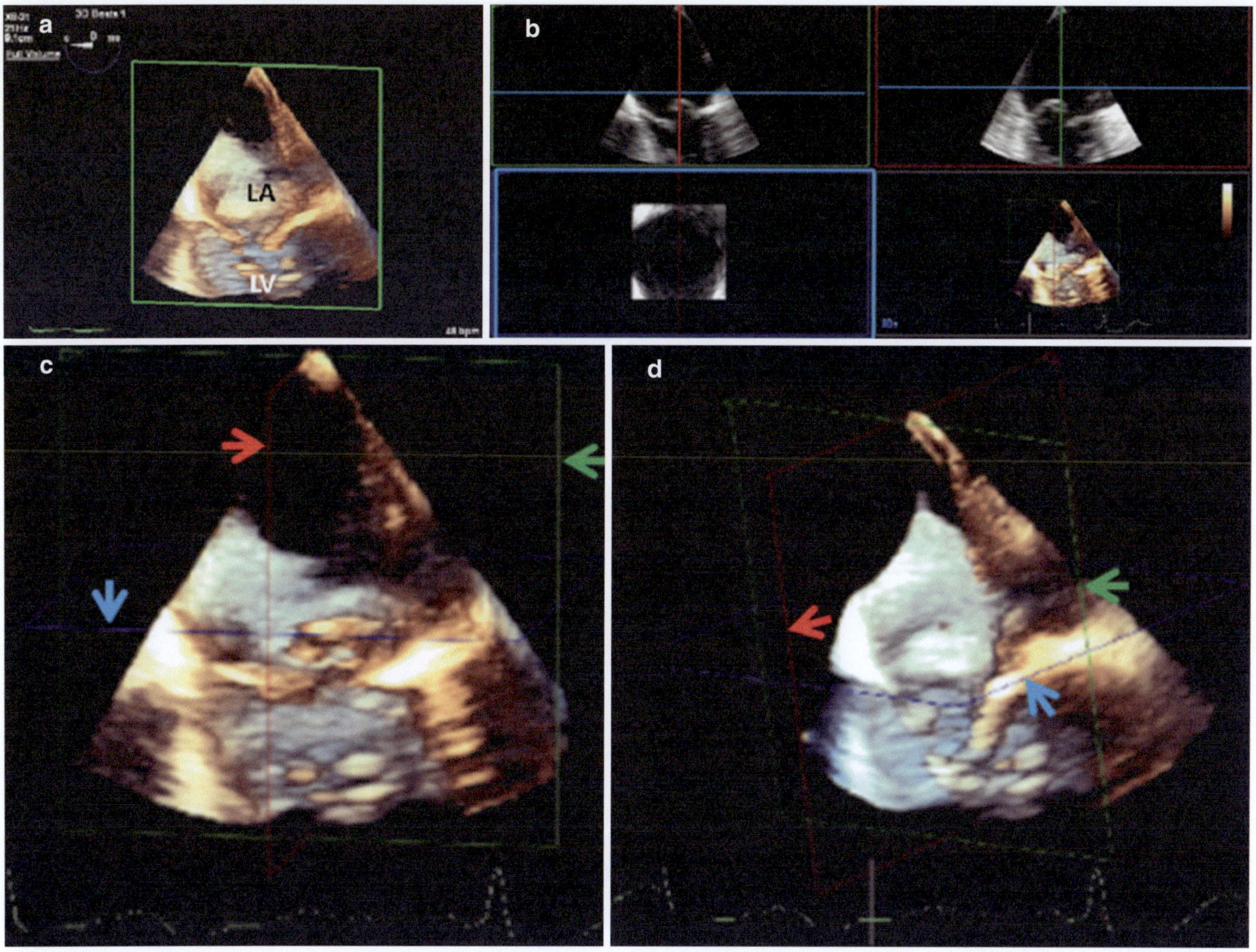

Fig. 2.19 **Top panel**: Default MPR; Philips Healthcare 3DQ (**b**) of volumetric 3D TEE data set (**a**) obtained from 2D 4 chamber (0°) mid-esophageal view. Blue lines and rectangle, Red line and rectangle, and Green line and rectangle refer to the transverse, sagittal, and coronal planes respectively as in Crop Box. The 2D TEE 4 chamber view is in the coronal plane (green rectangle) **Bottom panel**: Enlarged images of the default 3D data set (**c**) with tilted 3D volume to better show the crop planes (**d**). The same crop planes in MPR can be seen with the arrows color coded accordingly. Used with permission of Mayo Foundation for Medical Education and Research. All rights reserved. LA, left atrium; LV, left ventricle; MPR, multiplanar reconstruction

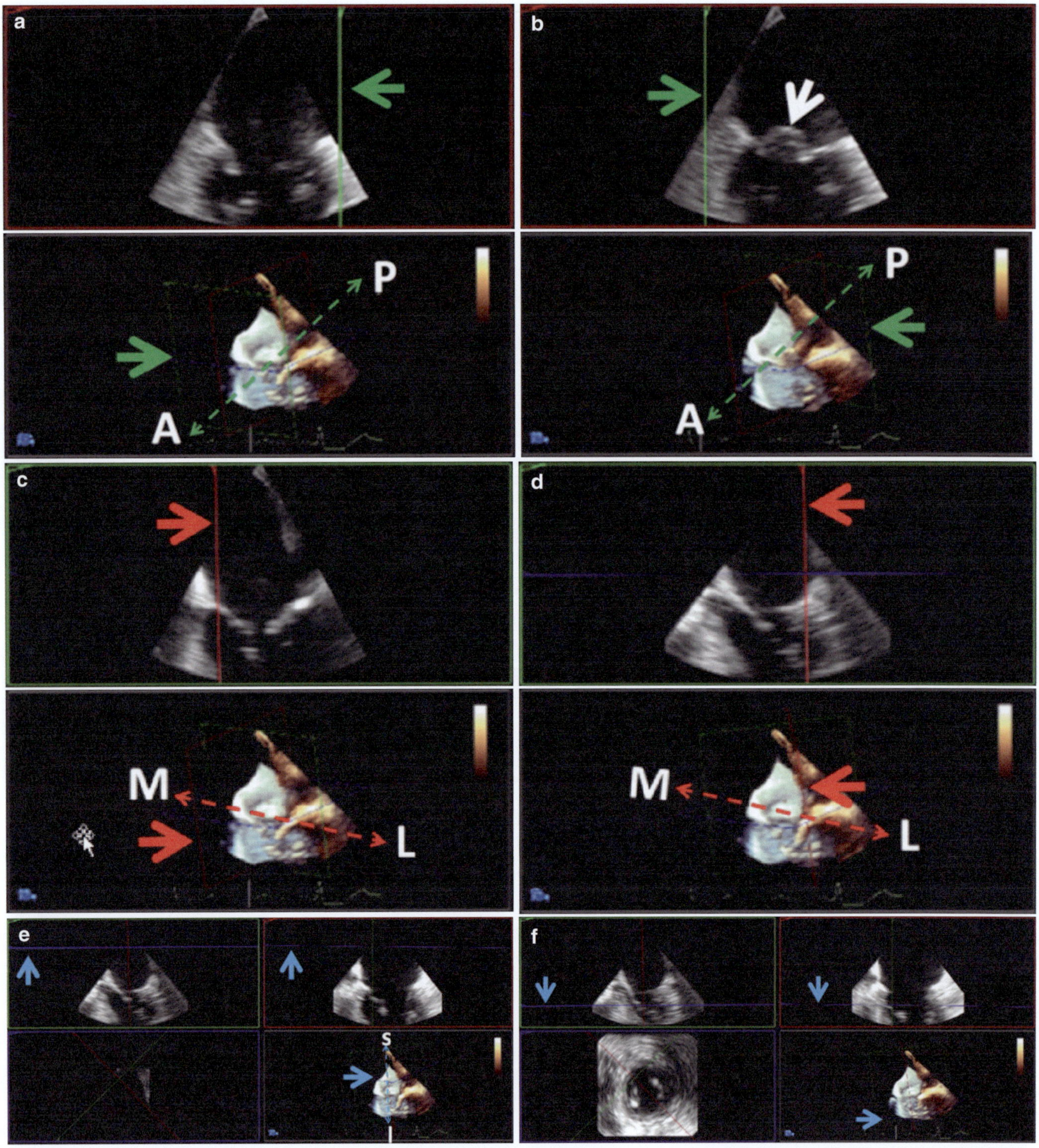

Fig. 2.20 Same MPR as in Fig. 2.19. (**a**, **b**) Green line/plane (green arrows) moved anteriorly (**a**) and posteriorly (**b**) in the tomographic 2D space with corresponding movements of the coronal plane (green arrows) in the 3D space. Note the P2 prolapse (white arrow) when the crop line/plane is posterior. (**c**, **d**) Red line (red arrows) moved from medial (**c**) to lateral (**d**) in the tomographic 2D space with corresponding movements of the sagittal plane in the 3D space (red arrows). (**e**, **f**) Blue line/plane moved in a superior (**e**, blue arrows) to inferior (**f**, blue arrows) direction. Used with permission of Mayo Foundation for Medical Education and Research. All rights reserved. A, anterior; I, inferior; L, lateral; M, medial; P, posterior; S, superior

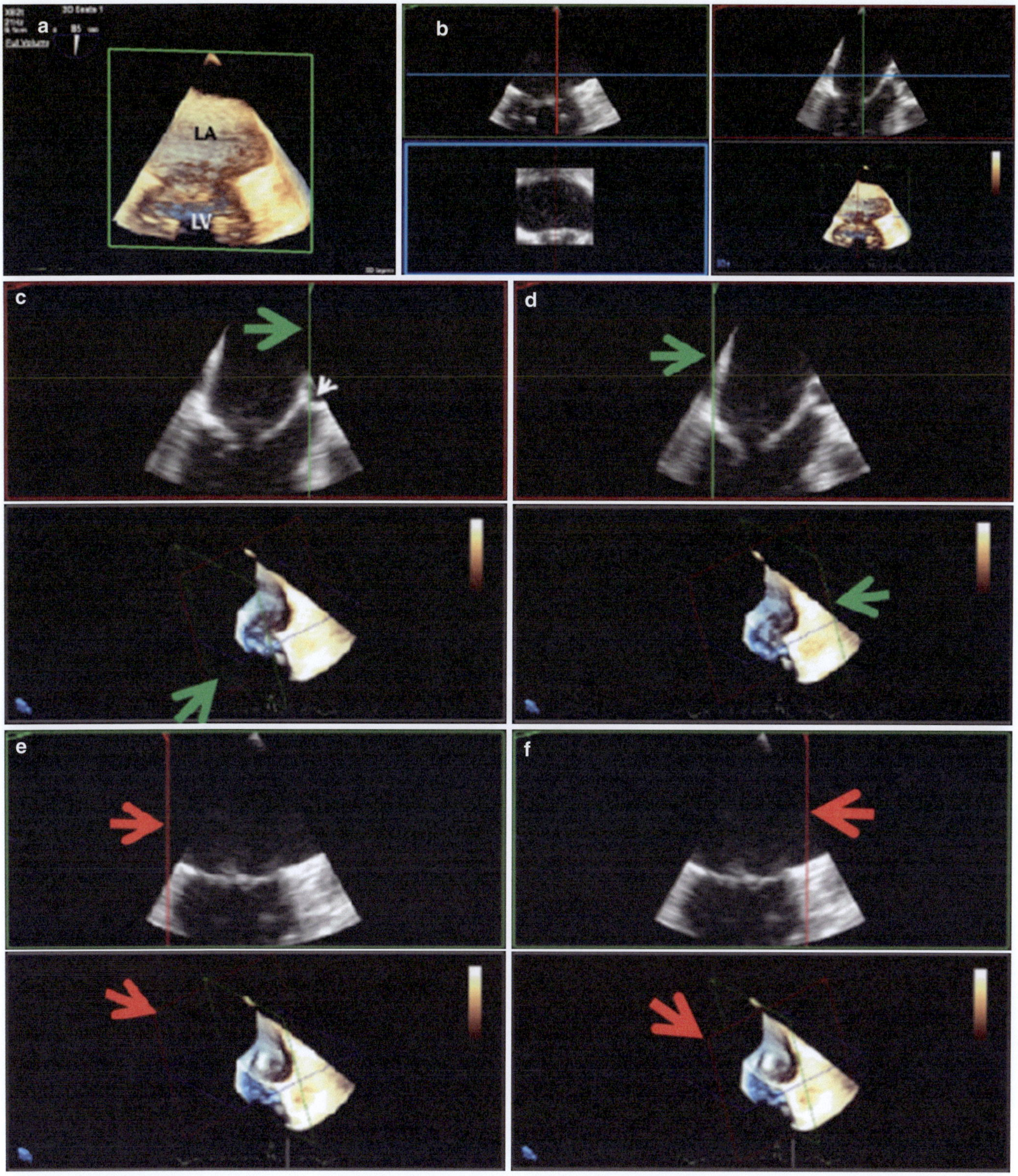

Fig. 2.21 **Top panel**: Default MPR; 3DQ Philips Healthcare (**b**) of volumetric 3D TEE data set (**a**) obtained in same patient in Figs. 2.19 and 2.20, from a nearly orthogonal mid-esophageal 2D view (85°). The 2D two chamber view is now in the coronal plane (green rectangle). (**c**, **d**) Green line/plane (green arrows) moved anteriorly (**c**) in direction of aortic valve (white arrow) and posteriorly (**d**) in the tomographic 2D space with corresponding coronal plane movement in the 3D space (green arrows). (**e**, **f**) Red or sagittal line/plane (red arrows) moved from medial (**e**) to lateral (**f**) in the two chamber tomographic 2D space with corresponding sagittal plane movements in the 3D space (red arrows). Used with permission of Mayo Foundation for Medical Education and Research. All rights reserved. LA, left atrium; LV, left ventricle; MPR, multiplanar reconstruction

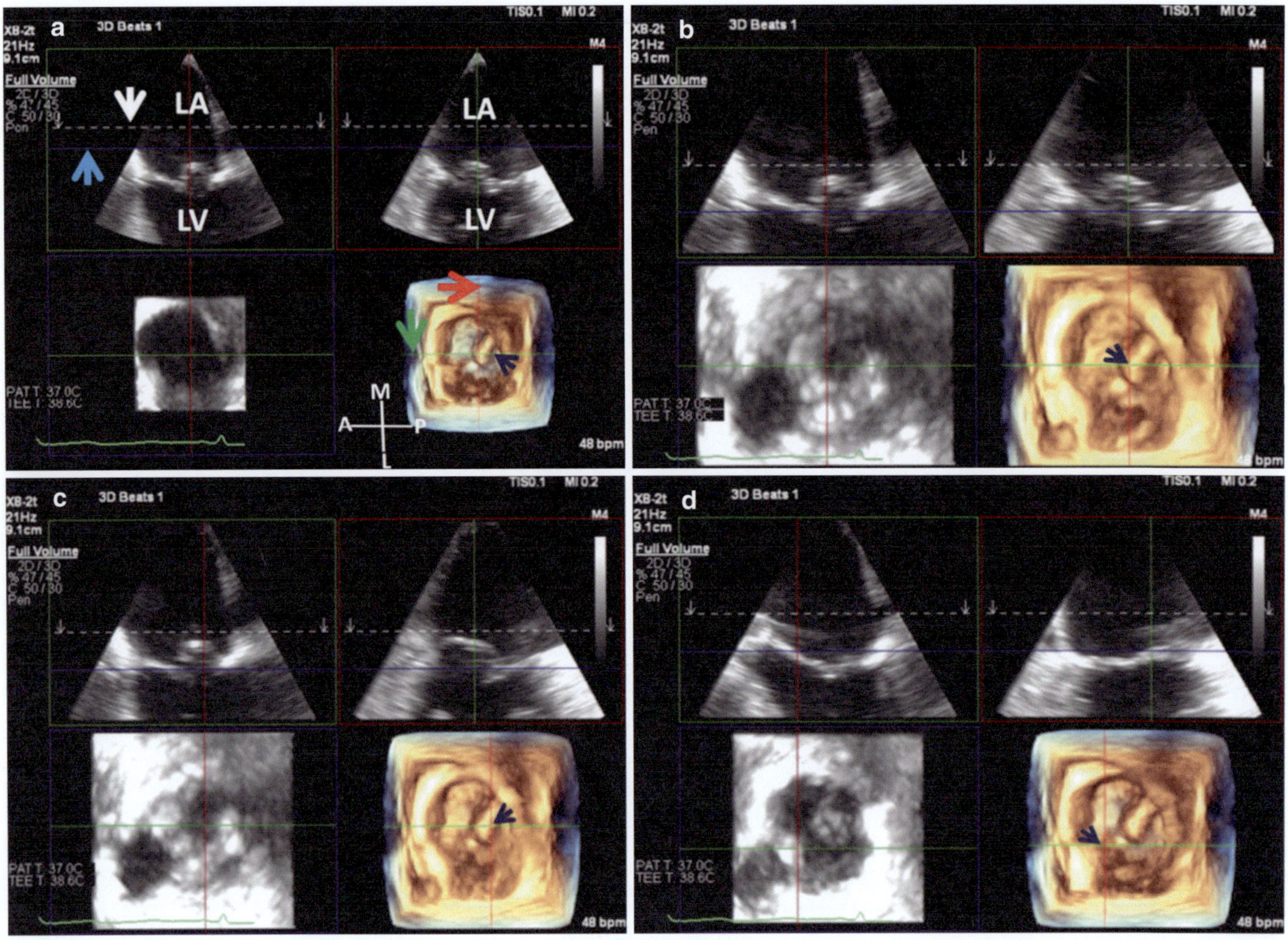

Fig. 2.22 RT FV MultiVue (Philips Healthcare). 3D TEE volumetric data set obtained from a midesophageal 2D four-chamber view (horizontal 0°) in a patient with a large prolapsing posterior mitral leaflet P2 segment. **Top panel**: (**a**) Default MPR. Crop planes are represented by lines or rectangles that are color coded green, red or blue. Direction of crop view is provided by the interrupted white line (white arrow). Light blue arrow points to blue line that represents the tail end of the crop plane reflected in the blue rectangle in left lower quadrant and the corresponding cropped 3D image. Dark blue arrow points to prolapsing P2 segment. Note the cross-hair intersection of the red line (red arrow) and green line (green arrow) in the blue rectangle tomographic 2D space and in the adjacent 3D space. (**b**) MPR enlarged by using zoom control after optimizing the image by adjusting position and size of the crop plane. **Bottom panel**: The cross-hair intersection of the red and green lines placed over the prolapsing P2 segment (**c**) and AML (**d**) and the corresponding changes in the MPR 2D tomographic space. Used with permission of Mayo Foundation for Medical Education and Research. A, anterior; AML, anterior mitral leaflet; FV, Full Volume; M, medial; L, lateral; LA, left atrium; LV, left ventricle; MPR, multiplanar reconstruction; P, posterior; RT, real time

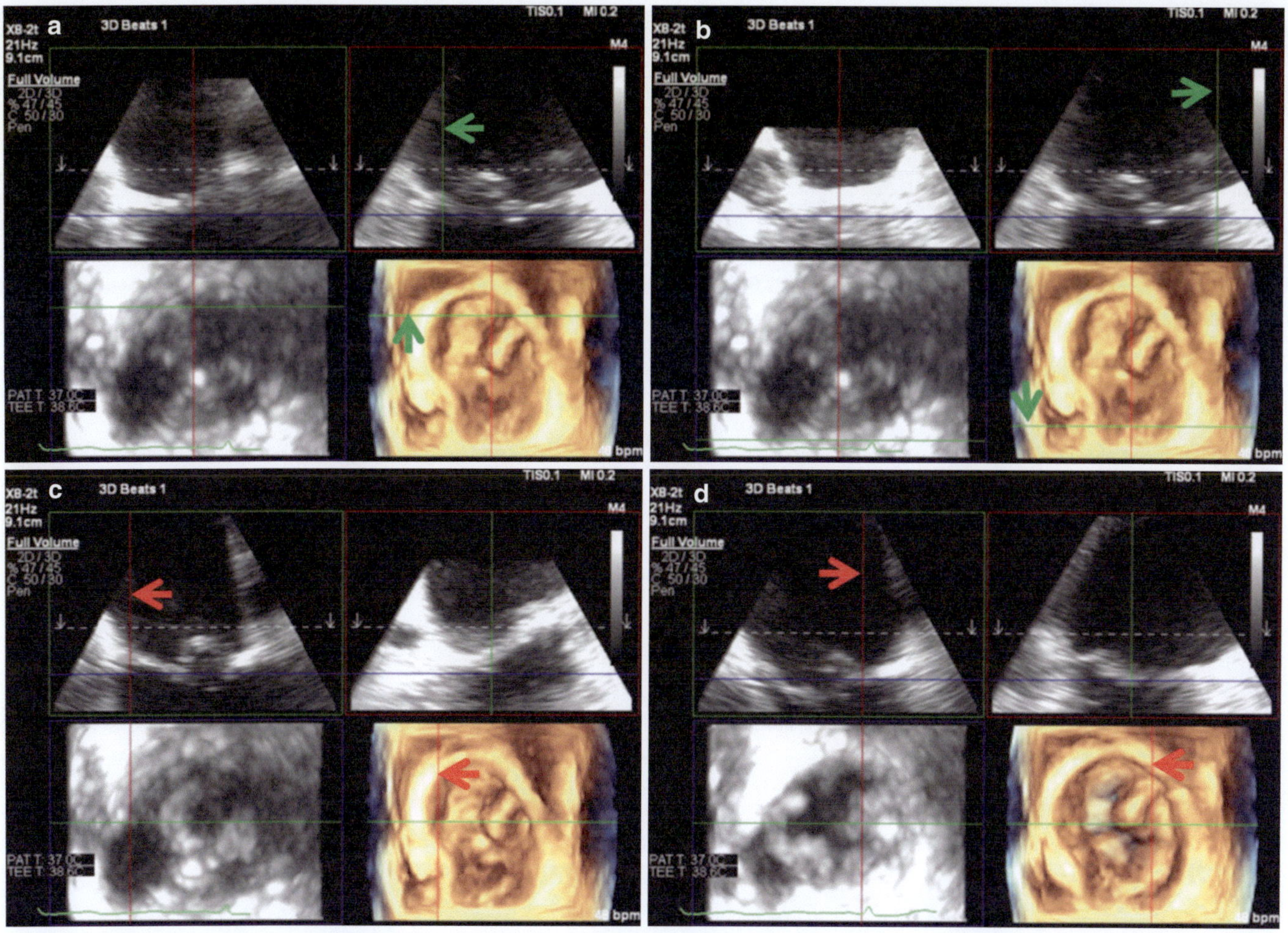

Fig. 2.23 Same MultiVue MPR of Fig. 2.22 to illustrate crop direction of the green and red lines that is clearly appreciated when viewed in the 3D space. Refer to 3D spatial coordinates legend in Fig. 2.21. **Top panel**: Green line (green arrows) moves in a medial (**a**) to lateral (**b**) direction in both the 2D tomographic and 3D space. **Bottom panel**: Red line (red arrows) moves in an anterior (**c**) to posterior (**d**) direction in both the 2D tomographic and 3D space. Used with permission of Mayo Foundation for Medical Education and Research.

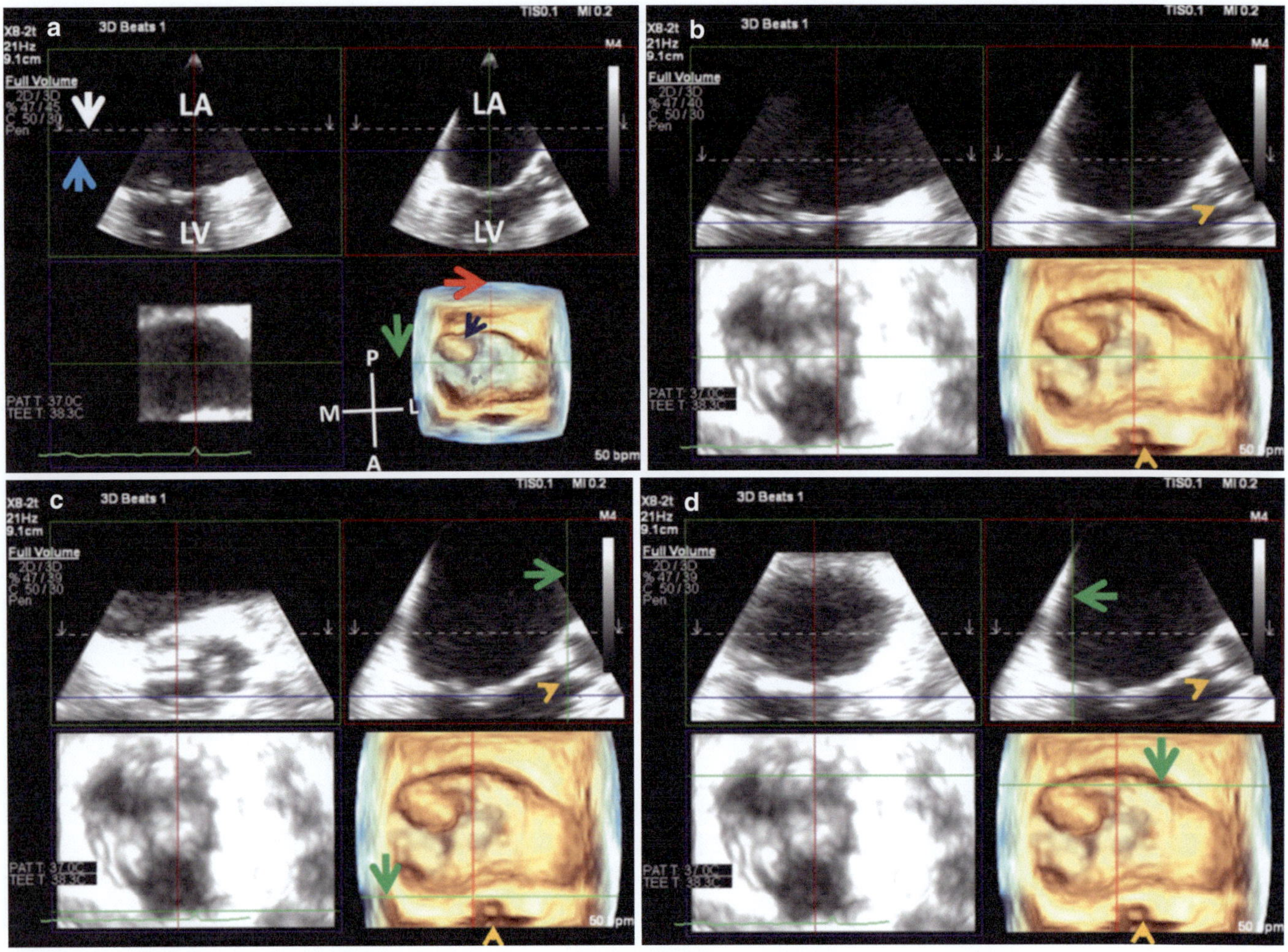

Fig. 2.24 **Top panel**: (**a**, **b**) 3D TEE MultiVue MPR from same patient but with 3D volumetric data set obtained from an orthogonal 2Chamber view. Legend same as for Fig. 2.22. Orange arrow heads point to aortic valve. **Second panel**: Green line (green arrows) moves in an anterior (**c**) to posterior (**d**) direction in both the 2D tomographic and 3D space. **Third panel**: Red line (red arrows) moves in a medial (**e**) to lateral (**f**) direction in both the 2D tomographic and 3D space. **Bottom panel**: (**g**, **h**) Tilting the green or red line provides a non-linear view of region of interest. Used with permission of Mayo Foundation for Medical Education and Research.

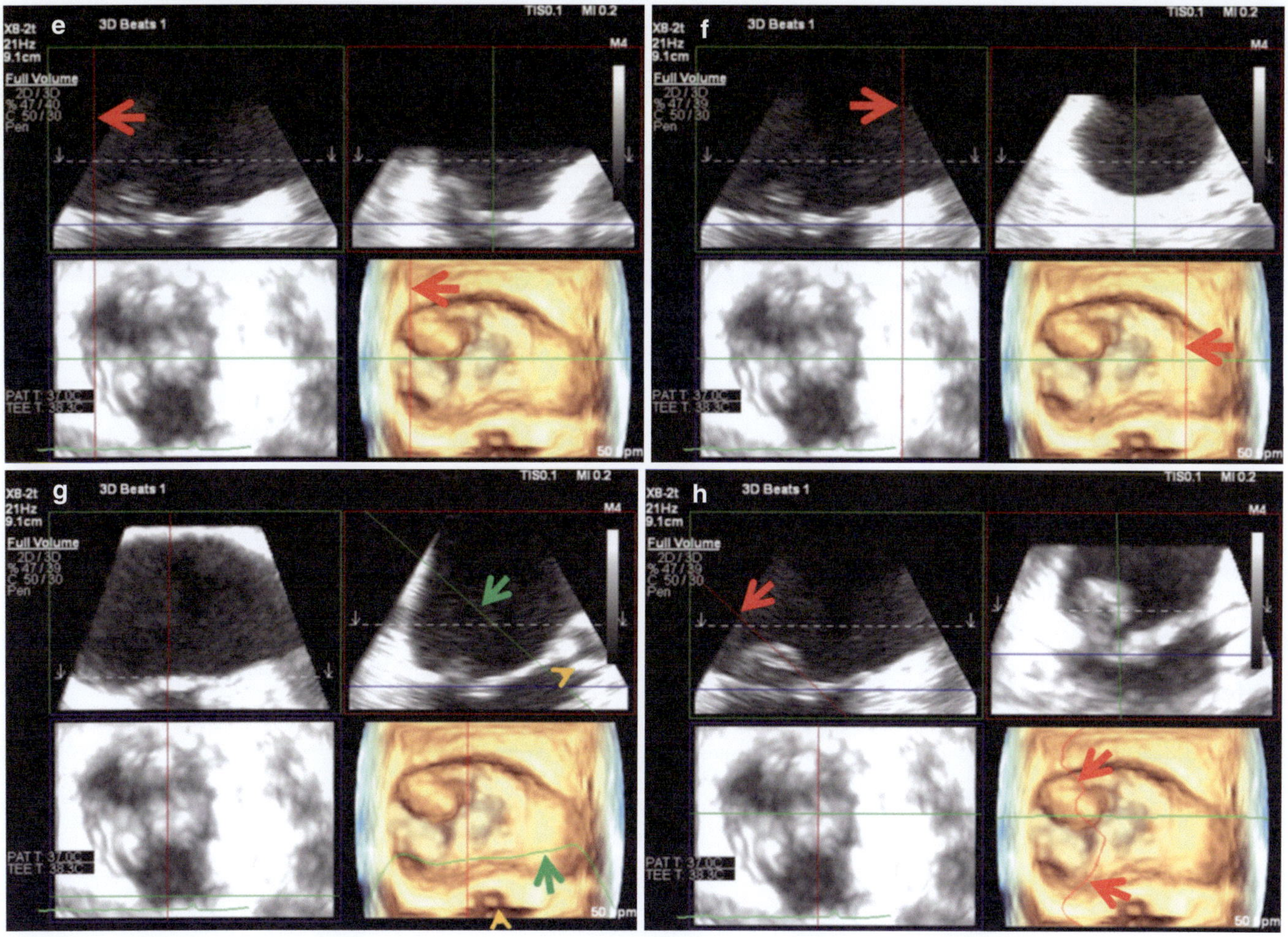

Fig. 2.24 (continued)

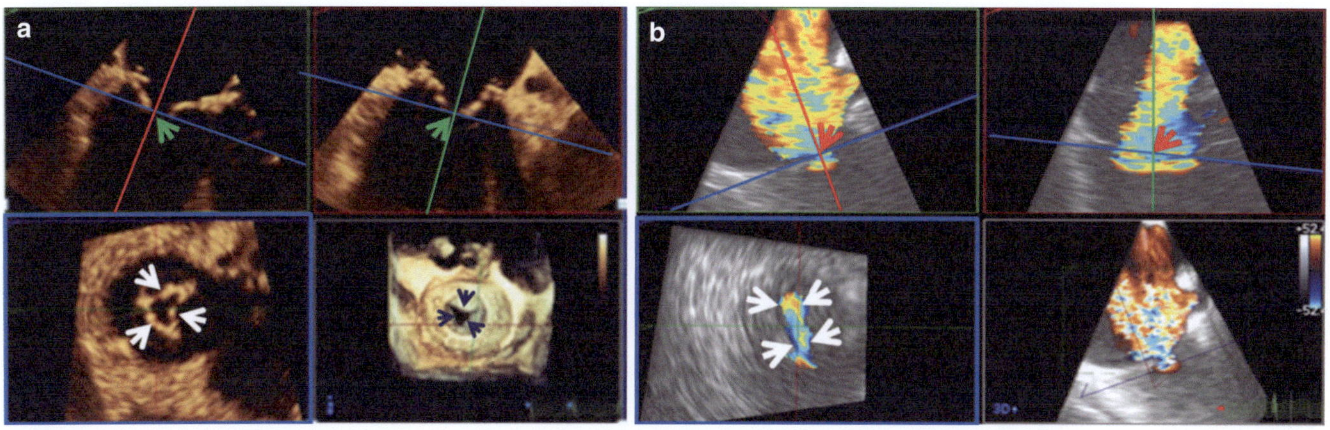

Fig. 2.25 Quantitative MPR of volumetric 3D data sets (3DQ, Philips Healthcare). Assessment of severity of mitral bioprosthesis stenosis (**a**, dark blue arrows), and MR severity (**b**). In both MPRs the intersection of two orthogonal crop planes (blue and red lines top left, and blue and green lines top right in each MPR) at LV tips of MV bioprosthesis leaflets (green arrows) and MR VC (red arrows) is displayed in the blue plane (blue box) at bottom left of each image (white arrows). Bioprosthesis stenosis severity and MR VC area can thus be quantified using the measurement software. Used with permission of Mayo Foundation for Medical Education and Research. All rights reserved. EROA, effective regurgitant orifice area; LV, left ventricle; MPR, muliplanar reconstruction; MR, mitral regurgitation; MV, mitral valve; VC, vena contracta

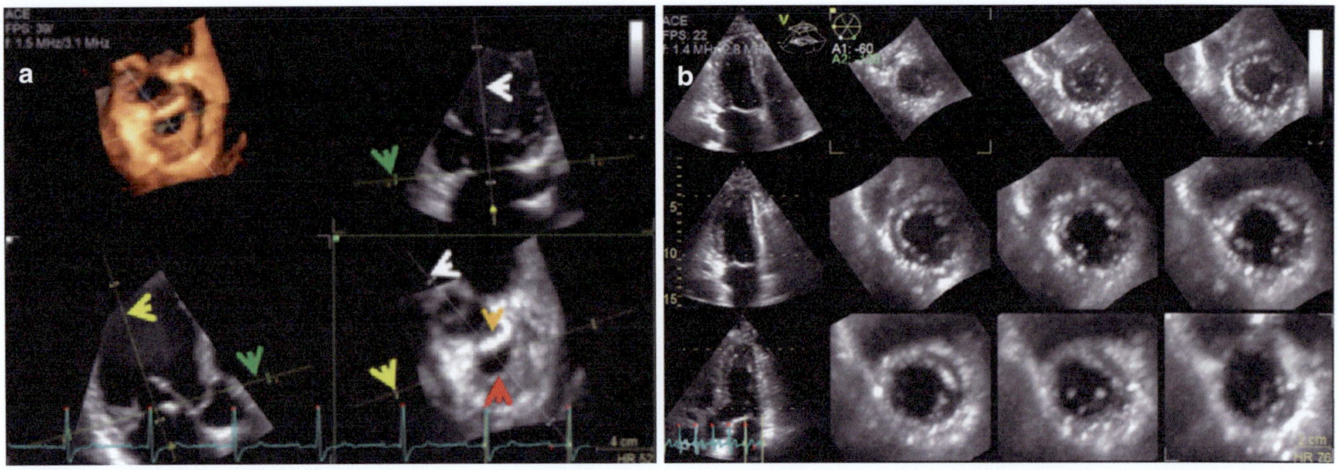

Fig. 2.26 (**a**) Post MV repair annuloplasty dehiscence quantitative MPR using **Flexi Slice** (GE Healthcare). The site and extent of dehiscence is clearly defined (red arrow) by the intersection of three arbitrary orthogonal planes (white, green, and yellow arrows). Orange arrow points to annuloplasty ring. (**b**) 3D TTE LV **Multi-Slice** acquisition (GE Healthcare) used for LV EF measurement and for regional wall motion analysis. Used with permission of Mayo Foundation for Medical Education and Research. All rights reserved. EF, ejection fraction; LV, left ventricle; MPR, multiplanar reconstruction; MV, mitral valve

References

1. Lang RM, et al. EAE/ASE recommendations for image acquisition and display using three dimensional echocardiography. Eur Heart J Cardiovasc Imaging. 2012;13:1–46.
2. Vegas A. Three-dimensional transesophageal echocardiography: principles and clinical applications. Ann Card Anaesth. 2016;19(Suppl 1):S35–43.

3DE Color Doppler Acquisition and Optimization and 3DE Artifacts, Caveats, and Pitfalls

3

Joseph F. Maalouf and Francesco F. Faletra

3D color flow Doppler (CFD) may be acquired in any of the available 3D acquisition modes [1], but the most commonly used modes are Philips Full Volume (FV) or 3D zoom (Fig. 3.1) or GE and Siemens 4D mode. As with any 3D acquisition, the 2D image must first be optimized before a 3D CFD image is obtained. If the volume rate or frame rate of a real time live single beat 3D CFD is too low, the frame rate can be increased by either decreasing the scanning density at the expense of decreased spatial resolution (Fig. 3.2), or through multi-beat acquisition as discussed in Chap. 1 thus maintaining spatial resolution.

3D color image size is optimized using the Lateral Size/Width and Elevation Width (Philips Healthcare) or Volume Size/Volume Shape (GE Healthcare) function controls (Fig. 3.3).

The initial 2D CFD image does not have to include the CFD region of interest (ROI) such as the origin of the jet of mitral regurgitation provided the entire CFD ROI is encompassed in the rendered 3D volume.

An alternate method to obtain a higher 3D CFD frame rate while maintaining the desired 3D volume size is to narrow the 3D color sector width to include only the CFD ROI within the larger 3D volume data set. If the CFD ROI is central, this is achieved using the lateral width button only. However, if the CFD ROI is not central, the narrowed 3D CFD beam can be directed to the ROI using the tilt lateral or elevation function, analogous to use of a torch light beam (Figs. 3.4 and 3.5).

Color filter when available, is a very useful tool to eliminate low velocity Doppler signals that may obscure the underlying pathology (Fig. 3.6). The transparency provided by GlassVue (Philips Healthcare) can bring to light the regurgitant jet origin and path (Fig. 3.7).

Quantitative assessment (see Chap. 2) of severity of regurgitant lesions is feasible using the multiplanar reconstruction software (Fig. 3.8).

3D Artifacts, Caveats, and Pitfalls

Although 3DE is subject to the same types of artifacts seen with 2DE [2, 3], some commonly shared artifacts such as dropout artifacts simulate a real defect such as an aortic valve perforation or atrial septal defect when displayed in a 3D format [3] (Fig. 3.9). And, the reduced spatial resolution compared with 2D may make thin structures such as suture material or chordae tendinae appear thicker than they are in reality and in comparison with 2D images which can affect resolution of adjacent structures [3]. This is referred to as blurring or amplification artifacts [3] (Figs. 3.10 and 3.11). Moreover, because 3D axial resolution is inferior to 2D, two adjacent ruptured chords may appear as a single thick chord on 3D images [3] (Fig. 3.10). Blurring artifacts may be minimized by reducing gain [3]

Additionally, there are artifacts that are unique to 3DE such as multibeat acquisition stitch artifacts (Fig. 3.12; see Chap. 1). And, in the setting of percutaneous transcatheter interventions that are guided by 3DE, artifacts caused by metallic components of wires, catheters and devices are particularly frequent and comprise a wide spectrum that includes acoustic shadowing (Fig. 3.13), blooming, railroad, and reverberation artifacts that may impact intraprocedural imaging [3].

Blooming and railroad-shaped artifacts (Fig. 3.14) are seen when the structure being imaged contains metallic components [3]. In addition to mechanical prostheses and

Supplementary Information The online version of this chapter (https://doi.org/10.1007/978-3-030-72941-7_3) contains supplementary material, which is available to authorized users.

J. F. Maalouf (✉)
Professor of Medicine, Mayo Clinic College of Medicine; Director, Interventional Echocardiography; Consultant, Department of Cardiovascular Medicine, Mayo Clinic, Rochester, MN, USA
e-mail: maalouf.joseph@mayo.edu

F. F. Faletra
Director of Cardiac Imaging Lab, Cardiocentro Ticino Institute, Lugano, Switzerland
e-mail: Francesco.Faletra@cardiocentro.org

J. F. Maalouf et al. (eds.), *Practical 3D Echocardiography*, https://doi.org/10.1007/978-3-030-72941-7_3

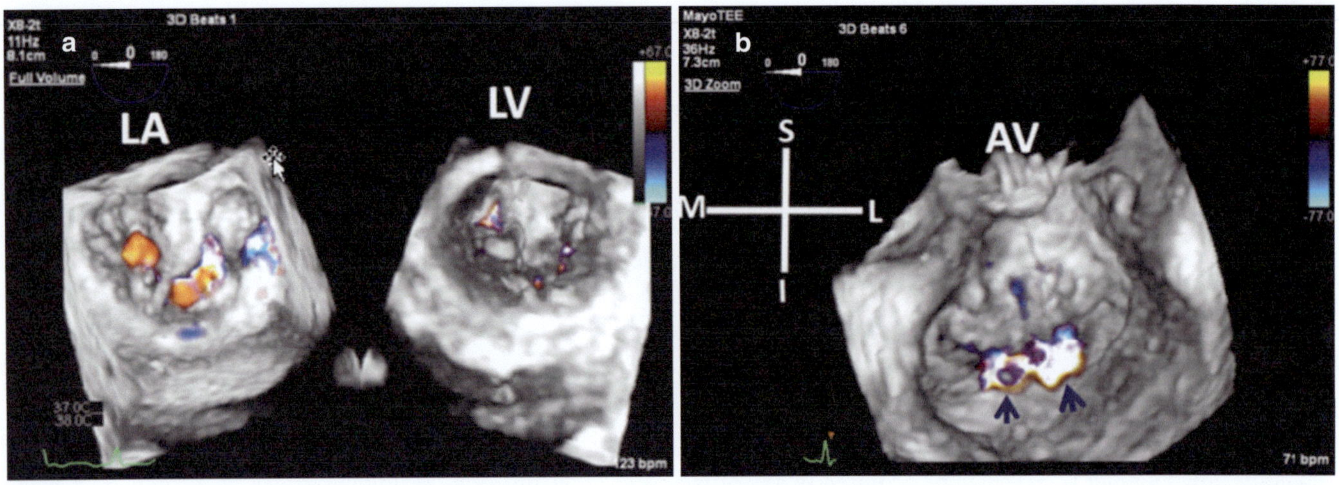

Fig. 3.1 (**a**) Dual LA and LV layout of FV CFD. (**b**) 3D Zoom enface LV view of MR (dark blue arrows). Used with permission of Mayo Foundation for Medical Education and Research. All rights reserved. AV, aortic valve; CFD, color flow Doppler; FV, Full Volume; I, inferior; L, lateral; LA, left atrium; LV, left ventricle; M, medial; MR, mitral regurgitation; S, superior

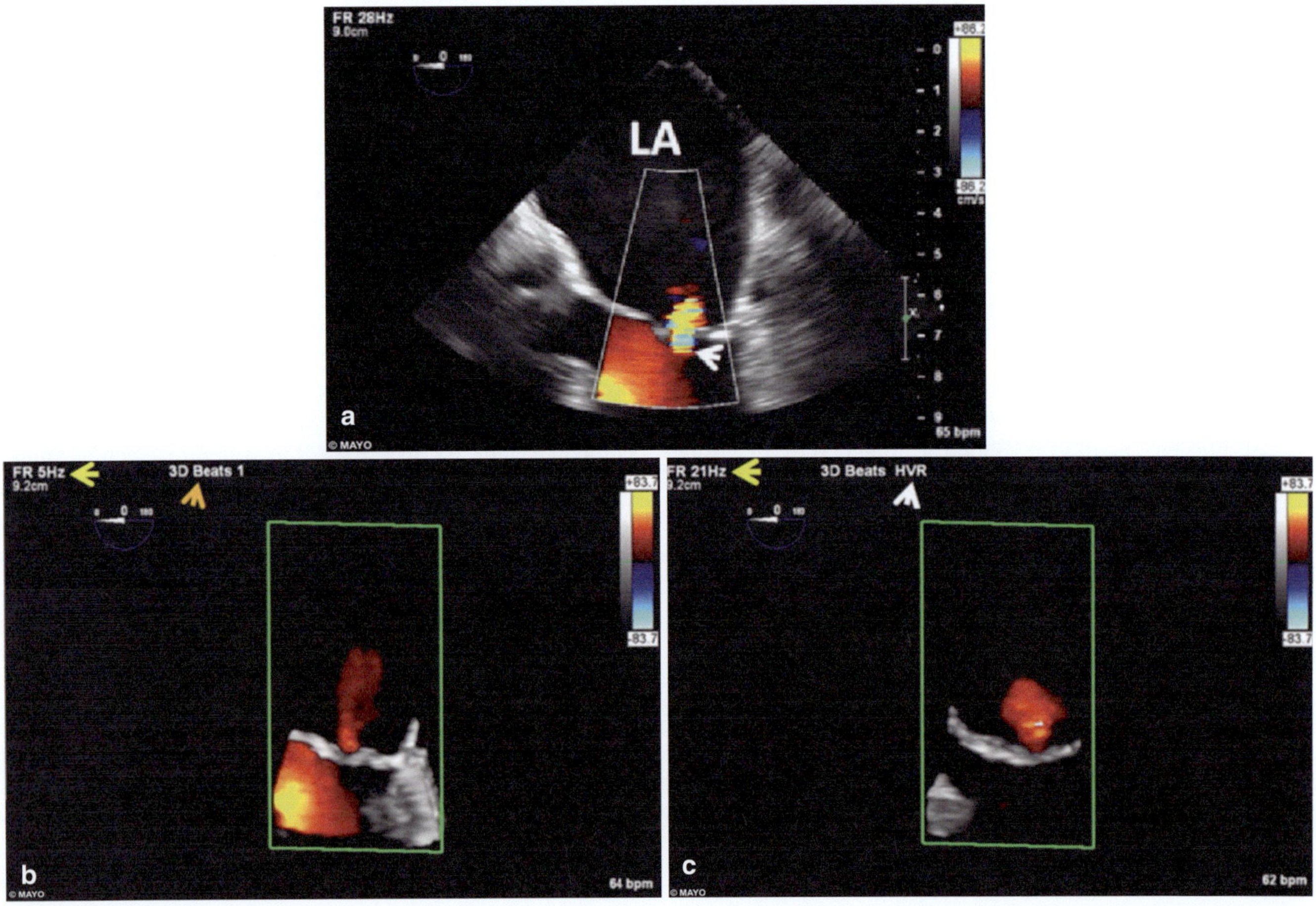

Fig. 3.2 (**a**) Optimized 2D TEE CFD view. (**b**) Same view, real time live single beat (orange arrow) FV 3D TEE CFD . The FR is only 5 Hz (yellow arrow). (**c**) The frame rate is increased to 21 Hz (yellow arrow) by changing the 3D TEE CFD acquisition mode to live single beat HVR (white arrow) at the expense of reduced spatial resolution. Used with permission of Mayo Foundation for Medical Education and Research. All rights reserved. CFD, color flow Doppler; FR, frame rate; FV, Full Volume; HVR, high volume rate, LA, left atrium

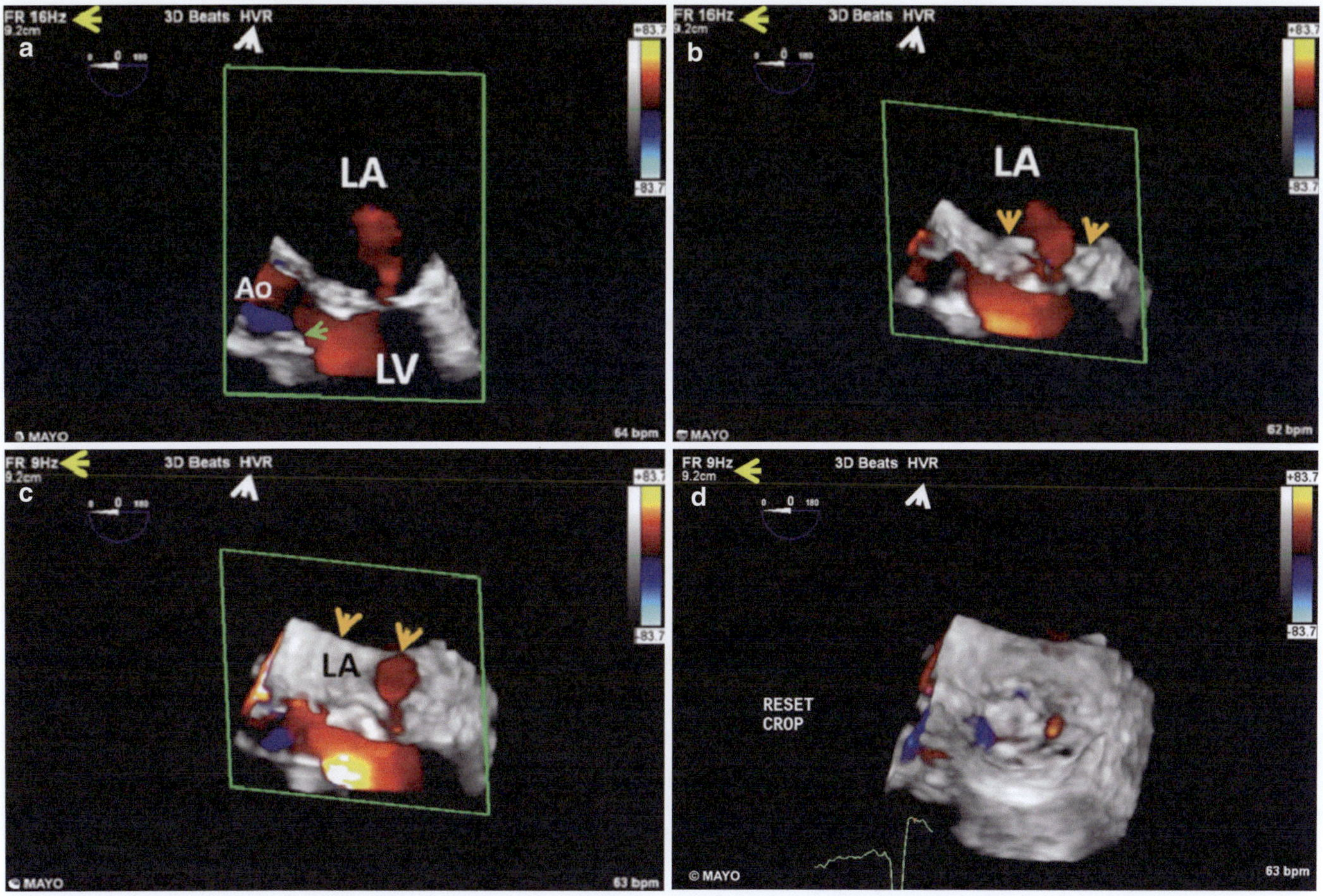

Fig. 3.3 Optimizing image size of the 3D CFD HVR (white arrows) shown in Fig. 3.1. **Top panel**: Increase in both lateral width (**a**) and elevation (antero-posterior) width (**b**). Note the greater posterior depth (orange arrows). Green arrow (left) points to AV RCC. **Bottom panel**: (**c**) Further increase in elevation width (orange arrows). (**d**) FV CFD after crop reset. Note the drop in FR (yellow arrows) with increase in 3D image dimensions. Used with permission of Mayo Foundation for Medical Education and Research. All rights reserved. Ao, ascending aorta; AV, aortic valve; CFD, color flow Doppler; FR, frame rate; FV, Full Volume; HVR, high volume rate; LA, left atrium; LV, left ventricle; RCC, right coronary cusp

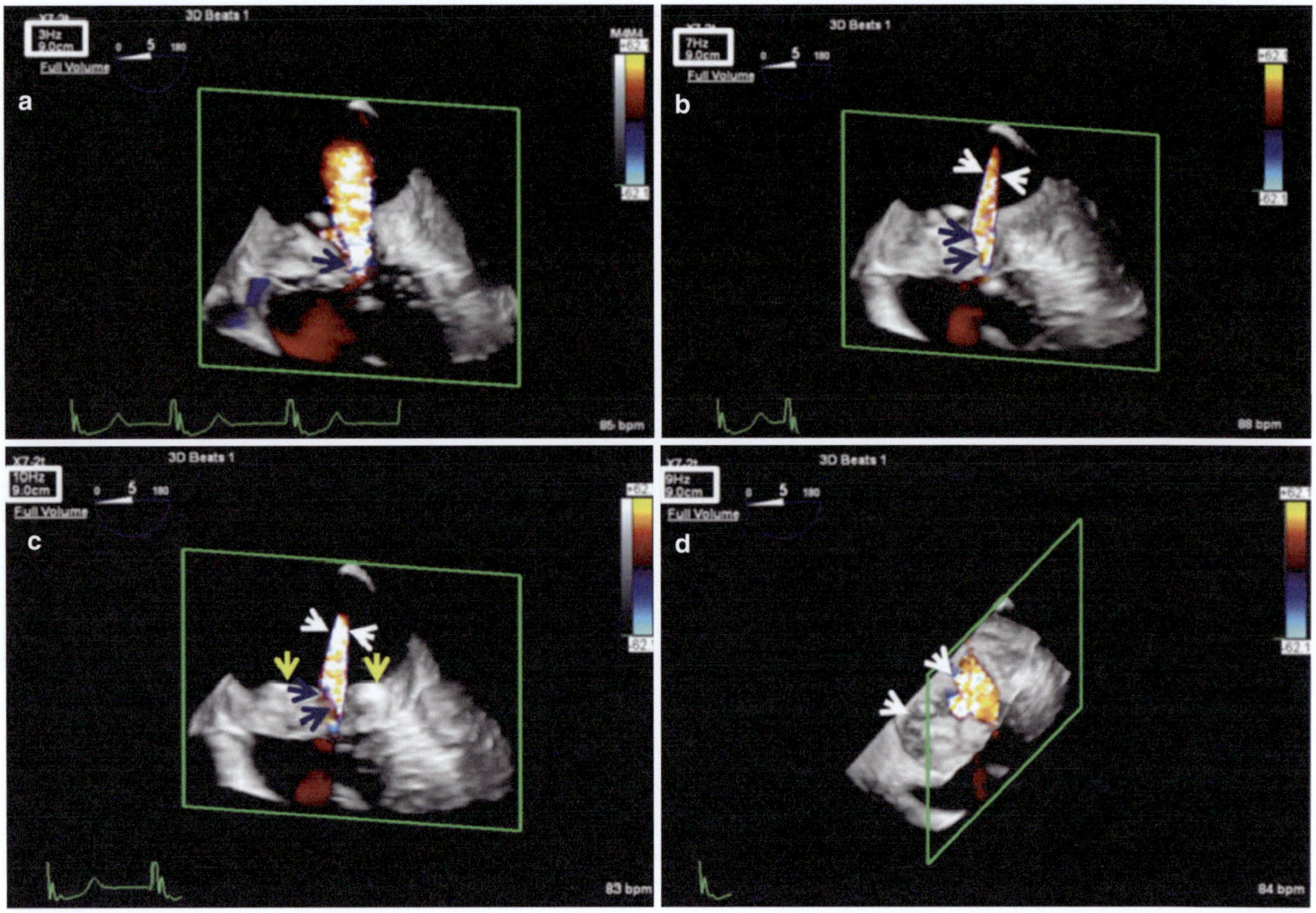

Fig. 3.4 Real time single beat autocropped FV TEE 3D CFD FR optimization (X7 Philips ultrasound platform) in a patient with MR (dark blue arrows). **Top panel**: (**a**) Baseline FV CFD. FR is only 3 Hz. (**b**) Same FV with reduced CFD sector width (white arrows) while maintaining 3D volume size the same. FR is slightly higher at 7 Hz. **Bottom panel**: (**c**) Further increase in FV CFD FR to 10 Hz by decreasing 3D volume size through a reduction in elevation width (Note the less posterior extension; yellow arrows). White arrows point to CFD sector size. (**d**) 3D volume size optimized to include the posterior mitral annulus (white arrows). FR is 9 Hz. Note that image depth and spatial resolution are maintained throughout. Used with permission of Mayo Foundation for Medical Education and Research. All rights reserved. CFD, color flow Doppler; FR, frame rate; FV, Full Volume; MR, mitral regurgitation

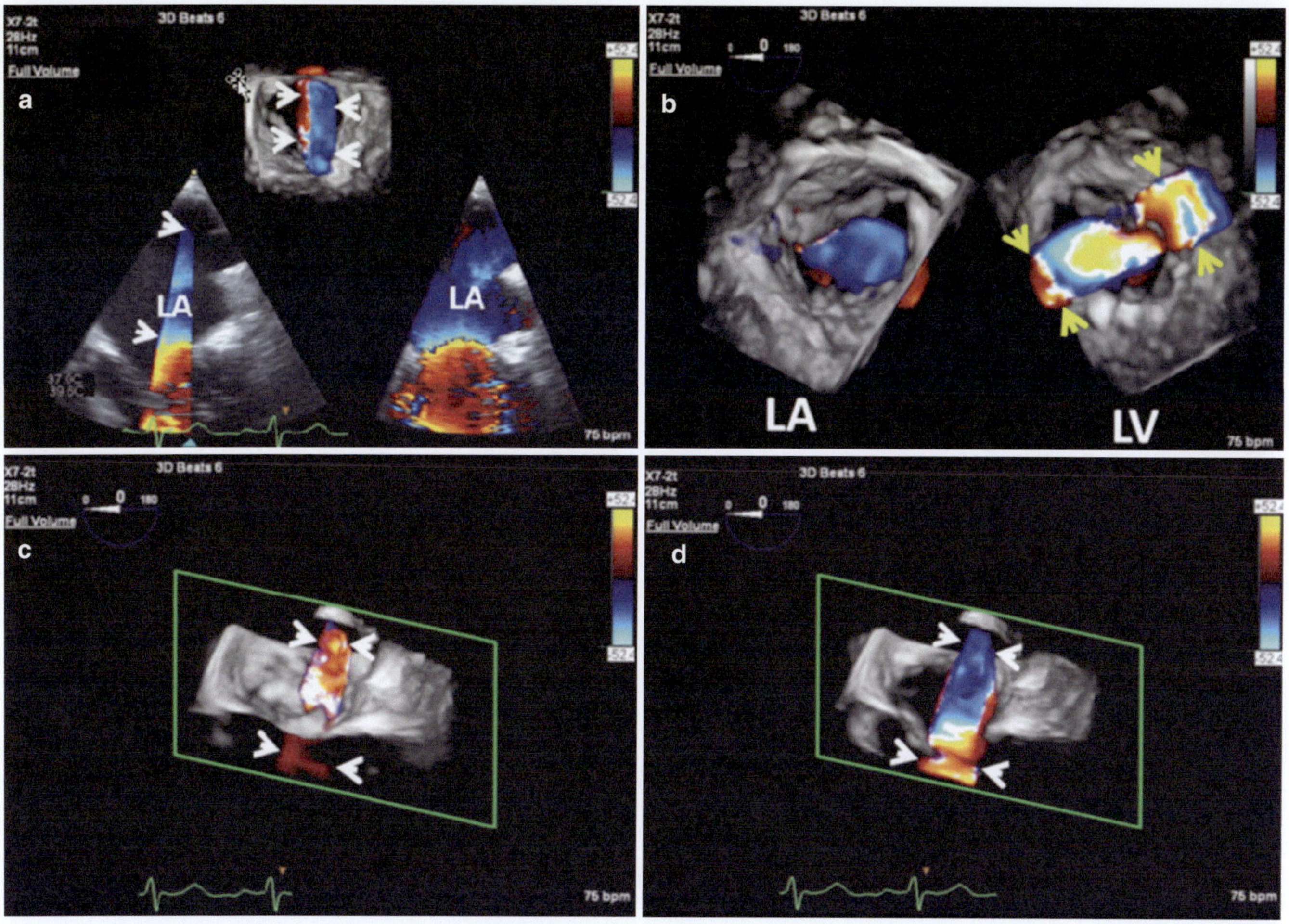

Fig. 3.5 FV multibeat (6) 3D TEE CFD acquisition with narrow CFD sector width (X7 Philips ultrasound). The FR of identical multibeat CFD of the entire 3D volume data set was only 6Hz. **Top panel**: (**a**) 3D-2D layout showing the narrowed CFD sector width (white arrows). (**b**) Dual layout highlighting the narrowed CFD sector width (yellow arrows) within the larger 3D volume data set. Note that the FR is high at 28 Hz despite no change in the 3D volume size. **Bottom panel**: Auto cropped FV 3D TEE CFD enface LA views from same patient highlighting the narrowed CFD sector width (arrows) in both systole (**c**) and diastole (**d**). Used with permission of Mayo Foundation for Medical Education and Research. All rights reserved. CFD, color flow Doppler; FV, Full Volume; FR, frame rate; LA, left atrium; LV, left ventricle

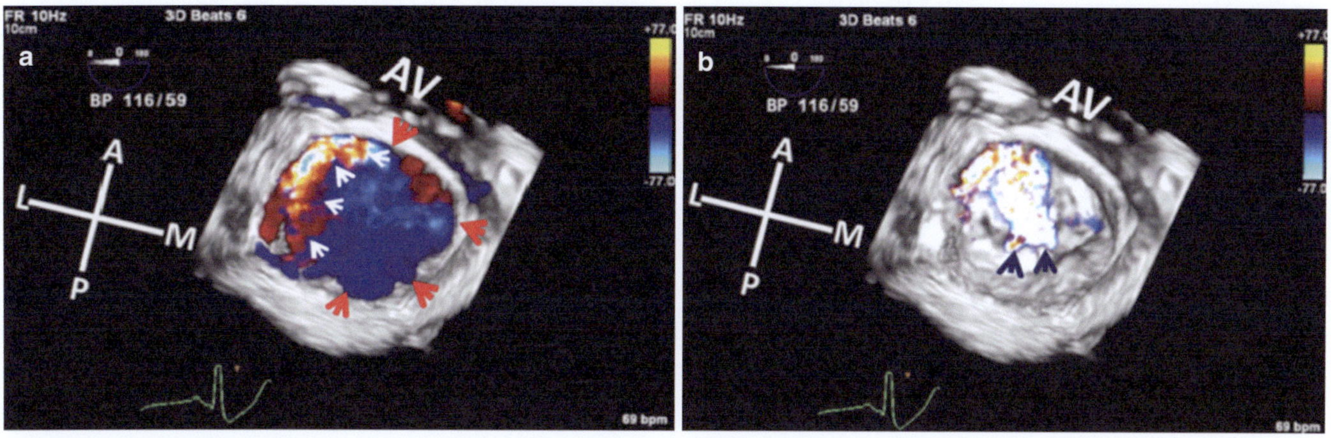

Fig. 3.6 Multibeat 3D FV CFD enface LA views in a patient with severe MR without use of color filter (**a**) and with high color filter setting (**b**). Note that without use of color filter, a cloud of low velocity flow (blue, red arrows) obscures the origin of the MR jet (white arrows). The central origin of the MR jet is clearly seen with use of color filter (dark blue arrows). Used with permission of Mayo Foundation for Medical Education and Research. All rights reserved. A, anterior; AV, aortic valve; CFD, color flow Doppler; FV, Full Volume; L, lateral; LA, left atrium; M, medial; MR, mitral regurgitation; P, posterior

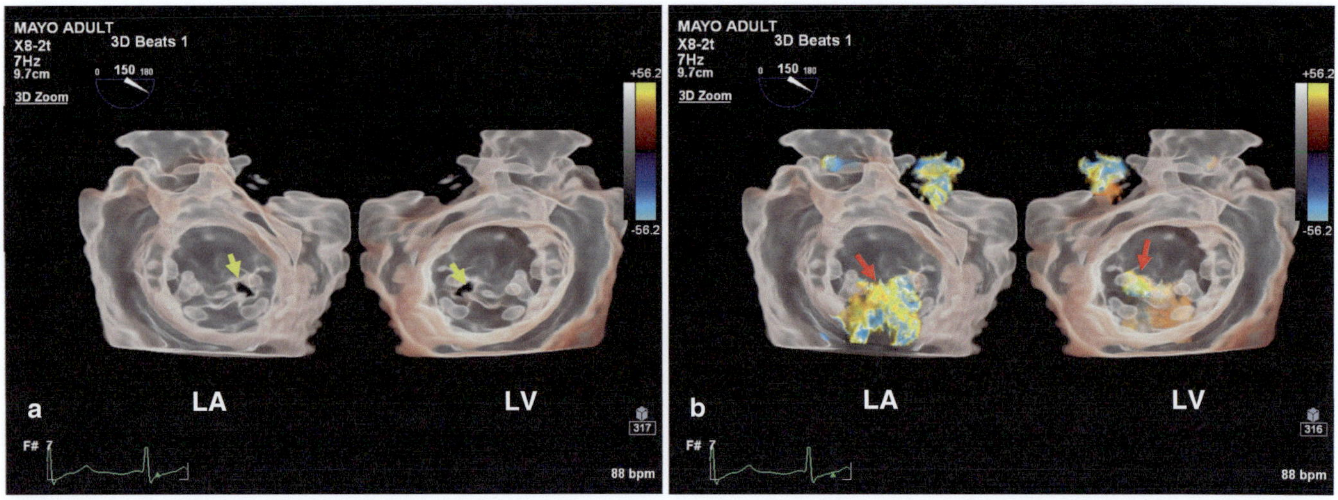

Fig. 3.7 3D Zoom Dual layout of MV in GlassVue (Philips Healthcare) without (**a**) and with (**b**) CFD showing the gap in leaflet coaptation in systole (**a**, yellow arrows) and MV regurgitation (**b**, red arrows). Note the discrete origin of the MR jet from the LV view and splaying of the MR jet in the LA. Images courtesy of Dr. Sari Padang. Used with permission of Mayo Foundation for Medical Education and Research. All rights reserved. CFD, color flow Doppler; LA, left atrium; LV, left ventricle; MR, mitral regurgitation

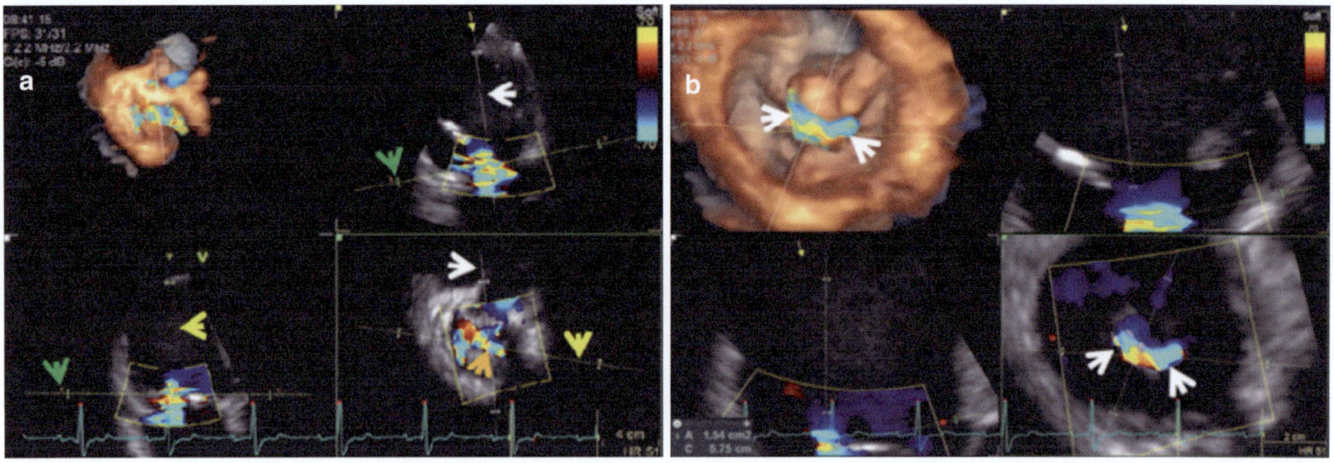

Fig. 3.8 Multiplanar reconstruction of 3D TTE CFD in a patient with MR using Flexi-Slice (GE Healthcare). (**a**) The 3D VC (orange arrow right lower quadrant) is obtained from the intersection of the three orthogonal crop planes (white, green and yellow arrows) at MR VC. (**b**) Measurement of VC area (white arrows). Note the elliptical shape of the EROA. Used with permission of Mayo Foundation for Medical Education and Research. All rights reserved. CFD, color flow Doppler; EROA, effective regurgitant orifice area; MR, mitral regurgitation; VC, vena contracta

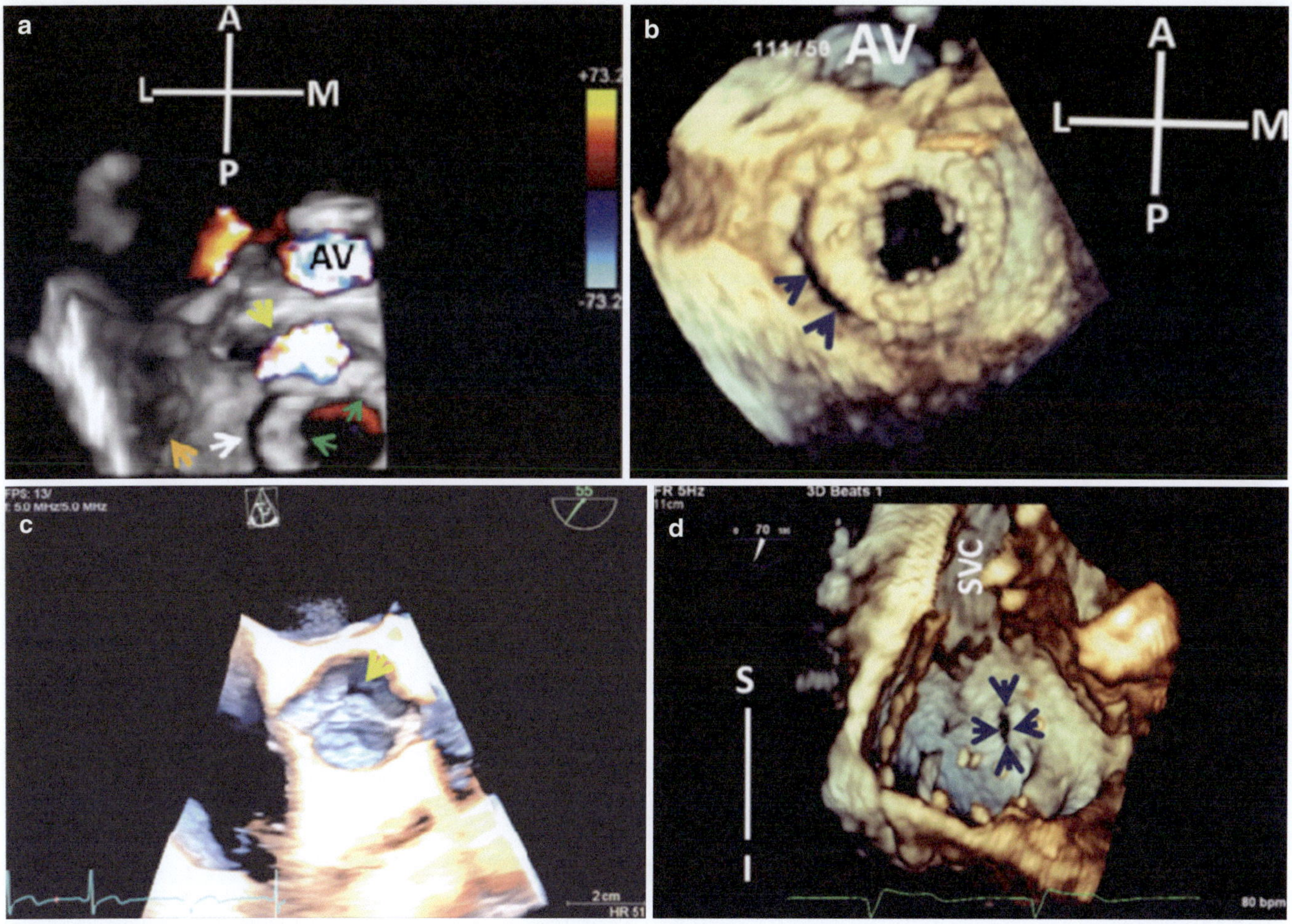

Fig. 3.9 Drop out artifacts. **Top panel**: (**a**) 3D TEE enface LA CFD of a mitral prosthesis PPL (yellow arrow). Note the drop out artifact (white arrow) lateral to the SR (green arrows). Orange arrow points to LAA. (**b**) Persistence of drop out artifact (dark blue arrows) after successful percutaneous closure of the PPL. **Bottom panel**: (**c**) Drop out artifact in AV LCC (arrow) simulating cusp perforation. (**d**) 3D TEE enface RA view of atrial septum showing a drop out artifact simulating a small ASD (dark blue arrows) at site of fossa ovalis. Patient had an intact atrial septum. As illustrated in these images, drop out artifacts appear as lack of tissue on 3DE. *Demonstration of flow through any 3D defect using color flow Doppler is therefore, a must to confirm that the defect is a true defect and not a drop out artifact.* Used with permission of Mayo Foundation for Medical Education and Research. All rights reserved. A, anterior; ASD, atrial septal defect; AV, aortic valve; CFD, color flow Doppler; I, inferior; L, lateral; LA, left atrium; LAA, left atrial appendage; LCC, left coronary cusp; M, medial; P, posterior; PPL, periprosthetic leak; RA, right atrium; S, superior; SR, sewing ring; SVC, superior vena cava

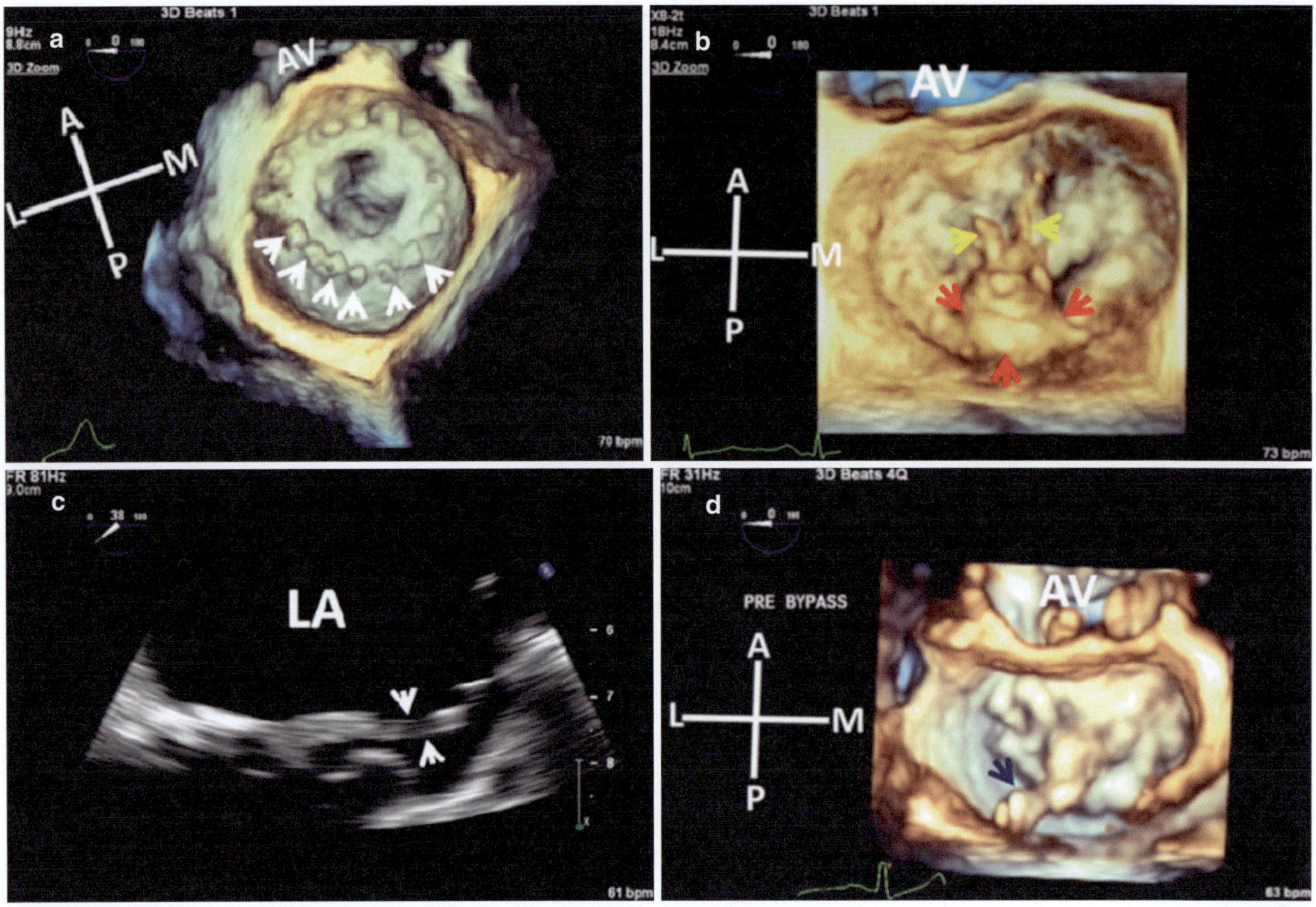

Fig. 3.10 Blurring artifacts. **Top panel**: 3D TEE enface LA views: (**a**) MV bioprosthesis. Arrows point to SR stitches/suture material that appear thick and blurred with indistinct edges. (**b**) Flail P2 (red arrows) with multiple ruptured chordae tendinae that appear thicker than they are in reality or when seen on 2DE (yellow arrows). **Bottom panel**: (**c**) 2D TEE of a flail AML. Two distinct ruptured chordae tendinae (white arrows) can be seen. (**d**) 3D TEE of same. The ruptured chords are indistinguishable and coalesced (dark blue arrow) because of blurring artifact. Used with permission of Mayo Foundation for Medical Education and Research. All rights reserved. A, anterior; AML, anterior mitral leaflet; AV, aortic valve; L, lateral; LA, left atrium; M, medial; MV, mitral valve; P, posterior; SR, sewing ring

devices, this includes wires and delivery catheters or sheaths used during percutaneous interventions [3]. Railroad-shaped artifacts are typically seen when imaging large catheters with wide lumens (Fig. 3.14), and may resolve with rotation of the 3D volume data set (Fig. 3.14), increase in compression which merges borders, and smoothing which reduces roughness [3]. Highly reflective metallic tips of catheters or sheaths can cause reverberation and side lobe artifacts [3] (Fig. 3.15). Reverberation artifacts may appear and disappear with catheter movement and usually form a sharp angle with the catheter tip [3] (Fig. 3.15). Gain artifacts were covered in Chap. 2.

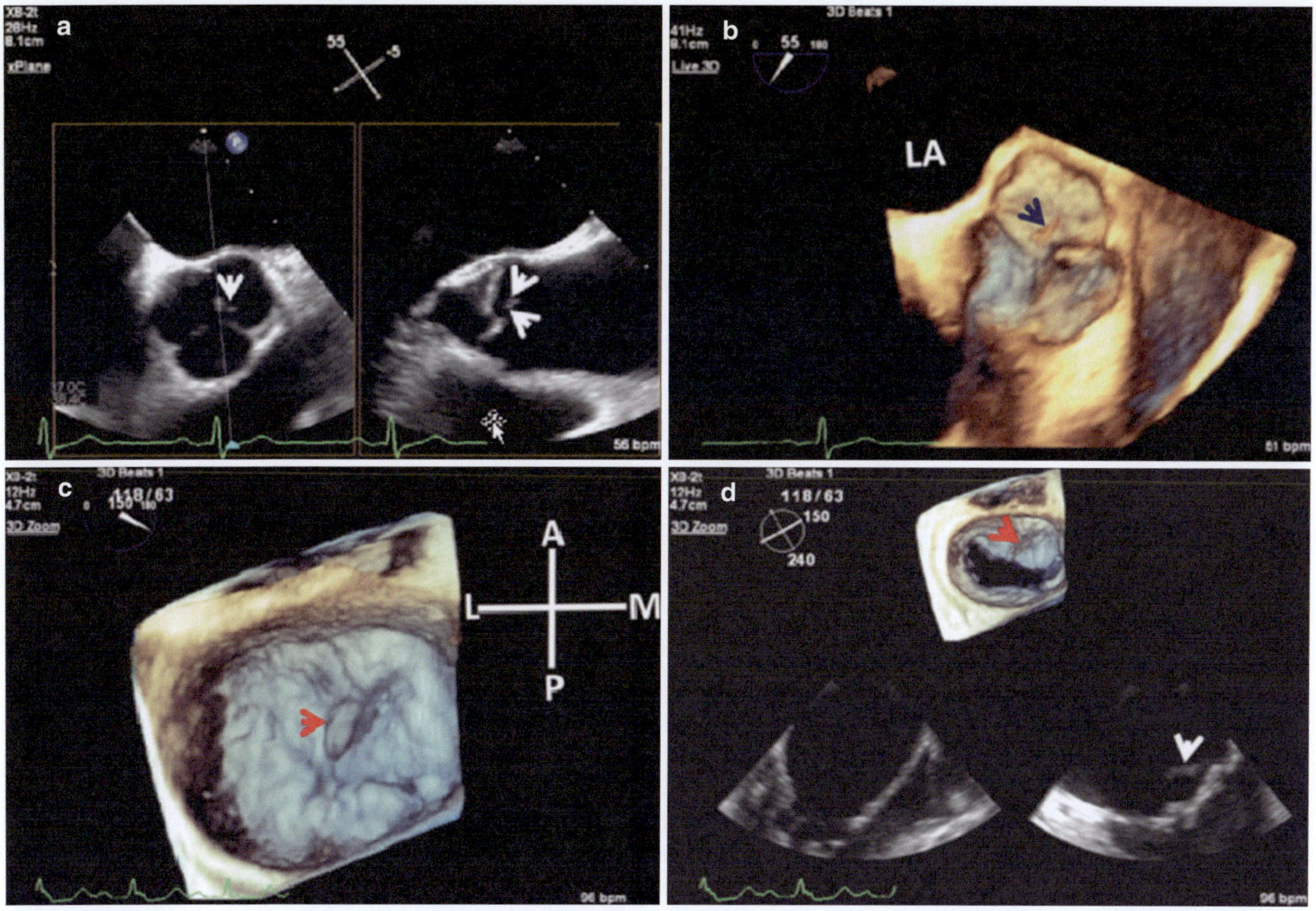

Fig. 3.11 Blurring artifacts. **Top panel**: (**a**) x-Plane of AV showing a tiny strand like structure (arrows). (**b**) Same strand (arrow) seen on 2DAV short-axis view appears thicker on real time 3D. **Bottom panel**: (**c**) 3D zoom enface LA view of MV shows a mass like lesion on AML (red arrow) simulating a vegetation. (**d**) 3D-2D layout of the same AML mass. The corresponding linear echo on 2D (white arrow) is much thinner and its appearance on multiple 2D views was consistent with artifact and not a real mass. Used with permission of Mayo Foundation for Medical Education and Research. All rights reserved. A, anterior; AML, anterior mitral leaflet; AV, aortic valve; L, lateral; LA, left atrium; M, medial; MV, mitral valve; P, posterior

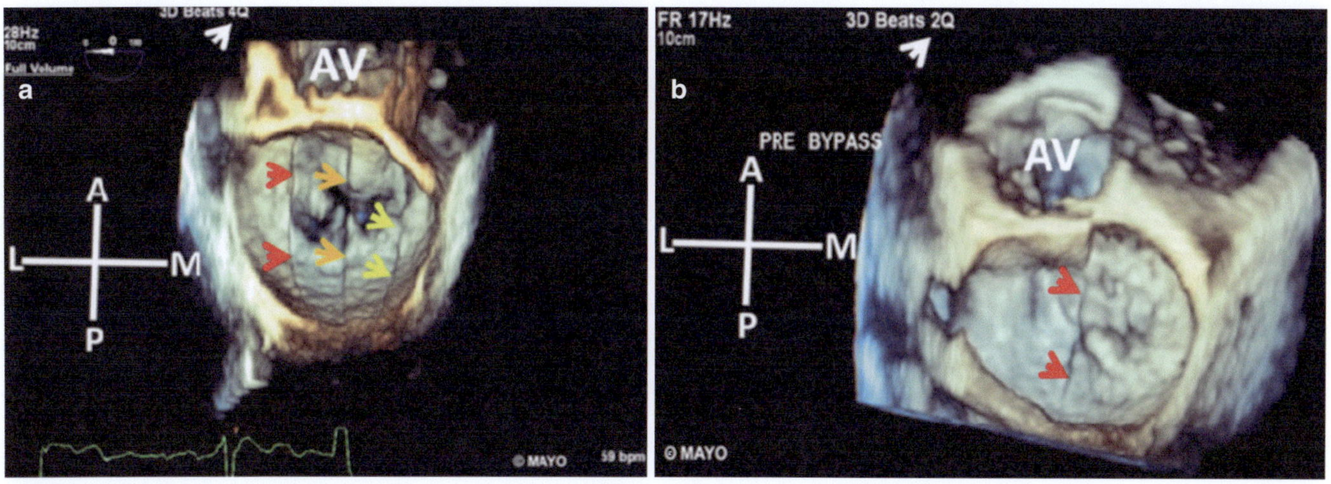

Fig. 3.12 Stitch artifacts caused by mutibeat FV acquisition. (**a**) Stitch artifacts (red, orange and yellow arrows) associated with 4 beat acquisition (white arrow) in a patient with atrial fibrillation. (**b**) Two beat acquisition (white arrow) stitch artifact (red arrows). Used with permission of Mayo Foundation for Medical Education and Research. All rights reserved. A, anterior; AV, aortic valve; FV, full volume; L, lateral; M, medial; P, posterior

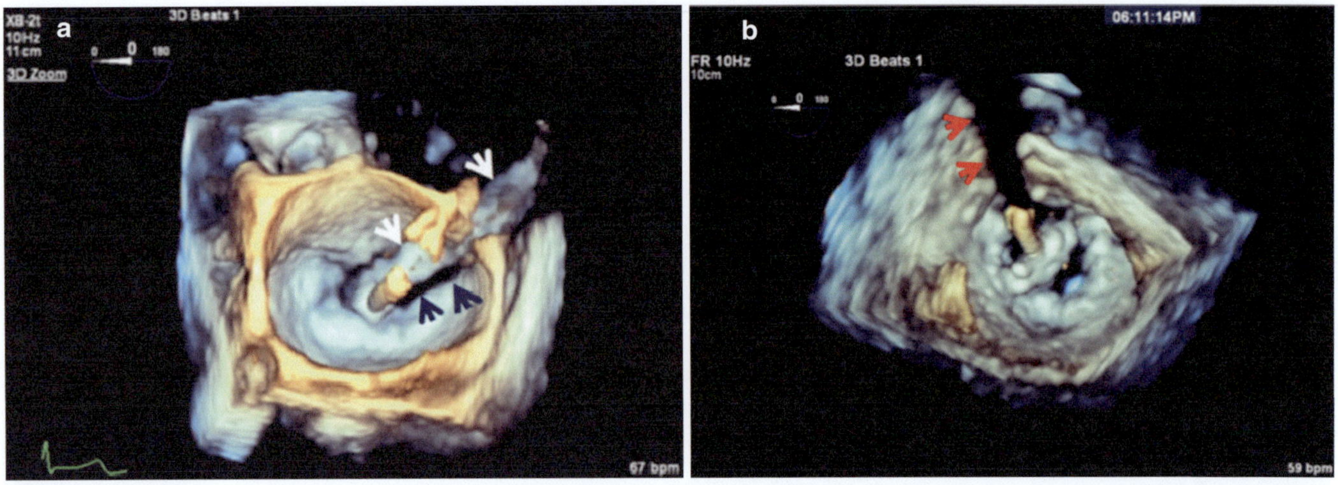

Fig. 3.13 Acoustic shadowing. Real time 3D TEE enface LA views of MV during transcatheter edge-to-edge MitraClip repair. (**a**) Acoustic shadowing (dark blue arrows) caused by overlying sheath in LA (white arrows). (**b**) Acoustic shadowing (red arrows) while advancing MitraClip in LA. Used with permission of Mayo Foundation for Medical Education and Research. All rights reserved. LA, left atrium; MV, mitral valve

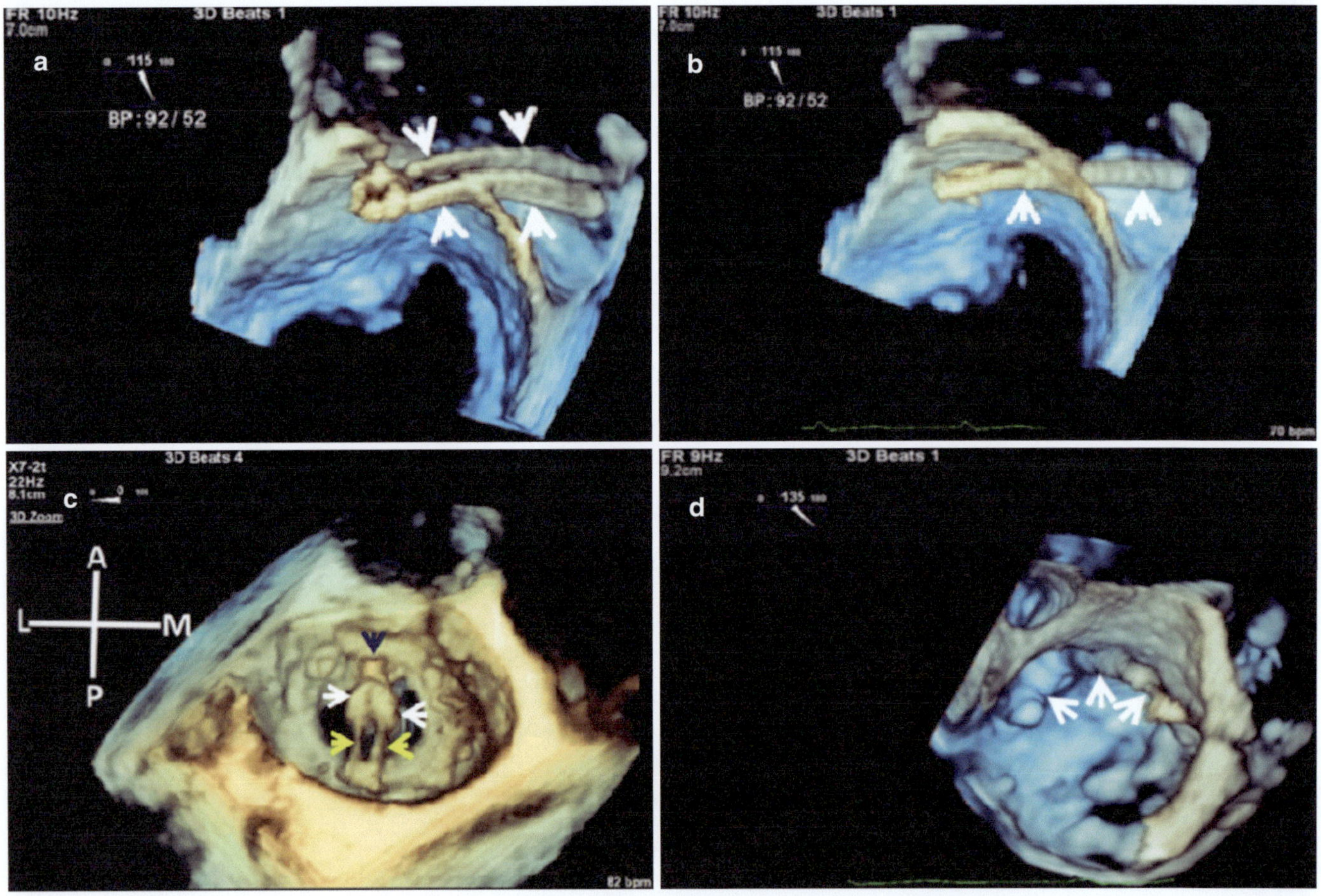

Fig. 3.14 **Top panel: railroad-shaped artifact**. (**a**) 3D TEE of SGC showing a railroad-shaped artifact (white arrows). (**b**) Resolution of artifact with slight rotation of 3D data set. The SCG now has a tubular appearance. **Bottom panel: blooming artifacts**. (**c**) Mechanical mitral valve bileaflet occluders. Compared with the posterior segments of the occluder leaflets (yellow arrows), the anterior segments (white arrows) appear much thicker with indistinct edges due to blooming artifacts. Note the typical "star artifact" due to blooming of the midline anterior hinge. (dark blue arrow). (**d**) Blooming artifacts creating uneven thickness of a stiff wire in LA (white arrows) depending on the angle of incidence of the ultrasound beam. Distinguishing wires from catheters on 3D echocardiography can therefore, be problematic. Used with permission of Mayo Foundation for Medical Education and Research. All rights reserved. A, anterior; L, lateral; LA, left atrium; M, medial; P, posterior; SGC, steerable guide catheter

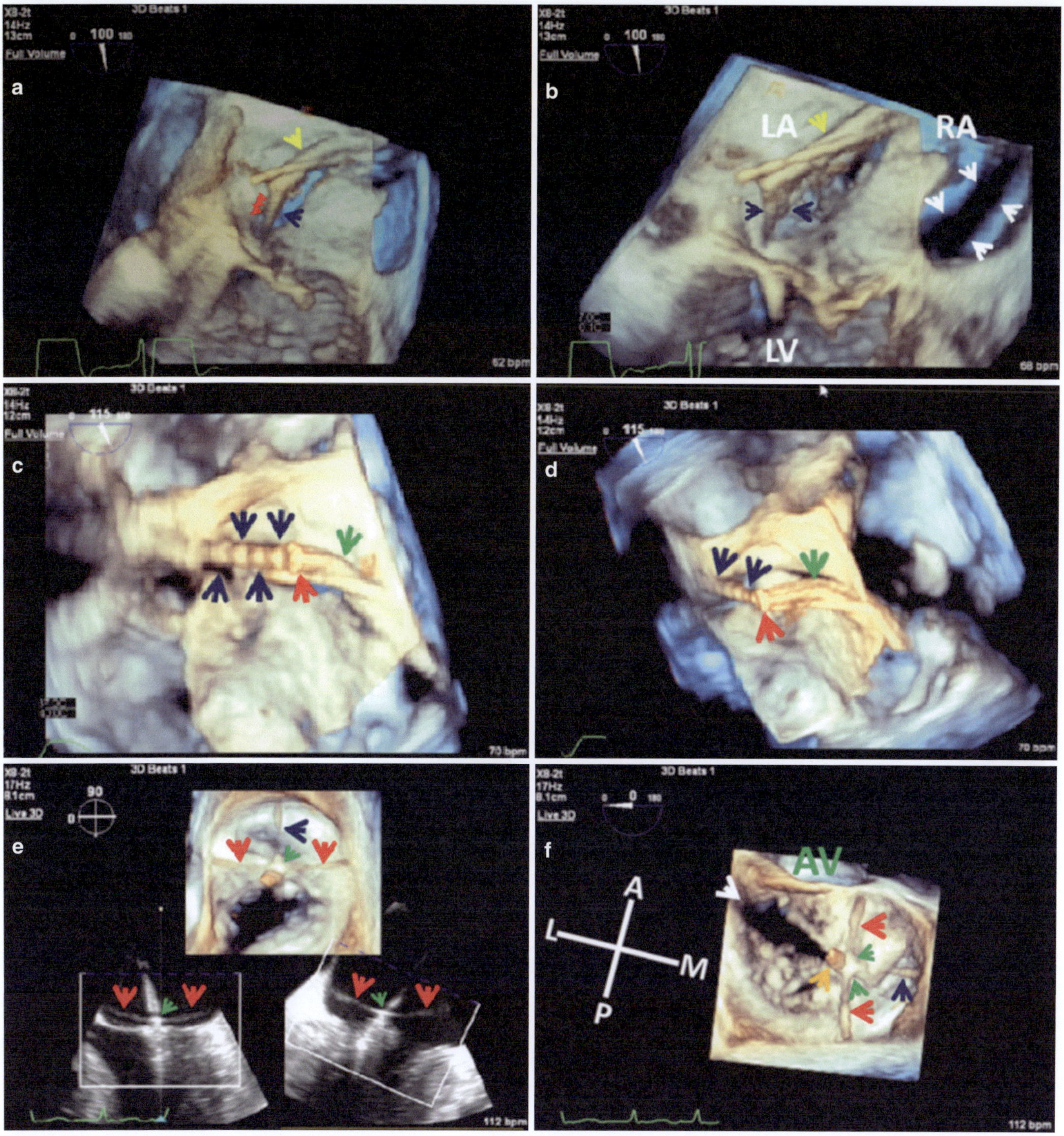

Fig. 3.15 (**a**, **b**) **Reverberation artifacts** (dark blue arrows) caused by metallic tip of delivery sheath (yellow arrow) in LA . Note the typical "comet tail/ring down" reverberations (red arrows) with successive reverberations gradually diminishing in intensity, and sharp angle of artifact in relation to catheter tip. Also, note the marked acoustic shadowing caused by the segment of the sheath in the RA (white arrows). (**c**, **d**) Another reverberation artifact (dark blue arrows) produced by metalic tip (red arrow) of a delivery sheath (green arrow). (**e**, **f**) Live 3D TEE LA views post MitraClip deployment showing **side lobe artifacts** (red arrows) caused by MitraClip: Note the linear arc-like artifact at both sides of the strong reflector (green arrows). Also note the acoustic shadowing (white arrow) caused by MitraClip (orange arrow). The same strong reflector produces another linear artifact (dark blue arrow) in the 3D space. Used with permission of Mayo Foundation for Medical Education and Research. All rights reserved. A, anterior; AV, aortic valve; L, lateral; LA, left atrium; LV, left ventricle; M, medial; P, posterior; RA, right atrium

References

1. Lang RM, et al. EAE/ASE recommendations for image acquisition and display using three dimensional echocardiography. Eur Heart J Cardiovasc Imaging. 2012;13:1–46.
2. Bertrand PB, Levine RA, Isselbacher EM, Vandervoort PM. Fact or artifact in two-dimensional echocardiography: avoiding misdiagnosis and missed diagnosis. J Am Soc Echocardiogr. 2016;29(5):381–91.
3. Faletra FF, Ramamurthi A, Dequarti MC, Leo LA, Moccetti T, Pandian N. Artifacts in three-dimensional transesophageal echocardiography. J Am Soc Echocardiogr. 2014;27(5):453–62.

3DE Knobology: A Practical Guide to Use of the Available Vendor Platforms

4

Joseph F. Maalouf

Introduction

A major limitation of current 3D echocardiography equipment is the very complicated and often confusing "knobology" that has kept even the most experienced echocardiographer weary from embracing imaging with 3D. This chapter, therefore, is a practical guide to the 3D control knobs and tabs most commonly used for image acquisition and optimization on the Philips (Philips Healthcare) , GE (General electric Healthcare), and Siemens (Siemens Healthineers) platforms. For ease of use, we have listed the salient 3D function terms for each vendor in a glossary format, and we have included illustrative images of how the most commonly used 3D control knobs and buttons are displayed or clustered on the equipment consoles and, where applicable, the most recent dashboards. A complete review that includes 3D quantification tools is beyond the scope of this chapter, however, and the interested reader is referred to the vendor specific 3D platform user manual and to Chaps. 22 and 23 for more details.

Philips 3D Platforms

IE33

Although Philips IE33 has been replaced by the Epic platform, it remains in use in many centers worldwide. Philips IE33 (Figs. 4.1 and 4.2) consists of a console and two side by side dashboard touch screens.

J. F. Maalouf (✉)
Professor of Medicine, Mayo Clinic College of Medicine; Director, Interventional Echocardiography; Consultant, Department of Cardiovascular Medicine, Mayo Clinic, Rochester, MN, USA
e-mail: maalouf.joseph@mayo.edu

IE33 Dashboards (Figs. 4.3 and 4.4)

Philips Epic Platforms

Philips Epic platforms (Fig. 4.5) consist of a console and a two page touch scroll screens. Although the various upgrades in Epic platforms share most of the 3D control tabs, they may differ in the way they are displayed or clustered mainly on the touch screens. In this chapter, the latest Epic version touch screen images are shown (Figs. 4.6, 4.7, and 4.8).

Glossary of Terms: Philips 3D Platforms

3D Acquisition Modes

1. ***3D or Live 3D (Epic);Live 3D (IE33)***: This is the smallest preset 3D volume and activates Live 3D. The right and left select keys next to the console trackball can be used to change lateral or elevation position of the Live 3D image
2. ***3D Opt***: A control used to select the 3D acquisition method. the term beats here refers to how many sub-volumes are used to build the complete volume
   (a) ***3D Opt 1 beat***: This is live or in real time and applies to 3D (Live 3D), Full Volume and 3D Zoom acquisition modes. Single beat acquisition means that the 3D image is obtained from a single ECG gated volume
   (b) ***3D Opt multibeat (2, 4 or 6)***: can be used for any of the three 3D acquisition modes and refers to number of ECG gated sub-volumes to build the complete volume
   (c) ***3D Opt High VR (Epic) or HVR (IE33)***: refers to high volume rate and is a real time acquisition but with four times the frame rate compared with single beat real time 3D acquisition

J. F. Maalouf et al. (eds.), *Practical 3D Echocardiography*, https://doi.org/10.1007/978-3-030-72941-7_4

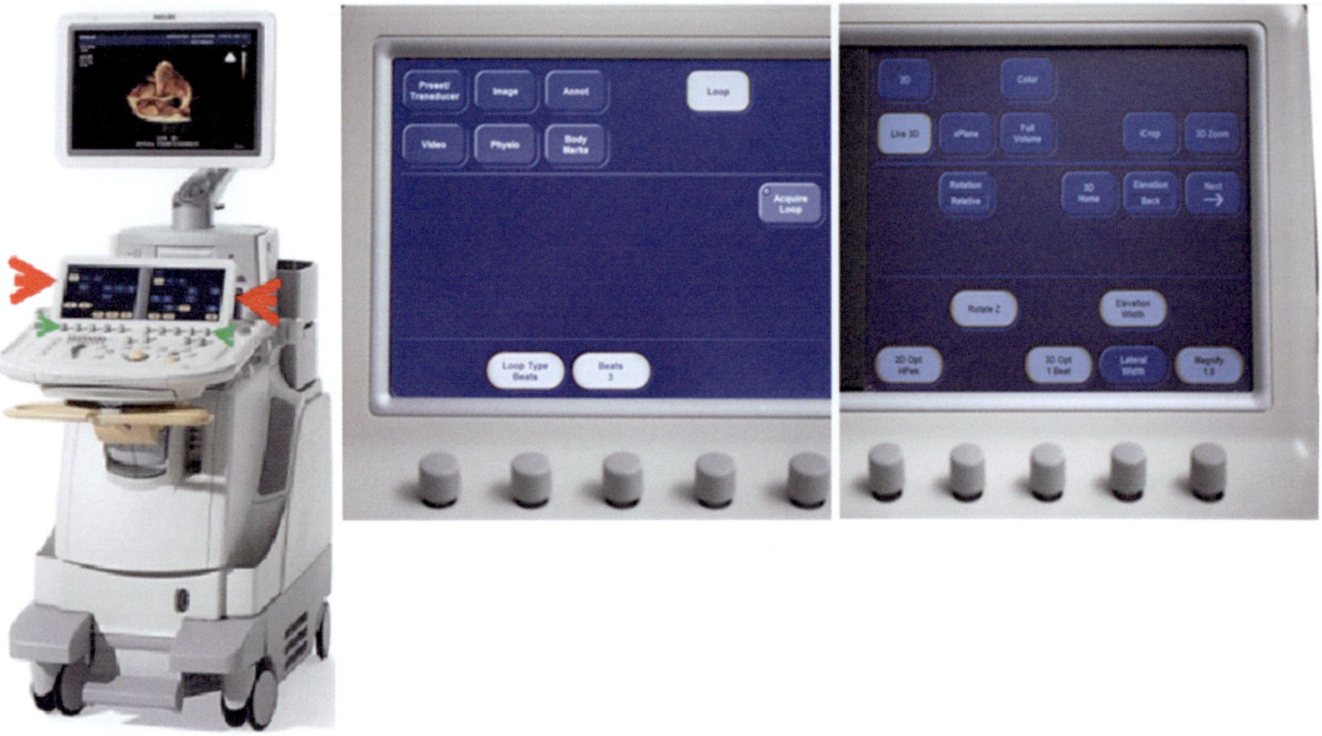

Fig. 4.1 **Left**: IE33 machine with two touch screen dashboards (red arrows) and control knobs (green arrows) on the machine console just beneath the dashboards that allow the operator to select from the different options at bottom of the dashboard. **Right**: Enlarged images of the right and left dashboards and corresponding control knobs. Note that the dashboard tabs that correspond to the control knobs vary in function depending on the dashboard page and image control mode selection. Courtesy of Philips

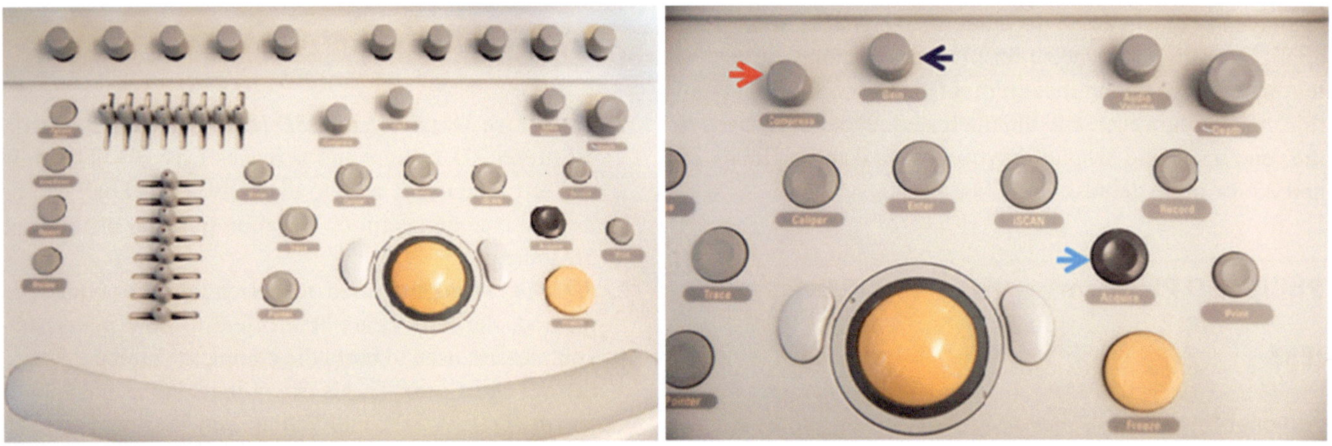

Fig. 4.2 IE33 console. The Gain (dark blue arrow) and Compress (red arrow) knobs, and Acquire (light blue arrow) button are highlighted in the enlarged image. Courtesy of Philips

3. ***3D Vision***: Provides different color hue displays of the 3D image and includes TrueVue
4. ***3D Zoom***: 3D Zoom is a truncated 3D pyramid with adjustable size and position.

   3D Zoom allows the user to configure the 3D volume based on a focused biplane (xPlane) region of interest (ROI). Using the right or left select key, box size and position frame the desired ROI within the left sided image in the 2D xPlane format, and the elevation width dial on the touch screen frames the desired ROI in the 2D plane on the right. Pressing 3D zoom again generates the desired 3D image

5. ***Auto view***: (for mitral and aortic valves). Available only in 3D Zoom and automatically rotates an image to a predefined view
6. ***Acquire***: The stored 3D clip will have a small gray square on the bottom right corner of the thumbnail image. Acquire allows manipulation of 3D data (post processing)
7. ***Color*** : adds color flow Doppler to the 3D volume
8. ***Full Volume***: Largest preset 3D volume, recognized by the autocrop green box
9. ***Loop Beats***: Refers to the number of cardiac cycles (also referred to as beats) of data that will be acquired
10. ***Retrospective versus prospective 3D acquisition***
    (a) ***Prospective*** captures the next completed 3D volume(s) ***after*** the **Acquire** button is pressed with the total number of acquired volumes being set by the number of beats in 3D Opt
    (b) ***Retrospective*** captures the last completed volume (s) ***before*** the **Acquire** button was pressed with the total number of acquired volumes being set by the number of beats
    (c) ***Selecting retrospective vs prospective 3D acquisition on IE33***
        I Press ***Setup*** tab on keyboard. A menu that includes System Settings, and Print/Network appears on the left monitor.
        II Press ***Print Network*** tab
        III Select Prospective or Retrospective under Live ***Capture Type*** menu
11. ***Save 3D***: 3D clip is saved but cannot be modified (i.e. post processed). The 3D clip will show a small circle at the bottom right hand corner of the thumbnail image
12. ***x-Plane***: Displays two simultaneous orthogonal views in grayscale and with color Doppler from the same heartbeat, utilizing one acoustic window. Using the track ball, a white line marker appears on the left image. Wherever the marker is placed using tilt function, the right image displays its orthogonal view

Image Optimization Tools

1. ***3D Vision***: A control used to set the contrast, transparency, lighting, and compositing values of the volume image. Provides different color hue displays of the 3D image and includes TrueVue
2. ***Auto view***: (for mitral and aortic valves) automatically rotates an image to a predefined view from ***3D zoom***
3. ***Bright***: Controls image brightness
4. ***Color Suppress/Hide Color***: Suppresses color on 3D CFD acquisition
5. ***Compress***: Adds soft echos, hence makes objects appear more opaque. Low compressions enhance edges of structures hence image details

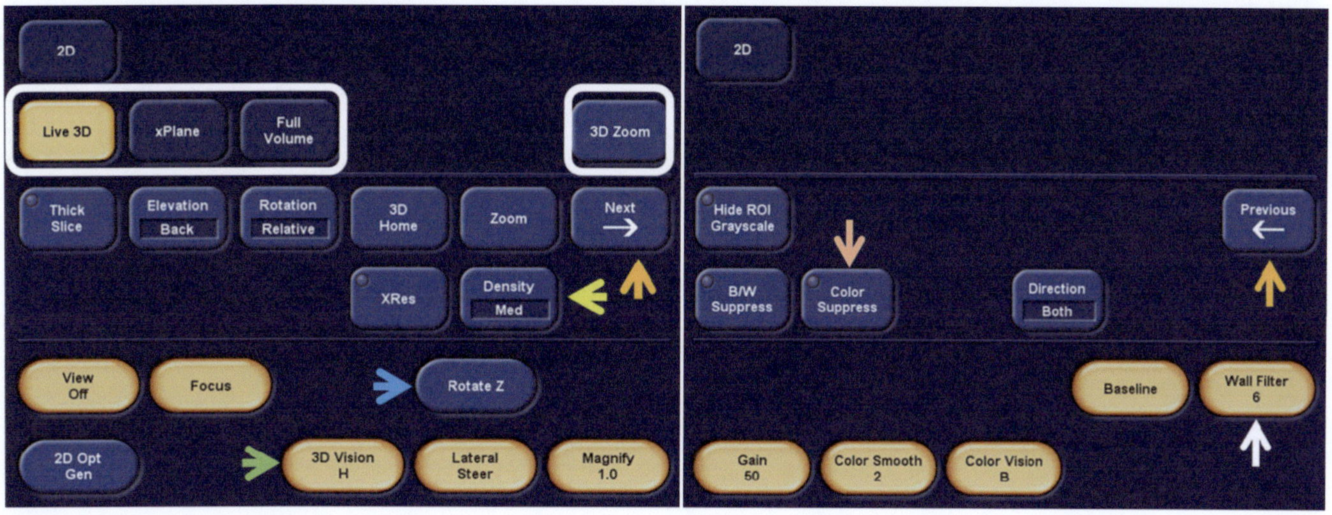

Fig. 4.3 **IE33 Right Screen dashboard. Top panel**: Two page touch screen controls (**Next** and **Previous**; orange arrows), **3D acquisition modes** (white rectangle), **Density** control (yellow arrow), **3D vision** (green arrow), **Wall Filter** (white arrow), **Color Suppress** (light orange arrow) and **Rotate Z** (blue arrow). **Second panel**: **Left**: **3D Opt 1 Beat** (yellow rectangle), **Live 3D** (orange arrow) with **Color** on (yellow arrow). White arrow points to the **Color Suppress** control. **Right**: **Live 3D** (orange arrow) with **3D Opt** at 2 beats. The **Elevation** and **Lateral Width** controls (white rectangle) and **iCrop** (yellow arrow) are also displayed. **Third panel**: **Left**: Cropping and image optimization tools including **Smoothing**, **3D Vision**, **Rotate Z** and **Magnify** (yellow rectangle), **Bright** (yellow arrow), **iCrop** and **iSlice** (white rectangle). White arrow points to **Save 3D Clip** control. **Right**: **Crop Adjust Off** (yellow rectangle), **Auto Crop** and **Reset Cropping** (white rectangle), and **Smoothing** (yellow arrow) are highlighted. **Fourth panel. Left**: **3D Opt HVR** (white arrow). **Right**: **Crop Adjust Box**, **Select Plane** set on **Green Max** and **Adjust Plane** (white rectangle), **Res/Spd** (white arrow), and **3D Vision** (yellow arrow). **Bottom panel**. **Left**: **Full Volume** with **Color** on (white rectangle), **Color Suppress** (yellow arrow), **Acquire** (white arrow) and **xPlane** (orange arrow). **Right**: **xPlane** on (white arrow) and selected 2D image component (**xP Image Left**; yellow arrow). Courtesy of Philips

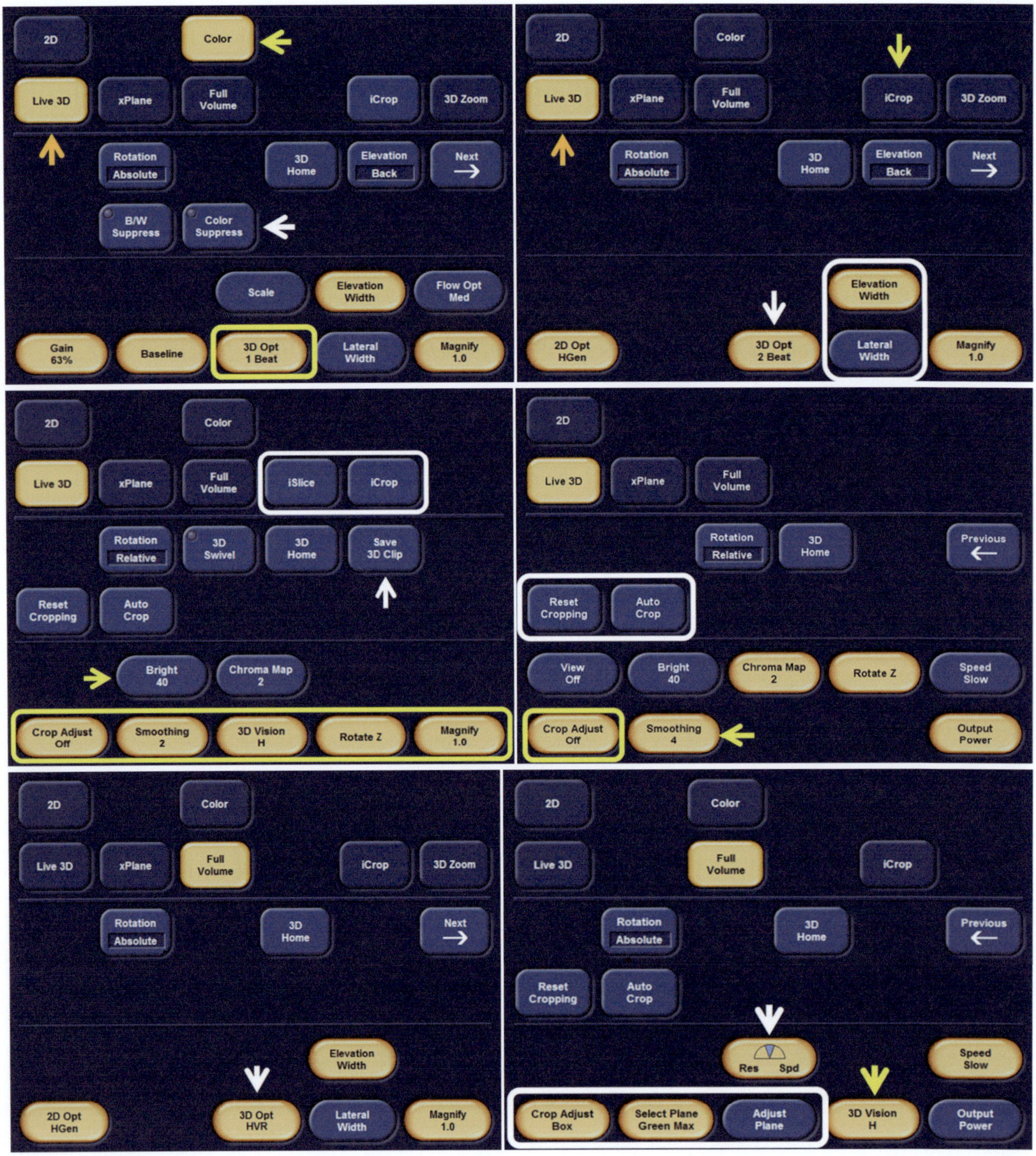

Fig. 4.3 (continued)

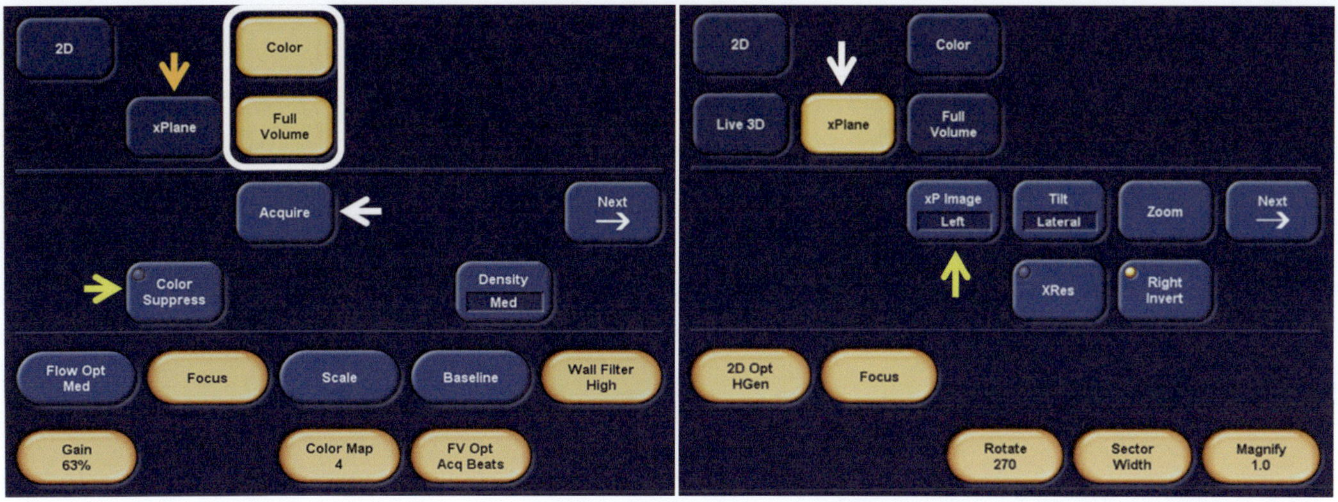

Fig. 4.3 (continued)

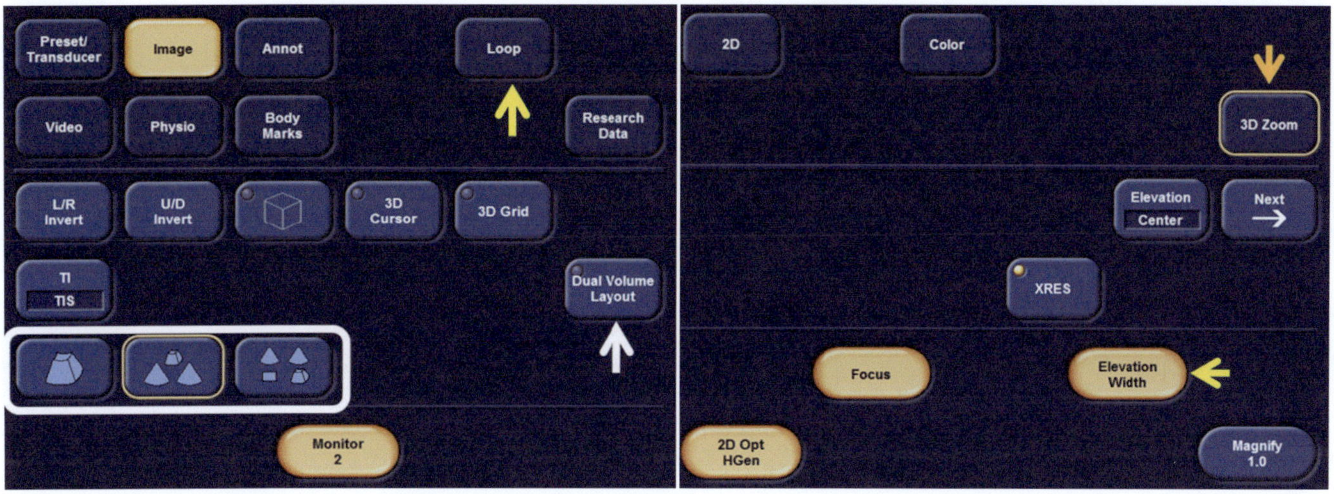

Fig. 4.4 **Left Screen dashboard** showing **3D layout display** modes (white rectangle), **Dual Volume Layout** (white arrow), and **Loop** (yellow arrow), and **Right Screen dashboard** showing **3D Zoom** (orange arrow) and **Elevation Width** control (yellow arrow). Courtesy of Philips

6. ***Dual or Dual volume layout***: Simultaneous display of two sides of the 3D volume acquired (e.g. atrial and ventricular surfaces of mitral valve or right and left atrial surfaces of atrial septum)
7. ***Elevation Width***: Controls antero-posterior dimensions of a 3D image regardless of 3D acquisition mode
8. ***Freeze button (control console)***: Images can be reviewed by pressing Cine Play on touch screen, and images can be edited as needed using the Trim keys (Trim Left and Trim right) in order to select the beat with best 3D volume to be acquired
9. ***Gain***: Adjusts for sound attenuation: Too high a gain produces noise. Too low a gain may create artefactual echo drop out. 3D gain is changed by turning the 3D knob. Image background should show a bluish gray for deep visualization. Overgain will show more gold in background with loss of definition
10. ***GlassVue***: Highlights edges in the image with the ability to control the transparency. It is a different way to setup TrueVue. GlassVue is accessed from the touchscreen when TrueVue is active
11. ***Layout***: A control to select the 3D display and includes three MPR modes. Note: If 3D image anatomy is not clear, the 2D reference images that make up the 3D image can be viewed using the Layout tab
12. ***Lateral Width***: Controls lateral (width)dimensions of a 3D image regardless of 3D acquisition mode
13. ***Smoothing***: Also referred to as persistence. Smoothing evens out the image surface. Too much smoothing will mask fine image details

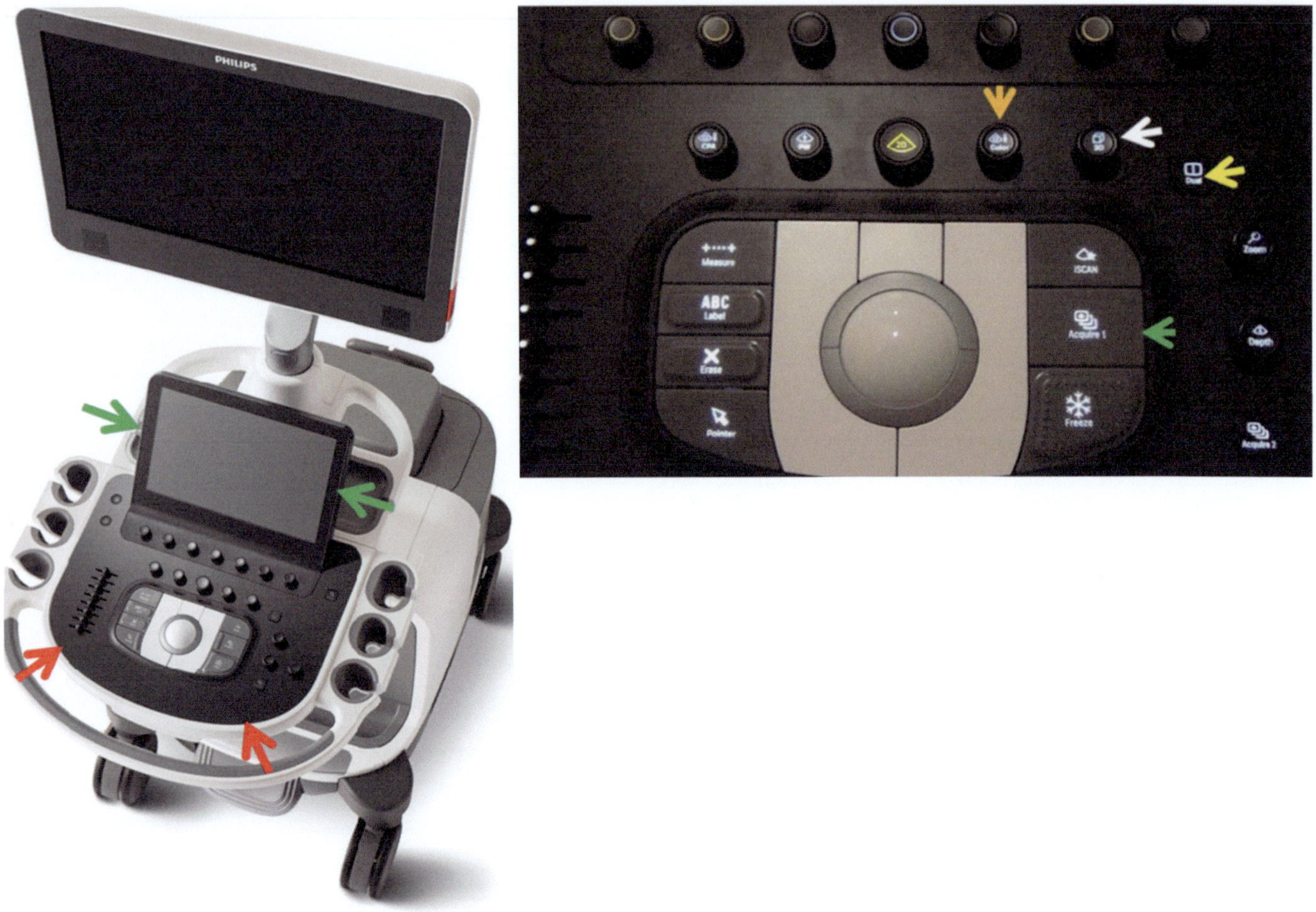

Fig. 4.5 **Left**: Philips Epic machine with console (red arrows) and two page touch scroll screens (green arrows), **Right**: Enlarged image of the console to highlight the **3D** knob (white arrow), **Dual** layout button (yellow arrow), one of the two **Acquire** tabs (**Acquire 1**; green arrow), and the **Color** control knob (orange arrow). Courtesy of Philips

14. ***TouchVue***: Allows use of hand or fingers instead of rotational knobs to manipulate a 3D image in all three planes (x, y or z)
15. ***TrueVue***: Allows light to be placed at various depths within the 3D image in order to provide unique shadows, tones/hues to a ROI
16. ***View Top/bottom/right/left***: refers to enface view desired
17. ***Wall Filter***: Range 0–9; Increasing this control suppresses lower color flow velocities. This is similar to the action of the Color Wall Filter in 2D

Cropping Tools

1. ***3DQ***: Provides post processing multiplanar reconstruction (MPR) of the acquired 3D data set. MPR creates 2D images from the 3D data set. Typically, they are placed orthogonal to each other with one plane parallel to the ROI for measurement purposes.
2. ***3D Auto LAA***: Rapid MPR guided automated method used to measure the area,circumference, and diameter of the left atrial appendage (LAA).
3. ***3D Auto MV***: provides for semi-automated analysis of MV anatomy.
4. ***Adjust Plane***: Moves selected cropping plane along its axis to achieve desired amount of cropping.
5. ***Auto Crop***: Automatically cuts the Full Volume pyramidal data set to the midpoint with the cut plane parallel to the reference plane. All Full Volume 3D data sets are generated auto cropped. Auto Crop is available in both 3D review (post-processed images) and live 3D acquisition.
6. ***Crop Adjust On/Off***: When switched on provides option to use Crop Adjust Box or Crop Adjust Plane.
7. ***Crop Adjust Box***: Allows cropping of 3D volume along color coded elevation, depth and lateral axes (Fig. 4.9): **Green** for elevation z-axis and plane. This is equivalent to a coronal or frontal plane which divides the heart into anterior and posterior portions; **Blue** for depth or axial (y-axis). This is equivalent to a transverse plane which

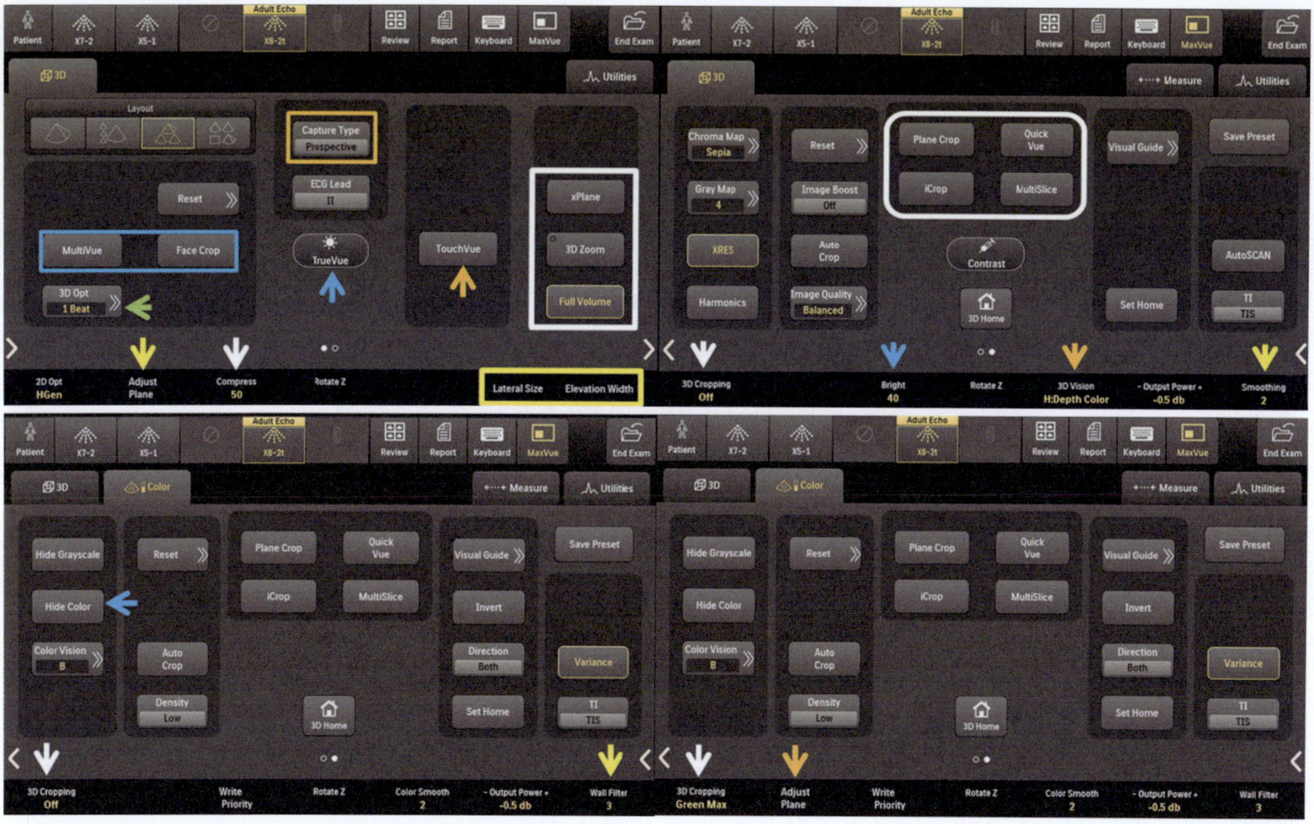

Fig. 4.6 **Touch scroll screen controls 1. Top panel. Left**: **3D acquisition** modes (white rectangle), **Lateral Size/Elevation Width** controls (yellow rectangle), **MultiVue** and **FaceCrop** (blue rectangle), **TrueVue** (blue arrow), **TouchVue**(orange arrow), **3DOpt** (1–6 beats, or HVR ; green arrow), and **Capture Type** (Prospective or Retrospective; orange rectangle) are all displayed. The **Compress** (white arrow) and **Adjust Plane** (yellow arrow) controls can also be seen. **Right**: Clustered cropping options (**Plane Crop**, **Quick Vue**, **iCrop,** and **MultiSlice**; white rectangle). **3D Cropping** (white arrow), **Bright** (blue arrow), **3D Vision** type (orange arrow) and **Smoothing** (yellow arrow) controls are also seen. **Bottom panel. Left**: The 3D Color **Wall Filter** control (1–9; yellow arrow) and **Hide Color** control (blue arrow) are seen. **3D Cropping** control (white arrow) is Off. **Right**: **3D Cropping** set on **Green Max** (white arrow) and **Adjust Plane** control (orange arrow) are seen. Courtesy of Philips

divides the heart into superior and inferior portions; and **Red** for lateral or azimuthal x-axis or plane. This is equivalent to a sagittal or vertical plane which divides the heart into right and left portions. Crop box allows cropping from six directions (two for each cropping plane referred to as Min and Max). Cropping is available in both Live 3D acquisition and 3D review (post processed images).

8. ***Crop Adjust Box on Min/Max*** Refers to location of selected crop plane from transducer.
9. ***Crop Adjust Plane (Plane Crop)***: Freely adjustable arbitrary cropping plane that has a purple color when in front the 3D volume data set in position for cropping and green when behind.
10. ***Face Crop***: Allows unidirectional cropping of 3D volume data (e.g. for Full Volume from apex to base of pyramidal data set). The trackball is used to position the 3D image so that the area to be cropped is facing the user (crop what you see directly in front of you), and rotating the plane adjust knob sets the crop depth. When not displayed as a separate touch screen tab, Face Crop is turned on by rotating the 3D Cropping knob 1 click counter clockwise.
11. ***HM ACQ***: Provides fast LV and LA quantification from a single Full Volume loop**.**
12. ***iCrop***: A control used to identify a ROI on two orthogonal MPR reference images within the 3D data set. MPR left or right on touch panel will allow operator to select the orthogonal reference volume on MPR to be cropped (using Box size, Box position, and Box rotation) and to toggle between the two orthogonal planes.
13. ***iSlice***: Provides multiple simultaneous 2D views by slicing the 3D volume on its short or long axis.
14. ***Light depth***: A control used to adjust the depth of the **TrueVue** light source on the 3D image.
15. ***Lock MPR***: Used with **MultiVue** (see later). Toggles to lock or unlock. When the MPRs are locked, all planes will remain orthogonal to each other. When the MPRs

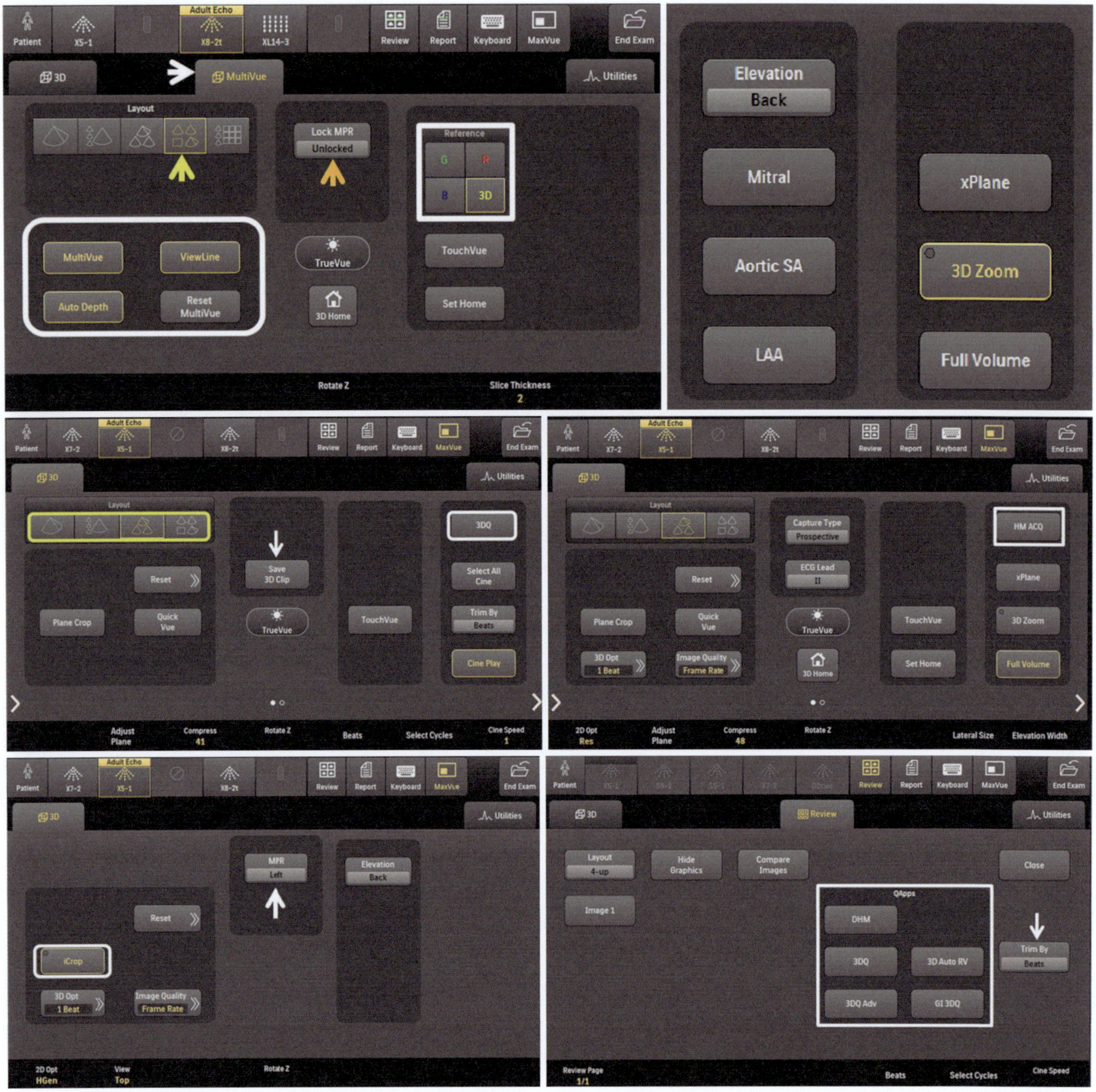

Fig. 4.7 **Touch scroll screen controls 2**: **Top panel**: **Left**: **MultiVue** (white arrow) control tabs (white rectangle) including color coded **Reference** planes (white square) and **Lock MPR** control (orange arrow). Yellow arrow points to 3D **Layout** selection. **Right**: **3D Zoom Mitral** , **Aortic SA** for short-axis, and **LAA** display options. **Middle panel**: **3DQ** (**left**) and **HMACQ** (**right**) MPR measurement packages are highlighted by the white rectangles. **Layout** selection options are highlighted by the yellow rectangle. White arrow points to **Save 3DClip** option. **Bottom panel**: **Left**: **iCrop** control (white rectangle) including **MPR** selection (white arrow). **Right**: Clustered MPR options (**QApps**; white rectangle) and **Trim** function (white arrow). Courtesy of Philips

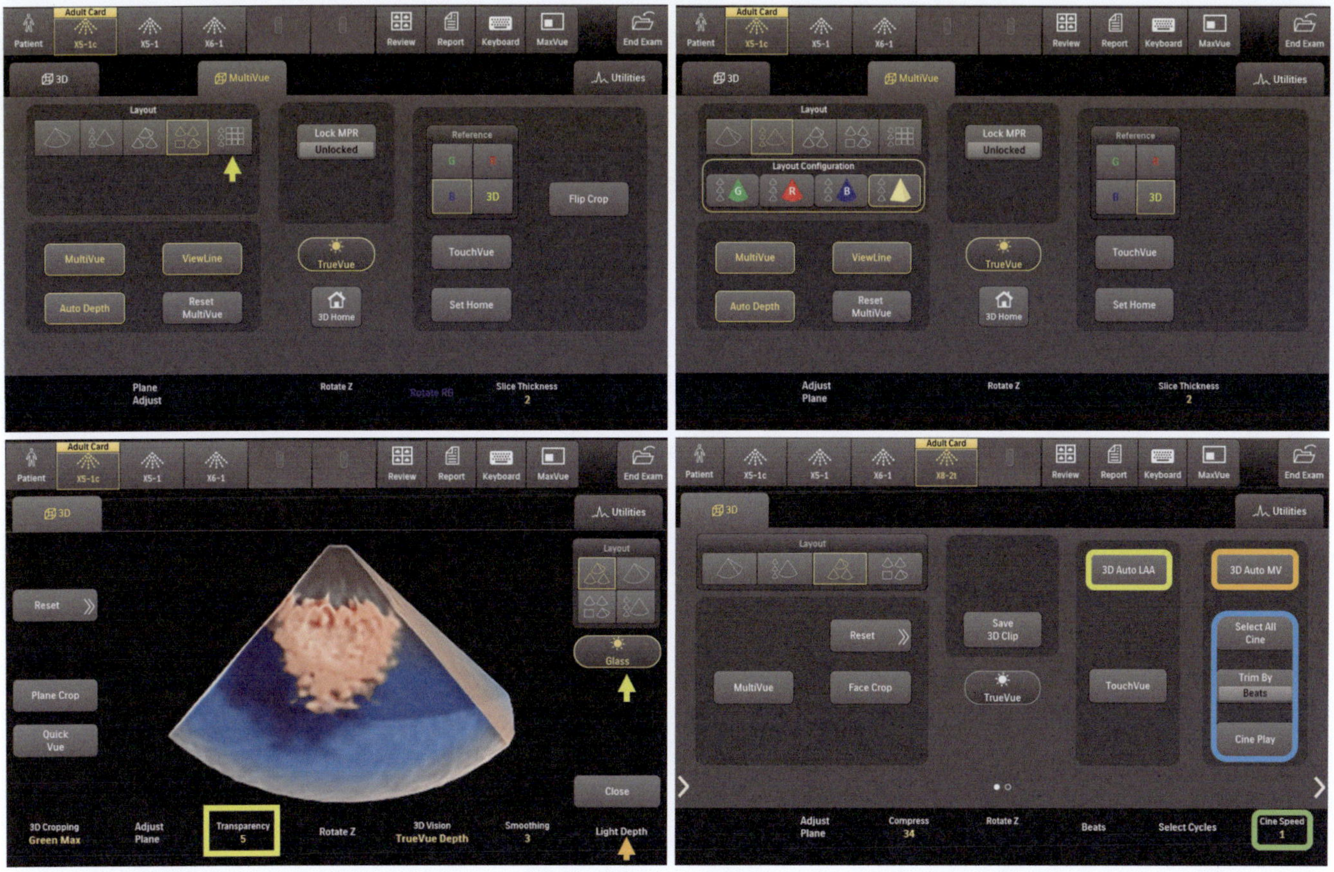

Fig. 4.8 Touch scroll screen controls 3. **Top panel. Left**: **Multislice** option in **MultiVue** (arrow). **Right**: Color coded crop planes **Layout Configuration** in **MultiVue. Bottom panel. Left**: **Glass Vue tab** (yellow arrow), **Transparency** (yellow rectangle), and **Light Depth** (orange arrow). **Right**: **3D Auto LAA** (yellow rectangle), **3D Auto MV** (orange rectangle), **Cine/Trim** functions (blue rectangle), and **Cine Speed** (light green rectangle). Courtesy of Philips

are unlocked, the planes can be freely manipulated and moved independently.

16. ***MPR Left/Right***: Necessary for iCrop and refers to left or right 2D crop box associated with each of the orthogonal 2D views.
17. ***MultiSlice***: Enables simultaneous display of multiple short axis views generated from a 3D volume acquisition.
18. ***MultiVue***: Used to orient and crop the 3D volume (regardless of mode of 3D acquisition) in real time by adjusting reference lines in the MPR views. The crop location is indicated by a white dashed line in the Green and Red MPRs. Arrows at the end of the crop line indicate the direction from which the 3D volume is being viewed. By clicking on the area of interest on the 3D volume, the MPR planes will automatically align to the area clicked. MultiVue can be used with **TrueVue** and **TouchVue.**
19. ***Quick Vue***: A control used to quickly crop a 3D volume from any MPR plane displayed in the 3D image Layout and is available in both 3D review (post-processed images) and Live 3D acquisition. Quick Vue requires only two steps to get the required view of the anatomy. On any MPR image, click where to view from to set the Tail and then click where to view to set the Tip (Fig. 4.10). Quick Vue is similar to 2-Click Crop on GE (see below) with easy to change the angle of view.
20. ***Reset Crop***: Restores anterior half of Full Volume data set.
21. ***Transparency***: Adjusts transparency level (range 0-20) when using GlassVue.
22. ***TrueVue***: Using a virtual light source, TrueVue makes it simpler to visualize the location of the defects and comprehend depth within the structures.
23. ***View Top/bottom/right/left***: Refers to enface view desired.

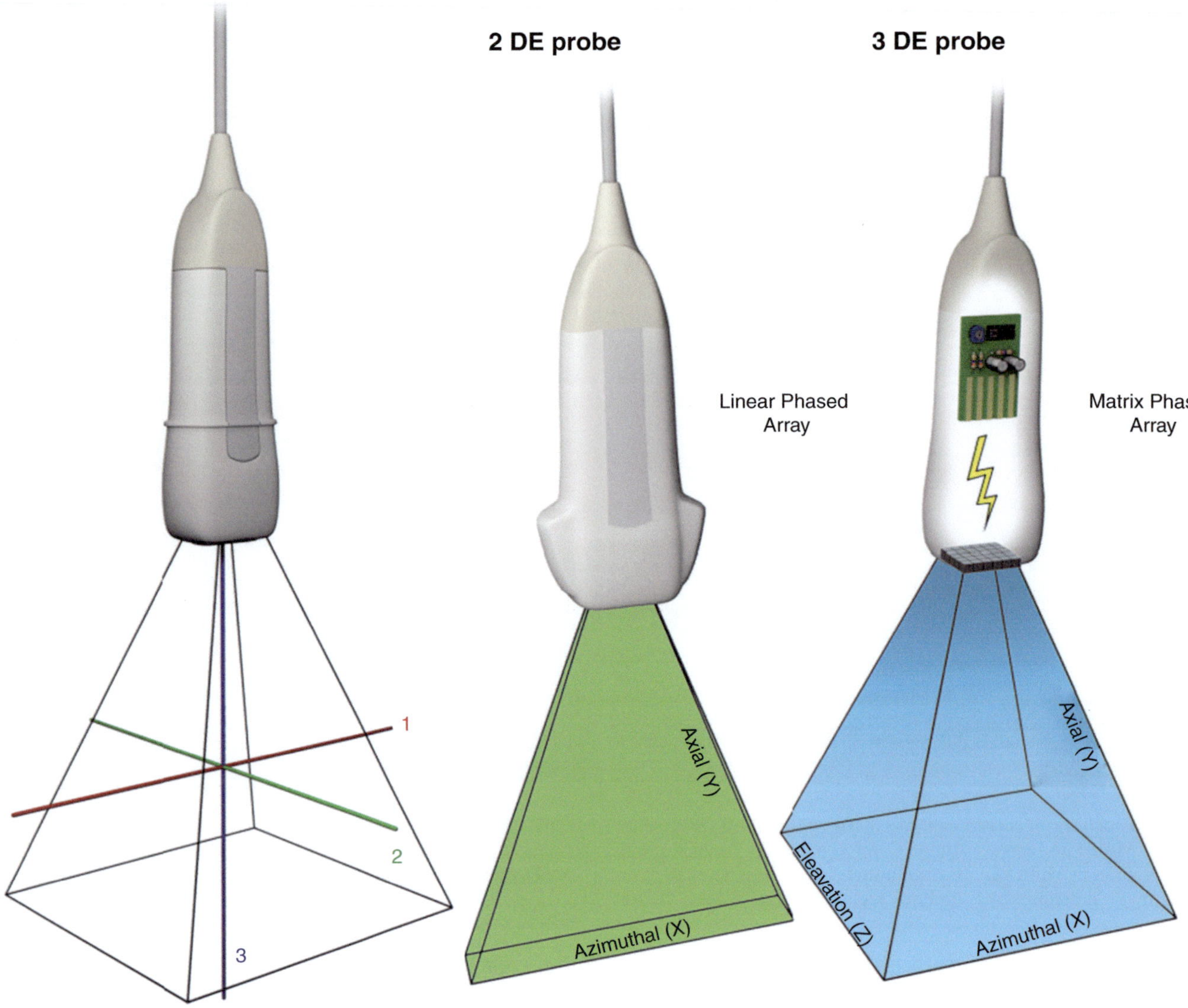

Fig. 4.9 Schematics of crop axes: **Left**: Pyramidal 3D. 1 (red) lateral or azimuthal x-axis, 2 (green) for elevation or z-axis, and 3 (blue) for height or axial y-axis. **Right**: schematic images as obtained by a 2D versus a 3D probe. Note the additional elevation (depth) z-axis dimension with 3D imaging. Courtesy of Philips

GE Healthcare E90/95

In this chapter, images from the more recent E95 model are shown. The console (Fig. 4.11) and dashboard/touch screen control displays (Figs. 4.12 and 4.13) of GE E90 and E95 models are very similar, however.

3D Acquisition Modes

1. ***Console 4D button*** (3D+ time as the fourth dimension) Switches on to single beat 3D imaging
2. ***Dashboard/Touch screen 4D***: provides three volume size options
   (a) ***Bird's view***: smallest preset 3D volume (50° lateral and 15° elevation)
   (b) ***Medium*** (35° lateral and 35° elevation)
   (c) ***Large*** (60° lateral and 60° elevation)
3. ***4D Zoom prepare***: Adjusts ROI within a biplane 2D image . Pressing the 4D button acquires the 3D data set. To start 4D Zoom prepare: From 4D or 4D Color Flow mode press the Zoom button on console (see Fig. 4.11, bottom right). Alternatively, from 2D, Color Flow or Biplane mode press 4D Zoom prepare

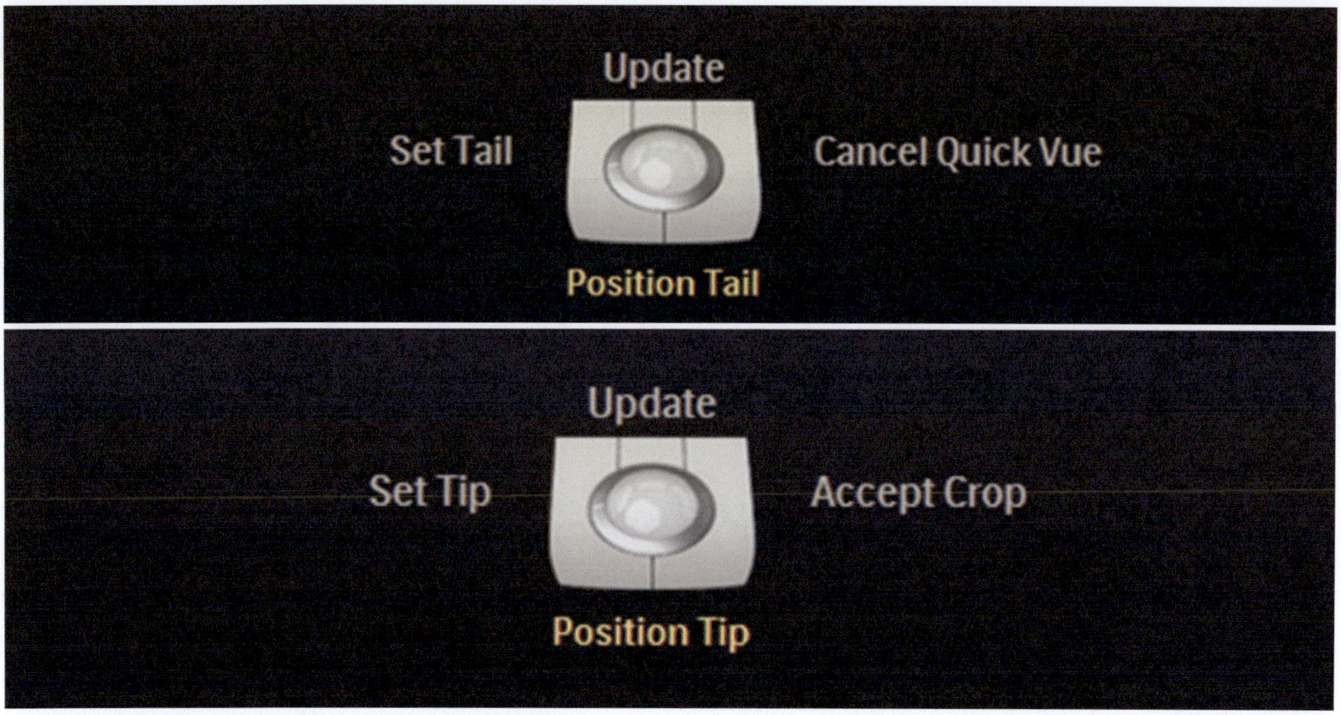

Fig. 4.10 QuickVue controls (see text). Courtesy of Philips

4. ***Color button*(console)**: Color flow can be enabled in 2D mode before entering 4D mode or when in 4D mode
5. ***Layout*** : Provides option to view the 3D data set with component 2D planes
6. ***Multi-Beat*** : number of subvolumes is selected by adjusting ***Num Beats*** (2, 3, 4, 6)
7. ***MultiD***: Provides ability to scan two planes (Bi-Plane) or three planes (Tri-Plane) from same heart cycle
8. ***Multi-Slice***: enables simultaneous display of multiple equidistant short axis views generated from a 3D volume acquisition

Image Optimization

1. ***2D button (console)*** : controls 4D ***gain*** settings and can be done in real time and also after image acquisition (post processing)
2. ***4D Clarity***: edge preserving specklke and noise reduction filter that reduces speckle while preserving or even enhancing significant boundaries in the volume data. Increasing 4D clarity will create images with less visible speckle noise and with a softer appearance
3. ***4D thickness***: allows adjusting crop slice thickness
4. ***Active Mode button (console)***: controls 4D image compression: This is accomplished by a twist rotation of the knob. Low compression provides better image details
5. ***Depth illumination***: Object illuminated by an imaginary light source, casting a shadow to help enhance depth/distance perception
6. ***Frame Rate***: increases or decreases the frame rate (temporal resolution) with concomitant opposite changes in spatial (detail) resolution
7. ***Gamma***: Affects only midtone values. Lower gamma is associated with brighter images whereas higher gamma with darker images
8. ***HD Live***: adds soft shadows and brightness to 3D volume by changing the direction and depth of a light source
9. ***Laser Lines***: may help improve visual linkage between 2D slices and 4D rendered images (the laser lines on a 3D image represent the displayed 2D tomographic slices within the 3D data; The laser lines can be color coded so as to easily identify them), and may aid depth visulazation, in live as well as replay
10. ***Multibeat***: Number of subvolume acquistion (range 2–6)
11. ***Shading***: Adjusts the shading effect on the volume rendering and may improve three dimensional perception
12. ***Smoothness***: Evens out image surface. Too much smoothing will mask fine image details

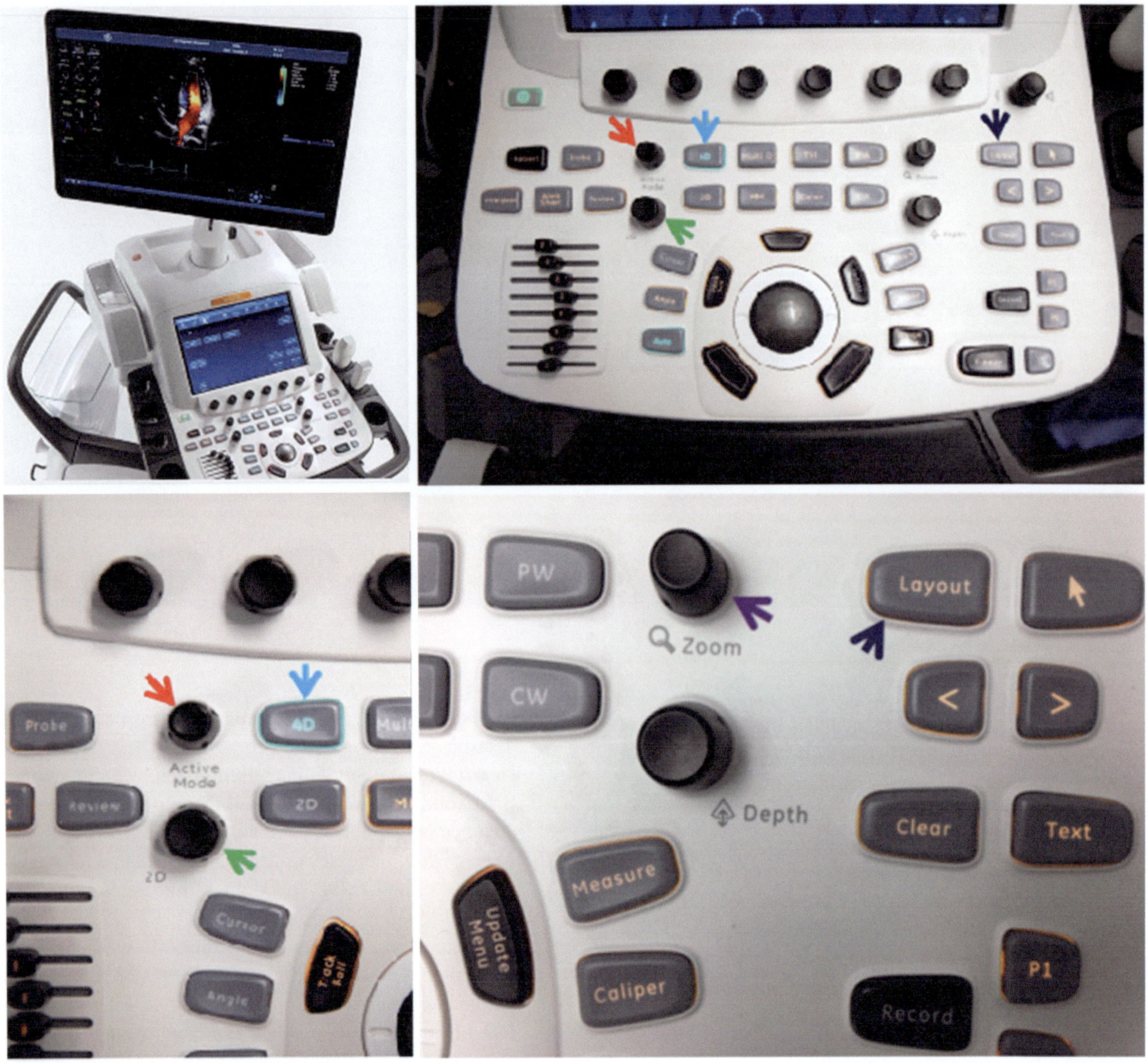

Fig. 4.11 GE Vivid 95 Machine and Console panels highlighting the **4D** button (light blue arrows), **Layout** button(dark blue arrows), **active mode** button (red arrows), **2D** (green arrows), and **Zoom** (purple arrows) on the console. Courtesy of GE Healthcare

13. ***Tissue Transp***: Serves to bring up tissue structures or flow information behind obscuring tissue structures
14. ***Transl***: Translates the crop plane into the volume
15. ***Volume Opt***: Optimizes volume rendering by adjusting several display controls simultaneously (e.g. shading, smoothness etc…)
16. ***Volume shape*** : Adjusts the ratio between the elevation (depth) and azimuth (width) in the 3D volumetric data set by primarily changing the amount of elevation
17. ***Volume size*** : Adjusts volume in both azimuthal (width) ***and*** elevation (depth) directions simultaneously

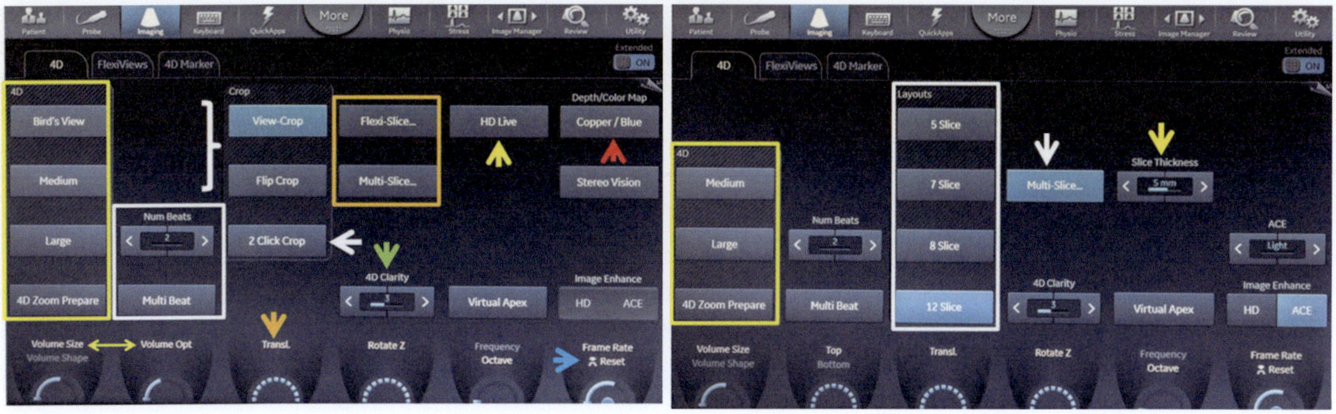

Fig. 4.12 **Vivid E95** Dashboard/Touch screen Panels **1. Left**: **4D** acquisition modes (**Bird's view**, **Medium**, **Large**, and **4D Zoom Prepare**; yellow rectangle), **Multi Beat** and **Num Beats** (white square), **Volume Size/Volume Shape** and **Volume Opt** (double headed yellow arrow), **Flexi Slice** and **Multi Slice** (orange square), **Transl** (orange arrow), **4D Clarity** (green arrow), **HD Live** (yellow arrow), **2ClickCrop** (white arrow), and **Crop** View/Flip options (white curly bracket). **Right**: **Multislice** (white arrow), Multislice **Layouts** selection (white rectangle), and **Slice Thickness** selection (yellow arrow). Note the associated **4D** selection (yellow rectangle). Courtesy of GE Healthcare

Cropping

1. ***2-Click Crop***: crop mode where two parallel crop planes are applied to the volumetric data set. The position and viewing direction are defined by clicking in two locations either in the 2D reference images or in the 3D volume
2. ***Flexi-Slice***: Customizes where 2D slices come from. Laser lines on 3D acquistion can be moved to desired ROI and the corresponding 2D images are displayed in three orthogonal planes. Flexi Slice displays 3 perpendicular cut planes and a volume rendering. The cut planes can be rotated and translated independently of each other or in combination. Flexi Slice mode is available in 4D, and 4D color flow modes in live and replay
3. ***Parallel Crop***: provides a slice of the 3D volume data set contained within two parrallel cropping planes that are advanced in tandem into the 3D data set

Siemens Healthineers Z6Ms

4D Controls (Figs. 4.14, 4.15, and 4.16)

1. ***Space/Time*** resolution control: Adjusts for temporal and/or spatial resolution. There are four settings: S1, S2, T1, and T2. The S settings optimize spatial resolution and the T settings optimize temporal resolution.
2. ***X, Y, and Z*** volume rotation controls rotate the volume rendered image along the different spatial axes.
3. ***Box Edit***: Allows cropping of the volume along the X, Y, and Z axes. Turn Box Edit on from soft keys and use X, Y, and Z controls to crop the box displayed around the volume.
4. ***Clip Store***: Acquires the 4D volume.
5. ***Dual V***: Simultaneously displays two views of the same 4D volume from opposite viewing angles by displaying two orthogonal reference planes and two opposing volume views.
6. ***Single V (Previously D'art)***: Crops the 4D image from a single viewing point. A reference point appears with an arrow, indicating viewing direction. The region of interest can be adjusted in size by selecting and moving the corners. The region of interest can also be rotated by selecting and moving the reference point or the view direction arrow.
7. ***Bi-plane+***: scans two imaging planes with different rotation and tilt angles in a side-by-side format, enabling individual manipulation of the planes.
8. ***RES enhanced resolution imaging***: Zoom function that re-optimizes and re-scans the selected region of interest, increasing temporal and spatial resolution. In 4D imaging, press RES and adjust ROI. Then press 4D to enter a focused viewing mode of selected anatomy.

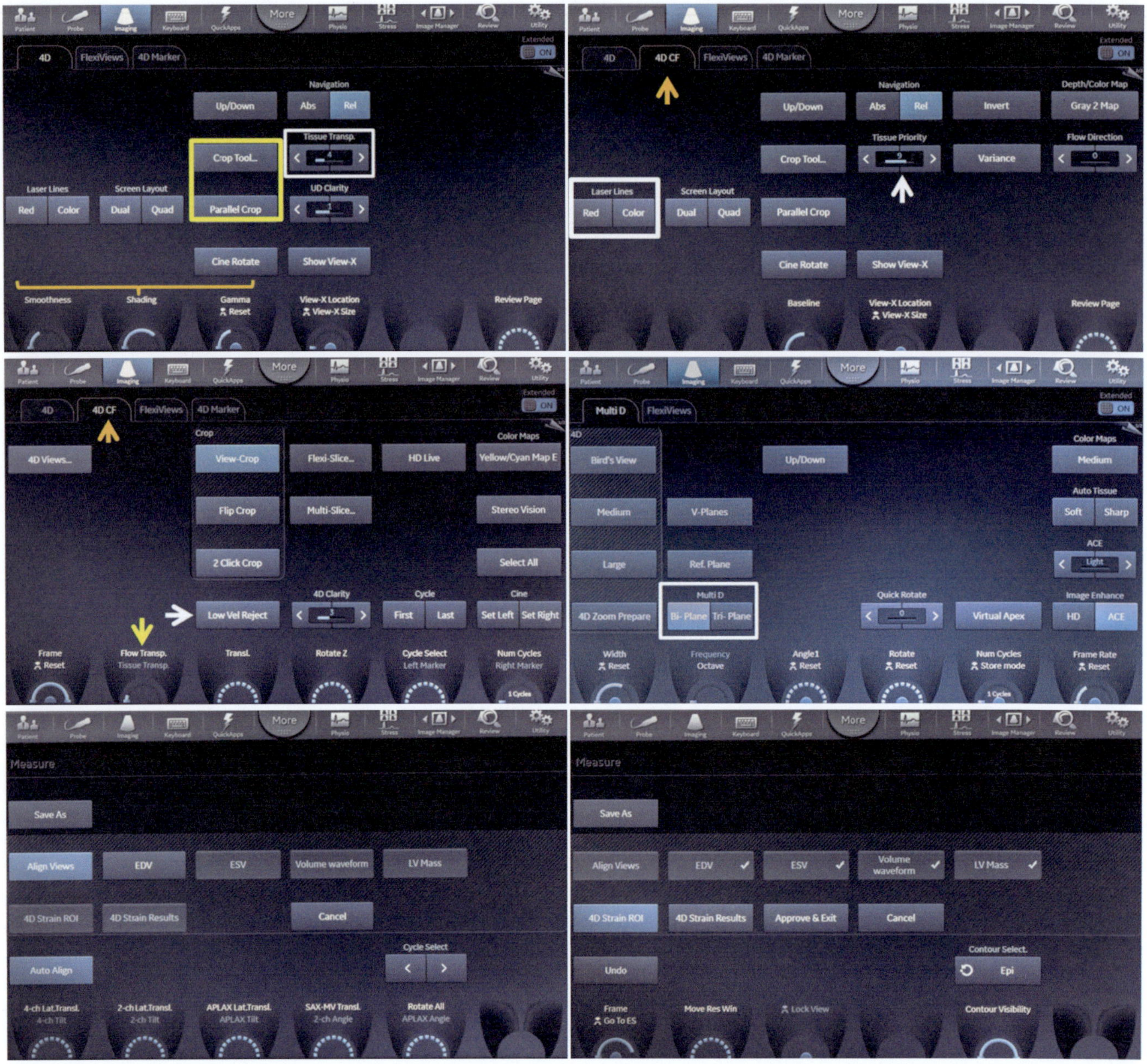

Fig. 4.13 **Vivid E95** Dashboard/Touch screen panels 2. **Top panel**: **Left**: **Parrallel Crop** (yellow rectangle), **Tissue Transp** (white rectangle), **Smoothness**, **Shading**, and **Gamma** controls (orange curly bracket) are highlighted. **Right**: **4D CF** (orange arrow), **Laser Lines** (white rectangle) and **Tissue Priority** (white arrow) are highlighted. **Middle panel**: 4D CF (orange arrow) **LowVelReject** (white arrow) and **Flow/Tissue Transp** (yellow arrow) controls are highlighted. **Right**: **MultiD Bi-Plane/Tri-Plane** selection option (white rectangle). **Bottom panel** shows 4D strain controls. Courtesy of GE Healthcare

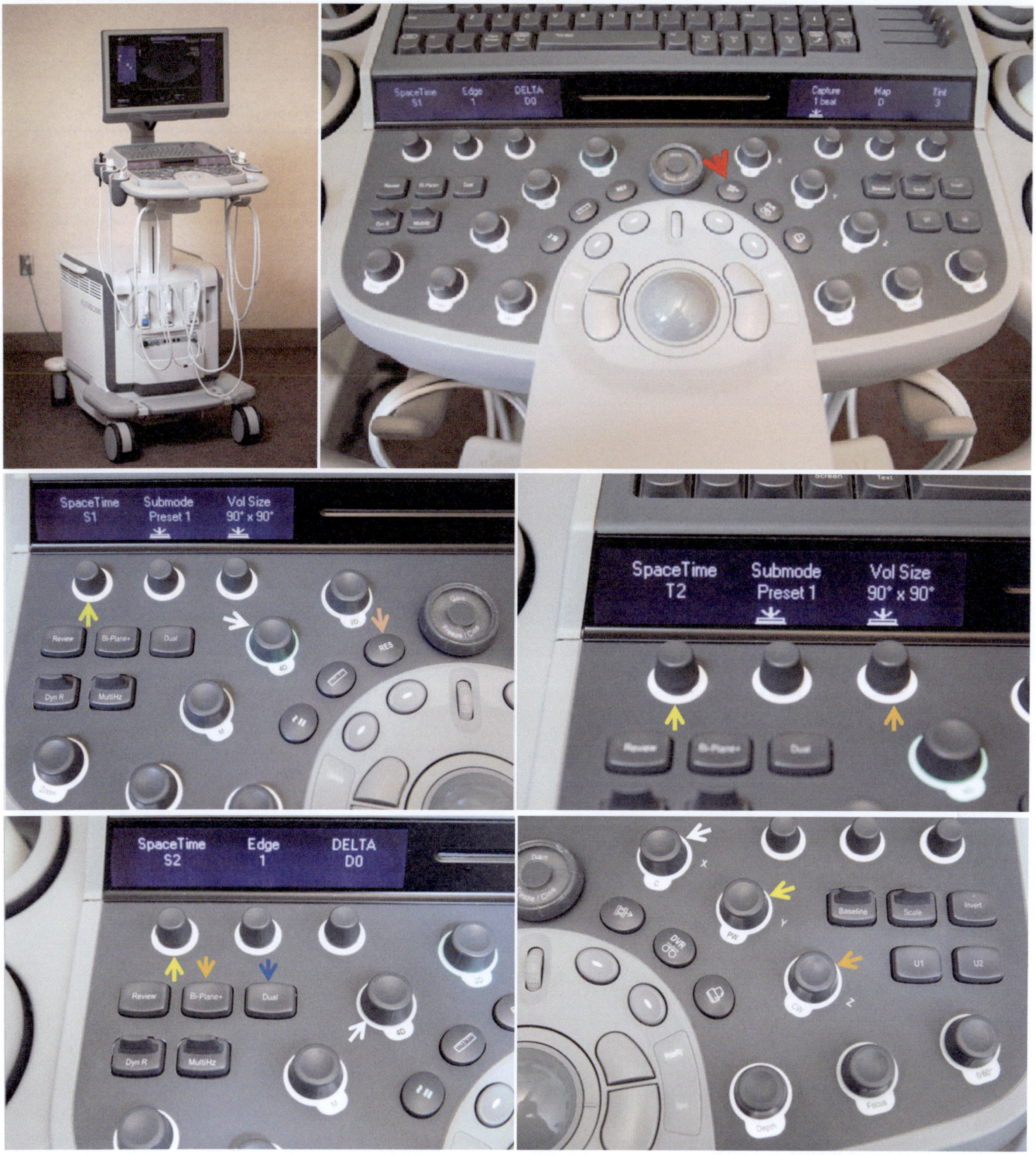

Fig. 4.14 **Top panel**: overview of Siemens machine and console. Red arrow points to **Clip Store** button**. Middle panel**. **Left**: Console **SpaceTime S1** setting (yellow arrow), **4D** control (white arrow), and **RES** control (light orange arrow)**. Right**: **SpaceTime T2** setting (yellow arrow) and **Vol Size** (orange arrow). **Bottom panel**. **Left**: **SpaceTime S2** setting (yellow arrow), **Bi-Plane+** (orange arrow), **Dual** (blue arrow) and **4D** control (white arrow)**. Right**: **X** (white arrow), **Y** (yellow arrow) and **Z** (orange arrow) 3D volume spatial axes rotation controls. Please note that these buttons also serve to provide color Doppler (**C**), pulse wave Doppler (**PW**) and continuous wave Doppler (**CW**) in that order. Courtesy of Siemens Medical Solutions USA, Inc.

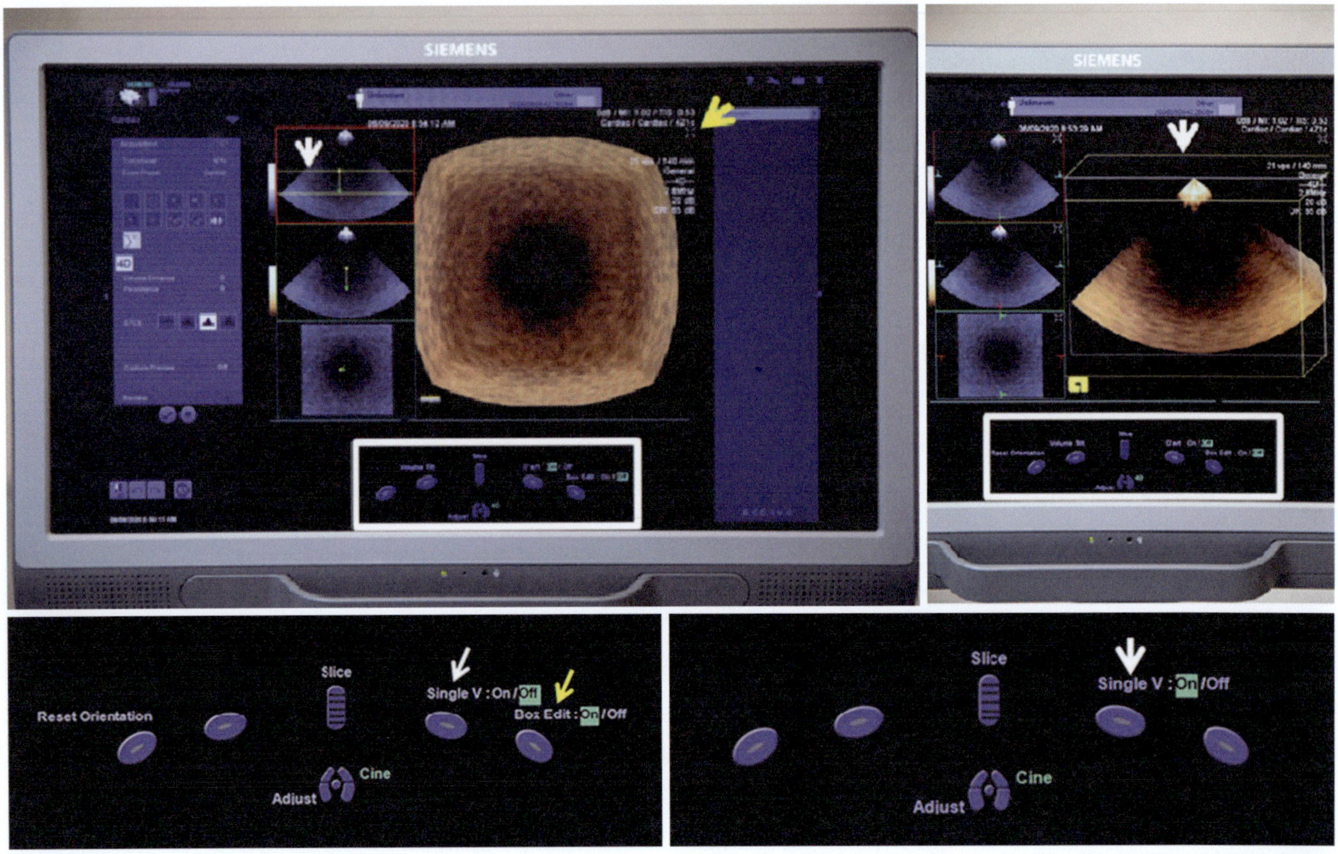

Fig. 4.15 **Top panel**: **Left**: Screen showing MPR of 3D image with component 2D planes. **Single V (D'art)** on and **Box Edit** off cropping tools are shown below (white rectangle). White arrow points to Single V (D'art) cropping viewing direction. Yellow arrow points to **icon** that allows viewing of the selected volume rendered image in full screen mode. **Right 3D** crop box on **(white arrow)**. **Bottom panel**: Enlarged views of **Single V** (white arrows) off (left) and on (right) and **Box Edit** on (yellow arrow)**.** Courtesy of Siemens Medical Solutions USA, Inc.

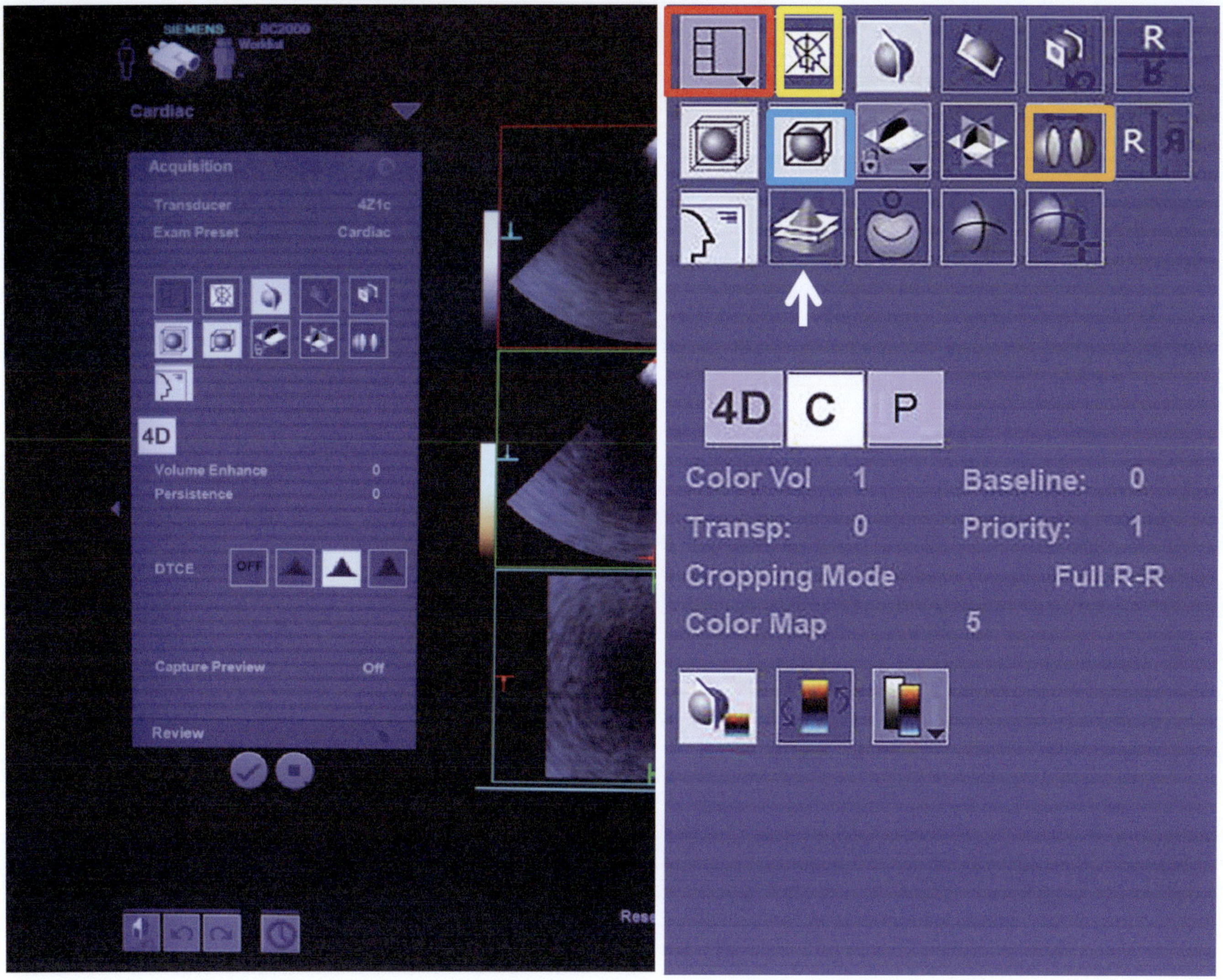

Fig. 4.16 4D volume review display options panel highlightighting the following: Dual V control (white arrow); Number of views including multislice (red square); no cross lines (yellow rectangle); box/wire frame (blue square); and split view (orange square) Courtesy of Siemens Medical Solutions USA, Inc.

Part II

Native and Prosthetic Heart Valves

3DE of Normal Mitral Valve: Image Display and Anatomic Correlations

5

Francesco F. Faletra, Laura A. Leo, Joseph F. Maalouf, and Joseph J. Maleszewski

Introduction

Cardiac anatomy is a fundamental part of the medical curriculum. Traditionally, pathologists illustrate cardiac structures using anatomic specimens derived from cadaver dissections. However, in the past two decades, technological advances in non-invasive imaging techniques have allowed acquisition of exquisite anatomical details of the heart in both two-dimensional (2D) and three-dimensional (3D) format. Thus, nowadays, students of cardiology may learn heart anatomy in the form of medical imaging to supplement and enhance the traditional teaching based on the observation of anatomical specimens. Understanding normal anatomy of the mitral valve (MV) is of paramount importance for a correct interpretation of the wide spectrum of MV diseases and for safe and effective surgery or percutaneous transcatheter procedures targeting the mitral annulus (MA) and leaflets. Three-dimensional transesophageal echocardiography (3D TEE), more than 3D transthoracic echocardiography, provides accurate images of the MV with a high temporal and spatial resolution. The particular ability of angulating and rotating the volumetric data set allows viewing the valve from several perspectives. Moreover, unlike anatomic specimens, this technique provides a never-seen-before three dimensional "dynamic" anatomy. Other non-invasive imaging techniques, in particular computed tomography (CT) and cardiac magnetic resonance (CMR), may visualize specific components of the mitral valve apparatus and surrounding structures with more details than 3D TEE, such as epicardial adipose tissue (EAT) in the atrio-ventricular groove, coronary arteries surrounding the MV or papillary muscles. These techniques are nowadays indispensable companions of 3D TEE for an accurate and complete description of the MV apparatus. In this chapter, we describe the salient anatomy of the mitral valve apparatus as it appears with the above-mentioned non-invasive imaging techniques.

As emphasized by Perloff and Roberts [1], the MV is a complex apparatus in which several components move in perfect spatial and temporal coordination to ensure effective valve competence. Key components are the annulus, leaflets, chordae tendineae and the papillary muscles (PMs) attached to the left ventricular free wall.

Mitral Valve Annulus

The perception that the MA is a continuous circular ring of dense connective tissue that encircles the atrioventricular junction, anchors the leaflets and divides the left atrium from the left ventricle, is rather incorrect. When an anatomic specimen or 3D TEE image of the MV is observed from an overhead perspective, the MA is seen as the hinge line of the mitral leaflets (the "transition zone" of the cardiac surgeons) and has a D-shaped configuration with two well distinct components: straight located anterior-medial and referred to as anterior MA, and curved located posterior-lateral and referred to as posterior annulus (Fig. 5.1a, b). This D-shaped

F. F. Faletra (✉)
Director of Cardiac Imaging Lab, Cardiocentro Ticino Institute, Lugano, Switzerland
e-mail: Francesco.Faletra@cardiocentro.org

L. A. Leo
Cardiac Imaging Lab, Cardiocentro Ticino Institute, Lugano, Switzerland
e-mail: lauraanna.leo@cardiocentro.org

J. F. Maalouf
Professor of Medicine, Mayo Clinic College of Medicine; Director, Interventional Echocardiography; Consultant, Department of Cardiovascular Medicine, Mayo Clinic, Rochester, MN, USA
e-mail: maalouf.joseph@mayo.edu

J. J. Maleszewski
Professor of Laboratory Medicine & Pathology, College of Medicine & Science; Professor of Medicine, College of Medicine & Science; Section Head, Cardiovascular Pathology; Consultant, Departments of Laboratory Medicine & Pathology, Cardiovascular Medicine, and Medical Genomics, Mayo Clinic, Rochester, MN, USA
e-mail: Maleszewski.Joseph@mayo.edu

J. F. Maalouf et al. (eds.), *Practical 3D Echocardiography*, https://doi.org/10.1007/978-3-030-72941-7_5

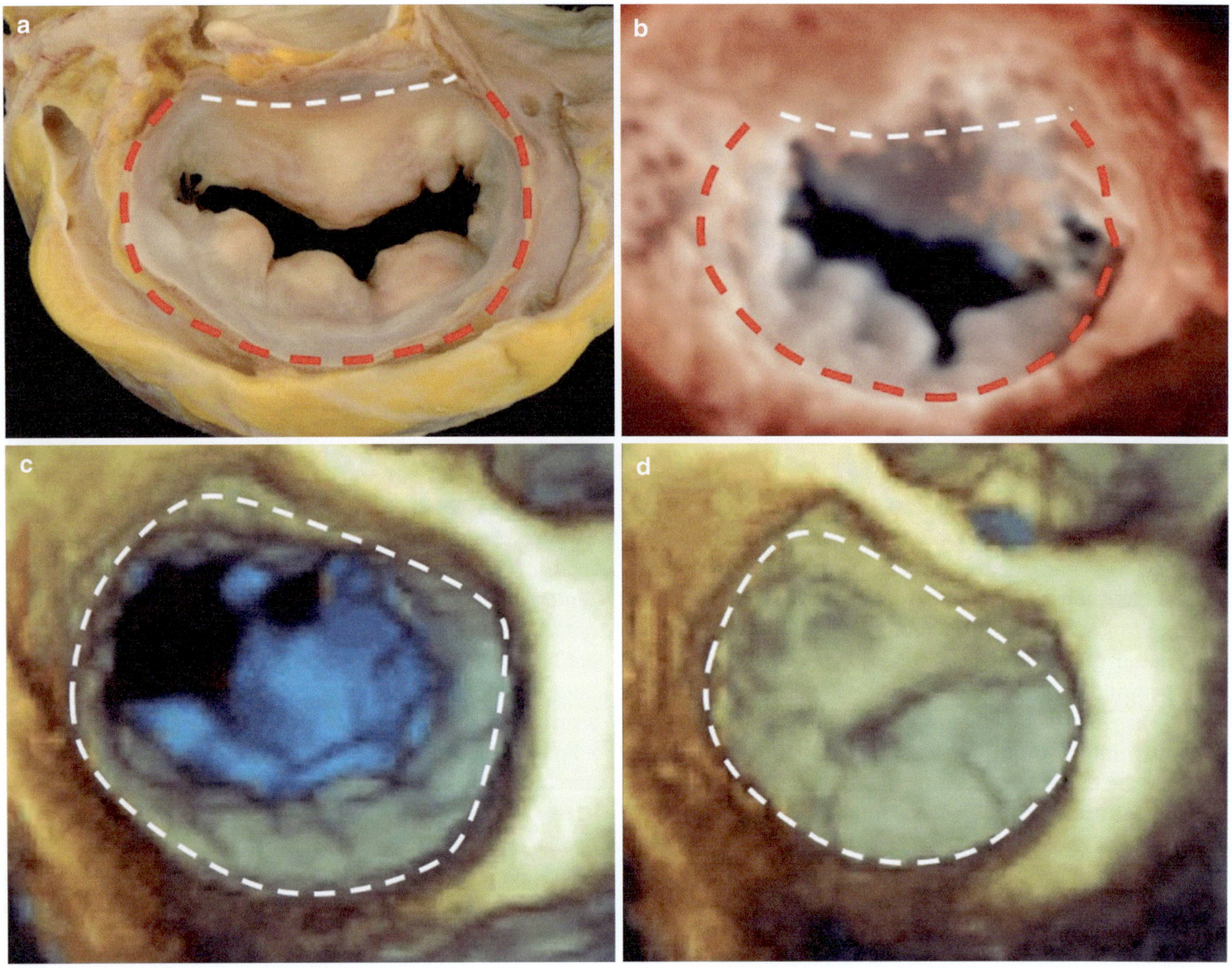

Fig. 5.1 (**a**) Anatomic specimen from an overhead perspective showing the D-shaped configuration of the mitral annulus. (**b**) 3D TEE image with a new volume rendering algorithm which provides a very realistic image. In both panels the white dotted line marks the anterior component of the mitral annulus and the curved red dotted line the posterior component. (**c**, **d**) 3D TEE still images in (**c**) diastole and (**d**) systole from overhead perspective showing that the annulus becomes more circular in early diastole

aspect of the MA varies throughout the cardiac cycle, becoming more circular in diastole (Fig. 5.1c, d). Because these components have different anatomical structure and function, they are described separately.

The Posterior MA

In cross-section the posterior MA appears as a juxtaposition of four components: the atrial wall, the ventricular wall, the hinge line of the posterior mitral leaflet, and the epicardial adipose tissue (EAT). These components are supposed to be "joined" together by a cord of fibrous tissue. It is undeniable that this fibrous cord, though attenuated, interspersed with fat and discontinuous, represents the posterior MA [2]. However, in areas in which it is absent, the posterior leaflet is attached directly on the ventricular muscular tissue. This specific anatomic structure explains the sphincteric action of the MA: segments of the hinge line of the posterior leaflet, attached directly to the muscular tissue, follow the contraction and relaxation of the left ventricle (see below). On the other hand, EAT penetrates deeply into the atrioventricular groove up to the base of the posterior leaflet. This particular arrangement provides a perfect electrical insulation between the left atrium and the left ventricle. Finally, the absence of a robust fibrous cord makes the posterior annulus rather "soft", explaining why dilatation of the MA affects prevalently this component.

Either 3D TEE or CT and CMR may illustrate the complex anatomical arrangement of the posterior annulus. 3D TEE distinguishes the atrial and ventricular myocardium and the hinge line of the posterior leaflet. However, the similar acoustic impedance between EAT and myocardium prevents a clear distinction between the two tissues (Fig. 5.2a, b). CT

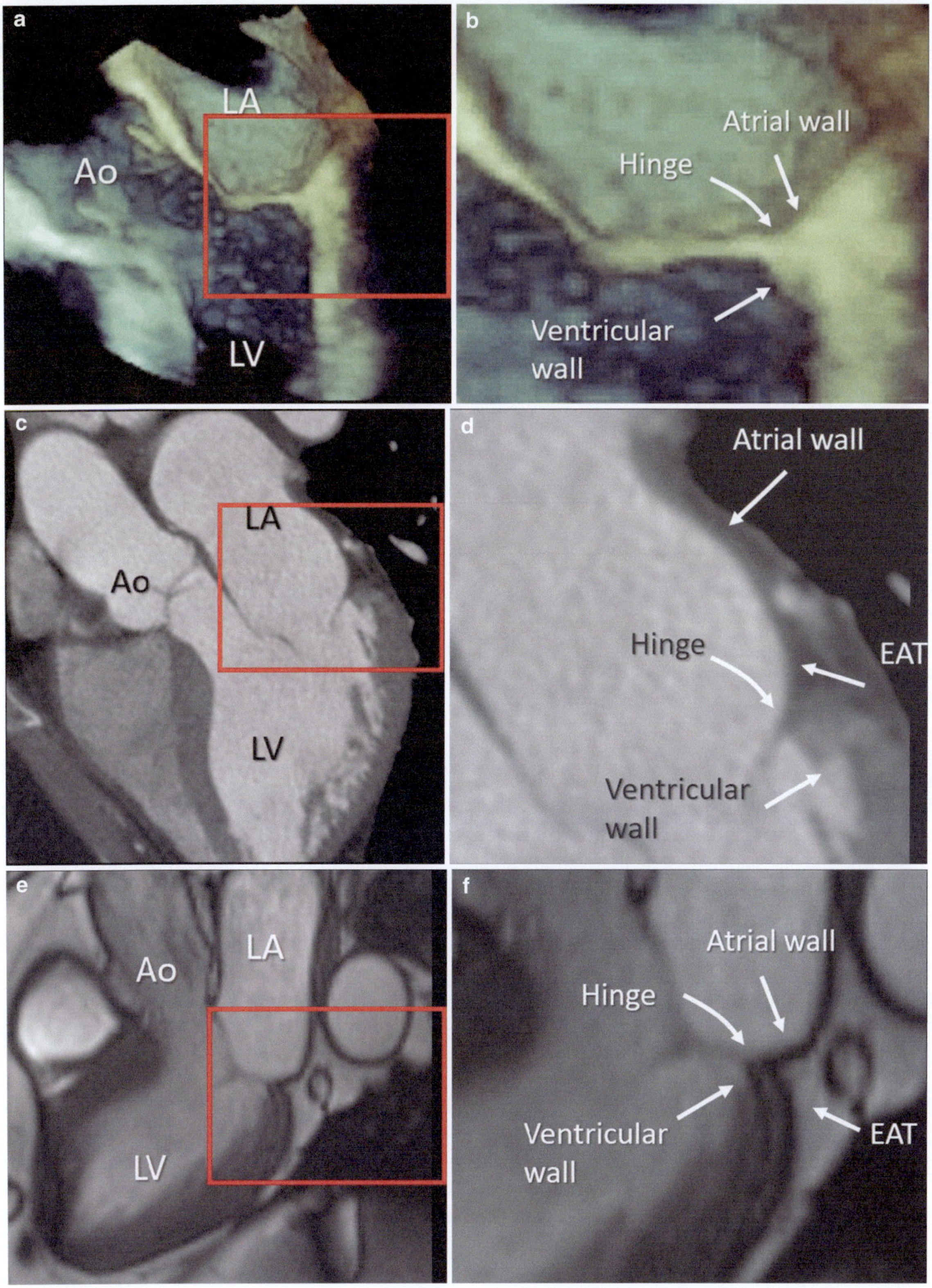

Fig. 5.2 (**a**) Cross-section image of 3D TEE in long axis view of the left ventricle (LV). (**b**) Magnified image of the area in the red box of panel **a**. Three components of the posterior MA can be distinguished: namely the atrial and ventricular walls and the hinge line of the posterior mitral leaflet. The epicardial adipose tissue (EAT) is not recognizable. (**c**) Computed tomography scan showing the LV in cross section long axis view. (**d**) Magnified image of the area in the red box in panel **c**. All four components of the posterior MA can be distinguished though the boundaries between EAT, which is darker than that of the surrounding structures, and the muscular tissue is rather indistinct. (**e**) CMR balanced steady state free precession (SSFP) sequence showing a cross section long axis view of the LV. (**f**) Magnified image of the area in the red box in panel E. All the four components of posterior MA can be clearly distinguished

scan is able to differentiate the four components of the posterior mitral annulus: its high spatial resolution allows obtaining exquisite images of the hinge line, the atrial and ventricular wall. EAT appears darker than surrounding structures though the boundaries between EAT and muscular tissue are rather indistinct. Moreover, CT allows defining the anatomic relationships between the course of the circumflex coronary artery and its marginal branches and the posterior MA (Fig. 5.2c, d). Finally, the balanced steady state free precession (SSFP) sequences of CMR produce strong signals from the blood and EAT, and weak signals from the muscular tissue, making CMR probably the technique that more precisely visualizes all four components that form the posterior MA (Fig. 5.2e, f). Interestingly, none of these techniques enables visualizing the fibrous cord described in histological specimens and corresponding to the posterior MA.

The Anterior MA

The anterior MA from an atrial perspective is just the junction between the yellowish anterior leaflet and the pink-coloured atrial wall. This line lies in a more apical position than the hinge line of the aortic leaflets. Because of this arrangement, from a ventricular perspective, the hinge line of the anterior mitral leaflet and the crown-shaped insertion of aortic leaflets are separated by a smooth fibrous band called mitral-aortic curtain also referred to as the mitral-aortic intervalvular fibrosa or mitral-aortic continuity. This band extents laterally and medially up to two robust fibrous nodules called trigons, superiorly and inferiorly continues imperceptible with the interleaflet triangle between the non-coronary and left coronary sinuses and with the anterior mitral leaflet respectively. Thus, from a strict anatomical point of view the anterior mitral leaflet, the mitral aortic curtain and the interleaflet triangle, are a unique anatomic structure. Both CT and CMR in a cross-section long axis view of the left ventricle, can elucidate this complex arrangement of anterior MA, while 3D TEE from a left ventricle perspective is able to visualize the mitral-aortic curtain "en face" (Fig. 5.3).

The Saddle Shaped Arrangement of MA

The notion that the MA is not planar but rather has a three-dimensional saddle-shaped configuration goes back to the seminal work of Robert Levine et al. [3]. Their work has led to a profound conceptual reconsideration of the diagnostic criteria of mitral valve prolapse. The highest point (peak) is located at the midpoint of the anterior segment, followed by the midpoint of the posterior segment, and the lowest points (valleys) are located at the commissures (near the fibrous trigons). A digitally computerized reconstruction of 3D TEE images (using software available on most echocardiography machines) may clearly show this three-dimensional architecture (Fig. 5.4). Interestingly, either in their original paper or using the available dedicated software, the contour traced to reconstruct the saddle-shaped configuration follows the hinge line of leaflets. Thus, the three-dimensional saddle-shaped arrangement should be referred to as the hinge line rather than a true anatomical annulus, which as a complete ring does not exist at all.

Dynamics of MA

The MA has three fundamental motions:

(a) *Sphincteric-like contraction*, which depends exclusively on the contraction of the left ventricle that leads to an anterior motion of the posterior segment hinge line; this motion facilitates leaflet coaptation assuring effective valve competence and it is best appreciated with 3D TEE from an overhead perspective.
(b) *Translation motion toward the apex*. The apex of the heart is firmly attached to the diaphragm by robust connective bands; the contraction of sub-endocardial and subepicardial myofibers longitudinally/obliquely orientated produces a longitudinal systolic shortening of the left ventricle, which drags the MA towards the apex. This motion enlarges the left atrium and the consequent drop in left atrial pressure promotes pulmonary venous return. The best technique to appreciate this translation motion is CMR.
(c) *Annular infolding* (i.e. an increase of the saddle-shaped arrangement). Accentuation of the annular infolding produces several beneficial effects: reduces the systolic stress on the leaflets (by increasing leaflet curvature), balances the tension exerted on chordae, reduces radial and circumferential deformation of the posterior leaflet promoting a better inter-scallop coaptation and concentrates the peak stress on the two trigones [4].

Mitral Leaflets

Anatomists and surgeons describe the mitral valve as having two leaflets, the anterior (or aortic) and the posterior separated by two deep incisures (commissures). The anterior leaflet has a triangular shape. Its insertion on the MV annulus covers approximately 1/3 of the annular circumference. The posterior leaflet has a quadrangular shape covering the remaining 2/3. Because the anterior leaflet is wider than the posterior leaflet, the area of each leaflet is almost equal. 3D TEE provides superb images of the MV leaflets. In nearly 70% of normal valves, the posterior leaflet presents two indentations, which divide the leaflet into three segments (or

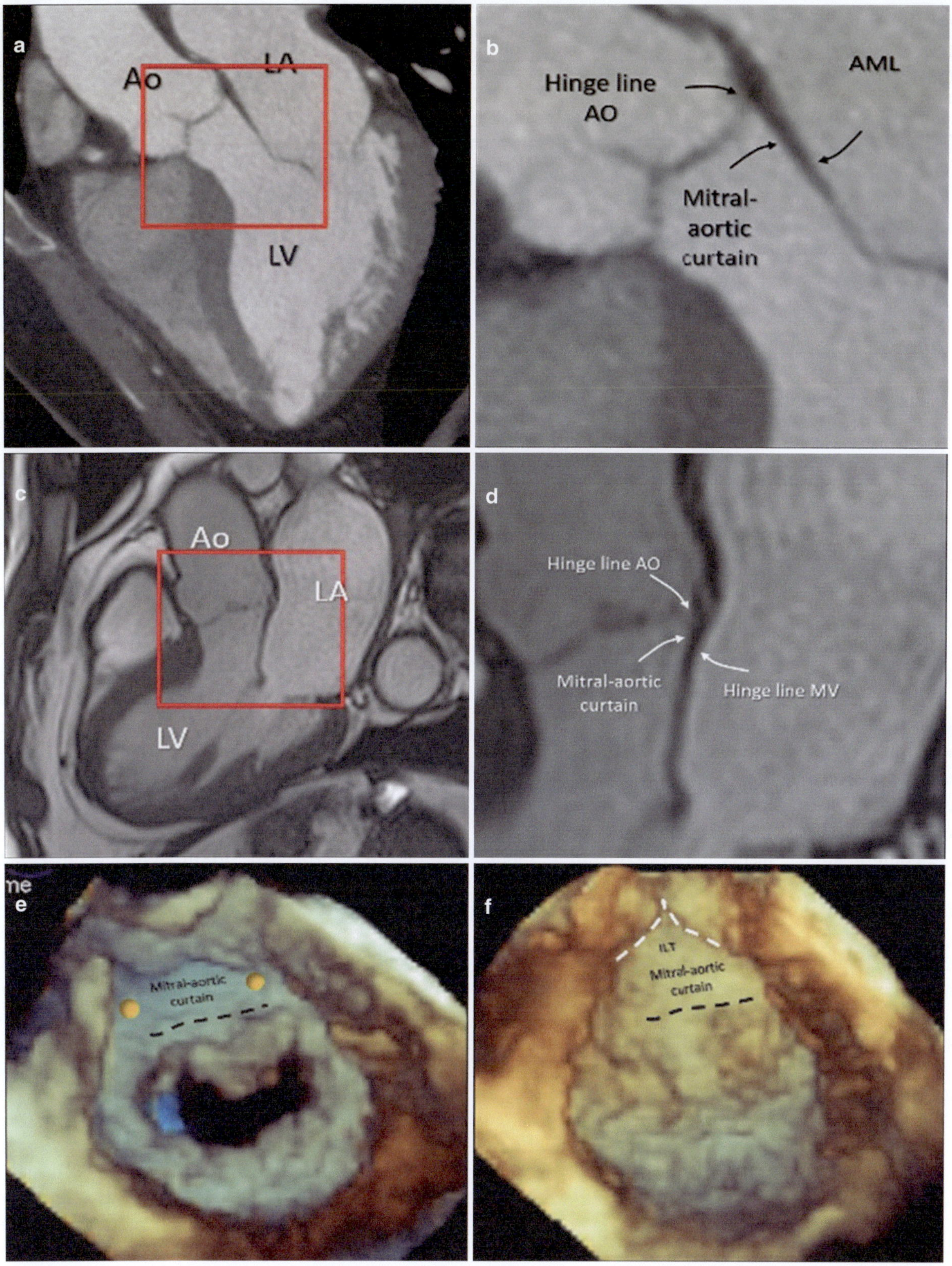

Fig. 5.3 (**a**) CT cross section long axis view of the left ventricle. (**b**) Magnified image of the area in red box in panel **a**. Arrows point to the hinge line of the aorta (AO), mitral aortic curtain and hinge line of the anterior mitral leaflet (AML). (**c**, **d**) Similar images obtained with CMR. (**e**, **f**) 3D TEE from a ventricular perspective in (**e**) diastole and (**f**) in systole showing the mitral-aortic curtain "en face". The two orange circles indicate the trigons. The black dotted line indicates the hinge line of the mitral valve, the triangular white dotted line indicates the interleaflet triangle (ILT). LV, left ventricle; LA, left atrium; MV mitral valve

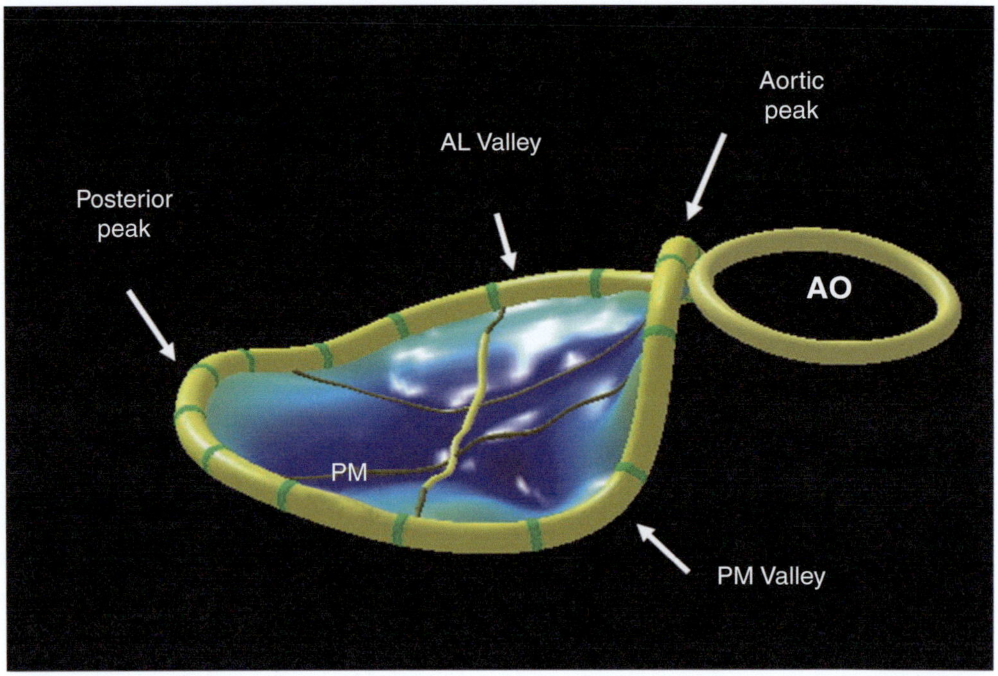

Fig. 5.4 Digitally computerized reconstruction of the saddle-shape aspect of the mitral annuls with peaks and anterior-lateral (AL) and posterior-medial (PM) valleys

scallops) P1 (lateral), P2 (central), P3 (medial). The anterior leaflet has no identifiable scallops. However, for practical reasons, surgeons divide the anterior leaflet into 3 segments, named A1, A2, and A3, indicating the areas opposite the corresponding scallops of the posterior leaflet (Fig. 5.5a, b). In contrast to other non-invasive imaging techniques, 3D TEE offers the unique opportunity of visualizing leaflets and scallops in a countless number of perspectives. There are at least four basic perspectives: the perspective from above, the so-called "surgical view", because it is the same vantage point of surgical inspection in the operating room, the perspective from the left ventricle and the angled right-to-left and left-to-right perspectives. The angled perspectives [5] allow a better vision of the medial and lateral commissures. Moreover, when needed, slight angulations or rotations from these basic perspectives or selective cuts permits visualizing anatomic details (Fig. 5.5c, d).

Quite often, the commissures do not reach the hinge line leaving a strip of valvular tissue connecting the two leaflets. In such a case, from a strict anatomical point of view, the mitral valve may be considered a continuous veil inserted around the entire hinge line of mitral orifice and commissures. In some valves one or both commissures present small commissural scallops, which facilitate coaptation between leaflets (Fig. 5.6).

Inspection of the ventricular surface of both leaflets reveals two distinct areas: the rough and the clear zones. The rough zone receives the insertion of chordae tendineae and presents a "corrugate" and thicker surface while the clear zone, lacking chordal insertion, has a smoother, thinner and sometime translucent appearance. Interestingly the rough zones on their atrial aspect correspond to the coaptation surfaces, i.e. the area where leaflets juxtapose each other during systole. The vast majority of chordal attachment is therefore within the coaptation area sharing the mechanical stress with the leaflets. The resolution power of 3D TEE does not allow a clear distinction between rough and clear zones (Fig. 5.7).

Chordae Tendineae and Papillary Muscles

Chordae tendineae take origin from the tip of papillary muscles in a number of 6–10 and before reaching the rough zone of both leaflets, they split into numerous branches and interconnections. This chordal network ensures a balanced distribution of the mechanical stress. Chordae tendineae may be subdivided into marginal (or first order), strut (or second order), and basal chordae (or third order). This nomenclature reflects their function. Indeed, marginal chordae insert near the free margins of both leaflets and prevent eversion of leaflets during systole. Strut chordae, usually two in number, insert on the border between the rough and clear zone of the anterior leaflet. They are the thickest and strongest chordae and appear to ensure a sort of fibrous continuity between leaflet and ventricular wall, supporting the longitudinal contraction of the left ventricle. Moreover, by reducing the mobility of the lateral parts of the AML, these chordae determine a concave shape of the leaflet in diastole (favouring diastolic inflow) and a convex shape in systole (favouring systolic outflow). Finally, basal chordae originate directly from trabeculae of ventricular myocardium and insert only on the posterior leaflet (mainly on the middle scallop). The role of these chordae remains unclear. 3D TEE is not able to distinguish among the different types of chordae. The best approach is probably the transgastric (the same view used in 2D TEE) using multiplanar reconstruction with thick sections. This modality has been used to measure chordal length [6] (Fig. 5.8).

The papillary muscles (PMs) originate from the distal third of the ventricular wall in the posterior-medial and anterior-lateral position as a single entity or a group of two or three muscles. The original definition of Perloff and Roberts [1] "…single bodies emerging from the left ventricular wall..." is not entirely true. Indeed, CT scan has shown that PMs do not attach directly on the compact myocardium but arise from a network of ventricular trabeculations [7]. Spaces between trabeculae beneath the base of papillary muscles are visible in late diastole when the left ventricle cavity is at its largest. Both 2D and 3D echocardiography are able to show these spaces in late diastole (Fig. 5.9).

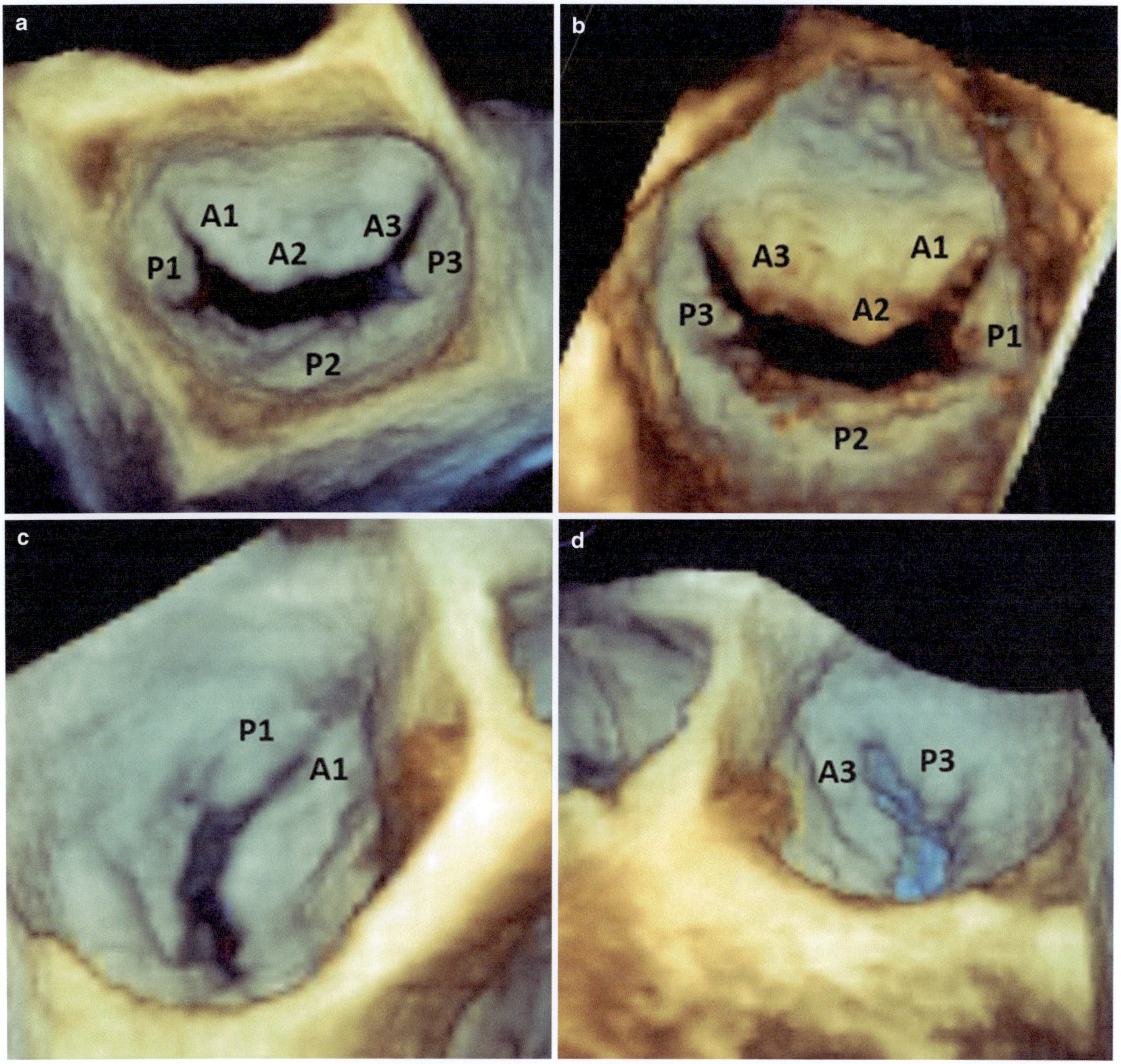

Fig. 5.5 The four basic perspectives of mitral leaflets. (**a**) An overhead (surgical) view showing the atrial surface of mitral leaflets and a well-defined image of the posterior leaflet scallops. (**b**) Same data set rotated to obtain a ventricular perspective. (**c**) Angled view right-to-left showing the lateral commissure and P1, A1 segments. (**d**) Angled left-to-right view showing the medial commissure and A3, P3 segments

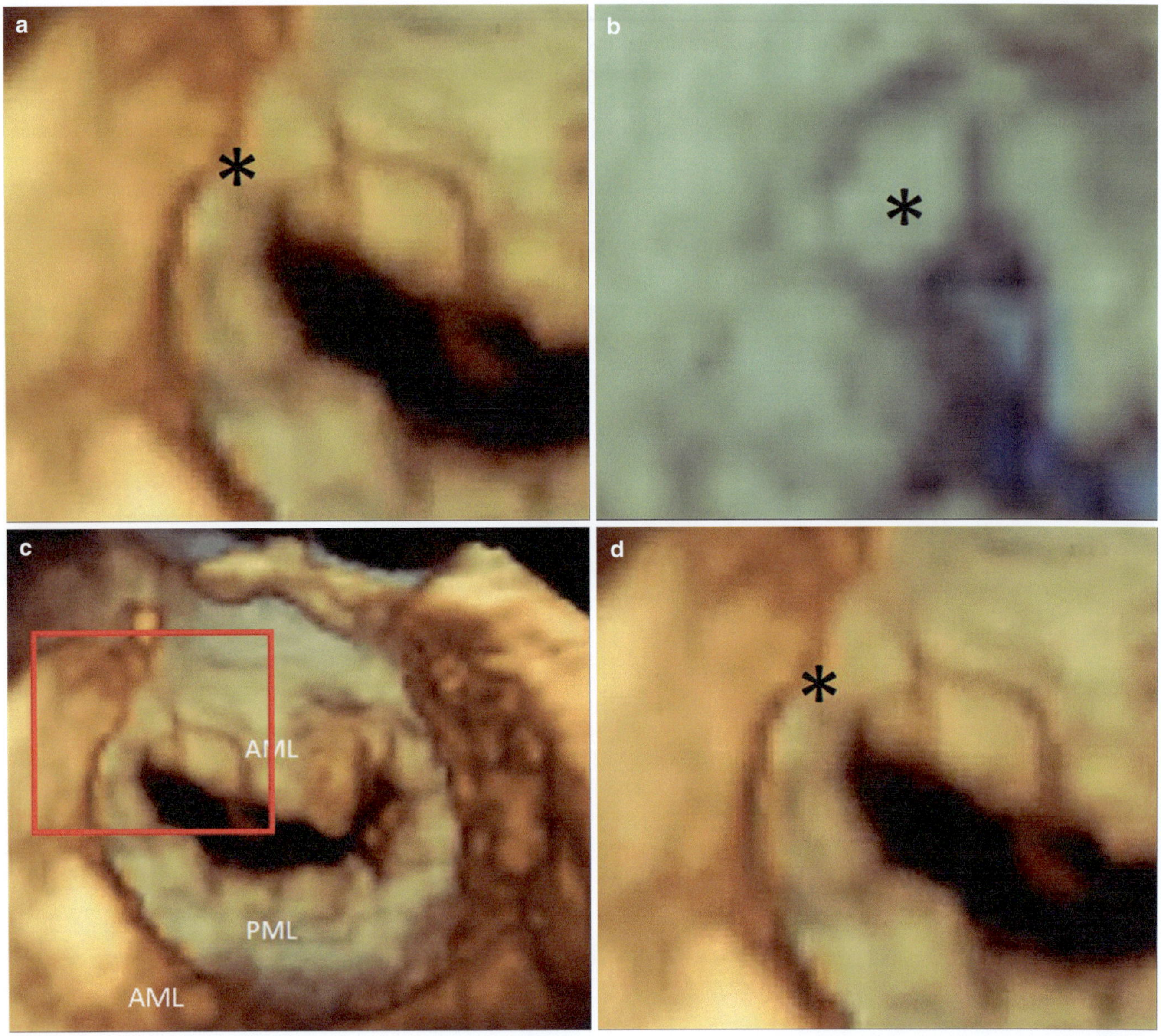

Fig. 5.6 (**a**) 3D TEE image of the mitral valve from an overhead perspective showing the anterior (AML) and posterior (PML) leaflets. (**b**) Magnified image of the area in the red box of panel **a** showing the lateral commissure. The asterisk points to a small lateral commissural scallop. (**c**) 3D TEE image of the mitral valve from a ventricular perspective. (**d**) Magnified image of the area in the red box of panel **c** showing the medial commissure. The asterisk is at the strip of commissural valvular tissue connecting the two leaflets

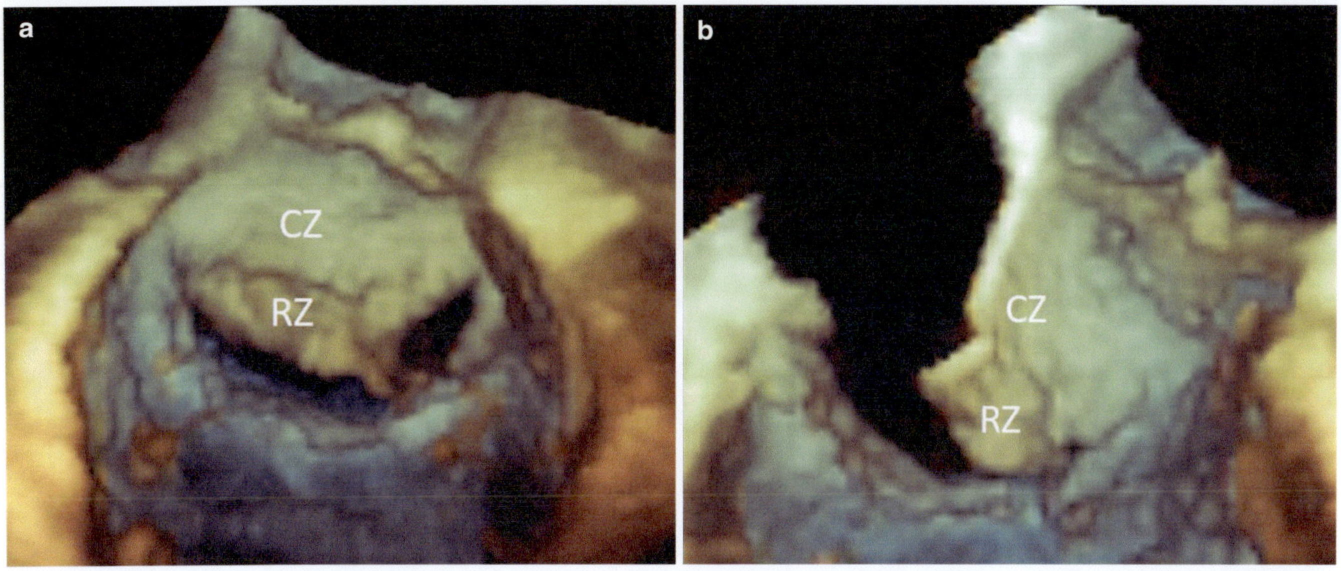

Fig. 5.7 (**a**) Mitral valve from ventricular perspective. The spatial resolution of 3D does not allow a clear distinction of the rough zone (RZ) from the clear zone (CZ). (**b**) Same data set partially cropped and angulated

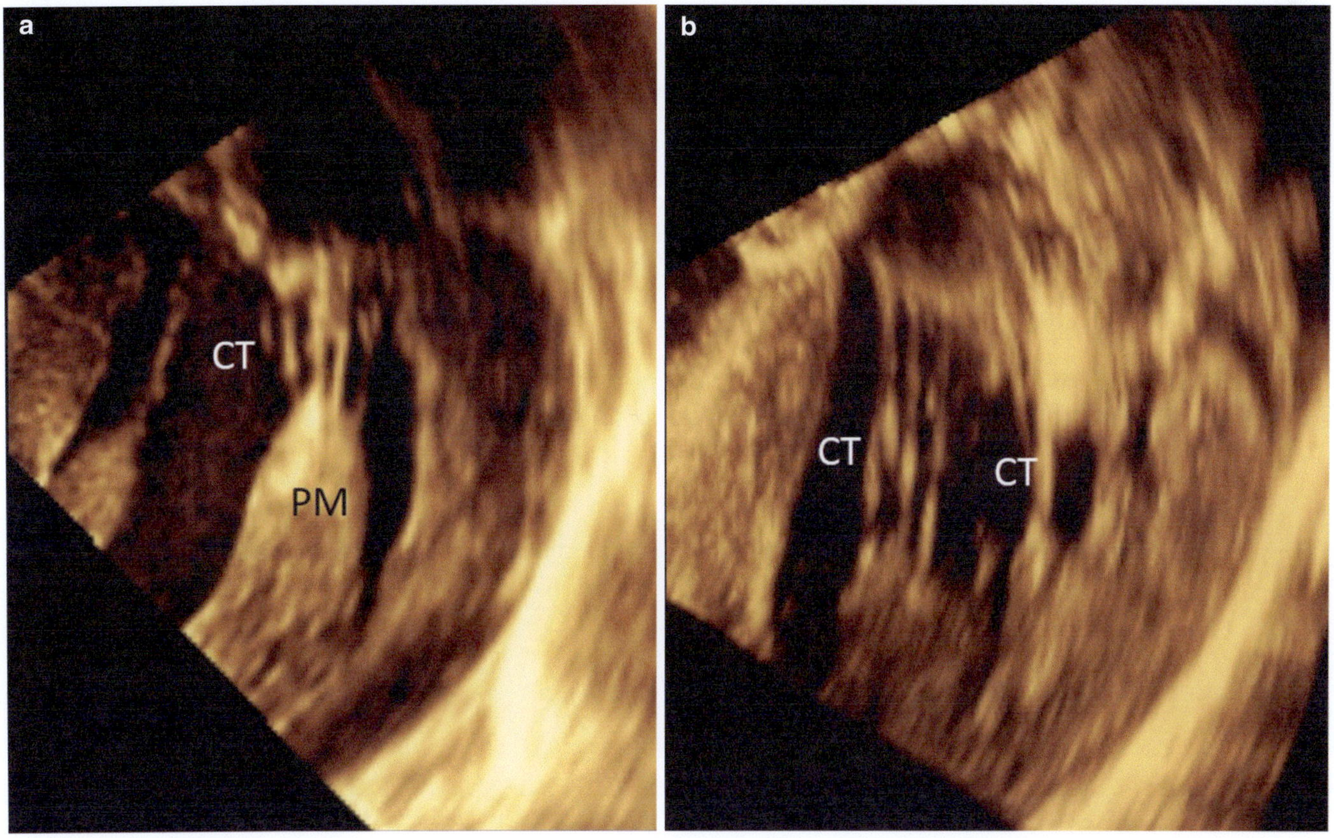

Fig. 5.8 (**a**) Multiplanar reconstruction from transgastric view showing the chordae tendineae (CT) arising from the tip of papillary muscle (PM). (**b**) Same view showing the entire length of CT

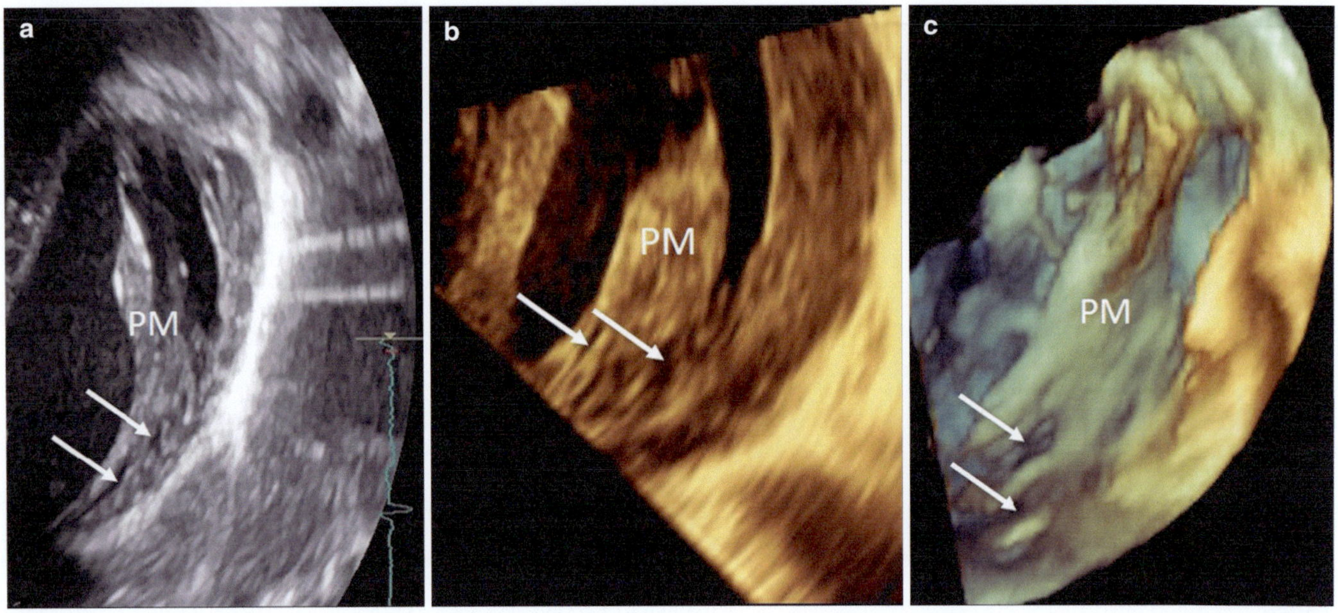

Fig. 5.9 (**a**) Transthoracic parasternal view, (**b**) 3D TEE transgastric view multiplanar reconstruction, (**c**) 3D TEE surface rendering. All three modalities show the spaces (arrows) beneath the body of papillary muscle (PM) in late diastole

References

1. Perloff JK, Roberts WC. The mitral valve apparatus: functional anatomy of mitral regurgitation. Circulation. 1972;46:227–39.
2. Angelini A, Ho SY, Anderson RH, et al. A histological study of atrio-ventricular junction in heart with normal and prolapsed leaflets of the mitral valve. Br Heart J. 1988;59:712–6.
3. Levine RA, Handschumacher MD, Sanfilippo AJ, et al. Three-dimensional echocardiographic reconstruction of the mitral valve, with implications for the diagnosis of mitral valve prolapse. Circulation. 1989;80:589–98.
4. Salgo IS, Gorman JH, German RC, et al. Effect of annular shape on leaflet curvature in reducing mitral leaflet stress. Circulation. 2002;106:711–7.
5. Biaggi P, Gruner C, Jedrzkiewicz S, Karski J, Meineri M, Vegas A, David TE, Woo A, Rakowski H. Assessment of mitral valve prolapse by 3D TEE: angled views are key. J Am Coll Cardiol Imaging. 2011;4:94–7.
6. Obase K, Jeevnandam V, Saito K, et al. Visualization and measurement of mitral valve chordae tendineae using three-dimensional transesophageal echocardiography from the transgastric approach. J Am Soc Echocardiogr. 2015;28:449–54.
7. Axel L. Papillary muscles do not attach directly to the solid heart wall. Circulation. 2004;109:3145–8.

3DE Spectrum of Mitral Valve Prolapse

6

Francesco F. Faletra, Laura A. Leo, and Joseph F. Maalouf

Introduction

Mitral valve regurgitation (MVR) is currently the most common disorder in developed countries affecting 2–3% of the general population (corresponding to nearly two hundred million people worldwide) [1]. Furthermore, due to aging and growth of the general population, the prevalence of MVR is likely to further increase in the coming decades.

The mechanism of MVR can be roughly classified as *primary or organic*, due to anatomical abnormalities of the mitral valve (MV) leaflets and chordae (such as degenerative, rheumatic, drug-induced, endocarditis, extensive annular calcifications, trauma, tumors, papillary muscle rupture in the setting of acute or subacute myocardial infarction) and *secondary* or *functional,* in which MVR is secondary to pathological remodeling of the left ventricle occurring in the setting of ischemic (i.e. adverse remodeling post myocardial infarction) or non-ischemic (i.e. idiopathic dilatative or hypertrophic cardiomyopathy) left ventricular (LV) disease. According to these definitions, while functional MVR may effectively be treated with pharmacological therapy, primary MVR clearly requires surgery or percutaneous replacement/repair. However, it is important to recognize that this dichotomous classification is not absolute and the two types are not mutually exclusive since both may coexist in a "mixed etiology". Moreover, recent data challenge the common belief that in secondary long-standing mitral regurgitation, leaflets and chordae remain completely normal. Indeed, stretching associated with tethering forces may lead to mitral leaflet remodeling which may be either "adaptive" (i.e. leaflet enlargement) which is supposed to reduce the regurgitation or maladaptive response (i.e. increased thickness and stiffness) that may exacerbate it.

Carpentier's Functional Classification

In the late 1970s, when surgical techniques of MV repair rather than MV replacement became available, it was clear that the classification of MV disease based on three main categories (i.e. mitral regurgitation, mitral stenosis and combined stenosis and regurgitation) was no longer inclusive of the multiform aspects of the disease. On the other hand, a comprehensive categorization purely based on the description of the individual valve pathoanatomy would have been clinically inapplicable.

The *Carpentier "functional" classification* based on leaflet motion, detected either by echocardiography or by direct surgical inspection had the merit of being at the same time exhaustive and practical and, currently, is one of the most used classifications [2]. The philosophy behind this "functional classification" is simple: the primary aim of mitral valve repair is to restore normal function rather than normal anatomy. Accordingly, four functional types of lesions have been described on the basis of leaflet motion: normal motion (Type I), increased motion (Type II), and restricted motion (Type III A and B).

In *Type I* leaflet excursion is normal. The regurgitation is caused either by leaflet perforation or by annular dilatation. *Type II* includes all the morphological anomalies in which the cause of MVR is excessive leaflet motion (i.e. prolapse of one or both leaflets, rupture of chordae or papillary muscles, or the rare papillary muscle elongation). In *Type IIIa, the* motion of the leaflets is reduced both in systole and in diastole (as in rheumatic mitral valve disease). Finally, in *Type III b* regurgitation is due to reduced motion predominantly during valve closure (due to the tethering of one or both leaf-

F. F. Faletra (✉)
Director of Cardiac Imaging Lab, Cardiocentro Ticino Institute, Lugano, Switzerland
e-mail: Francesco.Faletra@cardiocentro.org

L. A. Leo
Cardiac Imaging Lab, Cardiocentro Ticino Institute, Lugano, Switzerland
e-mail: lauraanna.leo@cardiocentro.org

J. F. Maalouf
Professor of Medicine, Mayo Clinic College of Medicine; Director, Interventional Echocardiography; Consultant, Department of Cardiovascular Medicine, Mayo Clinic, Rochester, MN, USA
e-mail: maalouf.joseph@mayo.edu

J. F. Maalouf et al. (eds.), *Practical 3D Echocardiography*, https://doi.org/10.1007/978-3-030-72941-7_6

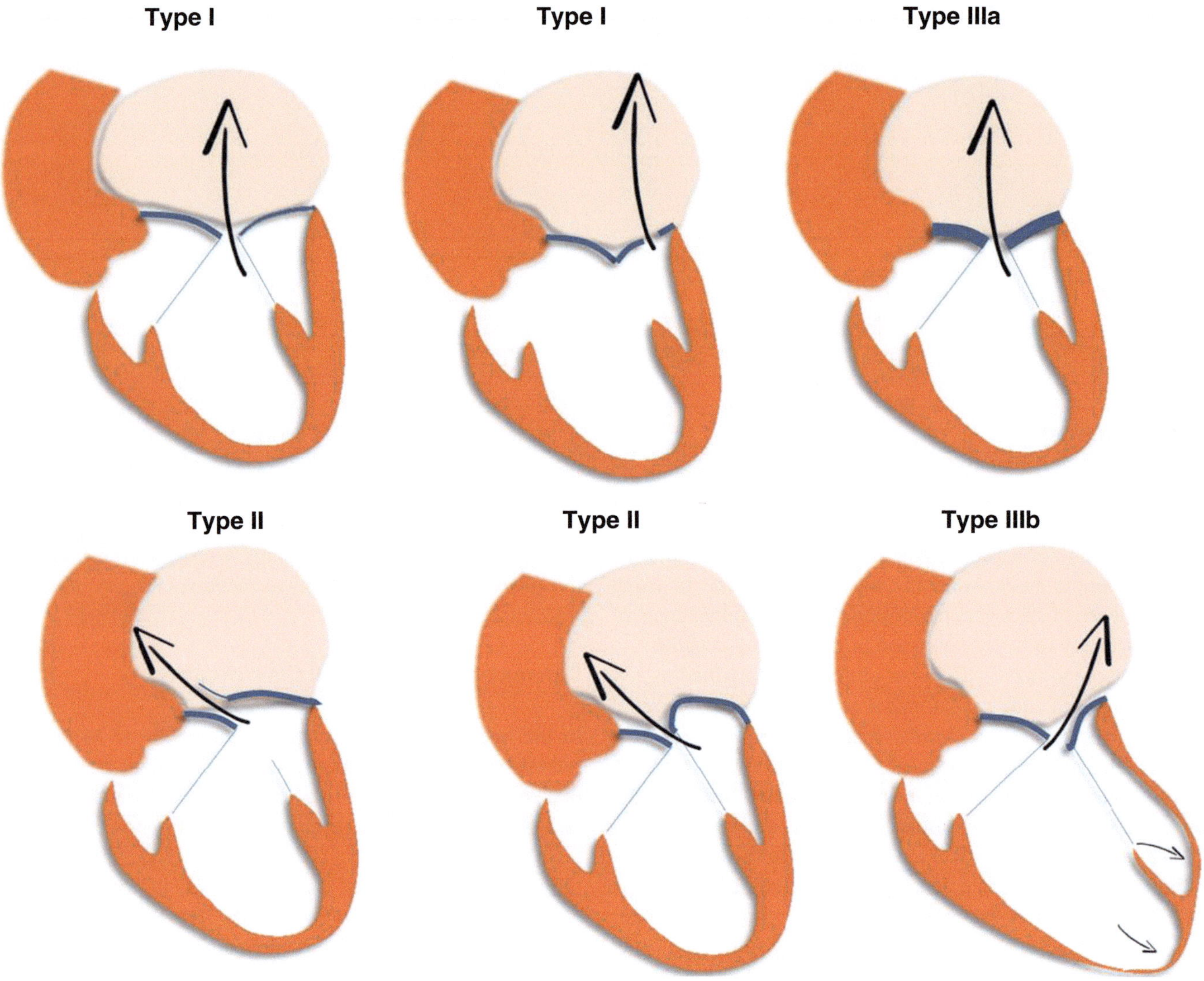

Fig. 6.1 Schematic representation of the Carpentier "functional classification" (see text)

lets) (Fig. 6.1). The following chapter will focus on type II and type III b valve mechanisms. Type I and type IIIa valve dysfunction will be described in Chaps. 7, 8, 17 and Fig. 17.3.

Mitral Valve Prolapse

The term "mitral valve prolapse" (MVP) describes a spectrum of pathological conditions affecting primarily MV leaflets and chordae tendineae. This condition, also called "degenerative" MV disease, includes different phenotypes. Preoperative differentiation of these phenotypes by both cardiologists and surgeons is important because the techniques, surgical skills, and expertise required to achieve an effective and durable repair vary among these different subsets [3].

Fibroelastic deficiency (FED) was first described by Carpentier [4] and it is characterized by connective tissue deficiency due to an impaired production of collagen, elastin and proteoglycans resulting in thin and fragile leaflet tissue. The leaflets preserve their own three layers architecture but at surgical inspection they appear translucent (pellucid) [2]. The etiology of connective tissue deficiency in FED is unknown but it has been suggested that it may be the result of an accelerated ageing process. The cause of regurgitation is rupture of one or more primary chordae tendineae which usually involves the central scallop of the posterior leaflet (P2) but can also affect the medial (P3) or lateral (P1) scallop. Patients with FED most commonly have a short history of MVR and symptoms appear suddenly in the sixth/seventh decade of life as a consequence of chordal rupture.

Barlow's disease is a result of abnormal accumulation of myxomatous substance (mainly proteoglycans) in the spongiosa layer with consequent destruction of the three-layered architecture of both leaflets. The characteristic appearance is that of thick, bulky, redundant leaflets, elongated chordae tendineae and annular dilatation. The excess in leaflet tissue leads to the displacement of both leaflets beyond the highest points of the valve hinge line with malcoaptation and consequent MR. This disease is generally diagnosed with echocardiography in early adulthood and followed up for several years until clinical and/or echocardiographic worsening mandates surgical repair/replacement. Interestingly, the term "*billowing mitral leaflets syndrome*" was coined after having seen the echocardiographic billowing of the leaflets.

Between these two well-defined entities there is a considerable variety of morphological features with varying degrees of myxomatous degeneration affecting one or more segments of the valve. Adams et al. [5] described two of these "***intermediate phenotypic morphologies***": FED+ and "form fruste". FED+ is a single scallop prolapse (as in FED), but the prolapsing tissue is redundant with myxomatous degeneration. It has been hypothesized that FED+ may be considered a "worsening stage" of FED where the regurgitant jet, over time, triggers myxomatous degeneration. Such a mechanism, if true, leads to the hypothesis that the myxomatous changes could also be secondary to jet lesions. The "form fruste" phenotype is probably an incomplete form of Barlow affecting the valve only partially (usually the posterior leaflet). Notably, MVP is not found in newborns, and its prevalence is low among children (0.3%), and young adults (0.6%). These findings suggest that MVP is a "progressive" degenerative disease affecting predominantly middle-aged individuals.

Finally, MVP can be defined as "*non-syndromic*" when sporadic or "familial and *syndromic*" MVP when it occurs in association with connective tissue disorders (such as Marfan syndrome, Ehler-Danlos syndrome, osteogenesis imperfecta, pseudoxanthoma elasticum and others).

A variable range of symptoms such as atypical chest pain, exertional dyspnea, palpitations, syncope, and anxiety and also several clinical findings (low blood pressure, slender habitus, and electrocardiographic repolarization abnormalities) have been associated with MVP and this constellation is called "MVP syndrome".

Echocardiographic Assessment

Rest Two-Dimensional Transthoracic and Transesophageal Echocardiography

In the early days of 2D transthoracic echocardiography (2D TTE), the diagnosis of MVP was made so frequently that its prevalence reached 35% of patients undergoing 2D TTE, thus gaining the reputation of "epidemic". This over-diagnosis was due to the erroneous assumption that the hinge line of mitral leaflets, i.e. the mitral annulus (MA), was planar. Thus, any echocardiographic cross section showing an excursion of leaflets superior to plane of the MA was considered pathological. In the 1980s Robert Levine et al. [6] redefined the tridimensional architecture of the MA, as a saddle-shaped configuration: concave upward anterior and posterior, and concave downward medial and lateral [6]. With this saddle shape annular geometry, leaflet excursion in the four-chamber view goes beyond the plane of the MA, creating the false appearance of prolapse. In this chapter we continue to refer to the mitral hinge line (i.e. the line at which the leaflets open and close) as MA. Indeed in the original paper of Levine et al. [6], the saddle-shaped architecture was based on hinge points and not on the anatomical fibrotic annulus. On the other hand, according to anatomists, a MA defined as a continuous ring of connective tissue does not exist, being formed by sparse fibrous strings on its posterior aspect and by a band of connective tissue (the mitral aortic curtain) in its anterior aspect (see Chap. 5 normal anatomy of the MV).

Nowadays two-dimensional (2D) transthoracic echocardiography (TTE) is the first line imaging technique for evaluating patients with degenerative MV disease. The 2D TTE criteria of MVP have been defined several years ago as a protrusion of >2 mm beyond the long axis antero-posterior hinge line plane. Prolapse associated with a leaflet thickening greater than 5 mm is termed "*classic*" prolapse, whereas prolapse with lesser degrees of leaflet thickening is regarded as "non-classic" prolapse. Importantly, TTE is used as a primary tool for a comprehensive assessment of patients with MVP, providing data on the pathoanatomy of the valve, the severity of regurgitation according to various methods, the left atrium (LA) and left ventricle (LV) dimensions and function, systolic pulmonary pressure and the size and function of the right ventricle (RV). Most of these echocardiographic parameters have a relevant prognostic impact. 2D transesophageal echocardiography (TEE) is generally used to better define the type of lesion, precisely identifying the prolapsing MV segment/s. Several cross-sectional TEE planes, intersecting different segments of the valve, have been described and standardized. In experienced hands a systematic approach (including long axis, two-chamber, four-chamber, trans-gastric short and long axis and off-axis sections) allows accurate description of the pathoanatomy of MVP (Fig. 6.2).

Until few years ago, 2D TEE was considered the most advanced technique to visualize degenerative MV disease and currently remains an indispensable tool for cardiologists and anesthesiologists in the setting of surgical (and nowadays percutaneous) mitral valve repair. However, some limitations of 2D TEE must be recognized. First, being a tomographic technique, 2D TEE is unable to provide a picture of the entire valve in one image. Thus, small lesions, especially those located near the commissures, may not be recognized [6]. Secondly, given the anatomical variants, visualization of one prolapsing segment in a given cross-section may not necessarily correspond to what we expect to see in that specific cross-section (for instance a large P3 prolapse can occasionally be intersected by the long axis view plane and misinterpreted as a P2 prolapse). Third, the same misinterpretation may also occur when a

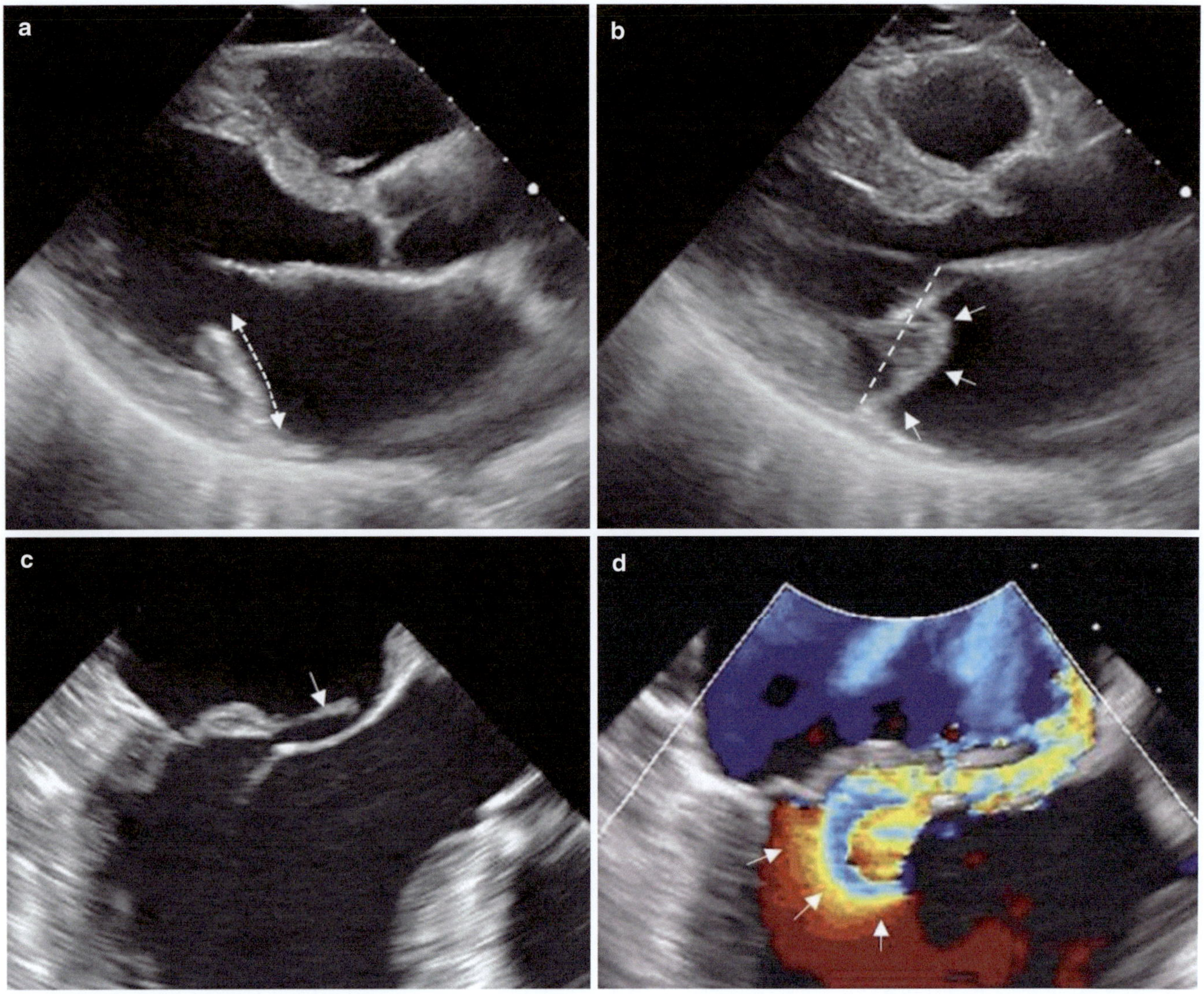

Fig. 6.2 (**a**) Two-dimensional transthoracic echocardiography in long axis view showing a classic prolapse of posterior leaflet in (**a**) diastole and (**b**) systole. The double-headed arrow in panel **a** delineates the length of the posterior leaflet. The arrows in panel **b** shows protrusion of the posterior segment beyond the hinge line (dotted line). (**c**) Two-dimensional transesophageal echocardiography in long axis view (approximately 120°) showing a flail middle segment of the posterior leaflet. The arrow points to the ruptured chorda (arrow). (**d**) Same image with color Doppler showing a large flow convergence area (arrows)

given cross-section plane foreshortens the left ventricle. Finally, reconstructing a mental 3D image based on the interpretation of multiple 2D cross-sections may be difficult, especially in the case of complex morphologies.

Three-Dimensional Transesophageal Echocardiography

Real-time three-dimensional (3D) echocardiography (3DE), initially applied to TTE and shortly thereafter to TEE, became available in the clinical arena almost 10 years ago. Since the very beginning, it was clear that 3DE, and especially 3D TEE, would become the ideal imaging technique for the MV, providing real time 3D images of extraordinary quality. This quality is achieved by an ideal, nearly perpendicular angle of incidence of the pyramidal beam to the mitral leaflets, as well as a short distance between the transesophageal transducer and the MV. For the first time it was possible to obtain "real-time" images of the MV with a visual perspective identical to the surgeon's view (aorta at 11–12 o'clock position) [7]. This so-called "surgical view" is the most intuitive and it was the first perspective historically to be reconstructed and analyzed. This view can be obtained by any echocardiographic cross-section that permits a full visualization of the MV (typically the horizontal four-five chamber view, long axis or bi-commissural view). Once the volumetric data set is acquired, the surgical view is obtained by rotating the image so that the aorta is at 11–12 o'clock and the left atrial appendage at 9–10 o' clock. From this perspective many details of valve pathology can be seen in vivo. In general, it can be said that this view allows visualization of almost any anatomical and functional data necessary for a comprehensive assessment of MVP (Fig. 6.3a).

Angled Views

Direct inspection of the MV in the surgical theater is limited to the view from above through the left atrium. In contrast, with 3D TEE, once the volumetric data set has been acquired, the valve can be viewed from a countless number of perspectives. Any segment of the mitral leaflets can therefore be analyzed independently from the vantage point which best shows the morphology (we call this approach "segment-oriented approach"). Over the years the use of the "non-surgical views" and in particular of the so called "angled or tangential views" have become widespread [8]. In fact, these "off axis" nonsurgical views have been shown to provide additional data in comparison to the surgical perspective alone. They may, for instance, better clarify the degree of protrusion above the annular plane (Fig. 6.3b, c) or show "de novo" secondary lesions. In particular an anterior perspective provides a picture of the anatomic regurgitant orifice seen "en face" (Fig. 6.3d).

To understand why angled or tangential views may occasionally be more informative, we must remember the modal-

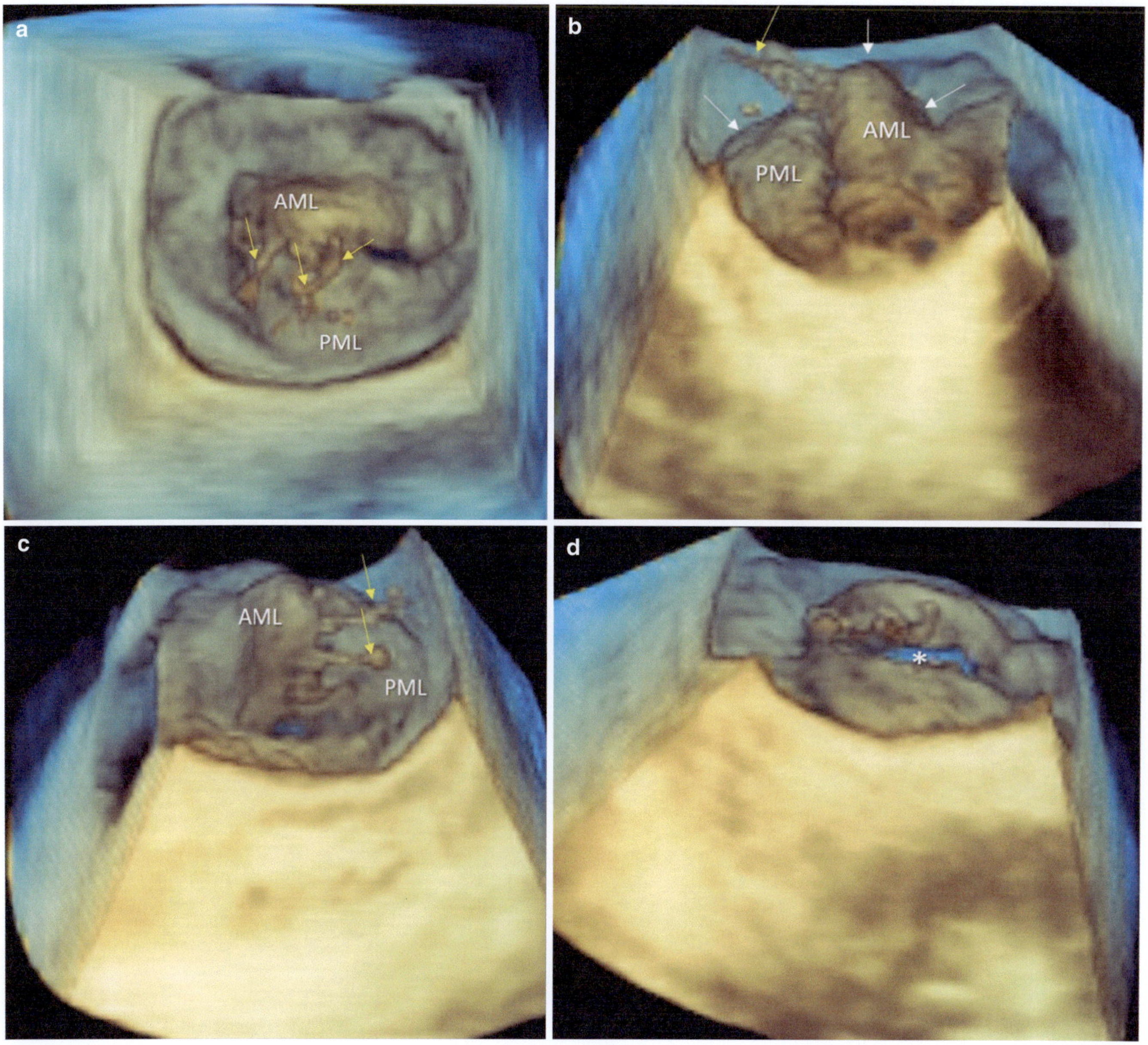

Fig. 6.3 (**a**) Barlow's disease with flail A2 and multiple chordal ruptures (yellow arrows). (**b**, **c**) Tangential medial to lateral (**b**) and lateral to medial (**c**) views showing the degree of protrusion into the left atrium (white arrows). (**d**) Tangential anterior view showing the anatomical regurgitant orifice (asterisk). AML, anterior mitral leaflet; PML, posterior mitral leaflet

ity by which 3D echocardiography allows a three-dimensional perception of an image projected on a 2D screen. In the most common display modality, the dual-color vision bronze/blue map, a specific algorithm that "illuminates" the valve with a fixed source of light is generated in proximity to the observer's head. Thus, structures closer to the observer appear brighter than structures located in a deeper plane. In the "surgical view", prolapsing segments moving in systole towards the observer appear therefore, brighter with a mixture of beige/yellow/white. Conversely, surrounding non-prolapsing segments, remaining at a deeper level, appear darker with a mixture of bronze/brown/blue. The surgical view has been shown to be very effective in identifying large prolapsing segments where the differences in shades are evident and easily appreciated. However, this difference may be less pronounced when the prolapse is small or is a secondary lesion close to the primary lesion. Conversely, in angled or tangential views the same algorithm produces shadows beyond the prolapsing segments, therefore enhancing their edges and making them visible. It is not surprising, therefore, that multiple studies have shown that, when compared with surgical data, 3D TEE is superior to 2D TEE in defining the multiform pathoanatomy of the MV. Moreover, there is now available a new volume rendering algorithm that uses a freely movable source of light, and is able to "illuminate" the MV from different perspectives. Particularly informative are 3D images obtained with the source of light located tangentially or beyond the valve leaflets. This new modality certainly will improve the identification of minor anatomical abnormalities (Fig. 6.4).

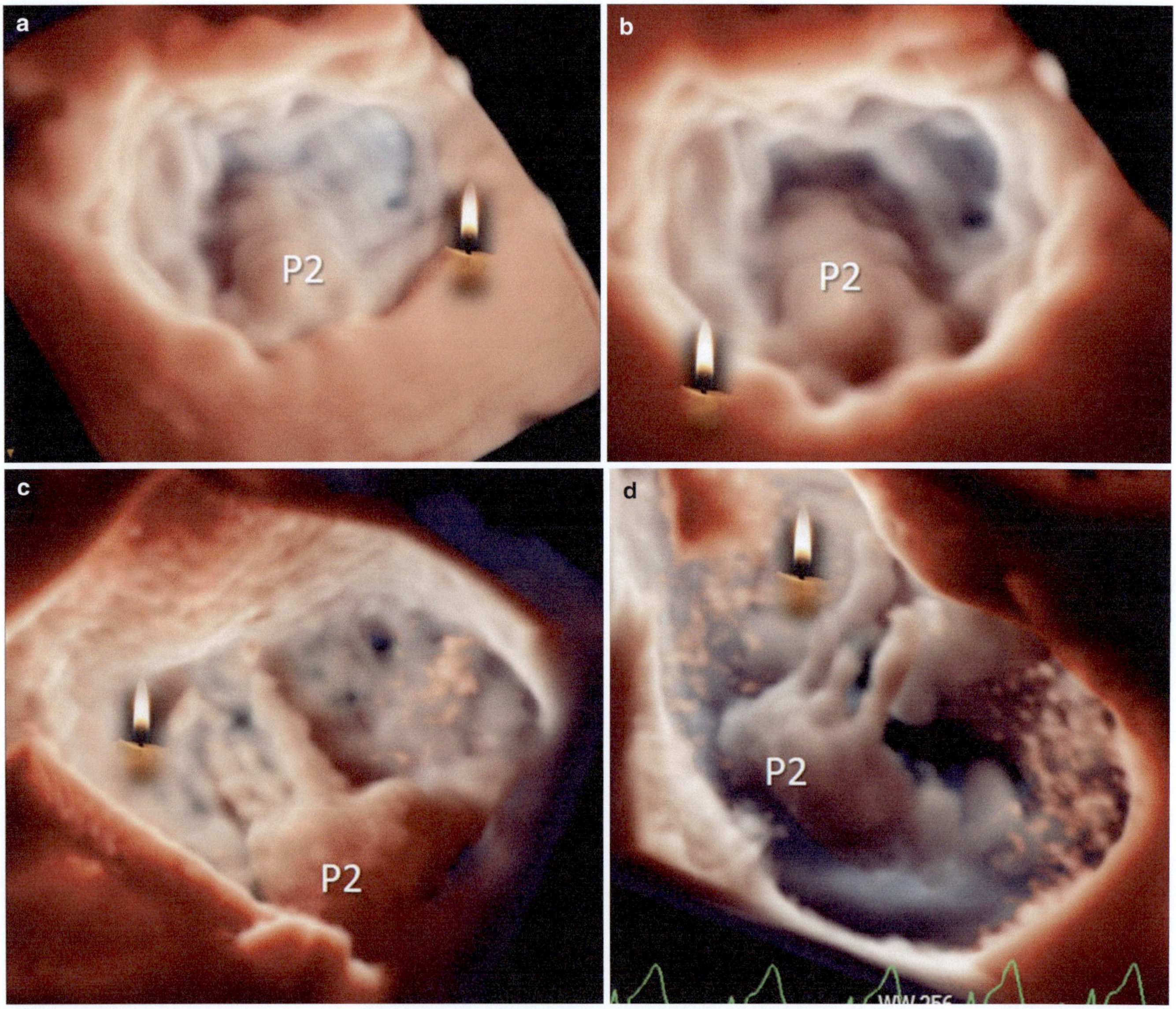

Fig. 6.4 (**a**, **b**) 3D TEE showing prolapse of the central segment of the posterior leaflet (P2) visualized with a new algorithm which uses a freely movable source of light. Candles indicate the source of light. In panel **a** the image is "illuminated" from the right and in panel **b** from the left. (**c**, **d**) 3D TEE showing a flail P2 with multiple ruptured chordae that appear as finger like projections

Acquisition of the 3D Data Set

The "dynamic" nature of prolapse/flail requires an imaging technique capable of a high spatial resolution (to identify fine morphological details of the valve) and a high temporal resolution (to allow an accurate frame-by-frame analysis). As discussed in Chap. 1, spatial resolution is a function of scanning density and temporal resolution is a function of scanning density and 3D volume size. Therefore, the narrower the acquired pyramidal data set, the higher the temporal resolution while maintaining or improving spatial resolution. There are two ways to acquire the MV volumetric data set. The first is single beat or real time which may be limited by the need to acquire a large pyramidal data set to encompass the entire MV, hence reduced temporal resolution with volume rates that may not exceed 10 volumes/s. The newly available 3D TEE platforms improve the volume rate/volume size ratio so that the entire MV can be acquired in a single beat volume rate of 20–24 volumes/s or much higher, but not infrequently at the expense of reduced spatial resolution.

The second is multi-beat acquisition that uses ECG-gating to capture narrow consecutive sectors up to six sequential cardiac cycles. Although the final images are not in "real-time" (the last sector is acquired five beats after the first) and may suffer from "stitching" artifacts (i.e. incorrect juxtaposition of sectors) due to respiration, irregular heart rhythm, or any transducer/patient movement, the multi-beat ECG gating acquisition being a summation of up to six sectors, remains the best modality to encompass a large volumetric data set such as that of the mitral valve while maintaining the highest temporal and spatial resolution equivalent to those obtained with a narrow sector acquisition. Finally, multi-beat acquisition can display 3D color Doppler with an acceptable volume/rate (up to 25–30 images/s), though in a typically narrower volume.

Quantitative Data

Generally, the pathoanatomy of degenerative MVR relies on qualitative description. Recently, a convincing amount of data has shown that a quantitative analysis of valve morphology may play a major role. Dedicated quantitative software can digitally reconstruct a precise three-dimensional parametric map of the entire valve with quantitative important parameters such as the circumference of the annulus, the height of its saddle-shaped configuration, the height, length, areas, and volumes of prolapsing tissue and the length of the chordae making 3D TEE probably the most complete and accurate imaging technique for the diagnosis of degenerative MVR. Moreover, 3D quantitative parameters may anticipate the complexity of valve repair and predict complex repair success. Because MV measurements are obtained by tracking the hinge line in cross section and the leaflets in 2D slices (derived from 3D data sets), this modality is, theoretically, the most reliable and reproducible quantitative method overcoming limitations of a visual interpretation/description. Indeed, the use of this multi-parametric map has been shown to improve the accuracy and reliability among novice readers, when compared with 2D echocardiography or visual 3D assessment. Finally, quantitative parameters (such as height, area and volume of prolapsing tissue) may differentiate normal findings from FED and from Barlow. New systems such as automated modeling of the valve may further improve quantitative analysis (Fig. 6.5).

Advantages of 3D TEE

Notwithstanding the merits of 2DTEE, 3D TEE further "refines" the diagnosis of MVP. The potential advantages of 3D TEE over 2D TEE are listed below:

(a) Any P2 prolapse appears unique and differs from any other owing to its width, length, site (more lateral or more medial). While these differences among P2 prolapses are easily visible with 3D TEE, they are not as appreciated with 2D TEE (Fig. 6.6).
(b) Secondary lesions near the main prolapsing area (such as deep cleft, or minor prolapse) which, if not recognized, may complicate surgical repair, are more likely to be detected with 3D than with 2D TEE. Moreover, since these "minor" dynamic prolapses are non-redundant and appear at the end of systole, they are easily missed by the surgeon in a still and flaccid heart. Notably, these lesions if not treated may deteriorate over time, thus becoming the cause of repeat surgery (Fig. 6.7).
(c) 3D TEE allows for easier distinction as compared to 2D TEE between an "ideal" pathoanatomy (i.e. single scallop prolapse/flail, tissue exuberance, absence of annular calcification, moderate annular dilation), a "challenging" pathoanatomy (i.e. FED, Barlow's disease, anterior leaflet flail), and a "very challenging" pathoanatomy (i.e. bileaflet prolapse, extensive posterior calcifications). These distinctions are of paramount relevance in planning mitral valve repair or replacement (Fig. 6.8).

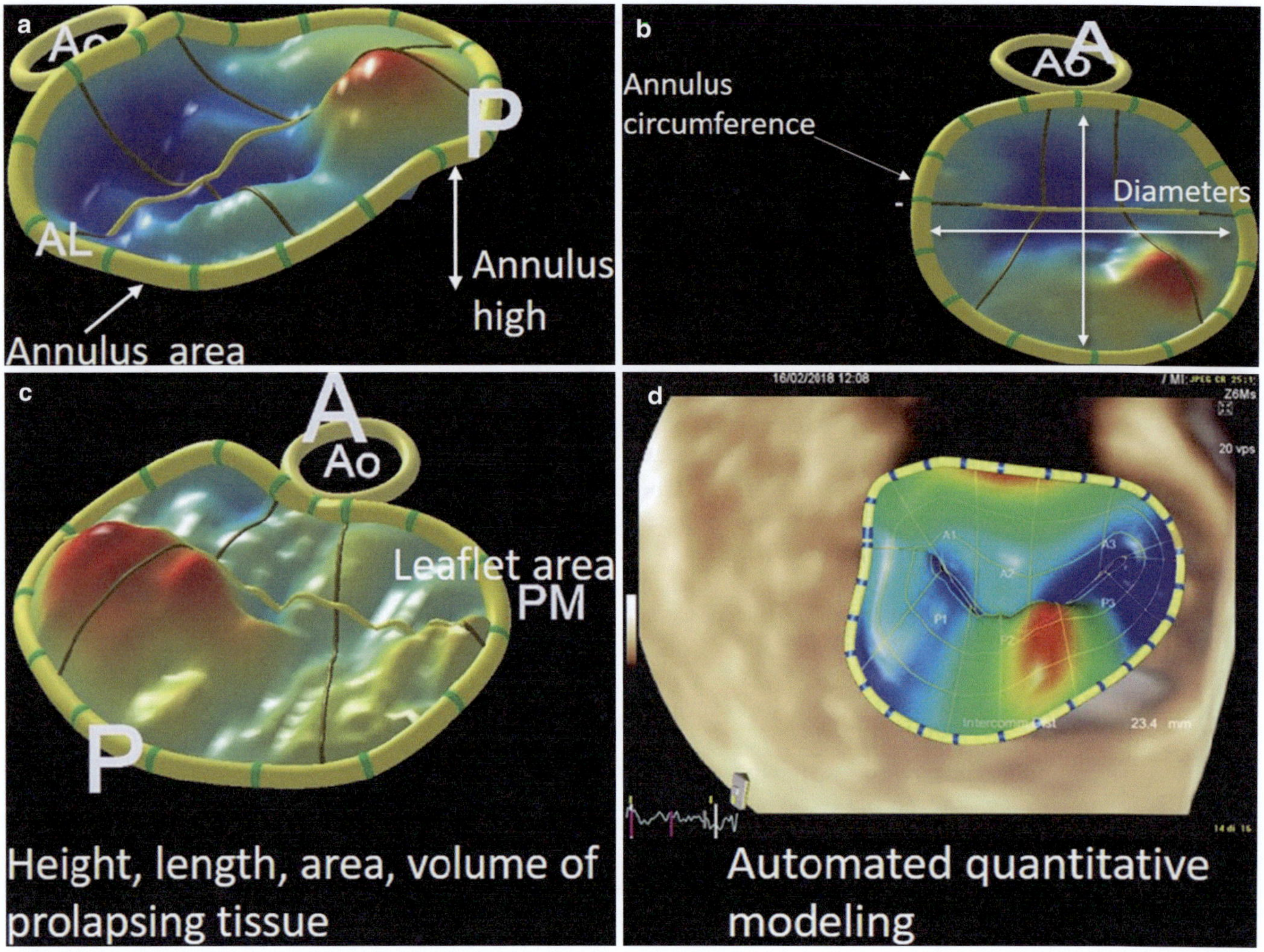

Fig. 6.5 (**a–c**) Quantitative software showing a precise three-dimensional parametric map of the entire valve with quantitative parameters such as the circumference of the annulus, the height of its saddle-shaped configuration, height, length, area, and volume of prolapsing tissue. (**d**) Automated quantitative modeling (see text). A, anterior; AL, anterolateral commissure; Ao, aorta; P, posterior; PM, posteromedial commissure

"Malignant" MVP

Since Barlow's seminal paper in 1966 [9], MVP has been suspected of being more than a benign entity. Severe mitral valve regurgitation, infective endocarditis, cerebrovascular events, and arrhythmias have been reported as major complications. Notably, in some patients MVP is associated with complex ventricular arrhythmias even in the absence of significant regurgitation. Arrhythmic MVP may be associated with a higher risk of sudden cardiac death (SCD) than patients with non-arrhythmic MVP.

These MVP complications were first emphasized by Devereux [10]. In 1988 Duren et al. [11] performed a prospective long term follow up of 300 patients with MVP and found several complications occurring in 100 patients (one/third of the population). Forty-seven percent of patients suffered from ventricular arrhythmias, 24% underwent mitral valve surgery, 15% suffered from infective endocarditis, 9% of cerebrovascular events and 2.5% died suddenly. Grigioni et al. [12] in a large cohort of patients with severe mitral regurgitation due to flail mitral leaflet followed conservatively, found that sudden cardiac death was relatively frequent (1.8% per year).

The perception that MVP is a perilous disease was challenged by Freed et al. [13] who found, in the Framingham Heart study, that MVP had a more benign profile than previously believed. More recently, Nordhues et al. [14] found that MVP is associated with ventricular arrhythmias, but not with an increased risk of cardiac arrest, ventricular fibrillation or ICD implantation.

From these data it seems reasonable to conclude that in the general population MVP can be considered a "benign"

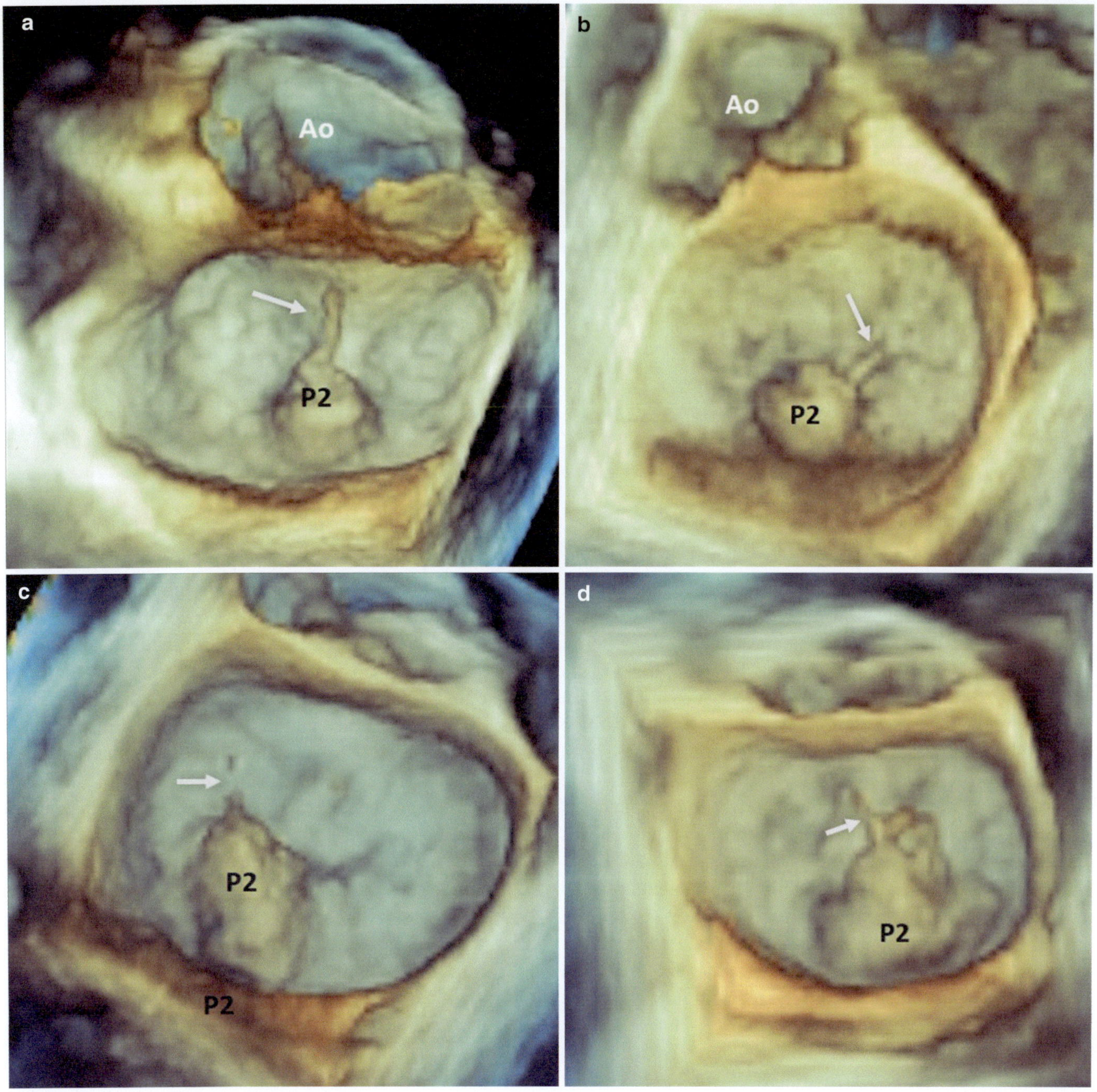

Fig. 6.6 (**a–d**) Four different P2 prolapse (see text). Ao, aorta

entity. However, a small but notable percentage of patients may develop complications including malignant arrhythmias and SCD. From the beginning, cardiologists focused their attention on specific patho-morphologic characteristics of the valve that could be associated with severe hemodynamic, infective, embolic and arrhythmic complications. Nishimura et al. in 1985 [15] noticed that in 97 patients with *redundant leaflets*, 10 suffered from major complications [sudden death (6), infective endocarditis (3) and cerebral embolic events (1)], while among 140 patients without redundant leaflets only 1 suffered from cerebral embolic events. They concluded that most patients with echocardiographic evidence of MVP had a benign course, but a subset of patients with redundant leaflets (i.e. leaflets longer and thicker than normal) were at risk of the above-mentioned complications. The "redundancy" of mitral leaflets as a risk

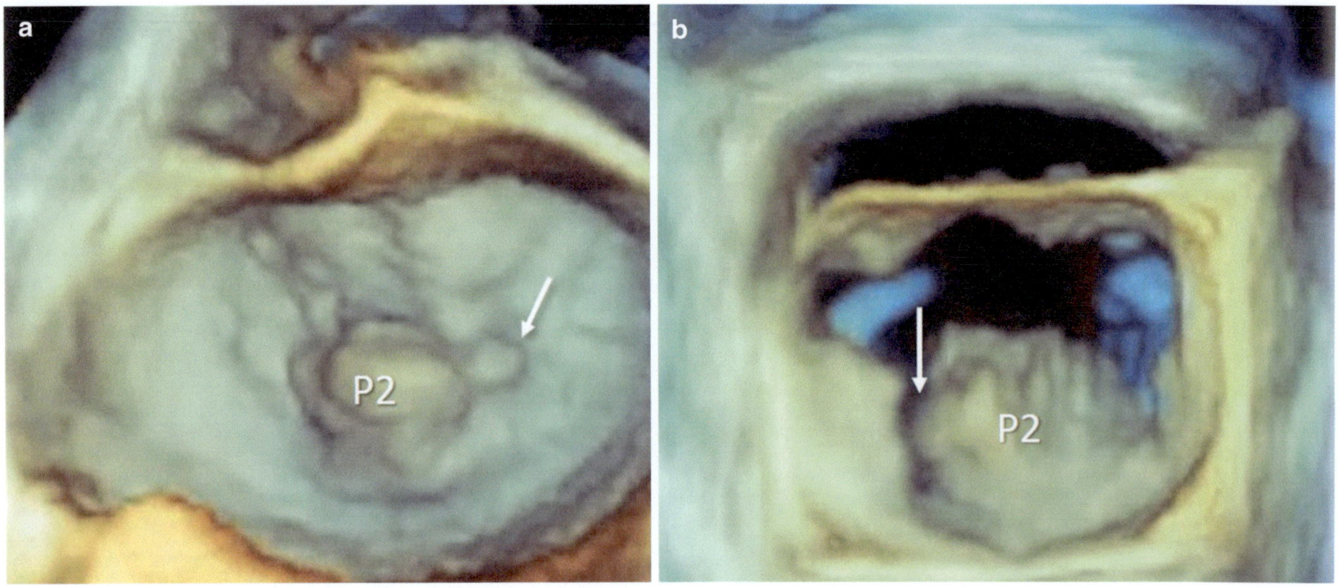

Fig. 6.7 (**a**) P2 flail with a secondary small prolapse laterally to the main lesion (arrow). (**b**) Cleft (arrow) adjacent to a P2 prolapse (see text)

factor for MVP complications was confirmed by Marks et al. in 1989 [16] using 2D echocardiography. They found that patients with bileaflet prolapse with redundant leaflets were at higher risk of complications than those without these patho-morphological features. More recently Sriram et al. [17] confirmed the presence of leaflet redundancy in patients with otherwise idiopathic out-of-hospital cardiac arrest. The authors described a "phenotype" associated with cardiac arrest: young woman with bileaflets MVP, biphasic or inverted T waves in the inferior leads and evidence of complex ventricular arrhythmias. While the association between MVP with leaflet redundancy (in other words Barlow's disease) and hemodynamic derangements (due to ruptured chordae tendinea and severe mitral regurgitation), infective endocarditis or embolism could be expected, the relation between such echocardiographic features and arrhythmias is still unclear although recently new data have become available (see below).

In 1992, Sanfilippo et al. [18] first hypothesized a connection between MVP and arrhythmias. They observed that MVP leads to a pathological "traction" on the papillary muscle and this traction may cause ischemia and electrical instability. This hypothesis was disregarded by cardiologists for several years. In 2008 Han et al. [19] studied patients with MVP with the aid of cardiovascular magnetic resonance and discovered late-gadolinium enhancement (LGE) at the tip of the papillary muscles (PMs) that was consistent with scar tissue. Notably, in their study the presence of scar tissue at the tip of the PMs was often present in a subgroup of patients with complex cardiac arrhythmias. Thus, the stretch-induced ischemia hypothesized by Sanfilippo, may over time cause fibrosis, a well-known trigger for arrhythmias.

In a pathological study from 1986 based on the analysis of 900 hearts, Hutchins et al. [20] described an anomalous attachment of the posterior leaflet directly on the atrial wall in 23 out of 25 patients with bileaflet MVP and leaflet redundancy. They called this anatomical variation mitral annulus disjunction (MAD). In this particular anatomical arrangement, the normal anatomical atrial-valvular-ventricular junction is lost and the insertion of the posterior leaflet takes place directly on the atrial wall *(atrial-valvular junction)*. The space between the hinge line of the posterior leaflet and the crest of the ventricular wall consists of fibrotic tissue that is stretched and curtain-like. After being ignored for almost 30 years, MAD was rediscovered recently by Marra et al. [21] in patients with arrhythmic MVP. This study extended the observations of Hans showing in the majority of these patient' small amount of fibrosis on the posterior basal left ventricular wall along with that on PM's tips.

Marra hypothesized a link between mitral valve prolapse associated with MAD, arrhythmias and scar tissue: the prolapsing myxomatous leaflets present a greater than normal surface area and a loss of coaptation surface, thus permitting an excessive pressure stress on the chordal apparatus, papillary muscles and basal posterior LV wall. Consequently, the tip of the papillary muscles as well as the posterior left ventricular wall are exposed to excessive traction with subsequent ischemia and fibrosis. Interestingly, in a recent 3D TEE study Lee et al. [22] demonstrated that MAD is more pronounced at the lateral and central segments of the annu-

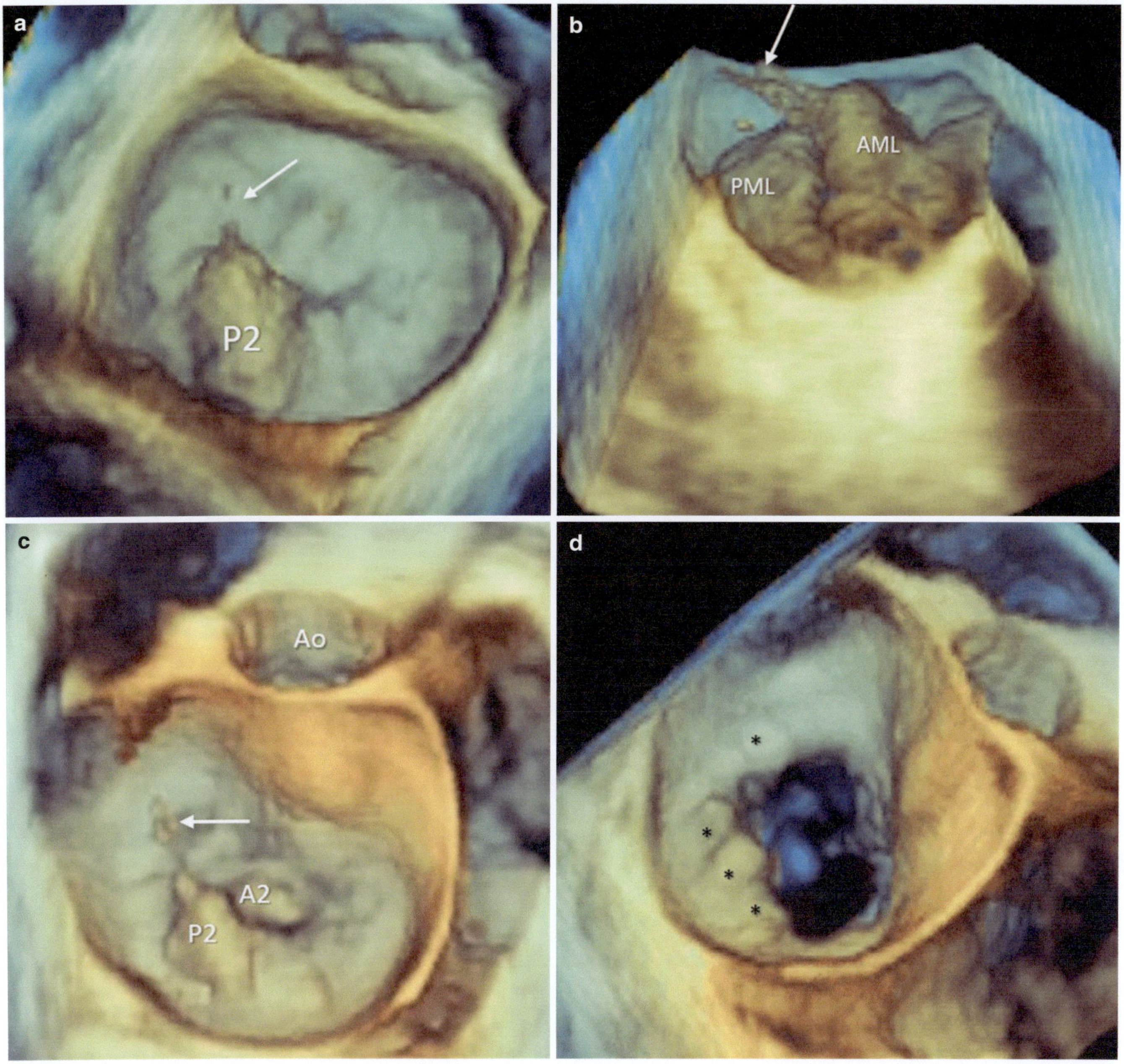

Fig. 6.8 (**a**) Ideal pathoanatomy: flail P2 with moderate tissue redundancy. The arrow points to a ruptured chorda tendinea. (**b**) A challenging pathoanatomy: Barlow's disease with rupture of multiple chordae (arrow). (**c**, **d**) Very challenging pathoanatomy: flail P2, A2 prolapse with scarce tissue redundancy, (**c**) Extensive annulus calcification (asterisks) (**d**). AML, anterior mitral leaflet; PML, posterior mitral leaflet; Ao, aorta

lus, thus leading to a paradoxical annular expansion in late systole, thus exacerbating MVR. This paradoxical motion of the leaflet's hinge line is perfectly comprehensible in that the leaflet is attached to the atrial wall that is well known to expand in systole (Figs. 6.9 and 6.10). Recently, an old hypothesis by Angelini et al. [23] that MAD is also present in individuals without prolapse was confirmed by Dejgaard et al. [24] Interestingly, they found that in patients with MAD without associated prolapse, the rate of malignant arrhythmias was higher than in patients with MAD associated with prolapse, supporting the intriguing hypothesis that MAD itself may be a generator of arrhythmias.

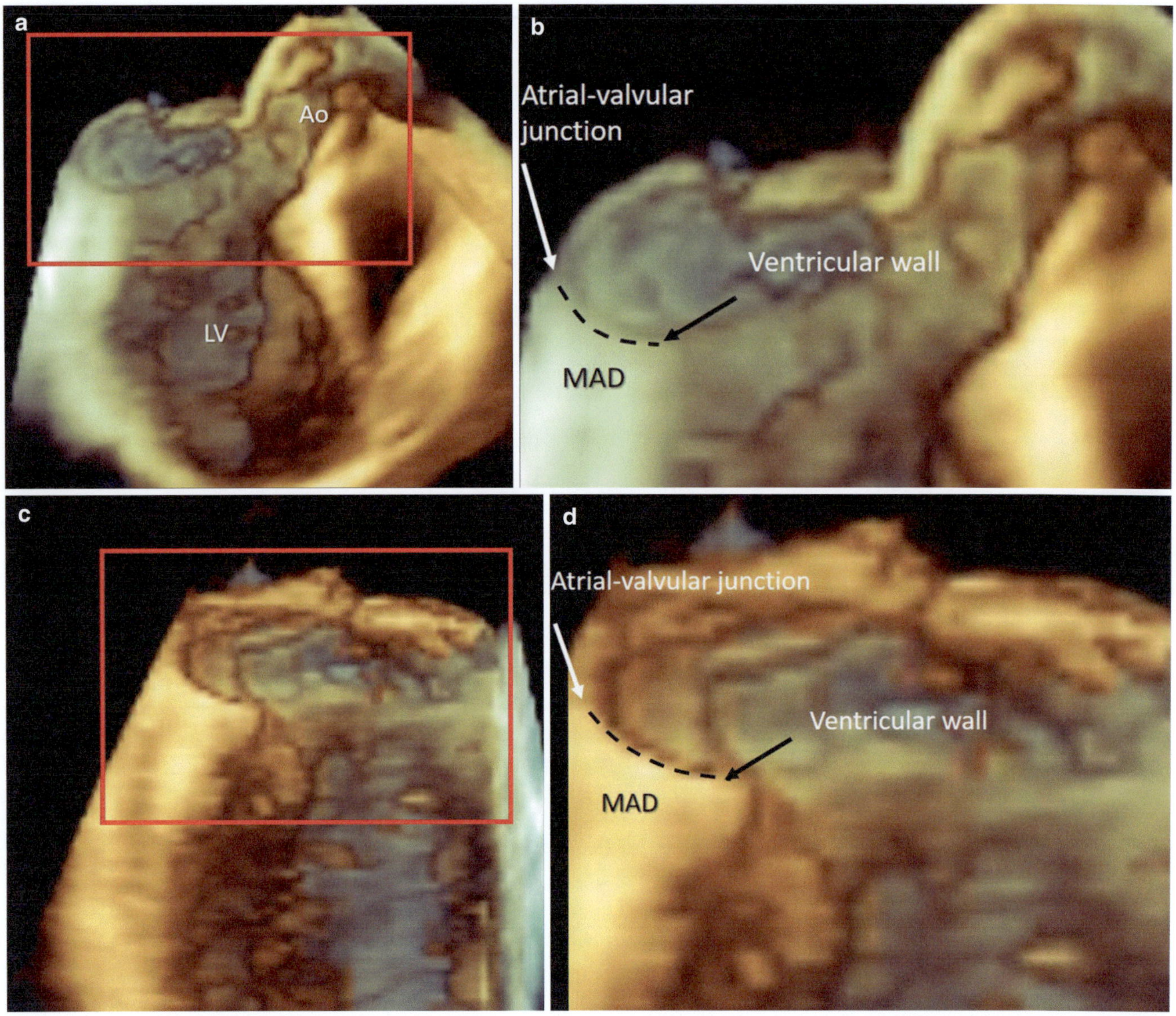

Fig. 6.9 (**a**) 3D TEE cropped image in "oblique" long axis view. (**b**) Magnified image (red square in panel **a**) showing mitral annulus disjunction (MAD). (**c**, **d**) Same patient. Oblique two-chamber view. The tissue space separating the atrial-valvular junction from the crest of the ventricular wall is made of fibrotic tissue, that is stretched and curtain-like (dotted line)

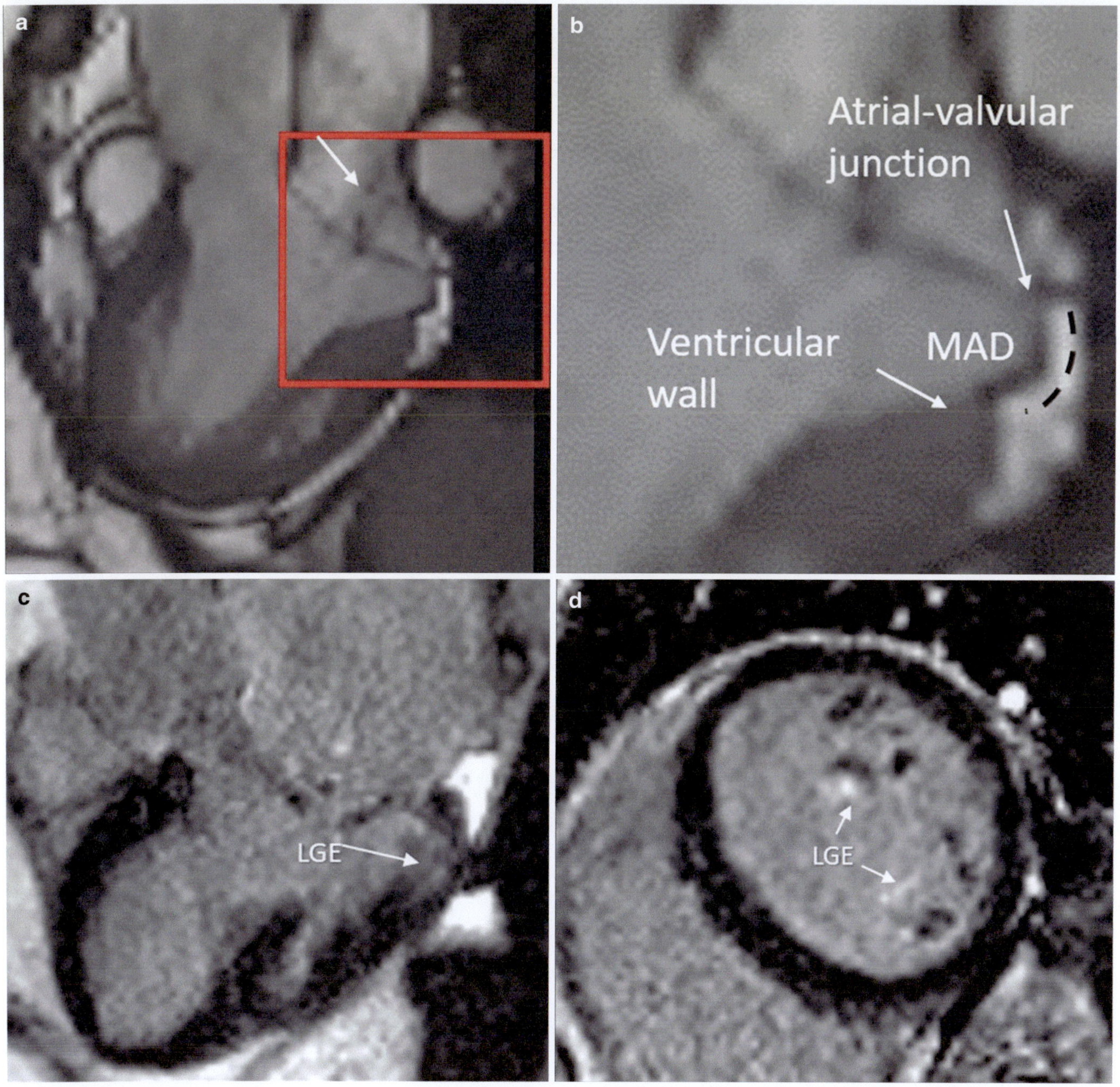

Fig. 6.10 (**a**) Still frame of cardiac magnetic resonance (CMR) cine imaging in long axis view showing prolapse with mild regurgitation (arrow). (**b**) Magnified image of the red box in panel **a**, showing the mitral annulus disjunction (MAD, curved dotted line). (**c**) CMR Late gadolinium enhancement (LGE) showing the presence of fibrosis (arrow) in the basal portion of the left ventricle and (**d**) at the tip of both papillary muscles

References

1. Lung B, Vahanian A. Epidemiology of valvular heart disease in the adult. Nat Rev Cardiol. 2011;8:162–72.
2. Carpentier A. Cardiac valve surgery—the "French correction". J Thorac Cardiovasc Surg. 1983;86(3):323–37.
3. Adams DH, Rosenhek R, Falk V. Degenerative mitral valve regurgitation: best practice revolution. Eur Heart J. 2010;31:1958–66.
4. Carpentier A, Chauvaud S, Fabiani JN, et al. Reconstructive surgery of mitral valve incompetence: ten-year appraisal. J Thorac Cardiovasc Surg. 1980;79:338–48.
5. Adams DH, Rosenhek R, Falk V. Degenerative mitral valve regurgitation: best practice revolution. Eur Heart J. 2010;31(16):1958–66.
6. Levine RA, Triulzi MO, Harrigan P, et al. The relationship of mitral annular shape to the diagnosis of mitral valve prolapse. Circulation. 1987;75:756–67.

7. Sugeng L, Shernan SK, Salgo IS, Weinert L, Shook D, Raman J, et al. Live 3-dimensional transesophageal echocardiography initial experience using the fully-sampled matrix array probe. J Am Coll Cardiol. 2008;52:446–9.
8. Biaggi P, Gruner C, Jedrzkiewicz S, Karski J, Meineri M, Vegas A, David TE, Woo A, Rakowski H. Assessment of mitral valve prolapse by 3D TEE: angled views are key. J Am Coll Cardiol Imaging. 2011;4:94–7.
9. Barlow JB, Bosman CK. Aneurysmal protrusion of the posterior leaflet of the mitral valve. An auscultatory-electrocardiographic syndrome. Am Heart J. 1966;71:166–78.
10. Devereux RB. Mitral valve prolapse and severe mitral regurgitation. Circulation. 1988;78(1):234–6.
11. Düren DR, Becker AE, Dunning AJ. Long-term follow-up of idiopathic mitral valve prolapse in 300 patients: a prospective study. J Am Coll Cardiol. 1988;11(1):42–7.
12. Grigioni F, Enriquez-Sarano M, Ling LH, Bailey KR, Seward JB, Tajik AJ, Frye RL. Sudden death in mitral regurgitation due to flail leaflet. J Am Coll Cardiol. 1999;34:2078–85.
13. Freed LA, Levy D, Levine RA, Larson MG, Evans JC, Fuller DL, Lehman B, Benjamin EJ. Prevalence and clinical outcome of mitral-valve prolapse. N Engl J Med. 1999;341:1–7.
14. Nordhues BD, Siontis KC, Scott CG, et al. Bileaflet mitral valve prolapse and risk of ventricular dysrhythmias and death. J Cardiovasc Electrophysiol. 2016;27:463–8.
15. Nishimura RA, McGoon MD, Shub C, Miller FA Jr, Ilstrup DM, Tajik AJ. Echocardiographically documented mitral-valve prolapse. Long-term follow-up of 237 patients. N Engl J Med. 1985;313(21):1305–9.
16. Marks AR, Choong CY, Sanfilippo AJ, Ferré M, Weyman AE. Identification of high-risk and low-risk subgroups of patients with mitral-valve prolapse. N Engl J Med. 1989;320(16):1031–6.
17. Sriram CS, Syed FF, Ferguson ME, Johnson JN, Enriquez-Sarano M, Cetta F, Cannon BC, Asirvatham SJ, Ackerman MJ. Malignant bileaflet mitral valve prolapse syndrome in patients with otherwise idiopathic out-of-hospital cardiac arrest. J Am Coll Cardiol. 2013;62:222–30.
18. Sanfilippo AJ, Harrigan P, Popovic AD, Weyman AE, Levine RA. Papillary muscle traction in mitral valve prolapse: quantitation by two-dimensional echocardiography. J Am Coll Cardiol. 1992;19(3):564–71.
19. Han Y, Peters DC, Salton CJ, Bzymek D, Nezafat R, Goddu B, Kissinger KV, Zimetbaum PJ, Manning WJ, Yeon SB. Cardiovascular magnetic resonance characterization of mitral valve prolapse. JACC Cardiovasc Imaging. 2008;1(3):294–303.
20. Hutchins GM, Moore GW, Skoog DK. The association of floppy mitral valve with disjunction of the mitral annulus fibrosus. N Engl J Med. 1986;314:535–40.
21. Perazzolo Marra M, Basso C, Lazzari D, Md Rizzo S, Cipriani A, Giorgi B, et al. Morphofunctional abnormalities of mitral annulus and arrhythmic mitral valve prolapse. Circ Cardiovasc Imaging. 2016;9:e005030.
22. Lee AP, Jin CN, Fan Y, Wong RHL, Underwood MJ, Wan S. Functional implication of mitral annular disjunction in mitral valve prolapse. A quantitative dynamic 3D echocardiographic study. JACC Cardiovasc Imaging. 2017;10:1424–33.
23. Angelini A, Ho SY, Anderson RH, Becker AE, Davies MJ. Disjunction of the mitral annulus in floppy mitral valve. N Engl J Med. 1988;318:188–9.
24. Dejgaard LA, Skjølsvik ET, Lie ØH, Ribe M, Stokke MK, Hegbom F, et al. The mitral annulus disjunction arrhythmic syndrome. J Am Coll Cardiol. 2018;72:1600–9.

Rheumatic Mitral Valve Diseases and Mitral Annular Calcification: Role of 3DE

7

Joseph F. Maalouf and Francesco F. Faletra

Introduction

Rheumatic mitral valve stenosis (MS) remains the most common valvular heart disease in developing countries [1]. Rheumatic heart disease (RHD) can also cause mitral regurgitation (MR) [1–3]. Echocardiography remains the main imaging modality for the diagnosis of RHD and to guide management. Commissural fusion is the main mechanism of rheumatic MS [1–3] (Fig. 7.1). Associated lesions are chordal shortening and fusion, and leaflet thickening [1–3] (Fig. 7.1). Mobility of the posterior mitral leaflet is reduced whereas mobility of the anterior leaflet is often preserved, but may be restricted due to superimposed calcification at a later stage in the disease [3] (Fig. 7.2). Echocardiography-Doppler techniques for assessment of MS severity include the mean gradient (MG) and both indirect and direct measurements of the mitral valve (MV) orifice area [4]. Although Doppler derived mitral MG is a reliable measure of MS severity in absence of significant regurgitation, it is highly dependent on the transvalvular flow and diastolic filling period and will vary greatly with changes in heart rate [1, 2, 4]. Indirect measurement of the MV orifice area using Doppler derived pressure half time (PHT) is heavily influenced by hemodynamic variables including changes in atrial and ventricular compliance [1, 4], and is not reliable in presence of more than mild aortic regurgitation, atrial septal defect or post mitral balloon valvuloplasty [1, 4]. Moreover, the continuity equation for assessment of MS severity has limited accuracy and reproducibility and the PISA method is technically demanding [1]. Accordingly, direct measurement of the MV orifice has emerged as the preferred method for assessment of rheumatic MS severity with a valve area less than 1.5 cm^2 denoting clinically severe MS [5, 6] and a valve area less than 1 cm^2 denoting very severe MS [5] according to the most recent valve guidelines.

Supplementary Information The online version of this chapter (https://doi.org/10.1007/978-3-030-72941-7_7) contains supplementary material, which is available to authorized users.

J. F. Maalouf (✉)
Professor of Medicine, Mayo Clinic College of Medicine; Director, Interventional Echocardiography; Consultant, Department of Cardiovascular Medicine, Mayo Clinic, Rochester, MN, USA
e-mail: maalouf.joseph@mayo.edu

F. F. Faletra
Director of Cardiac Imaging Lab, Cardiocentro Ticino Institute, Lugano, Switzerland
e-mail: Francesco.Faletra@cardiocentro.org

Rheumatic MS

Rheumatic MS is characterized by a funnel like narrowing of the MV orifice such that the narrowest orifice is at the tip of the mitral leaflets [1, 2, 7, 8]. With 2DE, the narrowest MV area is identified by slowly scanning from the papillary muscles towards the base of the heart in the transverse plane (parasternal short-axis view) [1] in order to visualize the narrowest valve orifice at the tip of the leaflets. The inner edge of the MV orifice is then traced in mid diastole [1]. A major limitation of this method is having the correct image plane orientation [1, 2, 7, 8]. High gain settings may also lead to underestimation of the MV area (MVA) [1]. Compared with other 2D echocardiography (2DE) MS assessment tools, planimetry has been shown to have the best correlation with anatomic MVA as assessed by explanted valves [1], but planimetry using 2DE tends to overestimate the MVA compared with 3D echocardiography (3DE) planimetry measurements [1] especially in patients with large left atria [1]. 3DE enface left ventricular (LV) views of the entire MV apparatus (Figs. 7.2 and 7.3) provide better alignment of the transverse 2D image plane with the mitral leaflet tips particularly on multiplanar reconstruction of the 3D volumetric data sets [1, 2, 7, 8] (Figs. 7.2 and 7.3). Compared with 2DE, 3DE MVA measurements are therefore, more accurate and reproducible, and post mitral balloon valvuloplasty, 3DE MVA measurements have the best correlation with invasively determined MV area [1].

J. F. Maalouf et al. (eds.), *Practical 3D Echocardiography*, https://doi.org/10.1007/978-3-030-72941-7_7

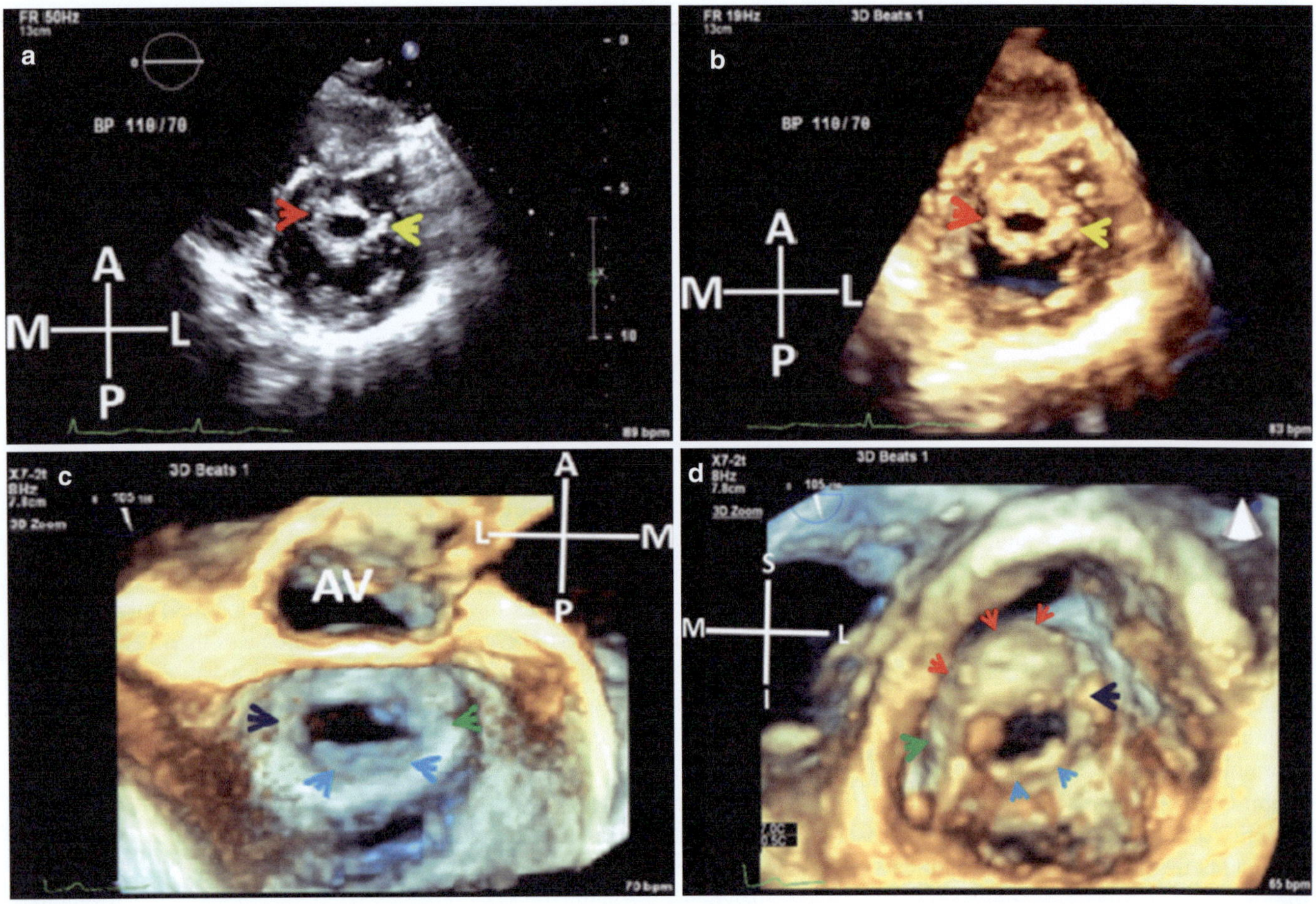

Fig. 7.1 3DE in MS. **Top panel**: 2D short-axis MV (**a**) in a patient with MS and RT 3D of same 2D view (**b**) for comparison. Yellow arrows point to lateral commissure and red arrows point to medial commissure. **Bottom panel**: RT 3D Zoom TEE enface LA (**c**) and LV (**d**) views from same patient. Note the fused and thickened medial (green arrows) and lateral (dark blue arrows) commissures. Light blue arrows point to thickened PML and red arrows point to thickened AML. Used with permission of Mayo Foundation for Medical Education and Research. All rights reserved. A, anterior; AML, anterior mitral leaflet; AV, aortic valve; I, inferior; L, lateral; LA, left atrium; LV, left ventricle; M, medial; MS, mitral stenosis; MV, mitral valve; P, posterior; PML, posterior mitral leaflet; RT, real time; S, superior

Percutaneous mitral balloon valvuloplasty (PMBV) remains the preferred treatment option for selected patients with rheumatic MS [1]. Chronic inflammation of the mitral valve leaflets as a result of rheumatic fever causes progressive leaflet thickening, calcification, commissural and chordal fusion [1] (Fig. 7.4). In absence of more than mild MR, these pathomorphological features are the basis for evaluation of suitability for PMBV by several echocardiography based scoring systems [1]. Anwar et al. [9], introduced a score based on real-time 3D transthoracic echocardiography (TTE) for the assessment of patients with MS before PMBV. This score includes the evaluation of both mitral leaflets and the subvalvular apparatus, and is both feasible and highly reproducible with good interobserver and intraobserver agreement in the assessment of MV morphology in patients with MS. Predictors of optimal PMBV results by the 3D scoring system are leaflet mobility and involvement of the subvalvular apparatus [1, 9]. The incidence and severity of post-procedural MR are associated with a high 3DE calcification score [1, 9].

Commissural splitting is the main mechanism of PMBV [1–3] (Fig. 7.4). Commissural calcification (Fig. 7.4) is a strong predictor of adverse PMBV outcomes including occurrence of severe MR, and severe or bicommissural calcification are contraindications to PMBV [1]. In addition to its incremental value over 2DE in assessing rheumatic MV stenosis severity, 3DE is better at assessment of the mitral commissures including extent of commissural thickening and detection of commissural calcification [1]. 3DE is therefore, the method of choice for assessment of impact of balloon valvuloplasty on the MV [1, 8, 10].

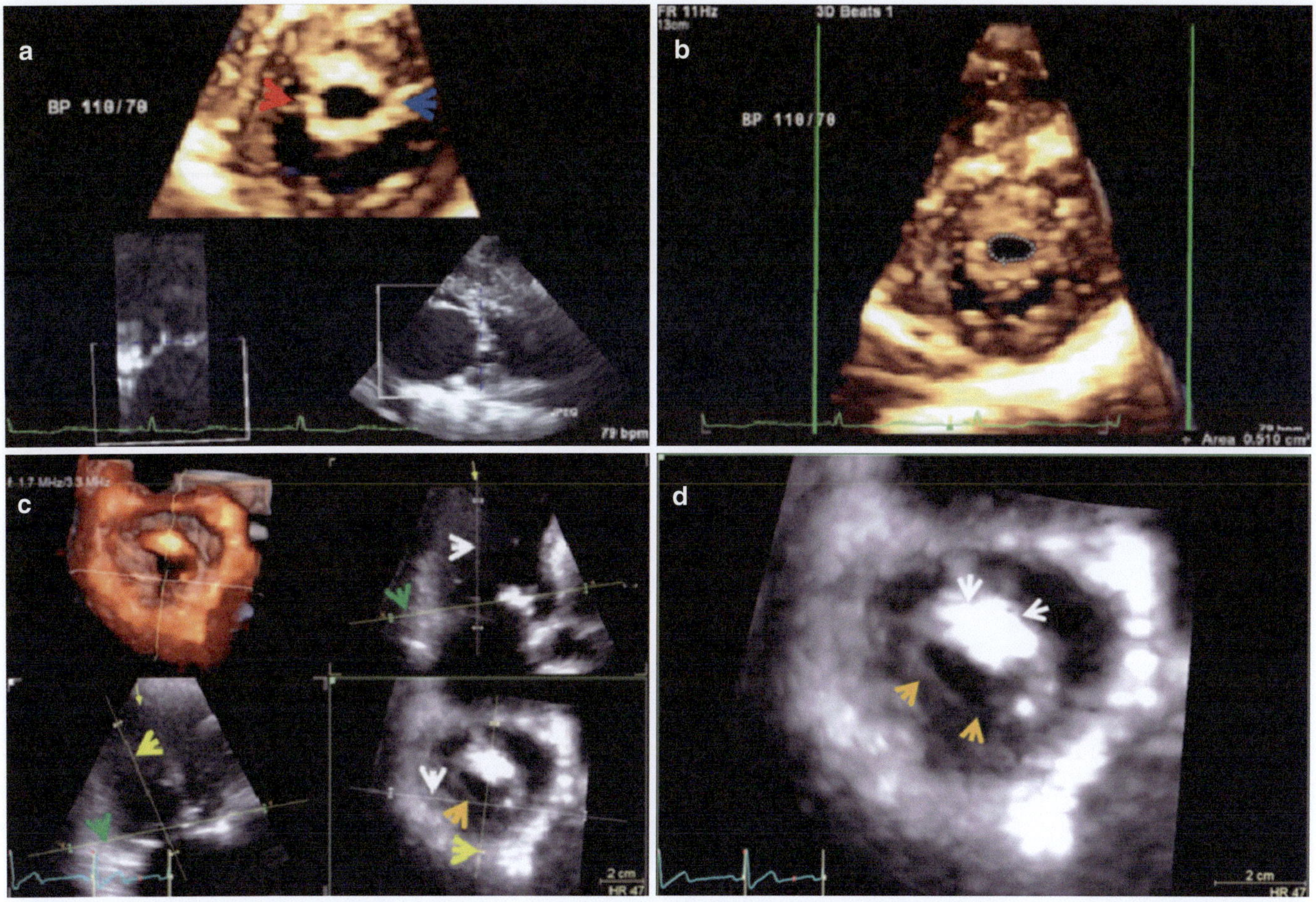

Fig. 7.2 3D TTE for assessment of MS severity. **Top panel**: (**a**) 3D guided placement of 2D tomographic plane using iCrop (Philips Healthcare) at tips of MV leaflets for accurate delineation of narrowest MVO in a patient with rheumatic MS. (**b**) Planimetry of 3D guided MV orifice area using on line calipers. Note that the validity of on line calipers for 3D measurements has been validated against calibrated phantoms. **Bottom panel**: MPR (GE Healthcare) of 3D MV short-axis volumetric data set (**c**) using three 2D tomographic planes (white, yellow and green arrows) to obtain the narrowest MV orifice area (**d**). Note the calcified AML(white arrows). Orange arrows point to PML. Used with permission of Mayo Foundation for Medical Education and Research. All rights reserved. AML, anterior mitral leaflet; MPR, multiplanar reconstruction; MS, mitral stenosis; MV, mitral valve; MVO, mitral valve orifice; PML, posterior mitral leaflet

Echocardiography plays a central role in guiding PMBV in the cardiac catheterization laboratory [1], and the transseptal puncture is usually guided using biplane imaging such as x-Plane (Philips Healthcare). Successful PMBV is contingent on achieving complete splitting of the commissures [1]. 3DE allows for enface imaging of the MV during balloon inflation (Fig. 7.5), and for rapid assessment of procedural success including extent of commissural splitting and MV area [1] (Fig. 7.6). Anatomic assessment of the results of valvuloplasty using 3DE is preferable to measuring mitral gradients because of the altered hemodynamic milieu due to general anesthesia or heavy sedation [1]. Real time 3DE can also guide positioning of the balloon away from chordal structures prior to balloon inflation [1]. Leaflet calcification including distribution of calcium is also better visualized with 3DE [1]. The presence of calcification can help predict adverse outcomes such as embolic stroke or conduction abnormalities [1]. A main concern during PMBV is worsening mitral regurgitation which may be caused by leaflet tear that is readily appreciated on 3D [1]. Guide-wires, catheters and devices used during the procedure may also be better appreciated on 3DE [1] particularly 3DTEE. Complications of PMBV include perforation of LA free wall, left atrial appendage, pulmonary veins, ventricular wall and aortic root. These complications can be diagnosed using real time (RT) 3DE [1]. In patients who develop restenosis following PMBV, 3DE can determine whether the mechanism of restenosis is commissural refusion or valve rigidity with persistent commissural splitting [2]. This is critical, because whereas repeat PMBV may be attempted for the former, it is of no use for the latter [2].

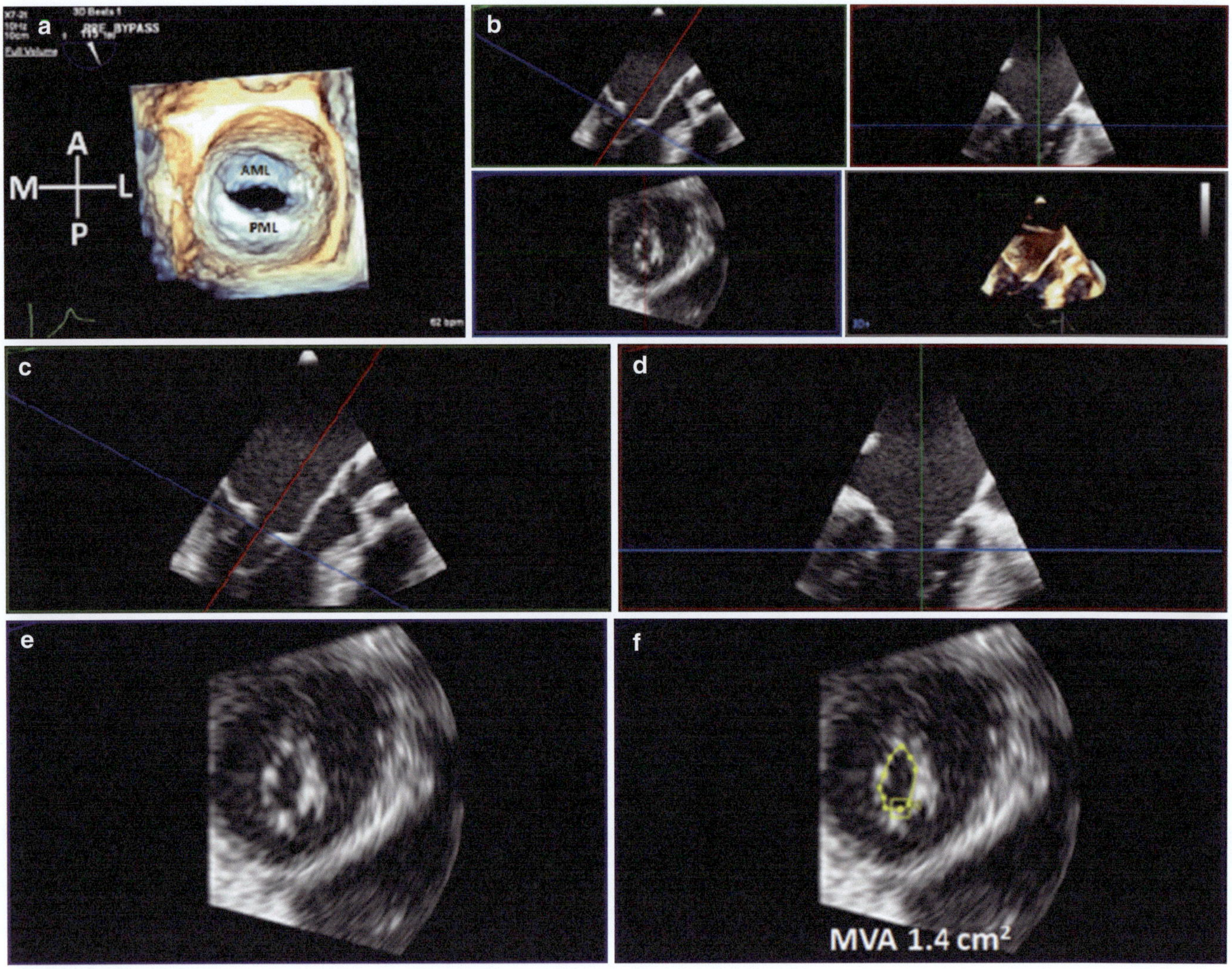

Fig. 7.3 (**a**) Live FV 3D TEE enface LA view of rheumatic MS. (**b**) MPR (3DQ, Philips Healthcare) with alignment of the blue line (transverse plane) at tips of the MV where the orifice is narrowest in both the coronal (green rectangle) and sagittal (red rectangle) planes and orthogonal to these two planes (i.e. green and red lines). The resulting MV orifice can be seen in the transverse plane at bottom left (blue rectangle). (**c, d**) Magnified images of the coronal (**c**) and sagittal (**d**) planes seen in MPR. (**e**) Magnified image of the MV orifice obtained using MPR. (**f**) Planimetry of the MV orifice using the measurement package. Used with permission of Mayo Foundation for Medical Education and Research. All rights reserved. A, anterior; AML, anterior mitral leaflet; FV, Full Volume; L, lateral; LA, left atrium; M, medial; MPR, multiplanar reconstruction; MS, mitral stenosis; MV, mitral valve; P, posterior; PML, posterior mitral leaflet

Acute mitral valvulitis [11] is a serious complication of rheumatic fever carditis. On echocardiography, the mitral leaflets are abnormally thick with restricted opening and incomplete leaflet closure in systole that can result in severe MR [11] (Fig. 7.7). Chronic rheumatic MR (Fig. 7.7) is characterized by a fixed posterior leaflet and anterior leaflet override resulting in a posteriorly directed jet of MR [1, 3]. In patients with predominantly rheumatic MR, the vena contracta anatomic regurgitant orifice area can be measured on 3DE using multiplanar reconstruction [12] (Fig. 7.8, see Chap. 3). The mitral valve has a saddle-shaped, nonplanar annulus and displays variation in size and shape during the cardiac cycle. RT3DE can also distinguish the differences in annular shape and function in various types of MR [2, 4].

Mitral Valve Disease Secondary to Mitral Annular Calcification

Mitral annular calcification (MAC) is a chronic degenerative process that, when severe, can result in MS and/or mitral regurgitation (MR) [13]. The prevalence of significant MS due to severe MAC is increasing in the developed world due

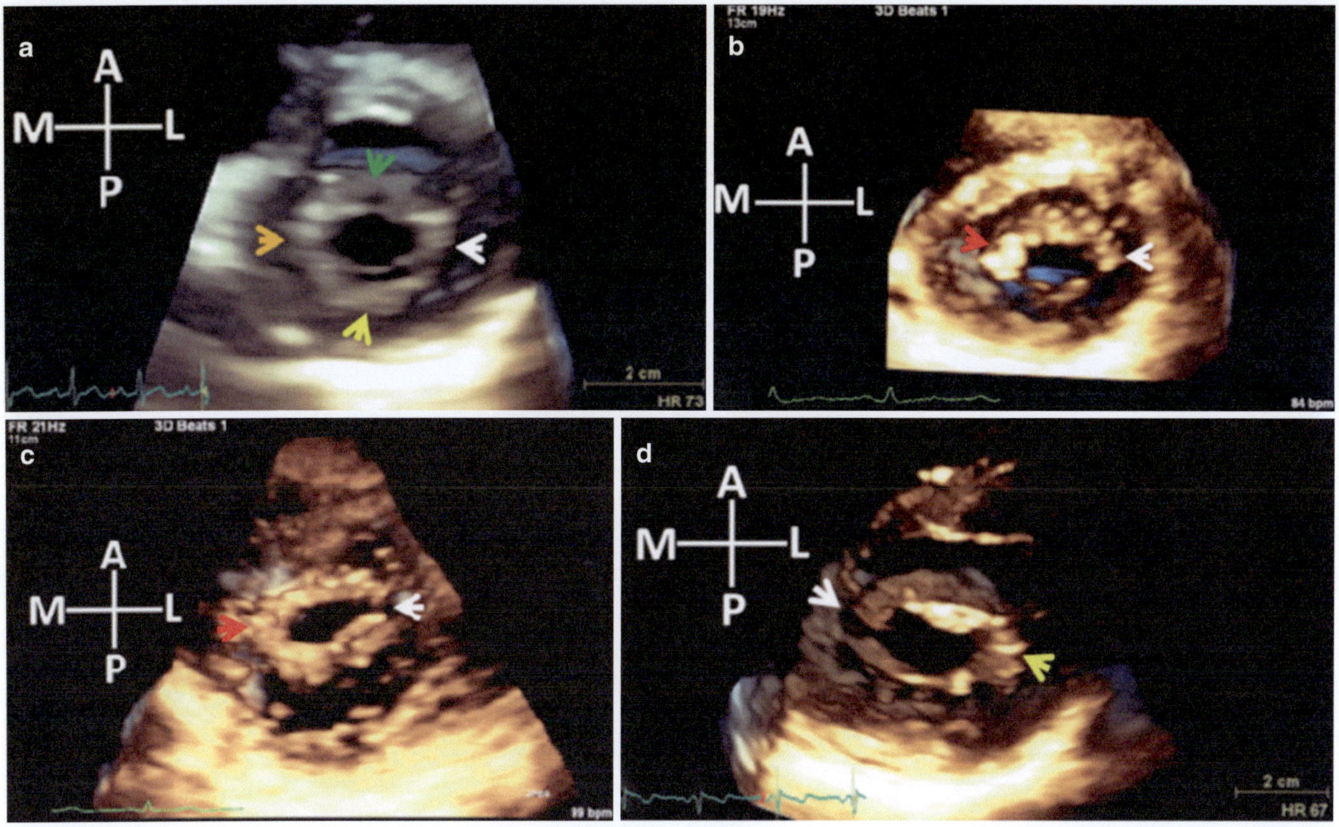

Fig. 7.4 3D TTE parasternal short-axis views of commissures in MS. **Top panel**: (**a**) symmetrical thickening of the medial (orange arrow) and lateral (white arrow) commissures. Note the thickened leaflets (PML; yellow arrow and AML; green arrow). (**b**) Calcified medial commissure (red arrow; white arrow points to lateral commissure). **Bottom panel**: Post PMBV. (**c**) Splitting of the lateral commissure (white arrow). Red arrow point to medial commissure. (**d**) Splitting of the medial commissure (white arrow). Yellow arrow points to lateral commissure. Used with permission of Mayo Foundation for Medical Education and Research. All rights reserved. A, anterior; AML, anterior mitral leaflet; L, lateral; M, medial; MS, mitral stenosis; P, posterior; PML, posterior mitral leaflet; PMBV, percutaneous mitral balloon valvuloplasty

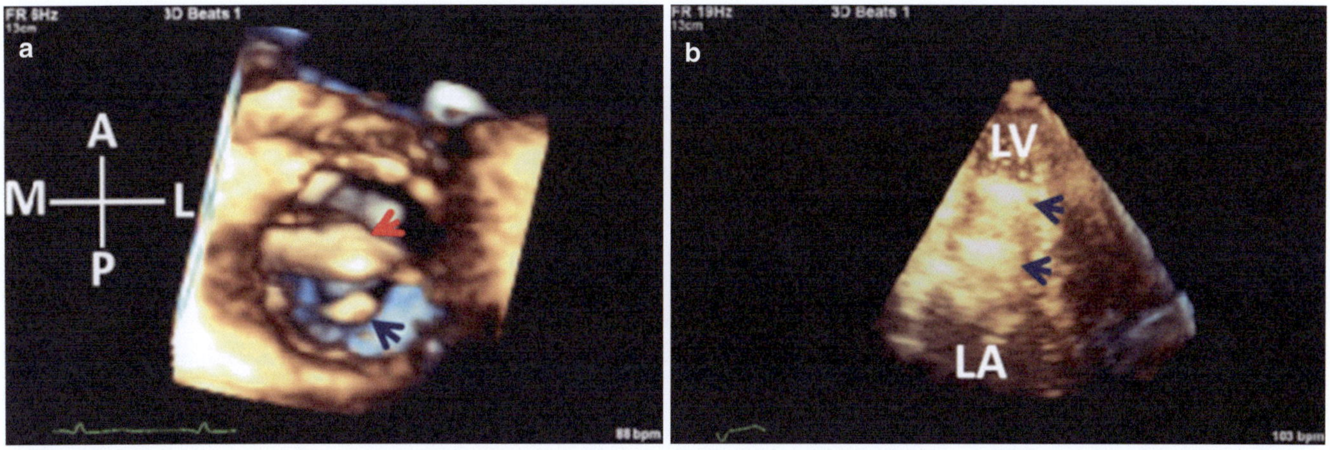

Fig. 7.5 3D TTE during PMBV. (**a**) Enface LV view showing balloon catheter (dark blue arrow) being advanced through the MV. Red arrow points to AML. (**b**) Apical view showing Inoue balloon inflation (dark blue arrows). Used with permission of Mayo Foundation for Medical Education and Research. All rights reserved. A, anterior; AML, anterior mitral leaflet; L, lateral; LA, left atrium; LV, left ventricle; M, medial; MV, mitral valve; P, posterior; PMBV, percutaneous mitral balloon valvuloplasty

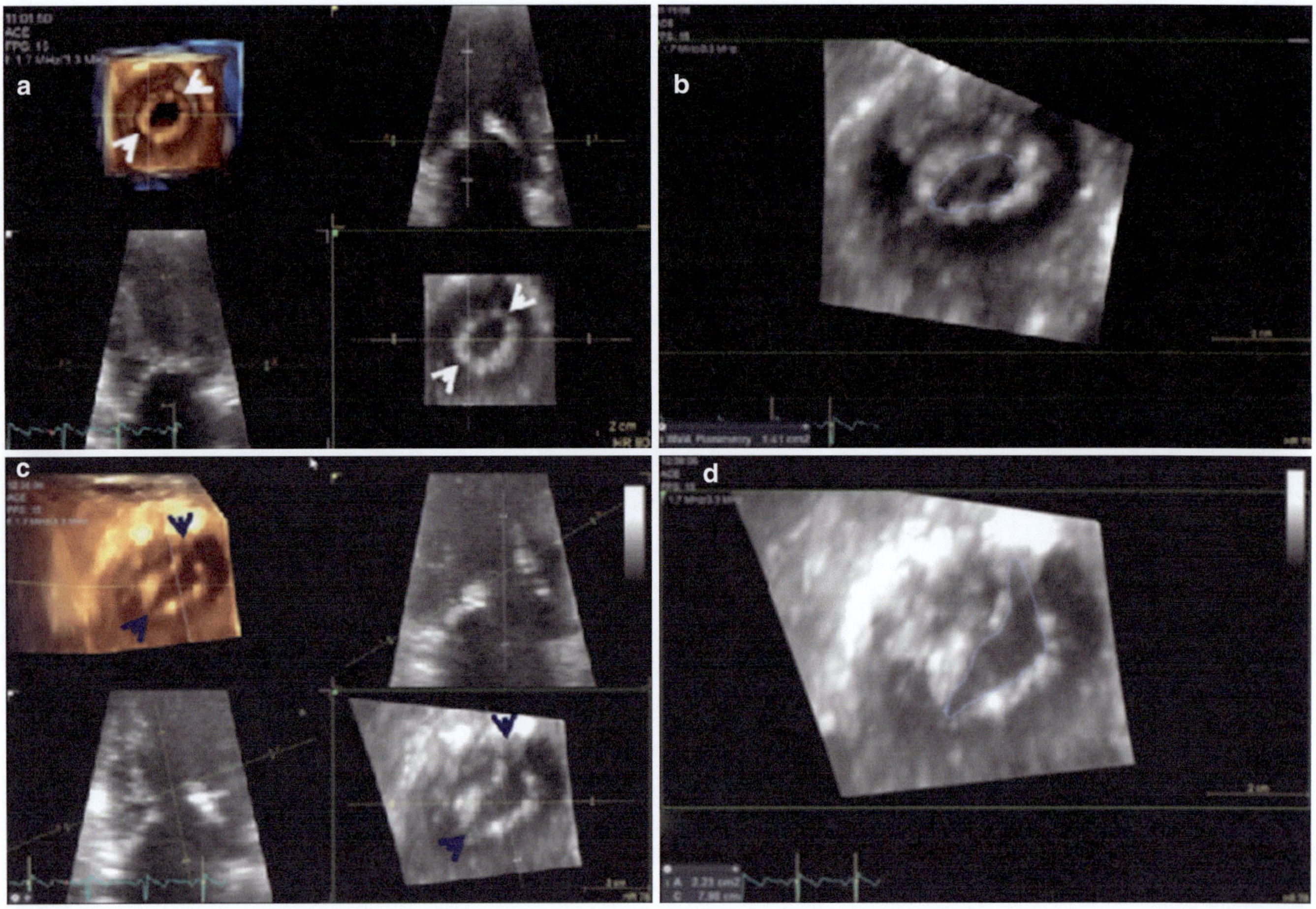

Fig. 7.6 3D TTE MS before and following PMBV. **Top panel**: pre PMBV images. (**a**) MPR showing thickened but intact commissures (white arrows). (**b**) MVA 1.4 cm² on planimetry of MV orifice in mid-diastole. **Bottom panel**: (**c**) post PMBV MPR showing bilateral commissural splitting (dark blue arrows) following mitral balloon valvotomy with a 26 mm Inoue balloon. (**d**) MVA increased to 2.2 cm². The mean left atrial pressure dropped from 27 to 6 mmHg. Used with permission of Mayo Foundation for Medical Education and Research. All rights reserved. MPR, multiplanar reconstruction; MS, mitral stenosis; MV, mitral valve; MVA, mitral valve area; PMBV, percutaneous mitral balloon valvuloplasty

to the growing population of elderly patients and risk factors such as hypertension, renal failure, and radiation heart disease [3, 13]. Although MAC is typically confined to the mitral annulus and the base of the leaflets, over time calcific degeneration tends to further expand into the body of both leaflets resulting in impaired leaflet mobility and geometric distortion of the mitral valve [3, 13]. These anatomic changes typically lead to development of both MS and MR. Either lesion may be dominant in a given patient, but more commonly there is mixed disease [3]. When MS or MR become severe, heart failure symptoms including dyspnea and exercise intolerance may ensue. Important distinctions compared to rheumatic MS is that in MS due to MAC, there is lack of commissural fusion and the narrowest valve area is usually at the mitral inflow orifice [1, 3]. *PMBV is therefore, not suitable for mitral stenosis due to MAC.*

The enface atrial and ventricular views of the MV on 3DE (Figs. 7.9, 7.10 and 7.14) provide the best information for topographical description of the MV including direct visualization of the extent and magnitude of MAC. Assessment of MS severity due to MAC with conventional echo-Doppler methods used to evaluate rheumatic MS is either not possible or not reliable. Direct planimetry with 2DE is very challenging and the pressure half-time method in this setting has limited utility in estimating the MVA. Planimetry of MVA using multiplanar reconstruction of the 3D volumetric data set is feasible in the majority of patients [13] (Figs. 7.11 and 7.13). By lowering the gain settings, 3DE and in particular 3D TEE also allows direct visualization of the circumferential extent of MAC (Figs. 7.9 and 7.10) which is important for determining the feasibility of a valve-in-valve procedure (see Chap. 30). 3D TEE is also excellent for detection and quantitation of MR [12] (Fig. 7.11), as the probe is located just behind the left atrium, with unimpeded views.

Quantitative 3DE also provides new insights into the dynamic consequences of MAC [14] (Fig. 7.12), and in

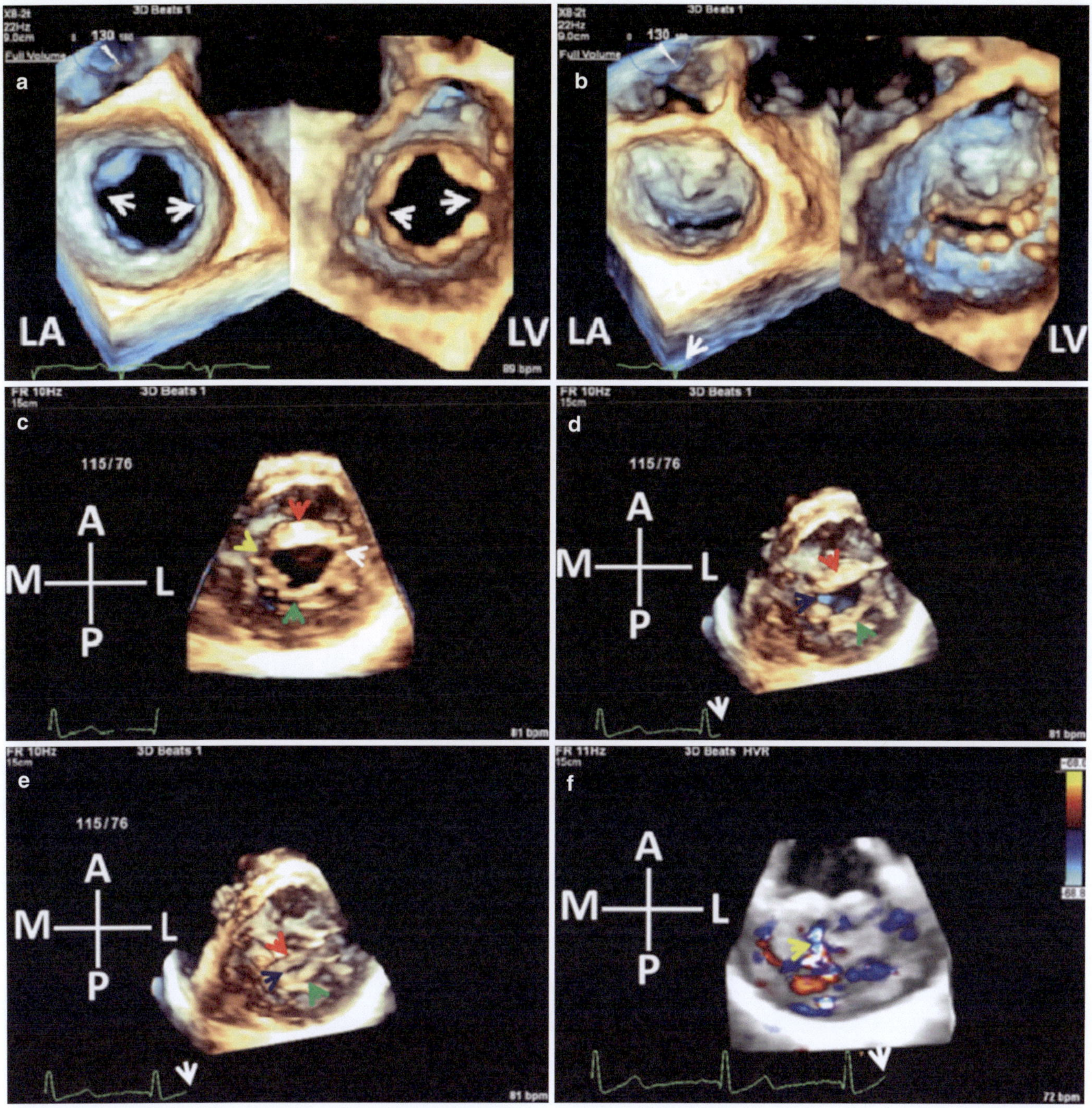

Fig. 7.7 3DE rheumatic MR. **Top panel**: 3D TEE in acute valvulitis. LA and LV dual layout views in diastole (**a**) and systole (**b**). Note the lack of commissural thickening (arrows) and incomplete leaflet coaptation in systole. **Middle panel**: 3D TTE MV in a patient with RHD and chronic MR. (**c**) End diastole. Note the thickened AML (red arrow) and thickened medial (yellow arrow) and lateral (white arrow) commissures. (**d**) Early systole(white arrow) showing leaflet malcoaptation (dark blue arrow). Red arrow points to AML and green arrow points to PML. **Bottom panel**: same patient: (**e**) persistent leaflet malcoaptation (dark blue arrow) in late systole (white arrow). (**f**) CFD late systole (white arrow) showing a posteriorly directed jet of MR (yellow arrow). On 2DE, the PML was immobile with AML override. Used with permission of Mayo Foundation for Medical Education and Research. All rights reserved. A, anterior; AML, anterior mitral leaflet; CFD, color flow Doppler; L, lateral; LA, left atrium; LV, left ventricle; M, medial; MR, mitral regurgitation; MV, mitral valve; P, posterior; PML, posterior mitral leaflet; RHD, rheumatic heart disease

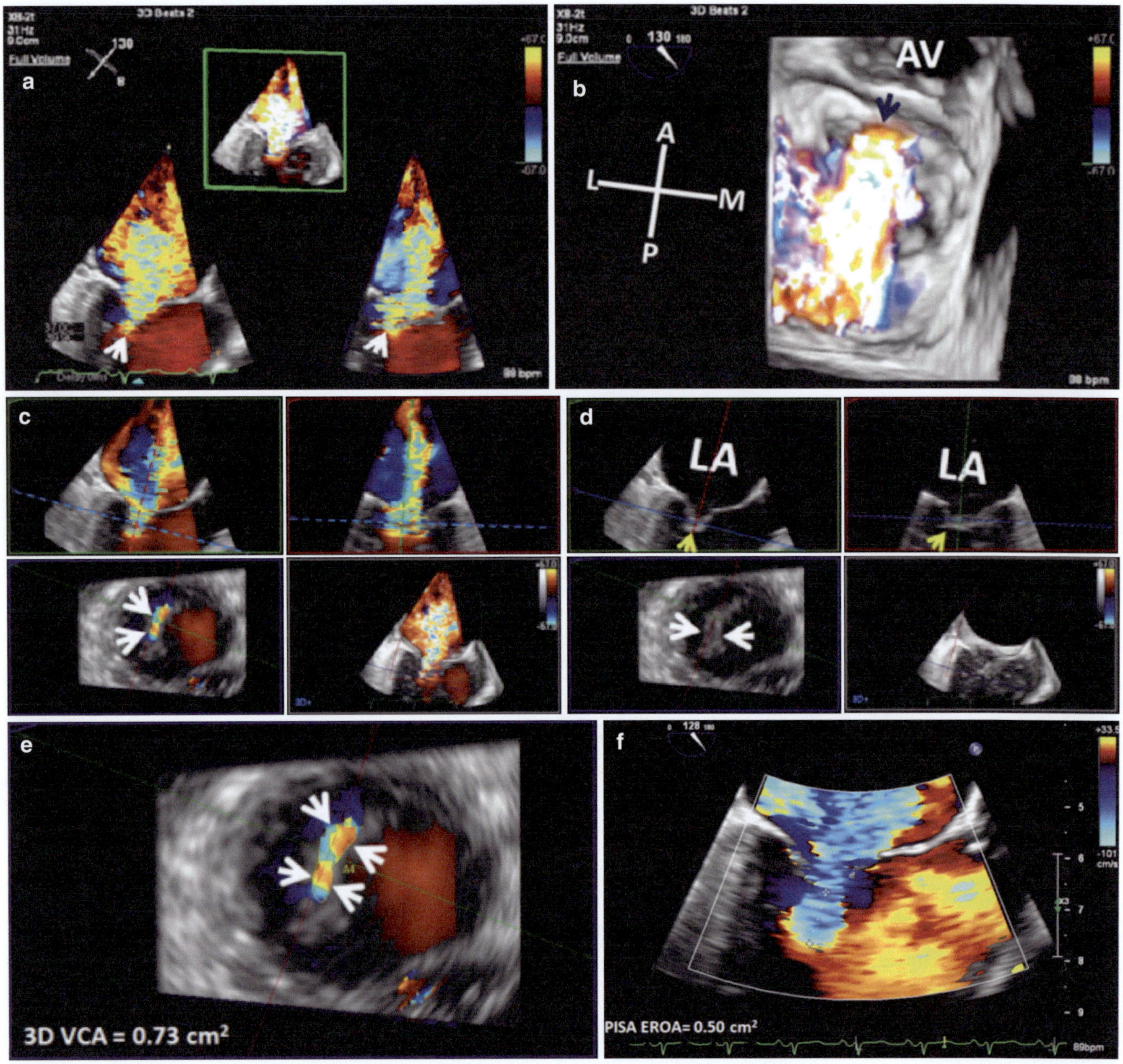

Fig. 7.8 3D TEE CFD in acute mitral valvulitis with severe MR . **Top panel**: (**a**) FV of MR (white arrows). (**b**) Enface LA view MV. Arrow points to posteriorly directed MR jet. **Middle panel**: MPR of the 3D CFD data set. (**c**) Intersection of three orthogonal planes: blue, red, and green lines at VC of MR jet delineates the VC area which represents the EROA (white arrows) in the transverse short-axis plane (left lower quadrant). (**d**) Same MPR with color suppress to highlight alignment of the transverse blue plane at site of VC just distal to leaflet coaptation (yellow arrows). The VC area with color on (**c**, white arrows) may be slightly larger than area without color (**d**, white arrows) because of color blooming artifact. **Bottom panel**: (**e**) elliptical shaped VC on 3D (arrows) and planimetered VC area. (**f**) By comparison, 2D CFD PISA derived EROA from same patient. Used with permission of Mayo Foundation for Medical Education and Research. All rights reserved. A, anterior; AV, aortic valve; CFD, color flow Doppler; EROA, effective regurgitant orifice area; FV, Full Volume; L, lateral; LA, left atrium; M, medial; MPR, multiplanar reconstruction; MR, mitral regurgitation; MV, mitral valve; P, posterior; PISA, proximal isovelocity surface acceleration; VC, vena contracta; VCA, vena contracta area

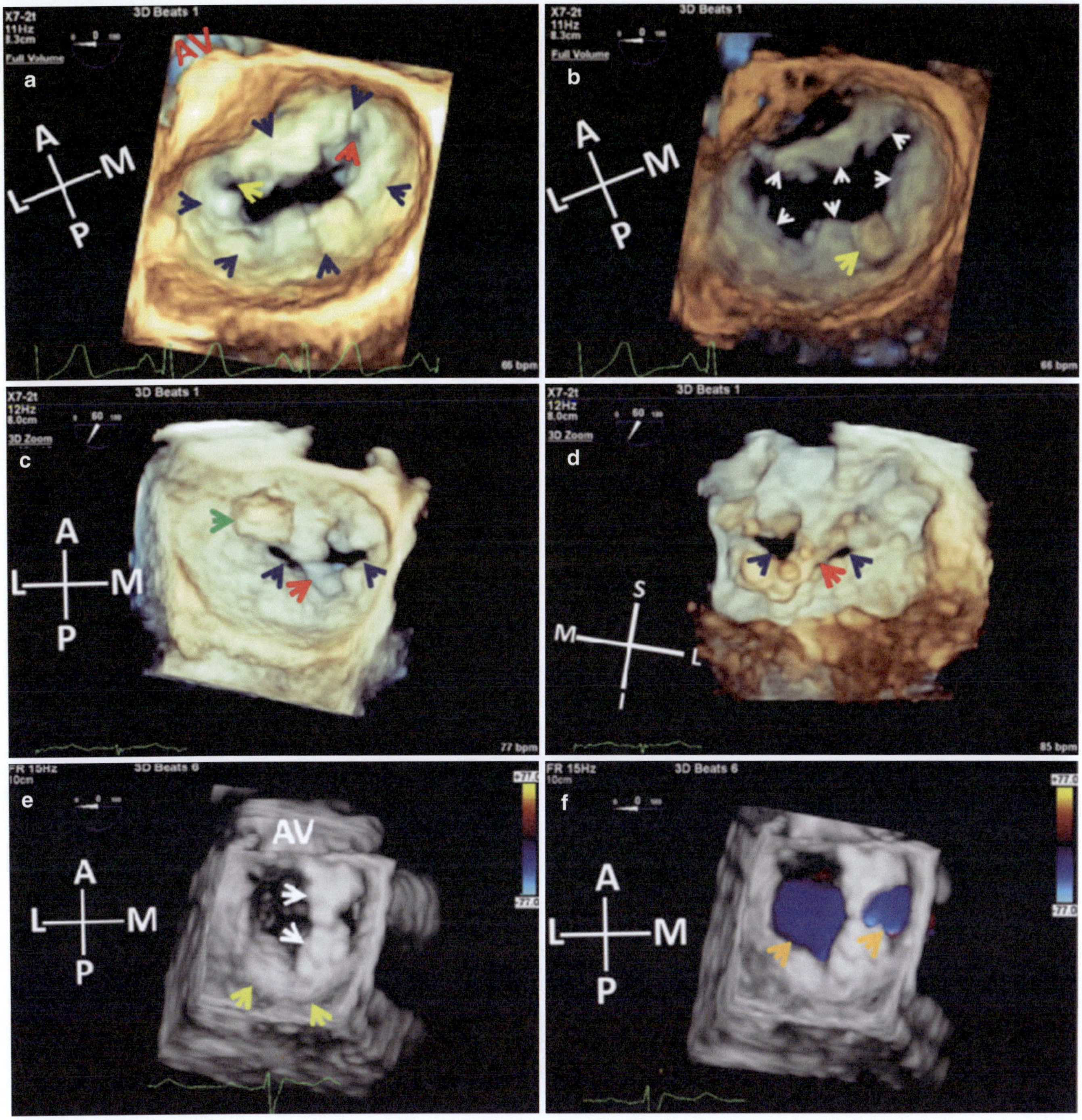

Fig. 7.9 3D TEE assessment of MAC. **Top panel**: enface LA views of the MV; (**a**) circumferential MAC (dark blue arrows). Red arrow points to medial commissure and yellow arrow points to lateral commissure. (**b**) By lowering the overall gain settings, the circumferential distribution of annular calcification (white arrows) is appreciated. Yellow arrow points to a calcified nodule on mid posterior annulus. **Middle panel**: LA (**c**) and LV (**d**) 3D TEE enface views of the MV in another patient with MAC showing a very narrow MV orifice (dark blue arrows) and a calcified mass (green arrow) at the lateral commissure. Note the calcium shelf that projects from posterior mitral annulus into the lumen towards the AML (red arrow). **Bottom panel**: Enface 3D TEE LA views with color suppress on (**e**) and CFD (**f**) showing posterior mitral annular calcification (yellow arrows) and a large calcium bridge between the posterior and anterior mitral annulus (white arrows) resulting in a double orifice MV (orange arrows). Used with permission of Mayo Foundation for Medical Education and Research. All rights reserved. A, anterior; AML, anterior mitral leaflet; AV, aortic valve; CFD, color flow Doppler; I, inferior; L, lateral; LA, left atrium; LV, left ventricle; M, medial; MAC, mitral annular calcification; MV, mitral valve; P, posterior; S, superior

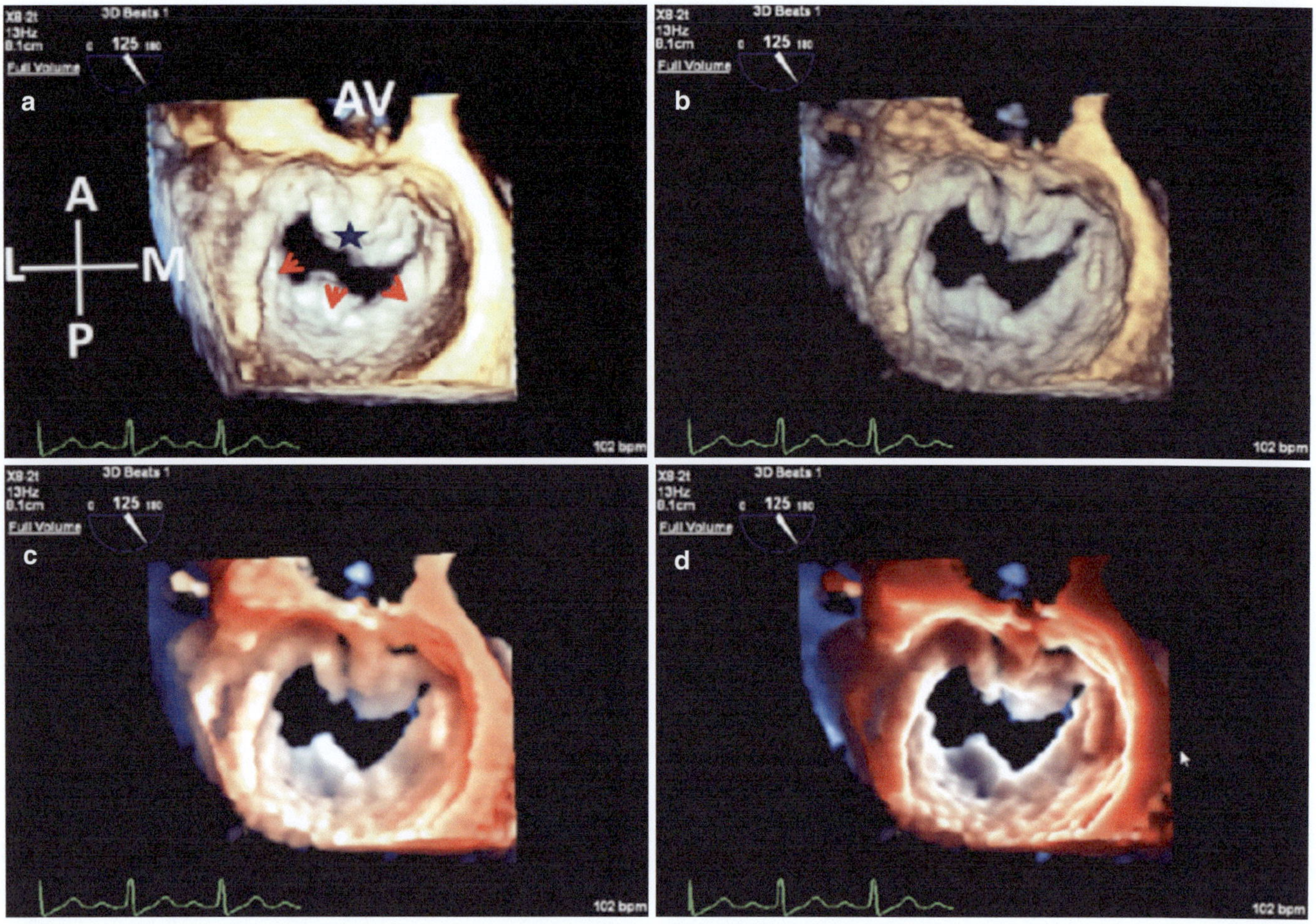

Fig. 7.10 Another patient with MAC. (**a**) Live FV 3D enface LA view of MV showing extensive posterior annular calcification (arrows) with MAC that extends anteriorly with calcium involvement of the AML (star). (**b**) Same frame, with lowered overall gain to appreciate the circumferential and AML calcification. (**c, d**) TrueVue (Philips Healthcare) of image in **b** at two different depths of the light source. Used with permission of Mayo Foundation for Medical Education and Research. All rights reserved. A, anterior; AML, anterior mitral leaflet; AV, aortic valve; FV, Full Volume; M, medial; MAC, mitral annular calcium; MV, mitral valve; L, lateral; LA, left atrium; P, posterior

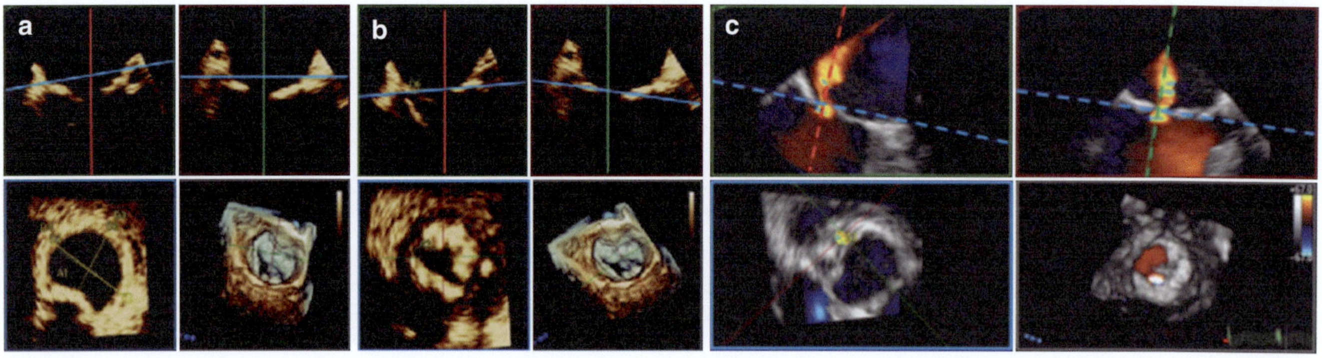

Fig. 7.11 (**a**) MPR in MAC with measurement of the mitral annular dimensions (blue square, lower left). (**b**) By careful translation of the transverse plane (blue lines) from the annulus towards the LV in two orthogonal planes (top right and left), the narrowest inflow area (blue square, lower left) is identified and measured using planimetry. (**c**) MPR of 3D CFD volumetric data set in another patient with MAC and MR. Note the circular orifice of the VC (lower left, blue rectangle). Used with permission of Mayo Foundation for Medical Education and Research. All rights reserved. CFD, color flow Doppler; LV, left ventricle; MAC, mitral annular calcification; MPR, multiplanar reconstruction; MR, mitral regurgitation; VC, vena contracta

patients with severe mitral stenosis due to MAC who are potential candidates for transcatheter mitral valve replacement (see Chap. 31), 3D-TEE assessment of mitral annular dimensions (Figs. 7.11 and 7.12) can be very useful in determining the transcatheter mitral valve implantation size [15].

Other rare causes of MS [1, 2] not to be confused with rheumatic MS include congenital MS, radiation induced heart disease (Fig. 7.14), inflammatory diseases, infiltrative diseases, carcinoid heart disease, and drug-induced MS (Fig. 7.14). The mitral leaflets in such patients are thickened with restricted mobility, but as with degenerative MS and unlike rheumatic MS, commissural fusion is rare. Radiation-induced valve disease typically involves both the mitral and aortic valves [3], and calcifications of the mitral aortic inter-valve fibrosa have been reported to be a highly suggestive finding [3].

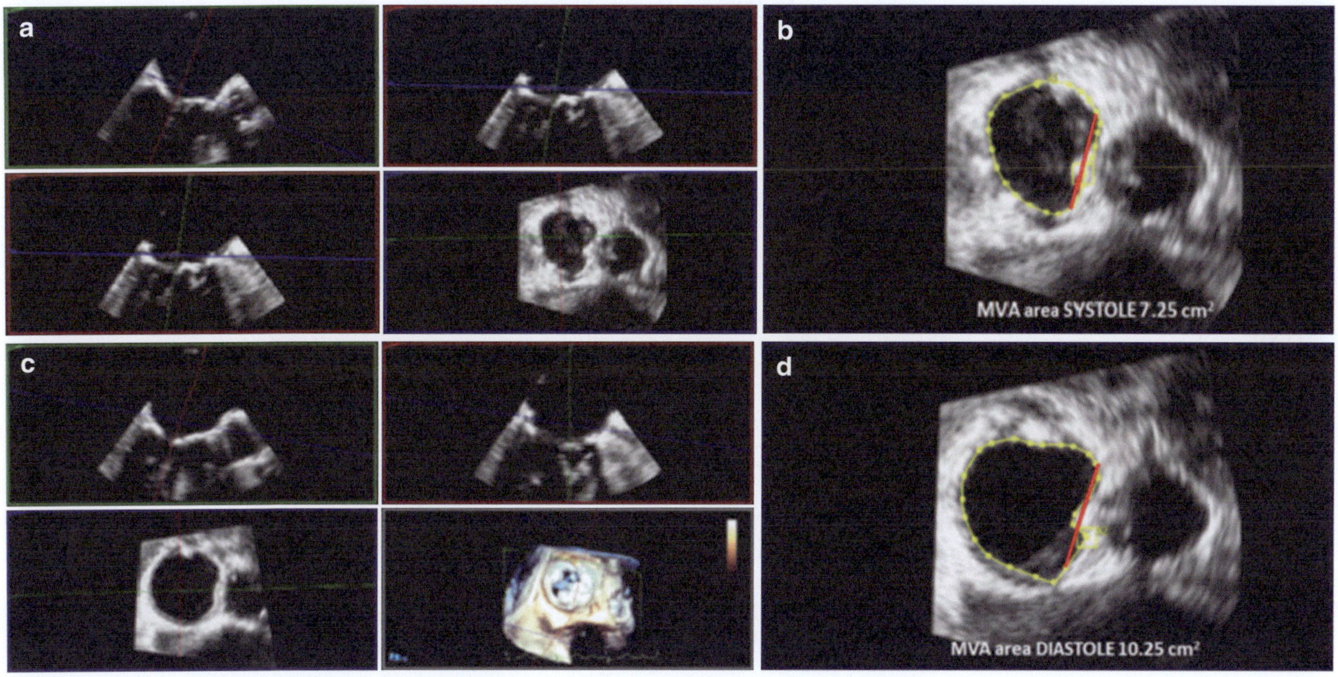

Fig. 7.12 MPR mitral annulus in same patient in Fig. 7.10 with annular area measurements in systole (**a**, **b**) and diastole (**c**, **d**). Red line indicates trigone-trigone distance. Used with permission of Mayo Foundation for Medical Education and Research. All rights reserved

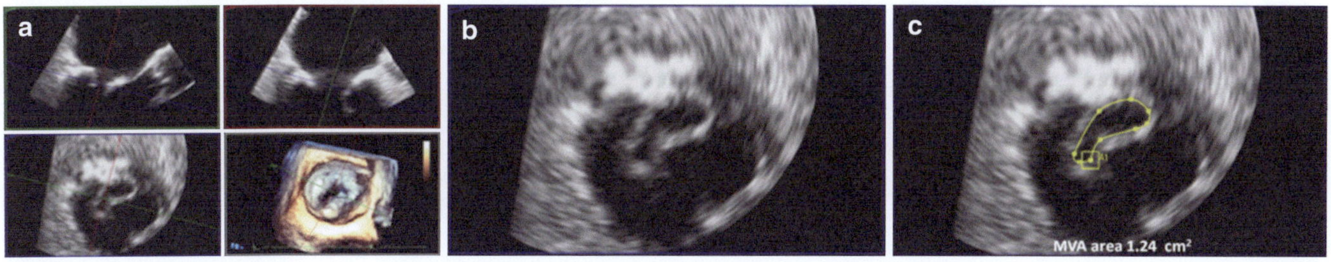

Fig. 7.13 (**a**) MPR of MV in another patient with severe MAC to detect narrowest MV area (**a**, **b**) and area measurement (**c**). Used with permission of Mayo Foundation for Medical Education and Research. All rights reserved. MAC, mitral annular calcium; MPR, multiplanar reconstruction; MV, mitral valve

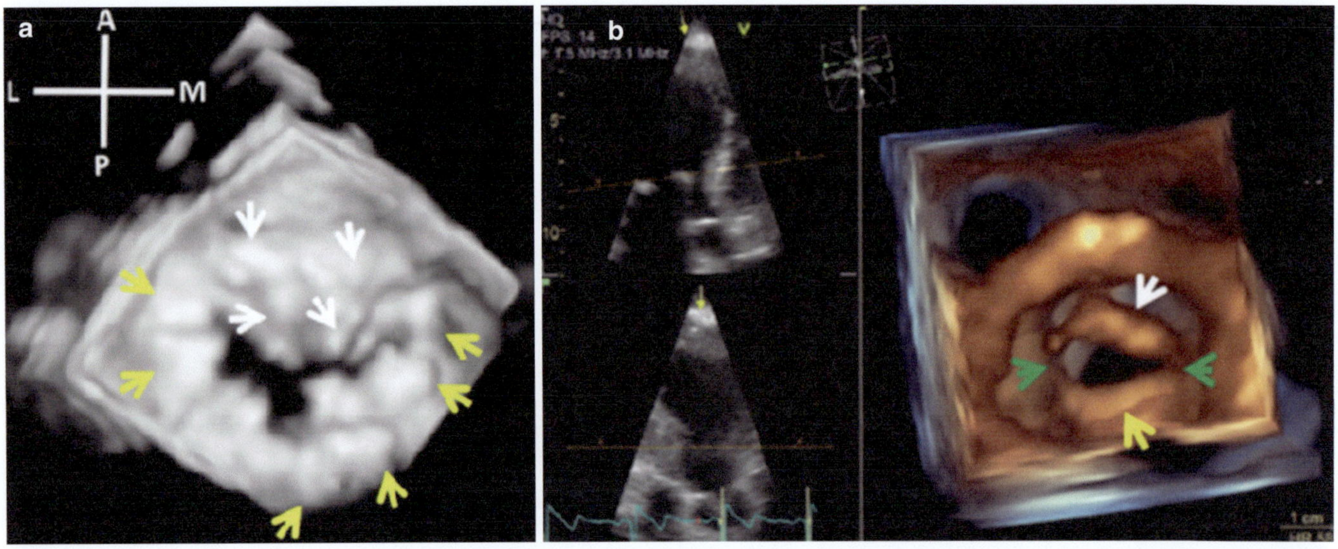

Fig. 7.14 (**a**) Radiation induced MVD. Note severe MAC (yellow arrows) and nodular calcifications AML (white arrows). (**b**) MV in a patient who was on the diet drug Fen-Phen. Both AML (white arrow) and PML (yellow arrow) are thick but the commissures (green arrows) are spared. Used with permission of Mayo Foundation for Medical Education and Research. All rights reserved. A, anterior; AML, anterior mitral leaflet; L, lateral; M, medial; MAC, mitral annular calcification; MV, mitral valve; MVD, mitral valve disease; P, posterior; PML, posterior mitral leaflet

References

1. Wunderlich NC, Beigel R, Siegel RJ. Management of mitral stenosis using 2D and 3D echo-Doppler imaging. JACC Cardiovasc Imaging. 2013;6(11):1191–205.
2. Gabriel V, Kamp O, Visser CA. Three-dimensional echocardiography in mitral valve disease. Eur J Echocardiogr. 2005;6(6):443–54.
3. Krapf L, Dreyfus J, Cueff C, Lepage L, Brochet É, Vahanian A, Messika-Zeitoun D. Anatomical features of rheumatic and non-rheumatic mitral stenosis: Potential additional value of three-dimensional echocardiography. Arch Cardiovasc Dis. 2013;106(2):111–5.
4. Oh JK, Kane GC, editors. The echo manual. 4th ed. Philadelphia: Wolters Kluwer; 2019.
5. Nishimura RA, et al. 2014 AHA/ACC guidelines for the management of patients with valvular heart disease. Circulation. 2014;129(23):2440–92.
6. Baumgartner H, et al. 2017 ESC/EACTS guidelines for the management of valvular heart disease. Eur Heart J. 2017;38(36):2739–91.
7. Bleakley C, Eskandari M, Aldalati O, Moschonas K, Huang M, Whittaker A, Monaghan MJ. Impact of 3D echocardiography on grading of mitral stenosis and prediction of clinical events. Echo Res Pract. 2018;5(4):105–11.
8. Chu JW, Levine RA, Chua S, Kian-Keong P, Morris E, Hua L, Ton-Nu TT, Hung J. Assessing mitral valve area and orifice geometry in calcified mitral stenosis: A new solution by real-time three-dimensional echocardiography. J Am Soc Echocardiogr. 2008;21(9):1006–9.
9. Anwar AM, Attia WM, Nosir YF, Soliman OI, Mosad MA, Othman M, Geleijnse ML, El-Amin AM, Ten Cate FJ. Validation of a new score for the assessment of mitral stenosis using real-time three-dimensional echocardiography. J Am Soc Echocardiogr. 2010;23(1):13–22.
10. Farrag HMA, Setouhi AM, El-Mokadem MO, El-Swasany MA, Mahmoud KS, Mahmoud HB, Ibrahim AM. Additive value of 3D-echo in prediction of immediate outcome after percutaneous balloon mitral valvuloplasty. Egypt Heart J. 2019;71:19.
11. Xu B, Rodriquez LL, Tan CD, Collier P. Rheumatic valvulitis—forgotten, but not gone. Int J Cardiovasc Acad. 2017;3(1–2):34–7.
12. Buck T, Plicht B. Real-time three-dimensional echocardiographic assessment of severity of mitral regurgitation using proximal isovelocity surface area and vena contracta area method. Lessons and clinical implications. Curr Cardiovasc Imaging Rep. 2015;8:38.
13. Eleid MF, Foley TA, Said SM, Pislaru SV, Rihal CS. Severe mitral annular calcification: multimodality imaging for therapeutic strategies and interventions. JACC Cardiovasc Imaging. 2016;9(11):1318–37.
14. Mak GJ, Blanke P, Ong K, Naoum C, Thompson CR, Webb JG, Moss R, Boone R, Ye J, Cheung A, Munt B, Leipsic J, Grewal J. Three-dimensional echocardiography compared with computed tomography to determine mitral annulus size before transcatheter mitral valve implantation. Circ Cardiovasc Imaging. 2016;9(6)
15. Pressman GS, Movva R, Topilsky Y, Clavel M-A, Saldanha JA, Watanabe N, Enriquez-Sarano M. Mitral annular dynamics in mitral annular calcification: a three-dimensional imaging study. J Am Soc Echocardiogr. 2015;28(7):786–94.

Role of 3DE in Assessment of Functional Mitral Regurgitation

8

Joseph F. Maalouf and Francesco F. Faletra

Functional mitral regurgitation (FMR) is defined as mitral regurgitation (MR) secondary to ischemic or dilated cardiomyopathy in the absence of structural abnormality in the mitral valve (MV) [1, 2]. The underlying cause of MR in this setting is regional or global left ventricular (LV) dysfunction and dilatation. The LV remodeling that ensues leads to apical and lateral papillary muscle displacement as a result of global LV enlargement or focal myocardial scarring, and can affect one or both papillary muscles [1, 2]. Additionally, the normal saddle-shape of the mitral annulus, important for maintaining low leaflet stress is lost [3], and annular flattening with LV remodeling results in increased leaflet stress and secondary MR [1–3]. Moreover, LV systolic dysfunction reduces the strength of MV closing. These aforementioned pathomorphologic changes result in leaflet tethering, tenting, and malcoaptation (Figs. 8.1 and 8.2) [1, 2].

In ischemic MR (the more frequent etiology of FMR), LV remodeling may be regional or global and symmetric or asymmetric mitral leaflet tethering may occur [1, 2]. Symmetric tethering typically causes mitral leaflet tenting and is associated with substantial LV systolic dysfunction, global remodeling with increased LV sphericity, and a central regurgitant jet. Asymmetric tethering typically involves the posterior leaflet and results from localized remodeling affecting the posterior papillary muscle and adjacent mid to basal myocardial segments, but global left ventricular ejection fraction (LVEF) does not have to be reduced [1, 2]. A characteristic feature of asymmetric posterior leaflet tethering is anterior leaflet override (Fig. 8.1) and secondary posteriorly directed jet of mitral regurgitation. Sufficient mitral leaflet tethering can result in severe MR. 3D echocardiography (3DE) is useful for assessing the morpho-anatomic changes associated with FMR, and for providing insight into the underlying mechanism of mitral regurgitation in this setting (Fig. 8.1). A better appreciation of the variability in mitral valve geometry due to differences in infarct location and size, and extent of left ventricular remodeling may help improve surgical planning [4].

Non-ischemic MR, most commonly due to longstanding hypertension or idiopathic dilated cardiomyopathy, is characterized by global LV dilation with increased sphericity and (typically) a centrally located regurgitant jet. Mitral annular dilation typically occurs late in the pathophysiology of secondary MR, and is often asymmetric, with greater involvement of the posterior annulus [3]. Symmetric mitral annular dilation correlates with the severity of LV dysfunction [3]. Isolated left atrial enlargement, with or without atrial fibrillation, is a relatively infrequent cause of severe secondary MR, due to dilated mitral annulus and reduced leaflet coaptation despite normal LV function and mitral leaflets [1].

Flow quantitation has emerged as the cornerstone for assessment of MR severity [5]. The smallest cross sectional area through which any regurgitant jet passes through before expanding into the receiving chamber is called its vena contracta (VC) [5]. Because regurgitant blood flow accelerates as it approaches the mitral valve orifice, conventional 2-dimensional (2D) Doppler derived quantitation of MR severity relies on the proximal isovelocity surface acceleration (PISA) method [5]. The PISA method assumes a circular regurgitant orifice geometry also referred to as the effective regurgitant orifice area or EROA for short [5]. However, the EROA is not circular in most patients, and MR severity may, therefore, be significantly underestimated when the orifice is elliptical as is typical in functional MR (Figs. 8.2 and 8.3), and this is compounded if multiple jets

Supplementary Information The online version of this chapter (https://doi.org/10.1007/978-3-030-72941-7_8) contains supplementary material, which is available to authorized users.

J. F. Maalouf (✉)
Professor of Medicine, Mayo Clinic College of Medicine; Director, Interventional Echocardiography; Consultant, Department of Cardiovascular Medicine, Mayo Clinic, Rochester, MN, USA
e-mail: maalouf.joseph@mayo.edu

F. F. Faletra
Director of Cardiac Imaging Lab, Cardiocentro Ticino Institute, Lugano, Switzerland
e-mail: Francesco.Faletra@cardiocentro.org

J. F. Maalouf et al. (eds.), *Practical 3D Echocardiography*, https://doi.org/10.1007/978-3-030-72941-7_8

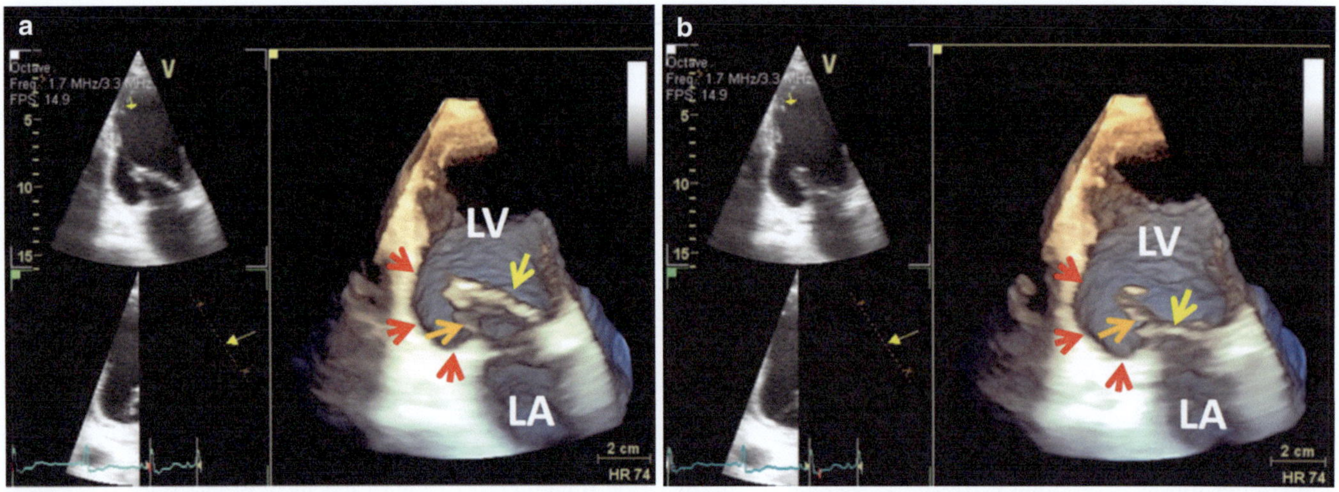

Fig. 8.1 Mechanism of IMR on 3D TTE; Orange arrow points to PML and yellow arrow points to AML (**a**) Valve tenting. (**b**) Tethered PML with AML override. Note the adjacent aneurysmal basal myocardial segment (red arrows). Used with permission of Mayo Foundation for Medical Education and Research. All rights reserved. AML, anterior mitral leaflet; IMR, ischemic mitral regurgitation; LA, left atrium; LV, left ventricle; PML, posterior mitral leaflet

are present [6–8]. 3DE overcomes this limitation by permitting direct planimetry of the vena contracta area (VCA) which in fluid mechanics corresponds to the EROA [7], regardless of orifice shape or number of jets (Figs. 8.3 and 8.4) [6, 7].

Compared with MRI, quantification of mitral EROA and regurgitant volume with 3D TEE is accurate and results in less underestimation of the regurgitant volume as compared with 2D TEE [9].

Notwithstanding the aforementioned merits of 3D, both 2D and 3D color flow Doppler tend to overestimate the regurgitant orifice area because of their inability to resolve the high velocity jet core due to aliasing and blooming artifacts (see Figs. 8.3 and 8.4) [6, 8]. FMR severity also varies during the cardiac cycle, and can peak in early or late systole, further complicating evaluation, which is traditionally done in mid-systole. There is also marked variability of shape, size, and number of VCAs on real time 3D color Doppler [6, 8]. Another important obstacle to 3D assessment of MR severity remains the limited temporal and spatial resolution of 3D color Doppler data.

For all the aforementioned reasons, 3D derived VCA has not yet become part of routine clinical practice, and there are no agreed upon cut off values for VCA for severe FMR. Therefore, more studies are needed, and because at present, no single parameter is sufficient to quantify the degree of FMR, multimodality assessment including both 2D and 3D echocardiography is optimal [5–8].

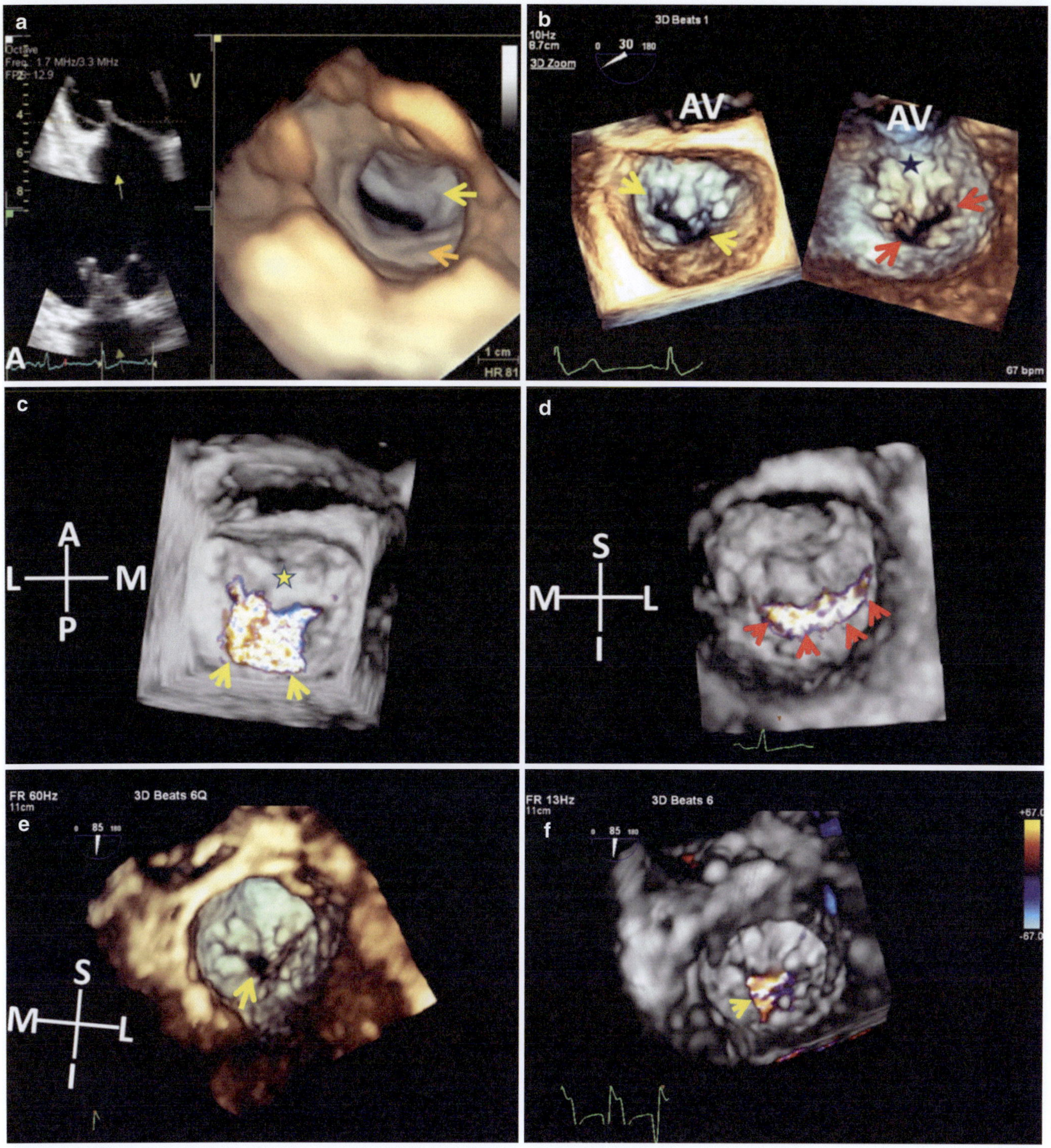

Fig. 8.2 **Top panel**: (**a**) Live 3D TTE LA view from patient with IMR in Fig. 8.1 showing lack of MV leaflet coaptation in systole (yellow arrow points to AML and orange arrow points to PML). (**b**) Live TEE 3D Zoom simultaneous dual layout enface LA (left) and LV (right) systolic views of MV in a patient with FMR due to non-ischemic cardiomyopathy. Note the lack of leaflet coaptation (arrows), star points to AML; **Middle panel**: 3D TEE CFD enface LA (**c**) and LV (**d**) views from another patient with FMR. (**a**) MR jet fans out in the LA (yellow arrows), star points to AML. (**b**) LV view shows that MR spans the entire mitral valve coaptation surface (red arrows). **Bottom panel**: (**e**) Multibeat 3D TEE FV enface LV views of FMR in a patient with a tethered P2 segment of the PML resulting in localized central malcoaptation of the MV (arrow). (**f**) 3D CFD in same patient showing MR through the localized malcoaptation site (arrow). Note the drop in volume rate or frame rate from 60 to 13 when color flow Doppler is added. Also note that regardless of etiology, the origin of MR is best appreciated from the enface LV perspective. Used with permission of Mayo Foundation for Medical Education and Research. All rights reserved. A, anterior; AML, anterior mitral leaflet; AV, aortic valve; CFD, color flow Doppler; FMR, functional mitral regurgitation; FV, Full Volume; I, inferior; IMR, ischemic mitral regurgitation; L, lateral; LA, left atrium; LV, left ventricular; M, medial; MR, mitral regurgitation; MV, mitral valve; P, posterior; PML, posterior mitral leaflet; S, superior; TEE, transesophageal echocardiography; TTE, transthoracic echocardiography

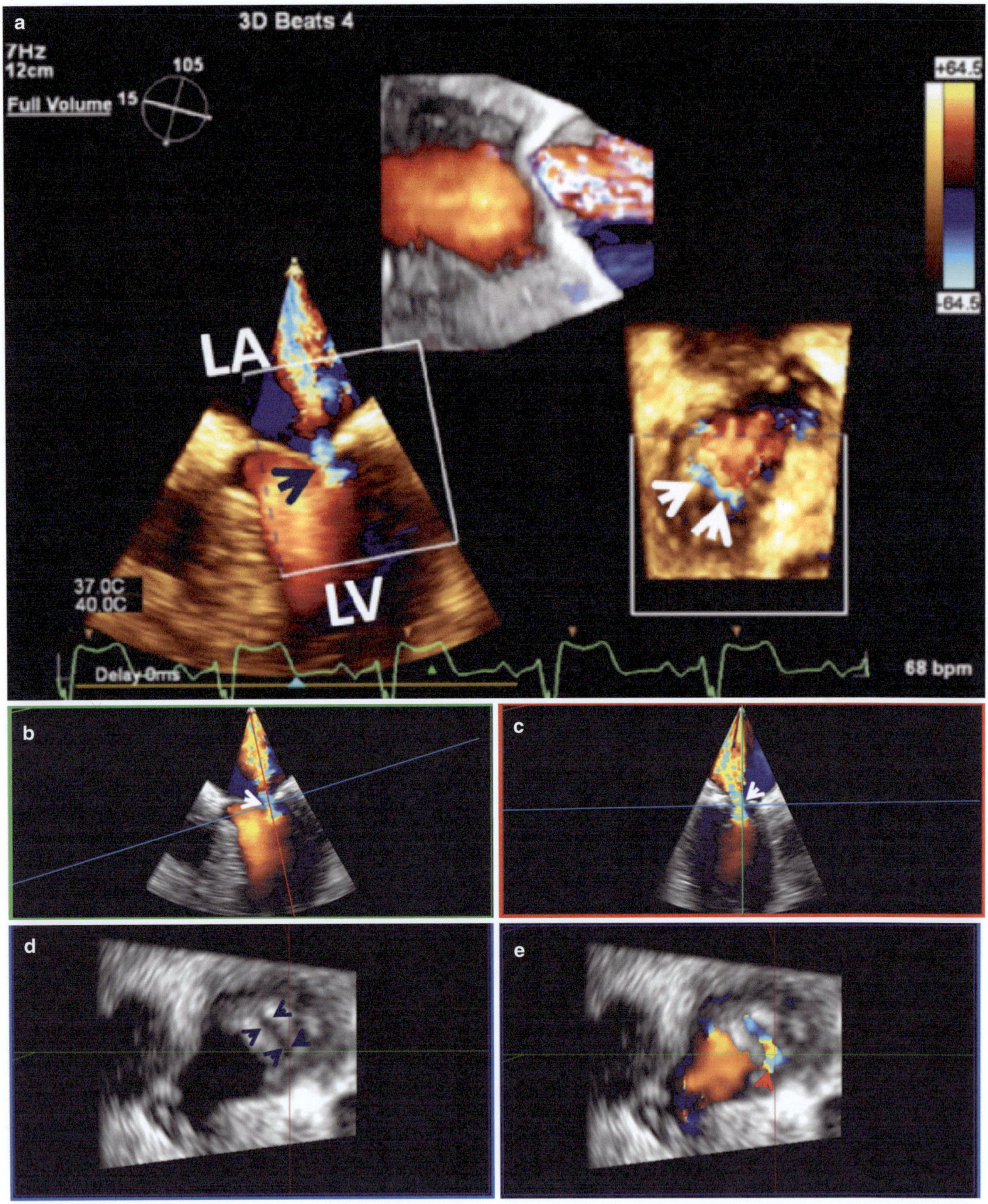
a
3D Beats 4
7Hz
12cm
105
15
Full Volume
+64.5
-64.5
LA
LV
37.0C
40.0C
Delay 0ms
68 bpm
b
c
d
e

Fig. 8.3 MR VC. (**a**) iCrop (Philips Healthcare) of multibeat 3D FV CFD showing a narrow VC when viewed sideways from the mid-esophagus (dark blue arrow) as opposed to a broad based VC that spans the entire MV coaptation surface (white arrows) when viewed enface from the LV perspective on the orthogonal MPR plane. (**b–e**) MPR of 3D CFD volumetric data set. (**b**) Alignment of the transverse plane (blue line) and orthogonal sagittal plane (red line) at VC (white arrow) in the coronal plane (Green rectangle). (**c**) Alignment of the transverse plane (blue line) and orthogonal coronal plane (green line) at VC (white arrow) in the sagittal plane (red rectangle). (**d**) elliptical shaped VC (dark blue arrows) as it appears in the transverse plane (Blue rectangle) with color Doppler off. (**e**) Same VC with CFD on. Note the slight color bleed beyond the anatomic boundaries of the VC cross-sectional area (red arrow) due to blooming artifact. Used with permission of Mayo Foundation for Medical Education and Research. CFD, color flow Doppler; EROA, effective regurgitant orifice area; FV, Full Volume; LA, left atrium; LV, left ventricle; MPR, multiplanar reconstruction; MR, mitral regurgitation; MV, mitral valve; VC, vena contracta

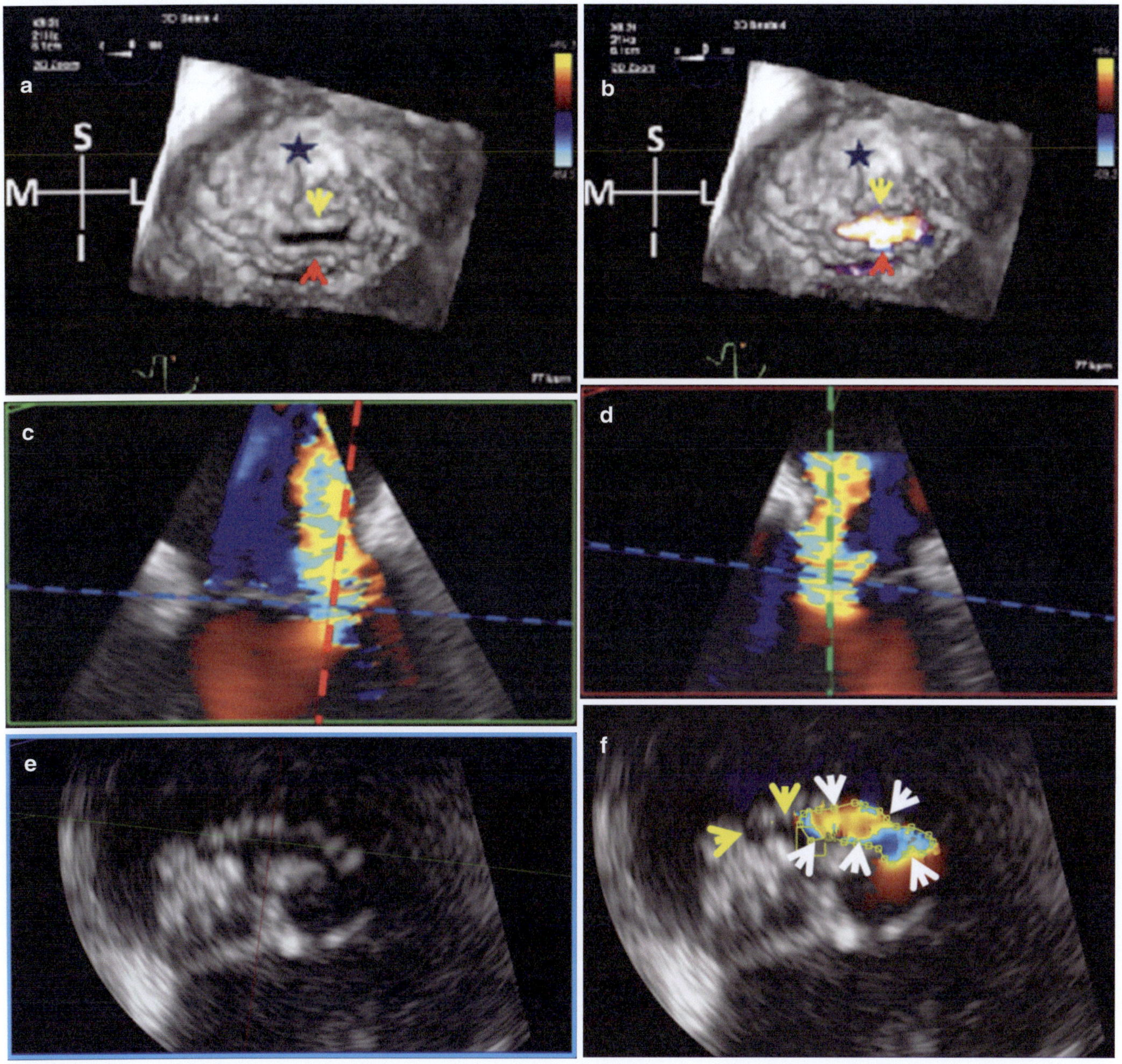

Fig. 8.4 (**a**) Multibeat TEE 3D Zoom enface LV views from a patient with FMR showing lack of anterior (yellow arrow) and posterior (red arrow) leaflet coapation. (**b**) secondary MR on CFD (star points to LVOT). (**c–f**) MPR of 3D CFD volumetric data set from same patient. (**c**) coronal plane (green rectangle) showing alignment of the transverse plane (blue line) and sagittal plane (red line) with the narrowest region of the MR jet just downstream to the orifice of the MV. (**d**) sagittal or vertical plane (red rectangle) and similar alignment of the transverse plane (blue line) and coronal plane (green line). (**e**) The resultant VC cross sectional area with color Doppler suppressed. (**f**) VC with CFD on. Note the dropout artifacts that are not covered by the CFD map (yellow arrows). Also note that the VC area measurement is limited to the high velocity core of the jet (white arrows). Used with permission of Mayo Foundation for Medical Education and Research. CFD, color flow Doppler; FMR, functional mitral regurgitation; I, inferior; M, medial; MPR, multiplanar reconstruction, MR, mitral regurgitation; L, lateral; LV, left ventricle, LVOT, left ventricular outflow tract; S, superior; VC, vena contracta

References

1. Asgar AW, Mack MJ, Stone GW. Secondary mitral regurgitation in heart failure: pathophysiology, prognosis, and therapeutic considerations. J Am Coll Cardiol. 2015;65(12):1231–48.
2. Saito K, Okura H, Watanabi N, et al. Influence of chronic tethering of the mitral valve on mitral leaflet size and coaptation in functional mitral regurgitation. J Am Coll Cardiol Imaging. 2012;5:337–45.
3. Silbiger JJ. Anatomy, mechanics, and pathophysiology of the mitral annulus. Am Heart J. 2012;164(2):163–76.
4. Buck T, Plicht B. Real-time three-dimensional echocardiographic assessment of severity of mitral regurgitation using proximal isovelocity surface area and vena contracta area method. Lessons we learned and clinical implications. Curr Cardiovasc Imaging Rep. 2015;8:38.
5. Oh JK, Kane GC, Seward JB, Tajik AJ. The echo manual. 4th ed. Philadelphia: Wolters Kluwer; 2019.
6. de Agustın JA, Marcos-Alberca P, Fernandez-Golfin C, et al. Direct measurement of proximal isovelocity surface area by single-beat three-dimensional color Doppler echocardiography in mitral regurgitation: a validation study. J Am Soc Echocardiogr. 2012;25:815–23.
7. Goebel B, Heck R, Hamadanchi A, Otto S, Doenst T, Jung C, Lauten A, Figulla HR, Schulze PC, Poerner TC. Vena contracta area for severity grading in functional and degenerative mitral regurgitation: a transoesophageal 3D colour Doppler analysis in 500 patients. Eur Heart J Cardiovasc Imaging. 2018;19(6):639–46.
8. Marsan NA, Westenberg JJ, Ypenburg C, Delgado V, van Bommel RJ, Roes SD, Nucifora G, van der Geest RJ, de Roos A, Reiber JC, Schalij MJ, Bax JJ. Quantification of functional mitral regurgitation by real-time 3D echocardiography: comparison with 3D velocity-encoded cardiac magnetic resonance. JACC Cardiovasc Imaging. 2009;2(11):1245–52.
9. Shanks M, Siebelink H-MJ, Delgado V, van de Veire NRL, Ng ACT, Sieders A, Schuijf JD, Lamb HJ, Ajmone Marsan N, Westenberg JJM, Kroft LJ, de Roos A, Bax JJ. Comparison between three-dimensional transesophageal echocardiography and magnetic resonance imaging. Circ Cardiovasc Imaging. 2010;3:694–700.

9 Incremental Value of 3DE over 2DE in Assessment of Mitral Clefts and Other Congenital Mitral Valve Diseases

Joseph F. Maalouf and Francesco F. Faletra

The mitral valve (MV) has only two leaflets. The anterior leaflet is large and semicircular and forms part of the outflow tract. The posterior mitral leaflet is more shallow and is typically divided into three scallops (i.e. P1, P2, and P3) with the middle scallop (P2) usually the largest of the three [1]. Commissural chords arise from each papillary muscle and extend in a fan-like array to insert into the free edge of both leaflets adjacent to the major commissures or into two adjacent scallops of the posterior leaflet (minor commissures) [1]. Normal posterior leaflet interscallop indentations formed by the minor commissures are superficial and do not affect mitral valve closure [1] (Fig. 9.1).

Congenital clefts divide one leaflet into two and may or may not reach the level of the annulus. Unlike commissures, congenital clefts have no papillary muscles beneath them and no chordal insertions along their edge [1]. Anterior mitral leaflet cleft is an unusual congenital lesion that may be a cause of severe mitral regurgitation (MR), and is most often encountered in association with other congenital heart defects [1, 2]. Isolated anterior leaflet cleft (Fig. 9.2) is a rare anomaly that can be wide and extend to the mitral annulus or only a few millimeters deep [2–4]. A similar congenital cleft has been rarely described in the posterior leaflet of the mitral valve [2] and even more rarely involving both leaflets [5]. The diagnosis of MV cleft using two- dimensional (2D) echocardiography is particularly challenging [6]. With three-dimensional (3D) echocardiography, the anatomy of congenital mitral valve clefts can be readily displayed in multiple views [6, 7] including the position, shape, longitudinal diameter, and width of the cleft as well as the spatial position between the chordae tendineae surrounding the cleft and the aortic valve [6, 7].

The term cleft is also commonly used to describe deep divisions or indentations between posterior leaflet scallops at site of minor commissures [1, 7] that may or may not be associated with MR, and are most commonly seen in myxomatous mitral valve disease [8, 9]. On 3D echocardiography, such clefts typically extend at least one half of the depth of the adjacent mitral leaflet and may be seen during systole and diastole [9]. Distinguishing these cleft like indentations from congenital posterior leaflet clefts on 3D echocardiography may not be possible, however, particularly when the MV is otherwise normal and there is no associated MR (Fig. 9.3). These anatomic differences notwithstanding, recognition of clefts causing MR (Figs. 9.4 and 9.5) is important prior to surgical or percutaneous MV repair because they are a relative contraindication to percutaneous MV repair and for patients undergoing surgical MV repair, such clefts can be easily missed in a flaccid non beating heart, and therefore, can be the cause of significant residual post operative MR.

Gaps (Fig. 9.6) are congenital abnormal spaces between two leaflets, often at the usual site of a major commissure [1].

3D TEE can also be very useful in the diagnosis of other more complex congenital MV pathologies (Fig. 9.7).

Supplementary Information The online version of this chapter (https://doi.org/10.1007/978-3-030-72941-7_9) contains supplementary material, which is available to authorized users.

J. F. Maalouf (✉)
Professor of Medicine, Mayo Clinic College of Medicine; Director, Interventional Echocardiography; Consultant, Department of Cardiovascular Medicine, Mayo Clinic, Rochester, MN, USA
e-mail: maalouf.joseph@mayo.edu

F. F. Faletra
Director of Cardiac Imaging Lab, Cardiocentro Ticino Institute, Lugano, Switzerland
e-mail: Francesco.Faletra@cardiocentro.org

J. F. Maalouf et al. (eds.), *Practical 3D Echocardiography*, https://doi.org/10.1007/978-3-030-72941-7_9

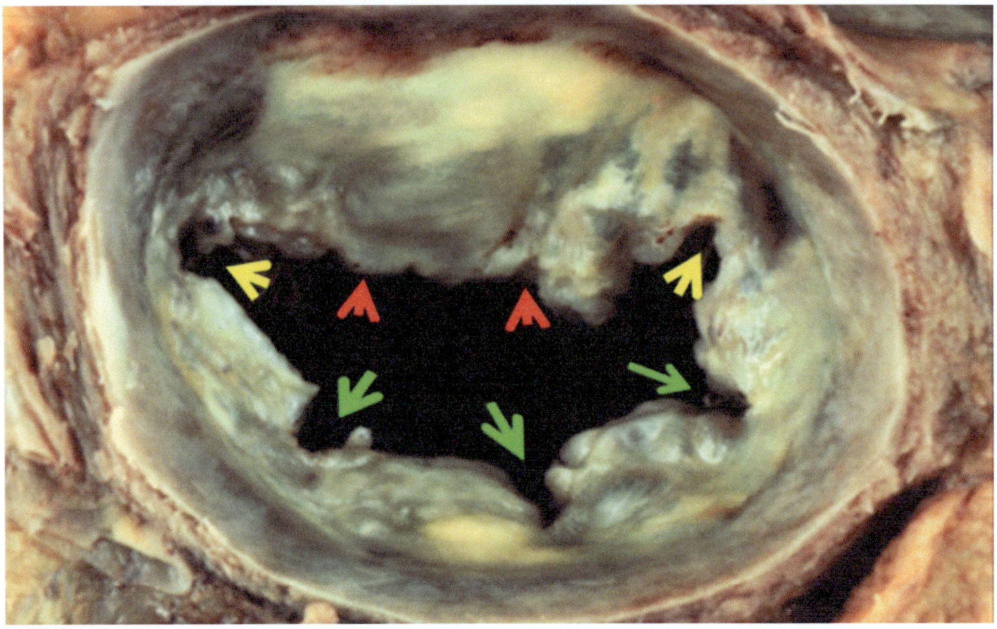

Fig. 9.1 Mitral valve, viewed from left atrium showing the two major commissures (yellow arrows) and three minor commissures between adjacent posterior leaflet scallops (green arrows). The red arrows point to the anterior leaflet. With permission from McGraw-Hill, Hurst's The Heart, 2017, Maalouf et al., Chapter 4 Functional Anatomy of the Heart

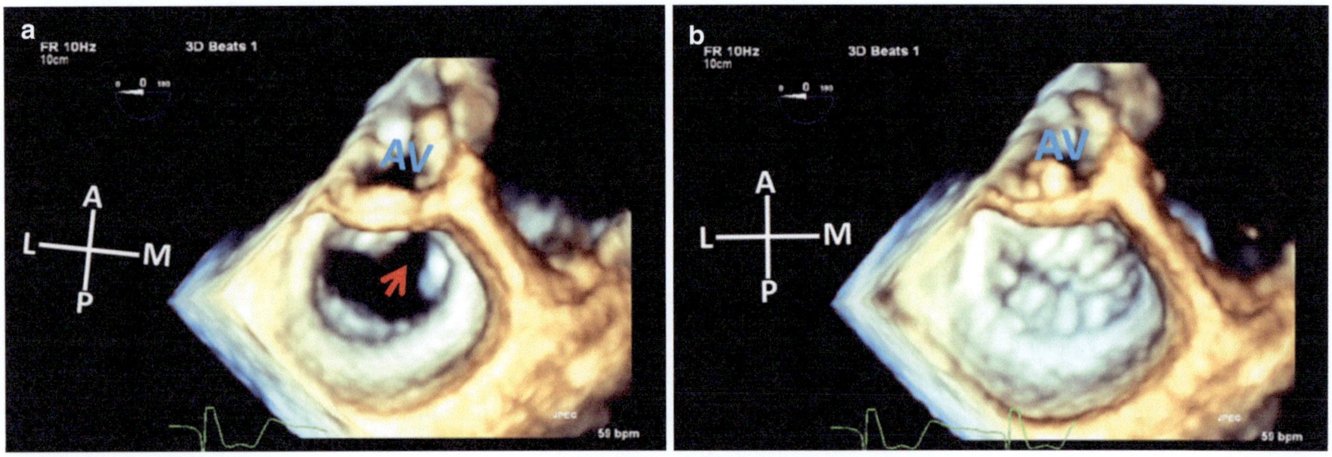

Fig. 9.2 Real time 3D TEE enface LA views of the MV in diastole (**a**) and systole (**b**). Red arrow points to a wide congenital AML cleft. Note that the cleft is not seen in systole and the MV was competent. A, anterior; AML, anterior mitral leaflet; AV, aortic valve; L, lateral; M, medial; MV, mitral valve, P, posterior. Used with permission of Mayo Foundation for Medical Education and Research.

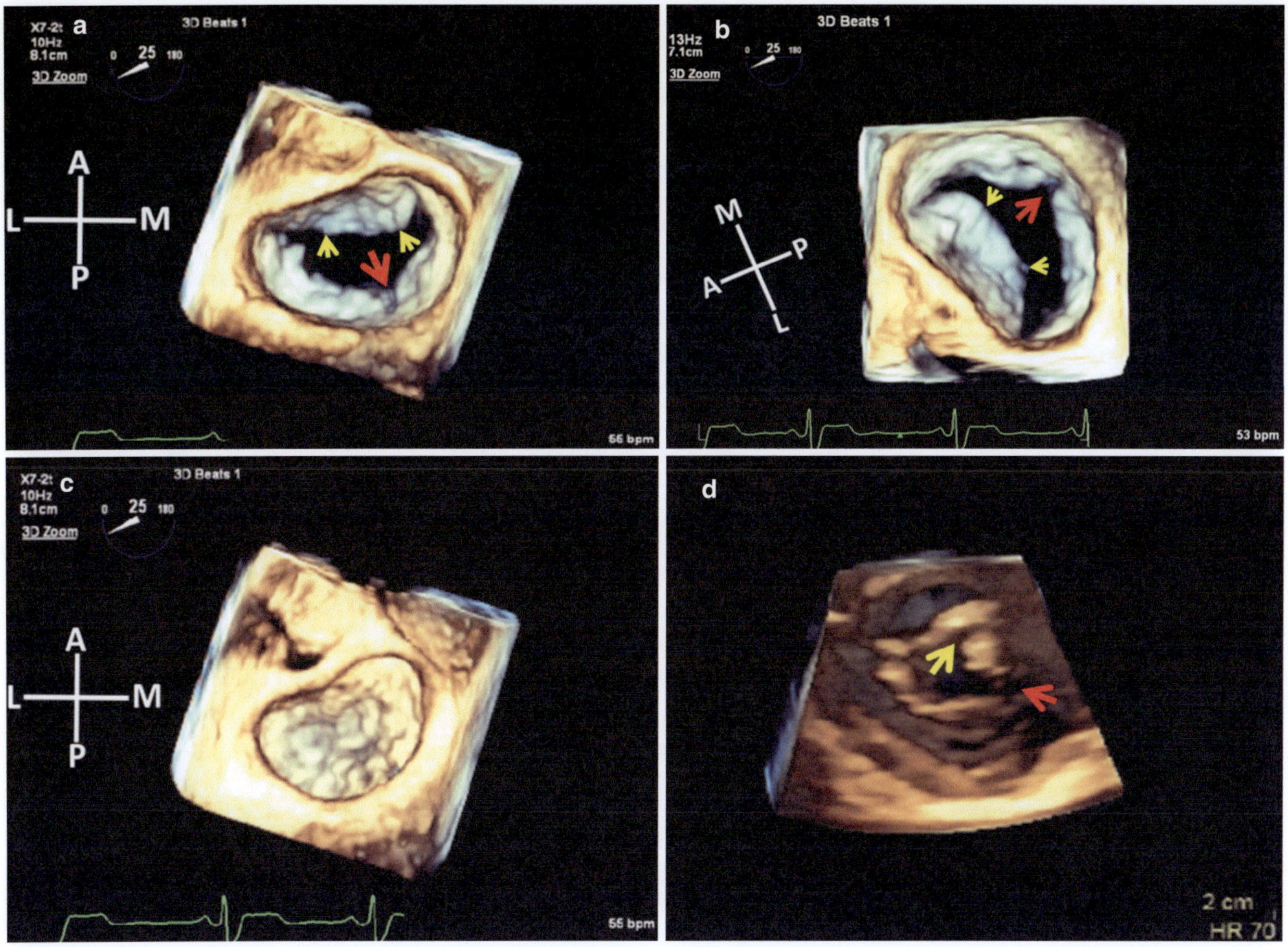

Fig. 9.3 (**a**, **b**) 3D zoom TEE enface LA views of a PML "cleft" in diastole. A deep indentation between P2 and P3 (red arrow) is seen in two views. Yellow arrows point to AML. (**c**) Same view in systole. The cleft like indentation is no longer seen. (**d**) 3D TTE LV view of mitral valve in another patient with an isolated PML "cleft" (red arrow). Yellow arrow points to the lateral commissure. The MV in both cases was otherwise normal. Used with permission of Mayo Foundation for Medical Education and Research. All rights reserved. A, anterior; AML, anterior mitral leaflet; L, lateral; LA, left atrium; LV, left ventricle; M, medial; MV, mitral valve; P, posterior; PML, posterior mitral leaflet

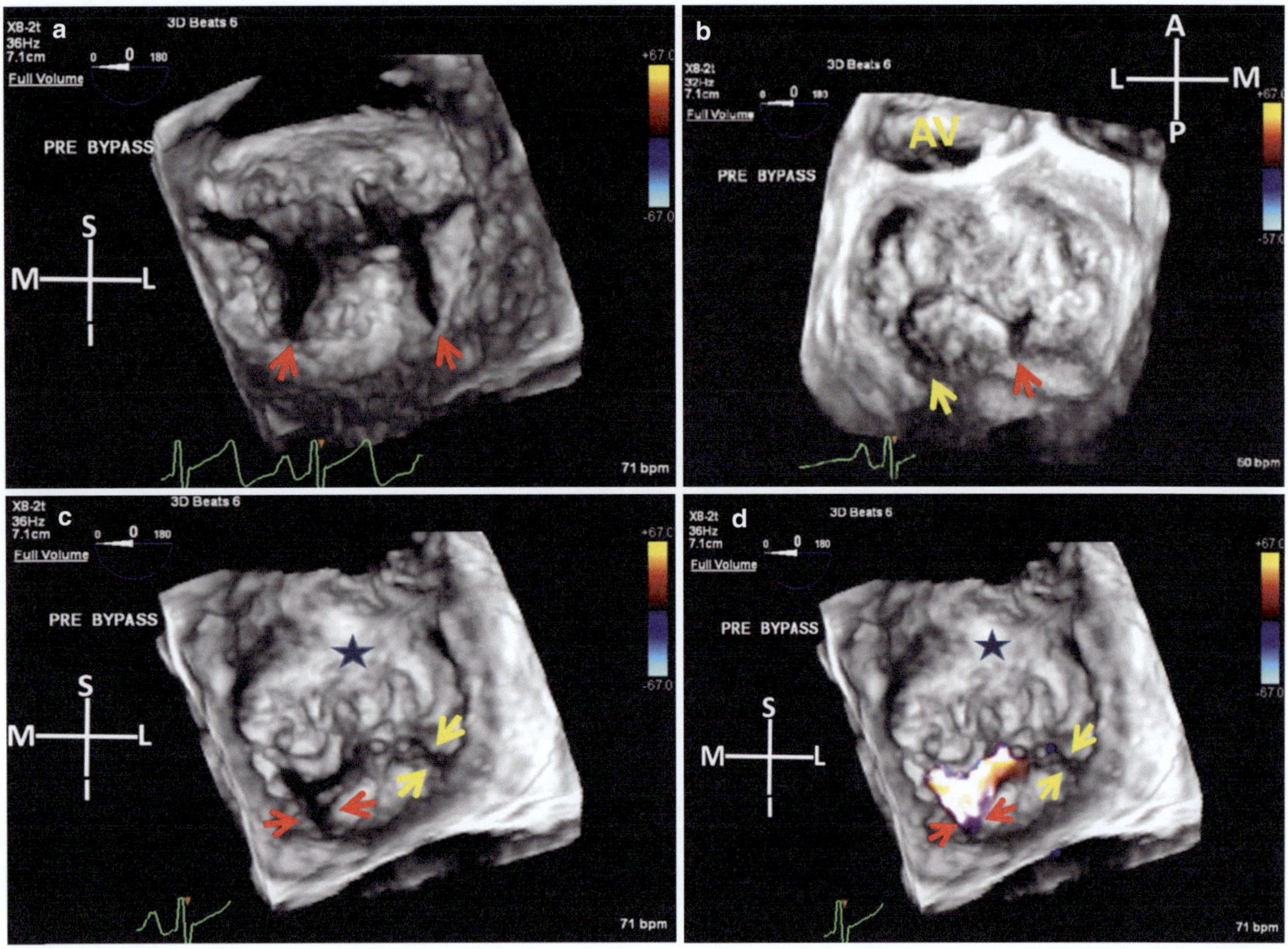

Fig. 9.4 **Top panel**: 3D TEE FV CFD with color suppress enface LV view of the MV in diastole (**a**) and LA view in systole (**b**) in a patient with severely myxomatous bileaflet MVP undergoing surgical MV repair. Two PML clefts at sites of minor commissures (red arrows) are clearly seen in diastole (**a**). In systole (**b**), the medial cleft (red arrow) is still seen but the the lateral cleft (yellow arrow) is less apparent. **Bottom panel**: Enface 3D CFD FV LV views of the MV in systole from same patient. With color suppress on (**c**) the medial (red arrows) and lateral (yellow arrows) clefts are delineated, but on turing color Doppler on (**d**) MR is only seen through the medial cleft (red arrows). Star points to the LVOT. Used with permission of Mayo Foundation for Medical Education and Research. All rights reserved. A, anterior; AV, aortic valve; CFD, color flow Doppler; FV, Full Volume, I, inferior; L, lateral; LA, left atrium; LV, left ventricle; LVOT, left ventricular outflow tract; M, medial; MR, mitral regurgitation; MV, mitral valve; MVP, mitral valve prolapse; P, posterior; PML, posterior mitral leaflet; S, superior

Fig. 9.5 **Top panel**: (**a**) 3D TEE FV enface dual lay out LA and LV views of the MV in systole in a patient with endocarditis complicated by windsock mycotic aneurysm of the AML (green arrow). A P2–P3 PML cleft, red arrows LA view, and blue arrows LV view is seen. (**b**) 3D TEE FV enface LV view with CFD from same patient in systole shows MR originating from within the cleft (red arrows). The stars in both images point to the LVOT. Images **a** and **b** used with permission of Mayo Foundation for Medical Education and Research. All rights reserved. **Middle panel**: (**c**) 3D TEE FV enface LA view in a patient with flail P2 segment (star) and two ruptured chords (yellow arrows) who on intraoperative TEE was found to have a deep cleft at P1–P2 that reached the annulus and that was missed on 2D TEE. (**d**) 3D TEE FV CFD showing significant MR originating within the cleft (red arrow). Yellow arrow points to regurgitation caused by the flail P2 segment. **Bottom panel**: The deep P1–P2 cleft (yellow arrows) as viewed by the surgeon intraoperatively when open (**e**) and closed (**f**). Permission for images **c**, **d**, and **e** from McGraw-Hill, Hurst's The Heart, 2017, Maalouf et al., Chapter 4 Functional Anatomy of the Heart. A, anterior; AML, anterior mitral leaflet; AV, aortic valve; CFD, color flow Doppler; FV, Full Volume; I, inferior; L, lateral; LA, left atrial; LV, left ventricular; LVOT, left ventricular outflow tract; M, medial; MR, mitral regurgitation; MV, mitral valve; MVP, mitral valve prolapse; P, posterior; P1, lateral posterior leaflet scallop; P2, middle posterior leaflet scallop; P3, medial posterior leaflet scallop; PML, posterior mitral leaflet; S, superior

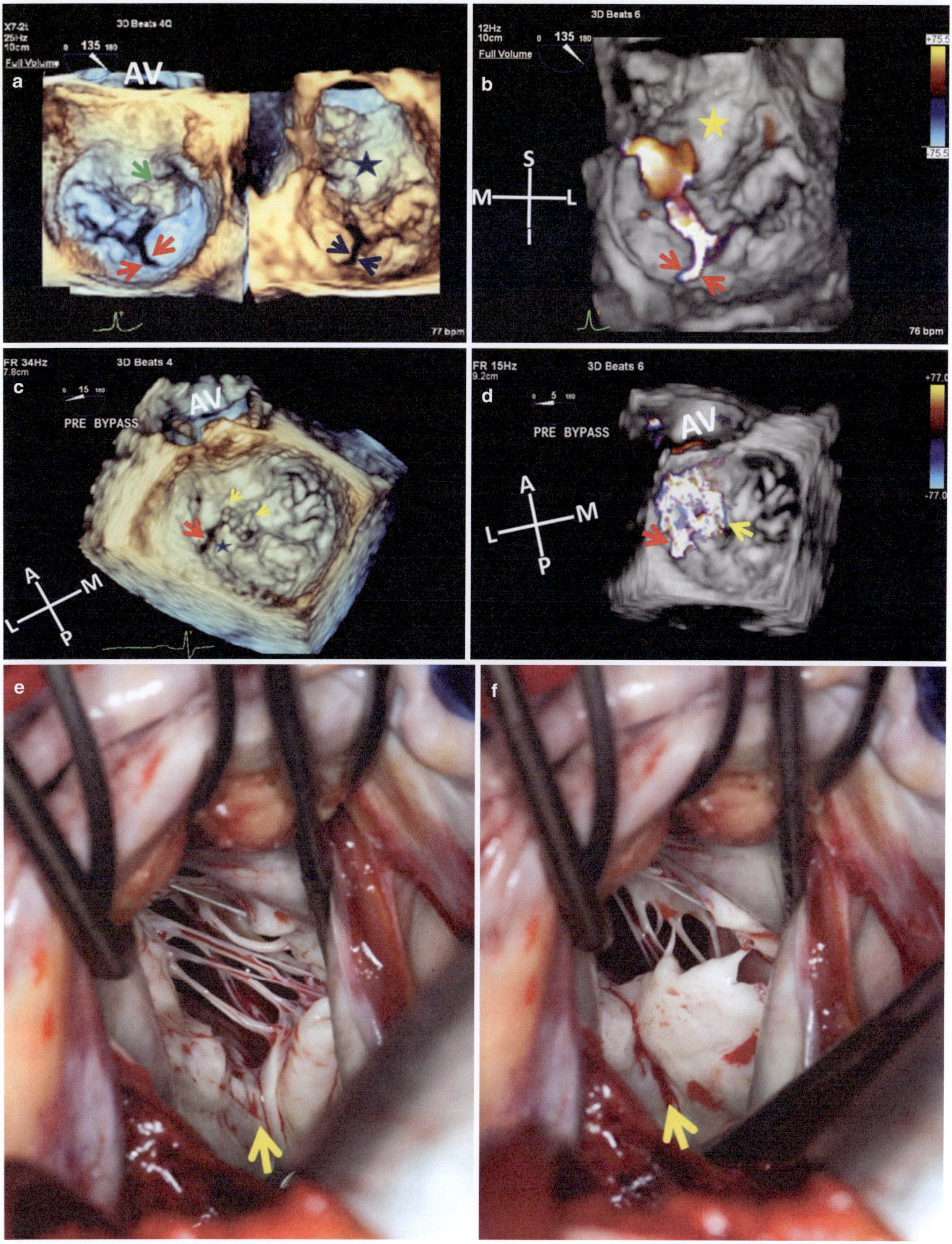
a
3D Beats 4Q
X7-2t
25Hz
10cm
Full Volume
0 135 180
AV
77 bpm
b
3D Beats 6
12Hz
10cm
Full Volume
0 135 180
S
M
L
I
+75.5
-75.5
76 bpm
c
FR 34Hz
7.8cm
3D Beats 4
0 15 180
PRE BYPASS
AV
A
M
L
P
d
FR 15Hz
9.2cm
3D Beats 6
0 5 180
PRE BYPASS
AV
A
M
L
P
+77.0
-77.0
e
f

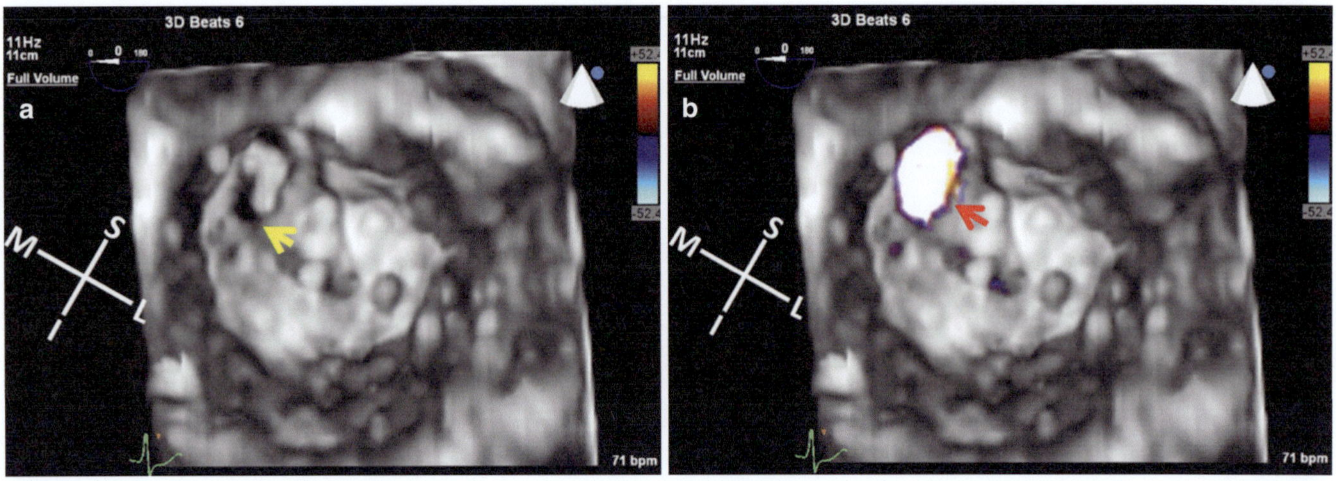

Fig. 9.6 3D TEE FV enface LV views of the MV in a patient with a medial gap at site of major commissure (**a**, yellow arrow). (**b**) MR through the gap on CFD (red arrow). Used with permission of Mayo Foundation for Medical Education and Research. All rights reserved. CFD, color flow Doppler; FV, Full Volume; I inferior; L, lateral; LV, left ventricular; M, medial; MR, mitral regurgitation; MV, mitral valve; S, superior

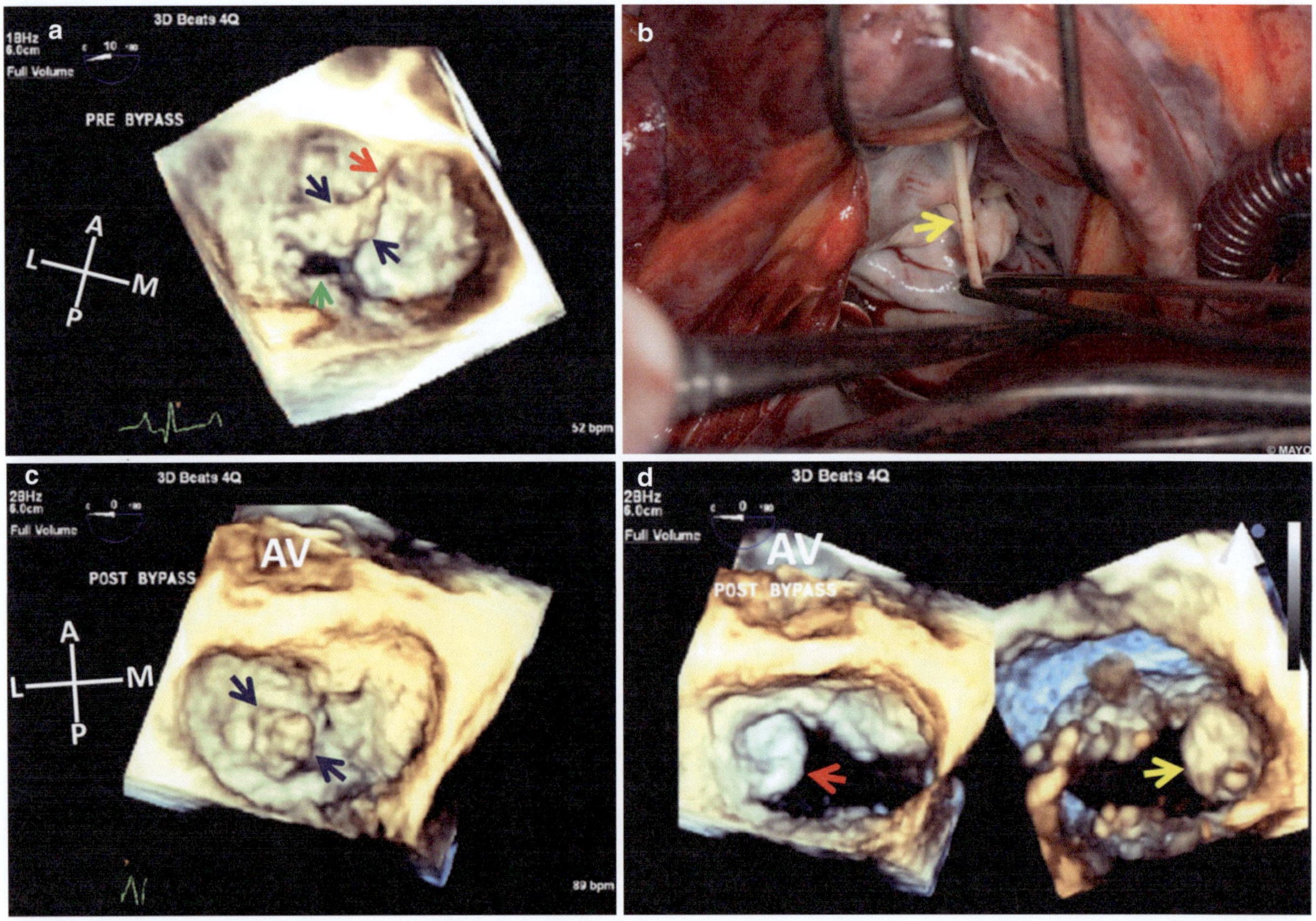

Fig. 9.7 **Top panel**: (**a**) 3D TEE FV enface LA view of the MV in a patient with AMVT [10] showing hammock-like appearance (blue arrows) of the AMVT at P1 scallop created by an anomalous chordal attachment (red arrow) with a resulting coaptation defect (green arrow). (**b**) Intraoperative photograph of the anomalous chord that extended from the PM papillary muscle through the MV, attaching to dome of the anterior wall of the left atrium. **Bottom panel**: (**c**) 3D TEE FV enface LA systolic view in same patient following resection of the anomalous chord showing retracted AMVT (blue arrows). (**d**) Post operative diastolic 3D TEE FV dual layout views showing the residual AMVT from the LA (red arrow) and LV (yellow arrow) perspectives. Images **c** and **d** used with permission of Mayo Foundation for Medical Education and Research. All rights reserved. A, anterior; AMVT, accessory mitral valve tissue; AV, aortic valve; FV, Full Volume; L, lateral; LA, left atrium; LV, left ventricle; M, medial; MV, mitral valve; P, posterior; P1, lateral posterior mitral leaflet scallop; PM, posteromedial

References

1. Malouf JF, Maleszewski JJ, Tajik AJ, Seward JB. Section 2: Foundations of cardiovascular medicine, Chapter 4: Functional anatomy of the heart. In: Fuster V, Harrington RA, Narula J, Eapen ZJ, editors. Hurst the heart. 14th ed. New York: McGraw-Hill; 2017.
2. Diqi Z, et al. Isolated cleft of the mitral valve: clinical spectrum and course. Texas Heart Inst J. 2009;36(6):553–6.
3. Minardi G, et al. An Isolated anterior mitral leaflet cleft: a case report. Cardiovasc Ultrasound. 2010;8:26.
4. Timoteo A, et al. Isolated cleft of the anterior mitral value leaflet. Eur Soc Cardiol. 2005;8(1):59–62.
5. Mohammadi S, et al. Mitral valve cleft in both anterior and posterior leaflet: an extremely rare anomaly. Ann Thorac Surg. 2006;82:2287–9.
6. Narang A, Addetia K, Weinert L, Yamat M, Shah AP, Blair JE, Mor-Avi V, Lang RM. Diagnosis of isolated cleft mitral valve using three-dimensional echocardiography. J Am Soc Echocardiogr. 2018;31(11):1161–7.
7. Xinchun Y, et al. Diagnosis of mitral valve cleft using real-time 3-dimensional echocardiography. J Thorac Dis. 2017;9(1):159–65.
8. Mantovani F, Clavel MA, Vatury O, Suri RM, Mankad SV, Malouf J, Michelena HI, Jain S, Badano LP, Enriquez-Sarano M. Cleft-like indentations in myxomatous mitral valves by three-dimensional echocardiographic imaging. Heart. 2015;101(14):1111–7.
9. Ring L, Rana BS, Ho SY, Wells FC. The prevalence and impact of deep clefts in the mitral leaflets in mitral valve prolapse. Eur Heart J Cardiovasc Imaging. 2013;14(6):595–602.
10. Gurrieri C, Nelson J, Wurm H, Cicek MS, Maalouf JF. An extremely rare cause of mitral regurgitation-accessory commissural mitral tissue with anomalous left atrial chordal attachment. CASE (Phila). 2019;3(5):200–3.

3D Color Flow Doppler Assessment of Mitral Regurgitation: Advantages over 2D Color Doppler

10

Jeremy J. Thaden and Joseph F. Maalouf

Introduction

Mitral regurgitation (MR) is among the most common valve lesions encountered in clinical practice [1]. Echocardiography remains the most common imaging modality for assessment. Multiple parameters are available for assessment of MR, but many are subjective resulting in uncertainty and variability in grading the severity of MR. Echocardiographic quantitation of MR by proximal isovelocity surface area (PISA) improves diagnostic certainty [2] and has important prognostic implications [3] but also has important limitations. In select cases, 3D TEE with color Doppler imaging can provide alternative or supplemental quantitative data that provides a better understanding of MR severity [4, 5]. In this chapter we will review the basic technique for calculation of 3D vena contracta area (VCA) using 3D TEE with color Doppler imaging and specific situations where there may be incremental value over 2DE techniques.

Measurement of 3D VCA

Acquisition of a high quality 3D with color Doppler acquisition is the first step for measurement of 3D VCA for assessment of MR. A minimum frame rate of 12–15 Hz is ideal for analysis depending on patient heart rate, faster heart rates may dictate the need for increased frame rates. Ideally, measurements should be performed on single beat or live acquisitions and not on multi-beat volumes. Multi-beat volumes and associated stitch artifacts have the potential to introduce error at the time of planimetry. Frame rate can ideally be optimized by reducing 3D sector width or height or by narrowing the 3D color box to the region of interest. Color Doppler aliasing velocity should be set to 50–70 cm/s. 3D gain should be set in the mid range because higher 3D gain can result in underestimation of the 3D VCA (Fig. 10.1). Color Doppler gain should generally be set just below the noise threshold. Figure 10.2 shows an example of a 3D VCA measurement using multiplanar reconstruction (MPR) in a patient with severe secondary MR.

Step-by-Step Instructions for 3D-Guided Measurement of VCA

1. Acquire a high quality 3D with color Doppler volume (single beat acquisition preferred).
2. Open the volume with available quantitative software package.
3. Select the frame for measurement, ideally around mid-systole for timing and using a frame where the regurgitant jet and orifice are well seen.
4. Designate the plane that will be used for planimetry of the VCA. Use the other two planes to align with the narrowest neck of the regurgitant jet (the vena contracta) in the two orthogonal views (Fig. 10.2). Note that arranging the two orthogonal views as a typical long axis view and commissural view is frequently helpful for orientation and to facilitate measurement (Fig. 10.2).
5. Perform planimetry of the VCA in the short axis view (Fig. 10.2).

J. J. Thaden (✉)
Assistant Professor of Medicine, Mayo Clinic College of Medicine; Co-Chair for Clinical Practice and Quality, Division of Cardiovascular Ultrasound; Consultant, Department of Cardiovascular Medicine, Mayo Clinic, Rochester, MN, USA
e-mail: Thaden.Jeremy@mayo.edu

J. F. Maalouf
Professor of Medicine, Mayo Clinic College of Medicine; Director, Interventional Echocardiography; Consultant, Department of Cardiovascular Medicine, Mayo Clinic, Rochester, MN, USA
e-mail: maalouf.joseph@mayo.edu

J. F. Maalouf et al. (eds.), *Practical 3D Echocardiography*, https://doi.org/10.1007/978-3-030-72941-7_10

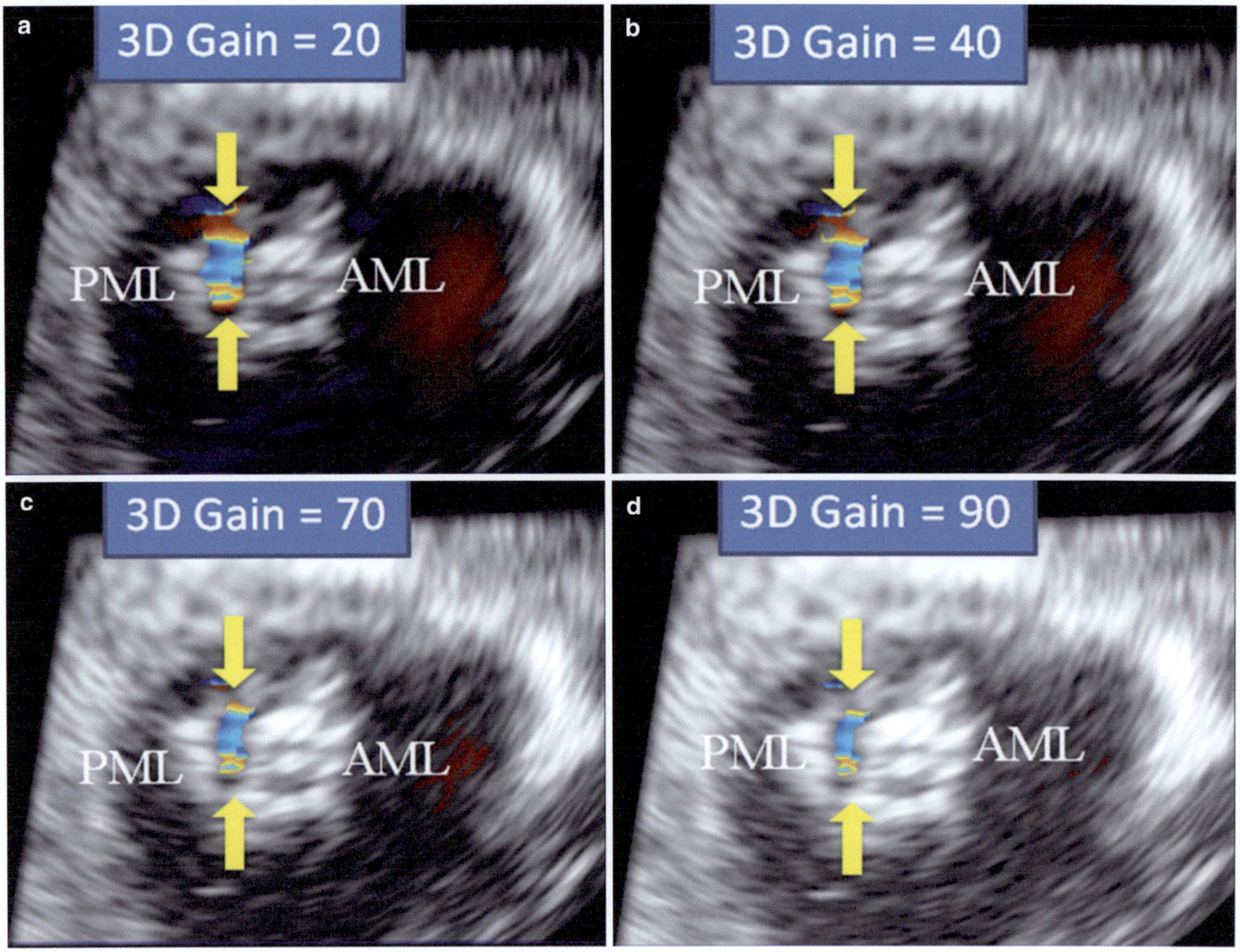

Fig. 10.1 Short axis view of the 3D VCA at various 3D gain settings. A short axis view in the same frame, mid-systole, is shown at progressively increasing 3D gain settings from panels **a** to **d**. Note the qualitative decrease in size of the vena contracta as 3D gain progressively increases (yellow arrows, panels **a**–**d**). 3D gain should optimally be set in the range of 40–60 for measurement of 3D VCA. Used with permission of Mayo Foundation for Medical Education and Research. All rights reserved. AML, anterior mitral leaflet; PML, posterior mitral leaflet

The Utility of 3D TEE with Color Doppler and VCA in Specific Clinical Scenarios

Correlation of Leaflet Pathology with Regurgitant Jet Origin

MR results from a heterogeneous group of pathologies. The entire mitral valve can be visualized by multiplanar 2D TEE, but particularly for complex mitral valve pathology 3D TEE frequently provides a more robust understanding of the underlying pathology [6]. 3D TEE often provides important incremental information, such as a more precise understanding of the regional leaflet pathology and how it correlates with the origin of the MR jet. Given the current emphasis on surgical mitral valve repair and percutaneous repair strategies, a precise understanding of the mitral valve pathology and the number and location of regurgitant jets is critically important. The left ventricular view of the mitral valve with color Doppler imaging provides a more precise understanding of the number and location of regurgitant jets (Fig. 10.3).

Cumulative 3D VCA in Patients with Multiple MR Jets

3D VCA, compared to PISA assessment, can be useful in patients with multiple MR jets [7]. The assessment of mul-

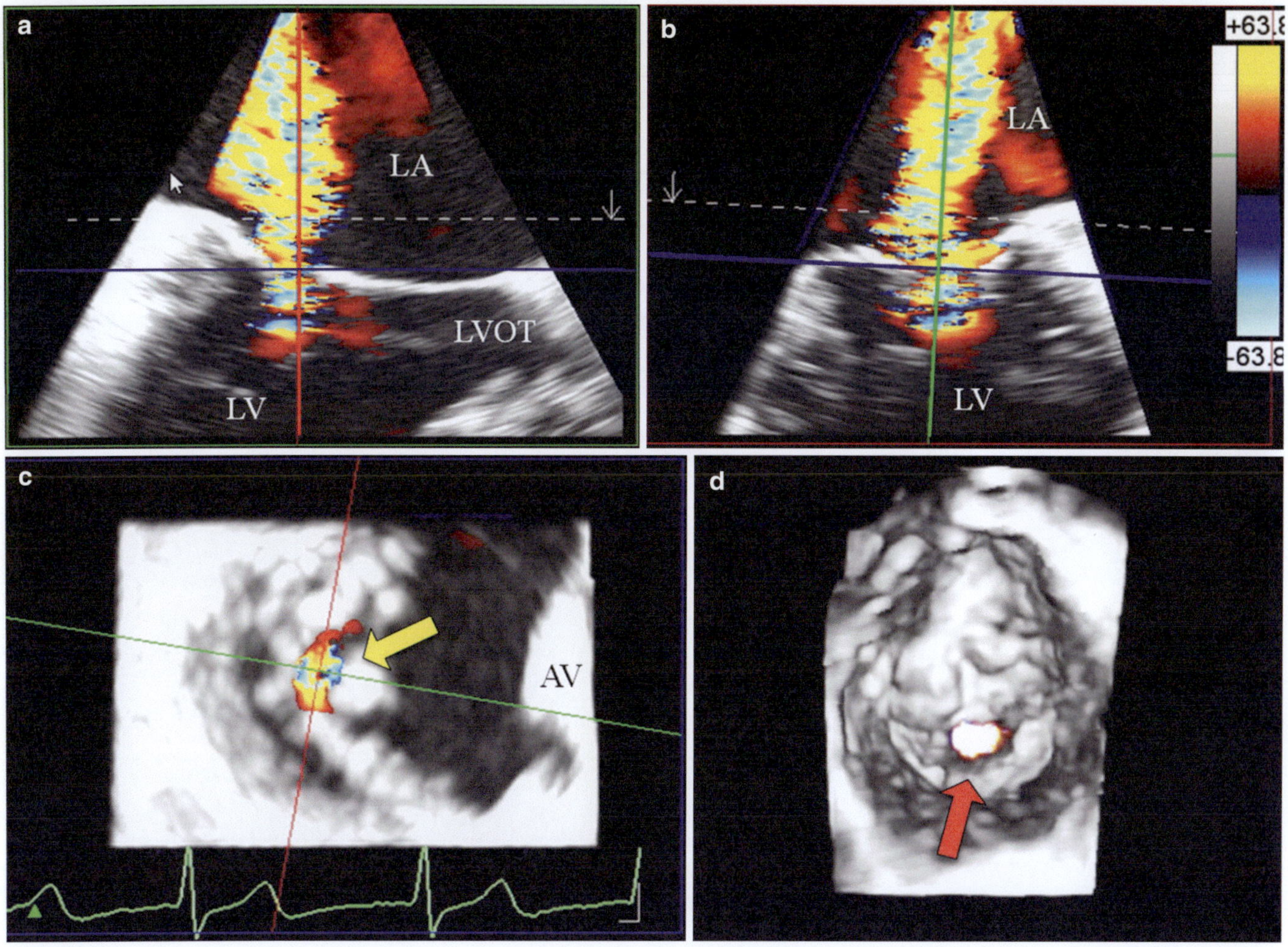

Fig. 10.2 Measurement of 3D-guided VCA using 3D color Doppler imaging with MPR. (**a**) typical long axis view of the mitral valve including a portion of the LVOT. (**b**) Typical commissural view showing the mitral valve in medial to lateral dimension. The blue line is aligned with the narrowest neck of the regurgitant jet (the vena contracta) in panels **a** and **b** to create a short axis image of the vena contracta (**c**, yellow arrow) for direct planimetry. (**d**) A view of the mitral regurgitation flow convergence (red arrow) from the ventricular perspective during systole. Measurement steps described in text. Used with permission of Mayo Foundation for Medical Education and Research. AV, aortic valve; LA, left atrium; LV, left ventricle; LVOT, left ventricular outflow tract

tiple MR jets by PISA can be technically challenging and time consuming. Multiple MR jets can be assessed on a single 3D TEE volume. Typically the 3D VCA of multiple jets are summed to determine the cumulative VCA as a measure of severity [7]. 3D VCA can also be a helpful measure in patients with multiple MR jets considered for percutaneous mitral valve repair, such as edge-to-edge repair, to help determine the dominant regurgitant jet. Note that frequently separate MR jets exist in different spatial planes and typically each jet must be aligned and measured in separate imaging planes to achieve accurate measurement (Fig. 10.4).

3D VCA in Patients with Eccentric MR Jets

Patients with flail mitral leaflet frequently present with very eccentric MR jets. Visual assessment may result in underestimation due to the Coanda effect and PISA quantification can be challenging due to suboptimal alignment of the CW Doppler beam. 3D VCA is frequently feasible in these cases as an objective marker of MR severity. Accurate measurement of the 3D VCA in such cases requires careful alignment with the regurgitant jet using MPR (Fig. 10.5). Toggling the color flow imaging can be helpful in some cases to visualize the flail leaflet itself and guide measurement (Fig. 10.5).

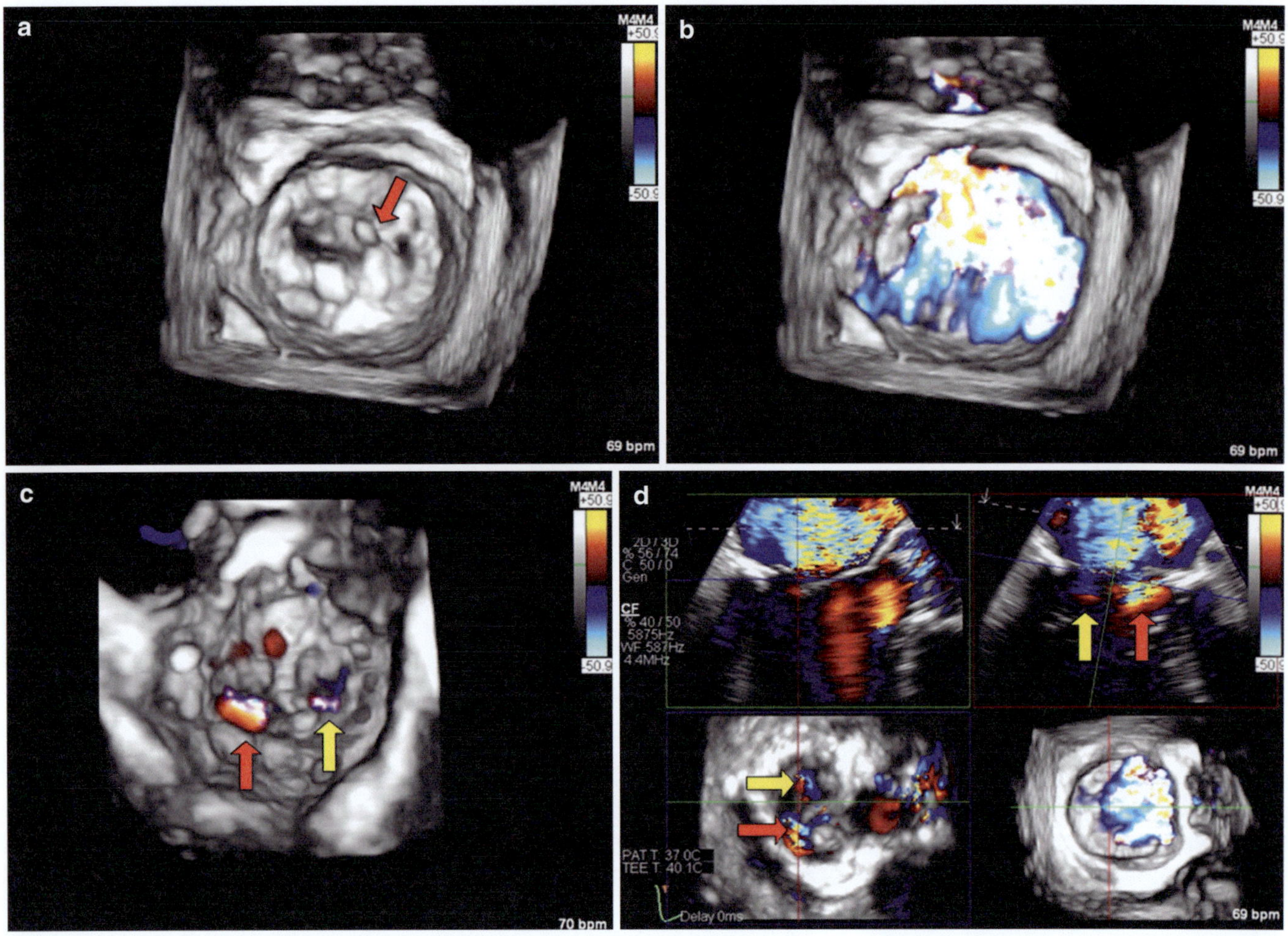

Fig. 10.3 Correlation between anatomic defect and jet origin by 3D TEE with color Doppler imaging. **Panel a** shows a 3D en face view of the mitral valve from the left atrial perspective with a flail P3 scallop (red arrow). **Panel b** shows live 3D color Doppler imaging from the left atrial perspective. Color flow fills the left atrium and obscures the jet origin. **Panel c** shows live 3D color Doppler from the left ventricular perspective, which confirms a regurgitant jet originating from the site of the P3 flail (red arrow) and a second jet arising from A1–P1 (yellow arrow). **Panel d** shows MPR using a 3D color Doppler volume, showing the two jets of mitral regurgitation in a typical commissural view (upper right panel, yellow and red arrows) and in a short axis view of the mitral valve (lower left panel, yellow and red arrows). Used with permission of Mayo Foundation for Medical Education and Research.

3D VCA in Patients with an Elliptical MR Orifice

PISA assessment of MR assumes a circular MR orifice shape and a hemispheric zone of flow convergence. However, particularly in patients with secondary MR, the regurgitant orifice area may be elliptical rather than circular (Fig. 10.6). In such cases PISA assessment may underestimate the severity of MR and 3D VCA may be a more accurate measure of true MR severity [5].

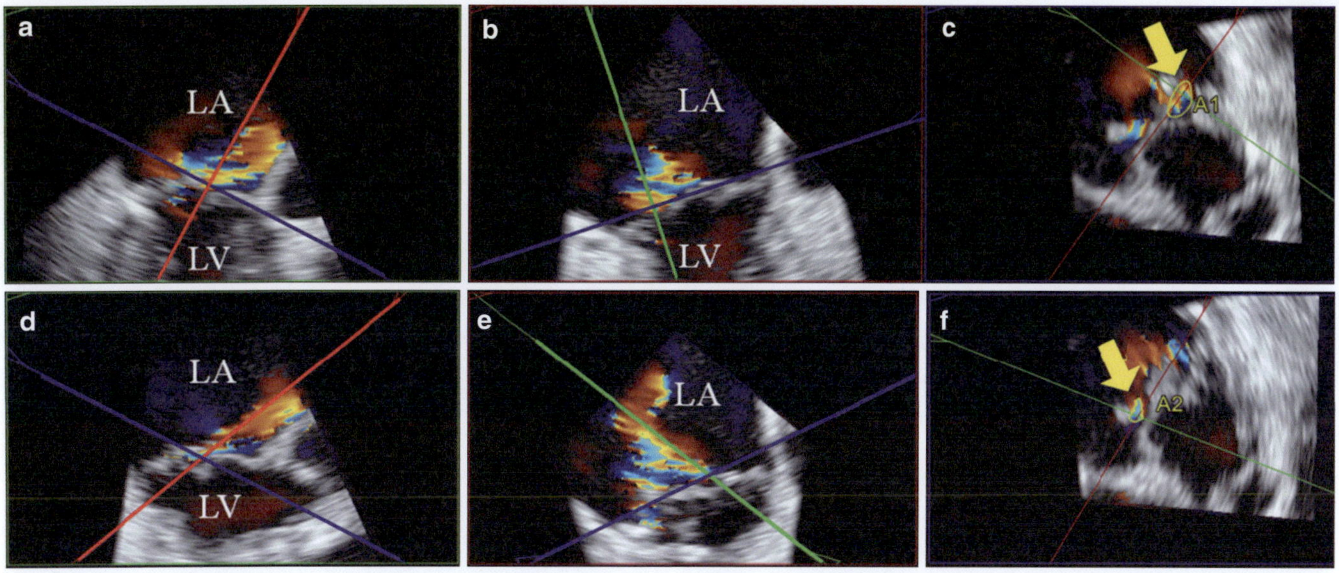

Fig. 10.4 Cumulative 3D VCA in a patient with two MR jets. **Panels a and b** show MPR alignment of the blue lines with the vena contracta of an eccentric regurgitant jet, creating a short axis view of the regurgitant jet in **panel c** (yellow arrow) for direct planimetry (A1). **Panels d and e** show MPR alignment with a second regurgitant jet in a different plane. Aligning the blue lines with the short axis of the regurgitant jet in panels **d** and **e** creates a short axis of the vena contracta in panel **f** for direct planimetry (A2). Used with permission of Mayo Foundation for Medical Education and Research. All rights reserved. LA, left atrium; LV, left ventricle

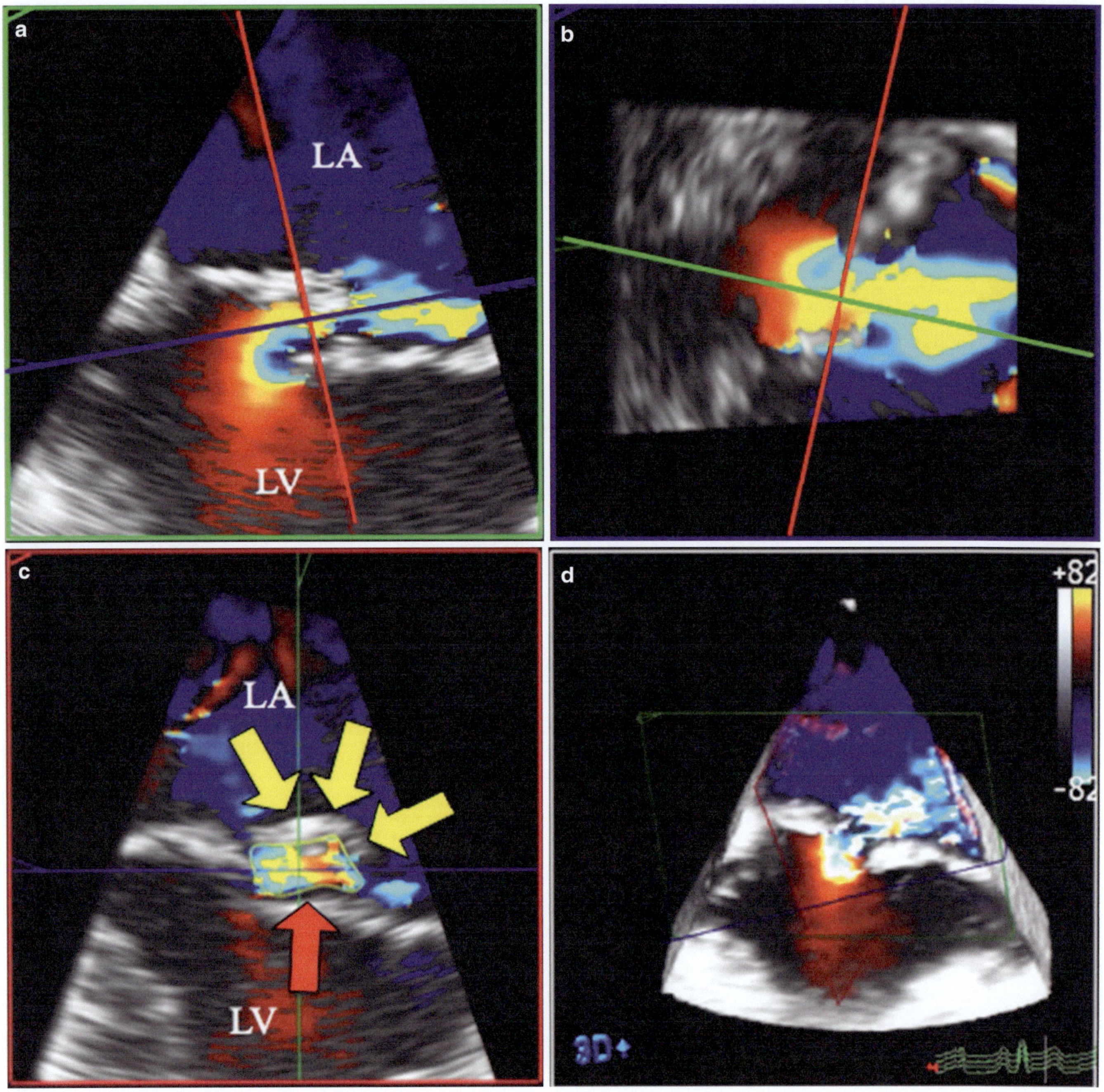

Fig. 10.5 3D VCA in a patient with a flail posterior leaflet and very eccentric MR. **Panel a** shows a typical long axis view zoomed on the mitral valve leaflets. **Panel b** shows an off axis commissural view due to the eccentric, anteriorly directed MR jet. **Panel c** shows the 3D VCA (red arrow) created by alignment of red lines in two orthogonal views with the vena contracta (panels **a** and **b**). Note that the flail scallop is frequently well visualized in its short axis (panel **c**, yellow arrows) which can be helpful to guide the measurement. **Panel d**: volumetric data set. Used with permission of Mayo Foundation for Medical Education and Research. All rights reserved. LA, left atrium; LV, left ventricle

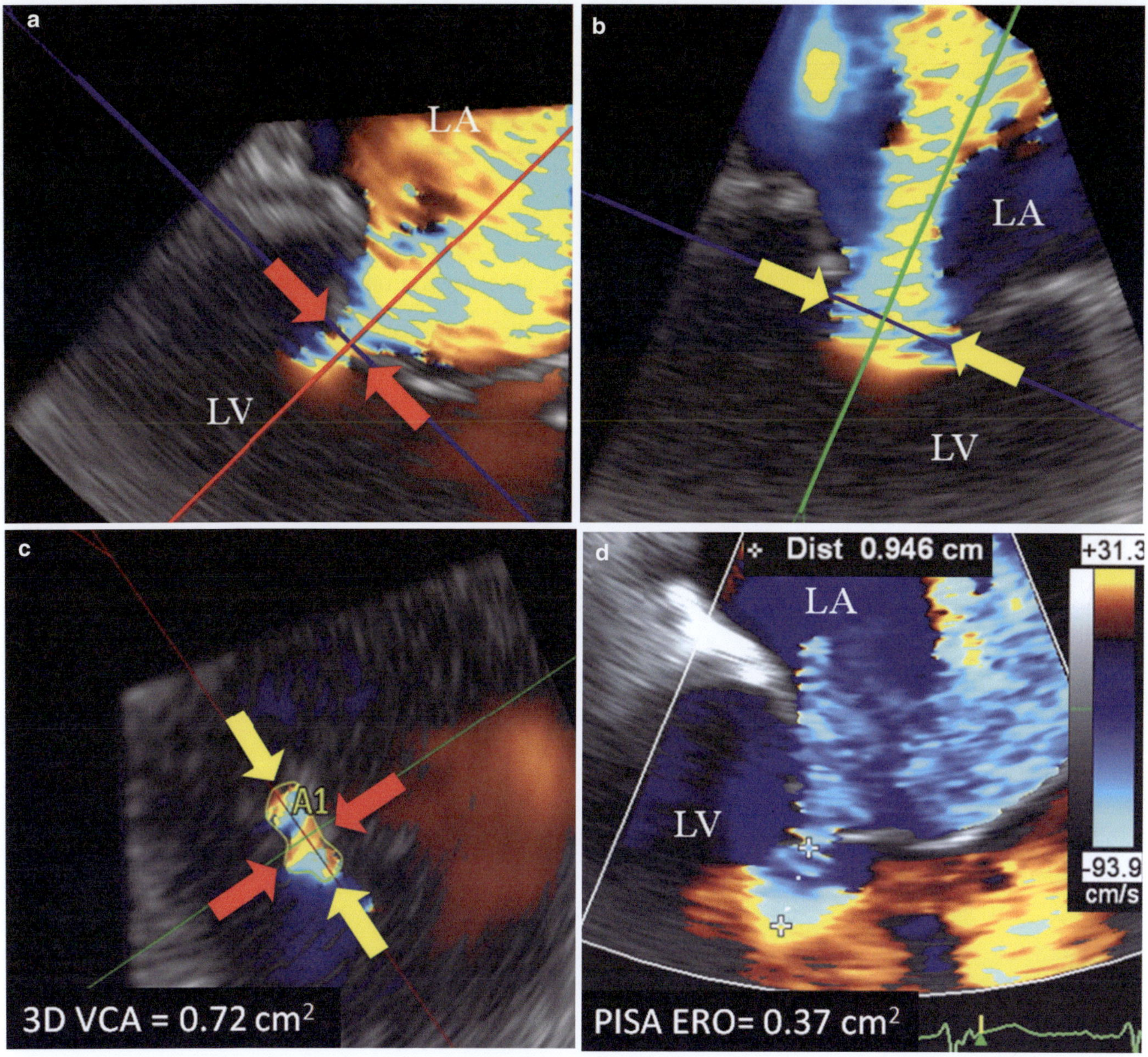

Fig. 10.6 3D VCA in a patient with secondary mitral regurgitation and an elliptical orifice area. **Panel a** shows a typical long axis view from a 3D color Doppler volumetric data set in a patient with severe, secondary MR. Note the relatively narrow dimension of the regurgitant jet in the anterior-posterior dimension (panel **a**, red arrows). **Panel b** shows a commissural view in the same patient showing an increased medial to lateral dimension of the regurgitant jet (yellow arrows). **Panel c** shows the 3D VCA in the transverse short-axis plane. Note the elliptical shape and the relatively small anterior-posterior dimension (red arrows) and the large medial-lateral dimension (yellow arrows). The 3D VCA by 3D-guided planimetry was 0.72 cm^2. **Panel d** shows a PISA measurement from a 2D long axis view. PISA quantitation of the ERO of this elliptical regurgitant jet was 0.37 cm^2. Used with permission of Mayo Foundation for Medical Education and Research. All rights reserved. LA, left atrium; LV, left ventricle

Conclusions and Future Directions

There is growing evidence that 3D VCA is useful in current clinical practice as an additional quantitative measure for MR severity or an alternative measure when PISA is not feasible. As 3D TEE image quality improves with each subsequent iteration of ultrasound machine we expect 3D VCA will be used more frequently in routine clinical practice. 3D PISA and 3D quantitative color Doppler are additional 3D color Doppler techniques that hold promise for the future. Each technique needs further study but has the potential to improve quantitation of MR severity by eliminating geometric assumptions inherent in current quantitative techniques.

References

1. Nkomo VT, Gardin JM, Skelton TN, Gottdiener JS, Scott CG, Enriquez-Sarano M. Burden of valvular heart diseases: a population-based study. Lancet. 2006;368:1005–11.
2. Thaden JJ, Tsang MY, Ayoub C, Padang R, Nkomo VT, Tucker SF, et al. Association between echocardiography laboratory accreditation and the quality of imaging and reporting for valvular heart disease. Circ Cardiovasc Imaging. 2017;10.
3. Enriquez-Sarano M, Avierinos JF, Messika-Zeitoun D, Detaint D, Capps M, Nkomo V, et al. Quantitative determinants of the outcome of asymptomatic mitral regurgitation. N Engl J Med. 2005;352:875–83.
4. Goebel B, Heck R, Hamadanchi A, Otto S, Doenst T, Jung C, et al. Vena contracta area for severity grading in functional and degenerative mitral regurgitation: a transoesophageal 3D colour Doppler analysis in 500 patients. Eur Heart J Cardiovasc Imaging. 2018;19:639–46.
5. Zeng X, Levine RA, Hua L, Morris EL, Kang Y, Flaherty M, et al. Diagnostic value of vena contracta area in the quantification of mitral regurgitation severity by color Doppler 3D echocardiography. Circ Cardiovasc Imaging. 2011;4:506–13.
6. Pisano C, Calia C, Ricasoli A, Fabio Triolo O, Argano V. Intraoperative transesophageal echocardiography for surgical repair of degenerative mitral regurgitation. J Heart Valve Dis. 2017;26:547–56.
7. Avenatti E, Mackensen GB, El-Tallawi KC, Reisman M, Gruye L, Barker CM, et al. Diagnostic value of 3-dimensional vena contracta area for the quantification of residual mitral regurgitation after MitraClip procedure. JACC Cardiovasc Interv. 2019;12:582–91.

3DE Anatomy of Normal Aortic Valve and Root. Image Display and Anatomic Correlations

11

Francesco F. Faletra, Laura A. Leo,
Susanne A. Schlossbauer, Vera L. Paiocchi,
Elisa Gherbesi, and Marco Valgimigli

Introduction

The first "scientific" report of the sophisticated architecture of the aortic root dates back to Leonardo da Vinci's writings and drawings. He described and superbly illustrated the three small bulges at the base of the aorta and correctly theorized their function picturing the "eddy currents" between leaflets and sinuses. Despite this "old" interest, anatomy of the aortic root was largely ignored by cardiologists until a few decades ago. Two main reasons behind this indifference towards this complex anatomical structure are: firstly, the aortic root was simply considered an inert unidirectional conduit between the left ventricle and the ascending aorta; secondly, because aortic valve leaflets do not have an extensive attachment with the ventricular myocardium, their motion was thought to be entirely passive, just driven by blood pressure gradients between the left ventricle and the ascending aorta. Tyron David, who first performed aortic valve sparing surgery in 1992 [1], and Alain Cribier, who first performed transcatheter aortic valve implantation (TAVI) in 2002 [2], renewed interest in the aortic root anatomy. Indeed, both procedures require a systematic and thorough analysis of the fine anatomy of the components of this valve apparatus.

There is no doubt that anatomic specimens remain the "gold standard" to illustrate the anatomy of the aortic root [3, 4]. Moreover, holding and dissecting a human heart is an excellent method to appreciate the complex "three-dimensional" interrelations between the different components of the aortic root. Accordingly, numerous studies have been published by anatomists and surgeons describing the fine details of the aortic root anatomy [3–6]. However, over the last 2 decades, sophisticated imaging technologies such as 3D transesophageal echocardiography (3DTEE) and computed tomography (CT), have undergone extraordinary developments providing exquisite images of the aortic root both in two and three dimensional formats. Being "intrinsically three-dimensional", 3D TEE and CT images can be displayed and analyzed in hundreds of cross-sections and perspectives. Importantly, at variance with anatomists, who explore dead hearts in a contracted state, and surgeons, who explore "still and empty" hearts, these techniques provide images of "beating" hearts with "live and dynamic" anatomical features.

Terminology

The term "aortic root" includes the aortic valve complex which extends from the ventricular-arterial junction to the sino-tubular junction. To fully appreciate the anatomy of the aortic root, a fundamental prerequisite is understanding the nomenclature. Indeed, there is remarkable variability in the everyday-used definitions of the aortic root components (Table 11.1).

Aortic Root and Surrounding Structures

When the base of the heart is viewed from an overhead perspective, the aortic root is the cardiac centerpiece, partially wedged between the orifices of the tricuspid and mitral valve. Viewed from an antero-posterior plane, the aortic root is positioned right and posterior with respect to the right ventricular outflow tract (RVOT). The angle between the aortic root and RVOT is approximately 60° while the line joining the nadir of the aortic sinuses lies in a plane that is tilted 30°

F. F. Faletra (✉)
Director of Cardiac Imaging Lab, Cardiocentro Ticino Institute, Lugano, Switzerland
e-mail: Francesco.Faletra@cardiocentro.org

L. A. Leo · S. A. Schlossbauer · V. L. Paiocchi E. Gherbesi
Cardiac Imaging Lab, Cardiocentro Ticino Institute, Lugano, Switzerland
e-mail: lauraanna.leo@cardiocentro.org; susanne.schlossbauer@cardiocentro.org; vera.paiocchi@cardiocentro.org; elisa.gherbesi@cardiocentro.org

M. Valgimigli
Professor, Division of Cardiology, Cardiocentro Ticino Institute, Lugano, Switzerland
e-mail: marco.valgimigli@cardiocentro.org

J. F. Maalouf et al. (eds.), *Practical 3D Echocardiography*, https://doi.org/10.1007/978-3-030-72941-7_11

Table 11.1 Definitions of aortic root components

Name	Meaning
Ventricular-arterial junction	The term describes the border between the ventricular myocardium and the fibro-elastic structure of the aortic root. This circular/elliptical border includes, along with muscular tissue, two fibrous components: the mitral-aortic curtain and the membranous septum
Cusps	Refer to the moving parts of the aortic root. The name is due to similarity between the aortic valve, viewed from a ventricular perspective in closed position, and the surface of a molar tooth (called cusp). The term is also used to describe the structure of the valve (i.e. unicuspidal, bicuspid, and tri-cuspid)
Leaflets	The term leaflet or "small leaf" has the same meaning as "cusp". The name describes a thin, pliable layer. This term perfectly fits the leaflet aspect
Commissures	The term generally means the angle between two lips or eyelids. In the anatomy of the aortic root it refers to the most distal insertions of the leaflets on the aortic wall where they abut
Aortic annulus	The term indicates the anatomical line where leaflets insert on the wall of the aortic root. This line of dense connective tissue, is not circular but has a crown-shaped morphology
Virtual annulus	Although neither anatomically or histologically recognizable, this term has become relevant in the TAVI era. Measurements of this virtual basal plane, allow for correct sizing of the valve. Since this region does not exist anatomically it is also called "virtual annulus"
Surgical annulus	Prosthetic heart valves are traditionally sutured to a sort of "*ring area*" lying between the nadirs of the sinuses and midway to the commissures. The term "*surgical annulus*" refers to this "ring area" and provides a precise reference point when the prosthesis is sutured in a "supra" annular position

to the left with respect to the horizontal line. Consequently, the left coronary sinus and its leaflet are at the highest position among the three sinuses. On its lateral aspect, the aortic root is wrapped up by the right atrial appendage, while posteriorly it is separated from the left and right atrial cavities by a space called "sinus transversum". The close proximity of the non-coronary sinus to the interatrial septum (IAS) is well known to interventionalists. Indeed, puncturing the IAS or implanting a devise for atrial septal defect closure, carries the risk of injuring the aorta, especially if it is enlarged (Fig. 11.1).

Function of the Aortic Root

The aortic root is a highly sophisticated and complex apparatus, forged by millions of years of evolution so as to allow for a lifetime of proper function in the most challenging physical environment. Indeed, the aortic root has several functions, including: (a) allowing the passage of a significant amount of blood across the aortic valve with a minimum gradient; (b) assuring a wide flow variation (up to five times); (c) preventing significant back flow and having at the same time a robust structural integrity to withstand the aortic pressure; (d) assuring optimal coronary perfusion and finally (e) preserving leaflets integrity. This latter function is probably the most relevant one. Although the leaflets are living structures subjected to natural biological turnover, such that their micro-architecture is continuously renovated and micro injuries self-repaired, there is no doubt, that working "inside" the aortic root, offers the leaflets an extraordinary "low-stress environment" that favors their life-long durability.

Components of the Aortic Root

The aortic root is composed of five key components, namely the ventriculo-arterial junction (VAJ), crown-shaped hinge-lines of semilunar leaflets (also called annulus), leaflets, sinuses and sinutubular junction (STJ).

The Ventricular-Arterial Junction

The VAJ refers to the virtual circumference where the muscular tissue of the left ventricular outflow tract (LVOT), abuts the fibro-elastic wall of the aortic root. Interestingly, the muscular component of the LVOT represents nearly 40% of the entire VAJ, with the remaining 60% being made up from connective tissue [3, 4]. The connective tissue component of the VAJ, includes the mitral-aortic continuity (between the left- and non-coronary sinuses) and the membranous septum (MS; between the non-coronary and the right coronary sinuses) (Fig. 11.2a, b). The muscular component extends above the nadir of the right and left sinuses, remaining enclosed in the lowest part of the sinuses, few millimeters above the hinge line of the leaflets. Left-sided ventricular arrhythmias may actually arise from this muscular "sinus" component (Fig. 11.2c, d). In humans, the MS connective tissue component of the VAJ and adjacent right fibrous trigone is a particularly delicate area because the bundle of His runs immediately below the inferior margin of the MS while the atrioventricular node is located within the muscular atrioventricular septum. Because of the muscular component, the VAJ expands during ventricular filling and isovolumetric contraction (together with the STJ), making the aortic root larger to accommodate the stroke volume. This expansion reduces the area of leaflet coaptation and at the time of their opening, the leaflets are in apposition only with their free edge, reducing the friction between them. During ejection, the VAJ contracts, while the STJ continues to expand. The shape of the aortic root becomes a truncated cone with the

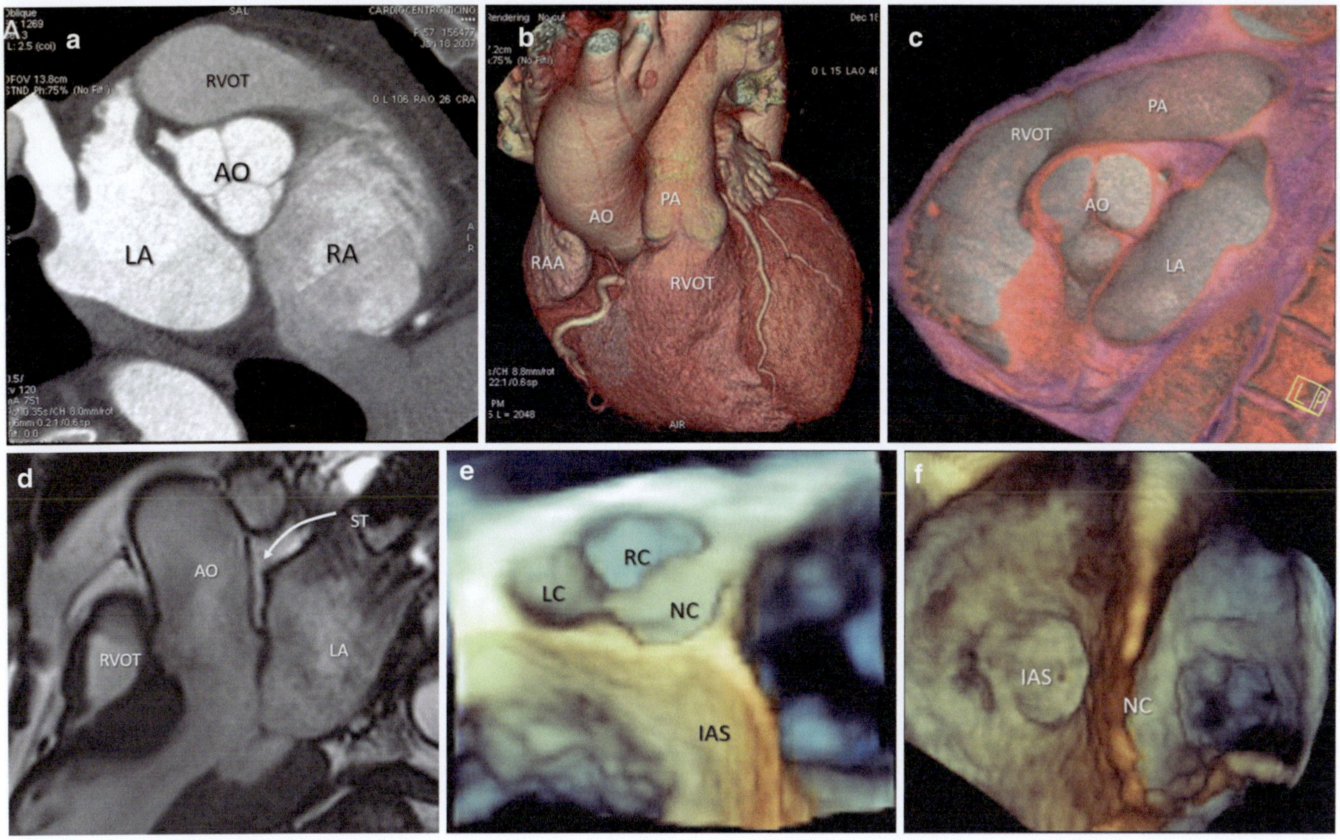

Fig. 11.1 (**a**) CT image in multiplanar reconstruction showing the aorta (AO) wedged between the right (RA) and left (LA) atrial cavities. (**b**) CT image in three-dimensional volumetric format showing the AO encased in the center of the heart immediately behind the right ventricular outflow tract (RVOT). The right atrial appendage (RAA) covers the lateral aspect of the AO. (**c**) CT cross section image along the long axis of the RVOT, showing the AO between the ROVT anteriorly and the LA posteriorly. (**d**) CMR image in long axis view showing the space between the AO and LA (curved arrow) called sinus transversum (ST) filled with epicardial adipose tissue. (**e**) Three-dimensional (3D) TEE image showing the proximity of non-coronary sinus (NC) to the interatrial septum (IAS). (**f**) 3D TEE image showing "en face" view of the IAS and the NC in cross-section

smaller opening toward the ventricle facilitating progression of the blood column towards the ascending aorta.

The Crown-Shaped Annulus

The insertion of the leaflets on the aortic wall has a crown-shaped arrangement, with the lowest part lying slightly below the ventricular-arterial junction (nadir) and the highest part joining the STJ [3]. This arrangement guarantees the flexibility that would not be possible in presence of a circular fibrotic ring. In fact, a fibrotic "ring-like" structure, must be robust and rigid enough to withstand the aortic pressure. Such type of annulus, would have probably resulted in a transvalvular gradient comparable to that present across mechanical or biological prostheses. Conversely, a crown-shaped configuration allows the VAJ to expand and twist during systolic isovolumetric contraction and the early ejection phase, minimizing the transvalvular gradient (Fig. 11.3).

The Interleaflets Triangle

Because of the particular crown-shape fashion of the annulus, the ventricular aspect of the aortic root is lined by three muscular/fibrous triangular extensions, filling the space between the hinge line of aortic leaflets and extending from the VAJ to the commissures [6]. The triangle between the left and right coronary leaflets is usually the smallest and is entirely muscular. The triangle between the left and the non-coronary leaflets is made up of fibrous tissue in continuity with the mitral-aortic curtain. The surgical relevance of this triangle lies in the fact that, in small aortic roots, the mitral-aortic continuity and the corresponding interleaflet triangle are the site of surgical aortic annulus enlargement to accommodate a larger valve prosthesis. Finally, the triangle between the non-coronary and right coronary leaflets, includes the MS which marks the site of the atrioventricular conduction bundle. Interestingly, all inter-leaflet triangles, while considered part of the aortic root, are subjected to ventricular

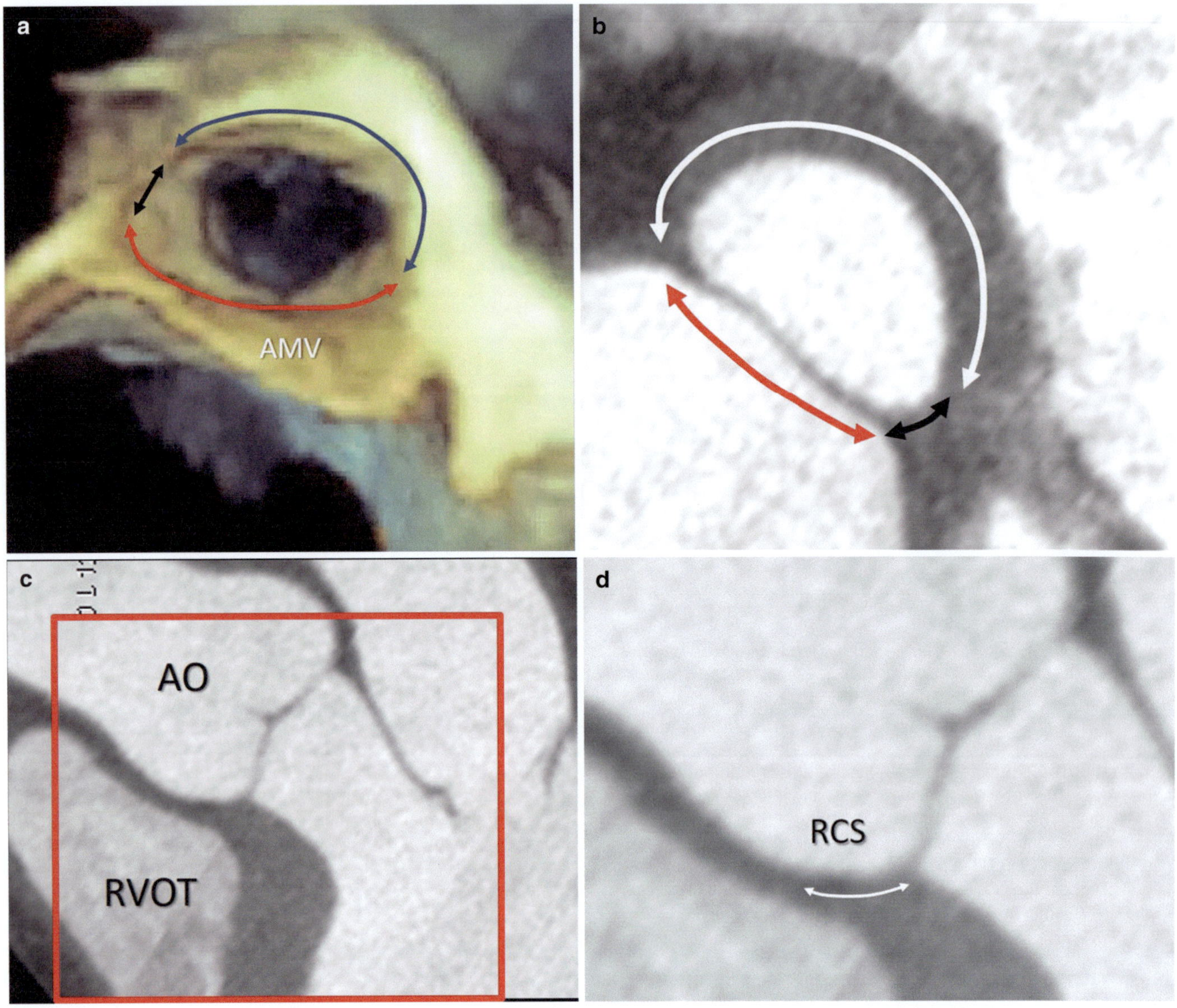

Fig. 11.2 **a** and **b**: 3D TEE (**a**) and CT scan (**b**) showing the ventricular-arterial junction with its muscular component (blue and white double-headed arrows respectively), the mitral-aortic junction (red double-headed arrow) and membranous septum (black double-head arrow). (**c**) CT scan image long axis view, showing the aortic root (AO) and the right ventricle outflow tract (RVOT). (**d**) Magnified image of the structures included in the red box of panel **c**. The white double-headed arrow marks the muscular portion extending above the nadir of the right coronary sinus (RCS)

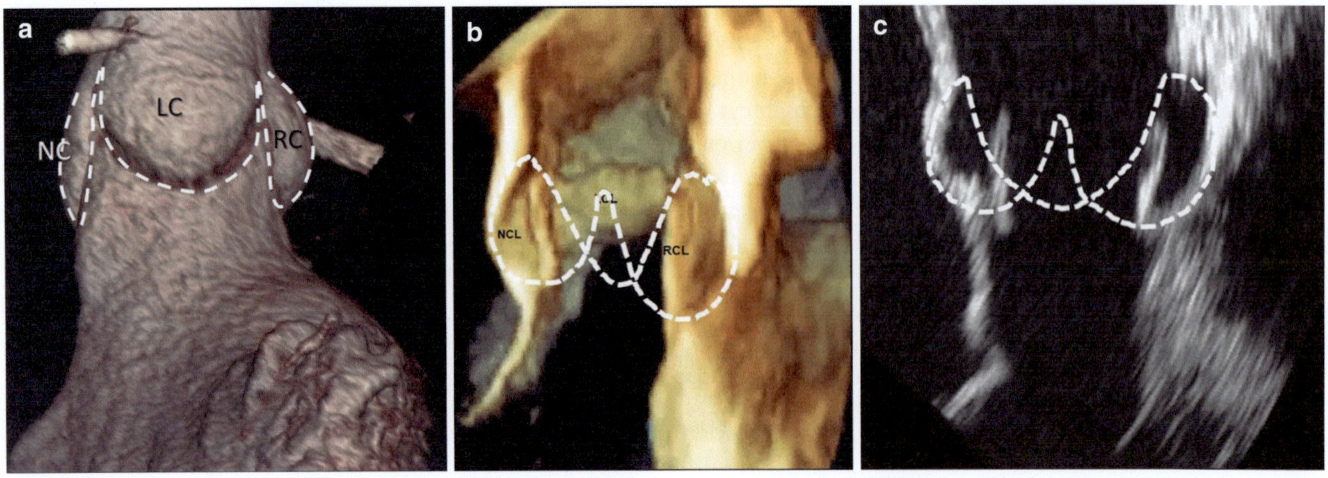

Fig. 11.3 The crown shaped arrangement (dotted lines) superimposed on images provided by (**a**), CT "electronic cast" (**b**) 3D TEE and (**c**) 2D TEE

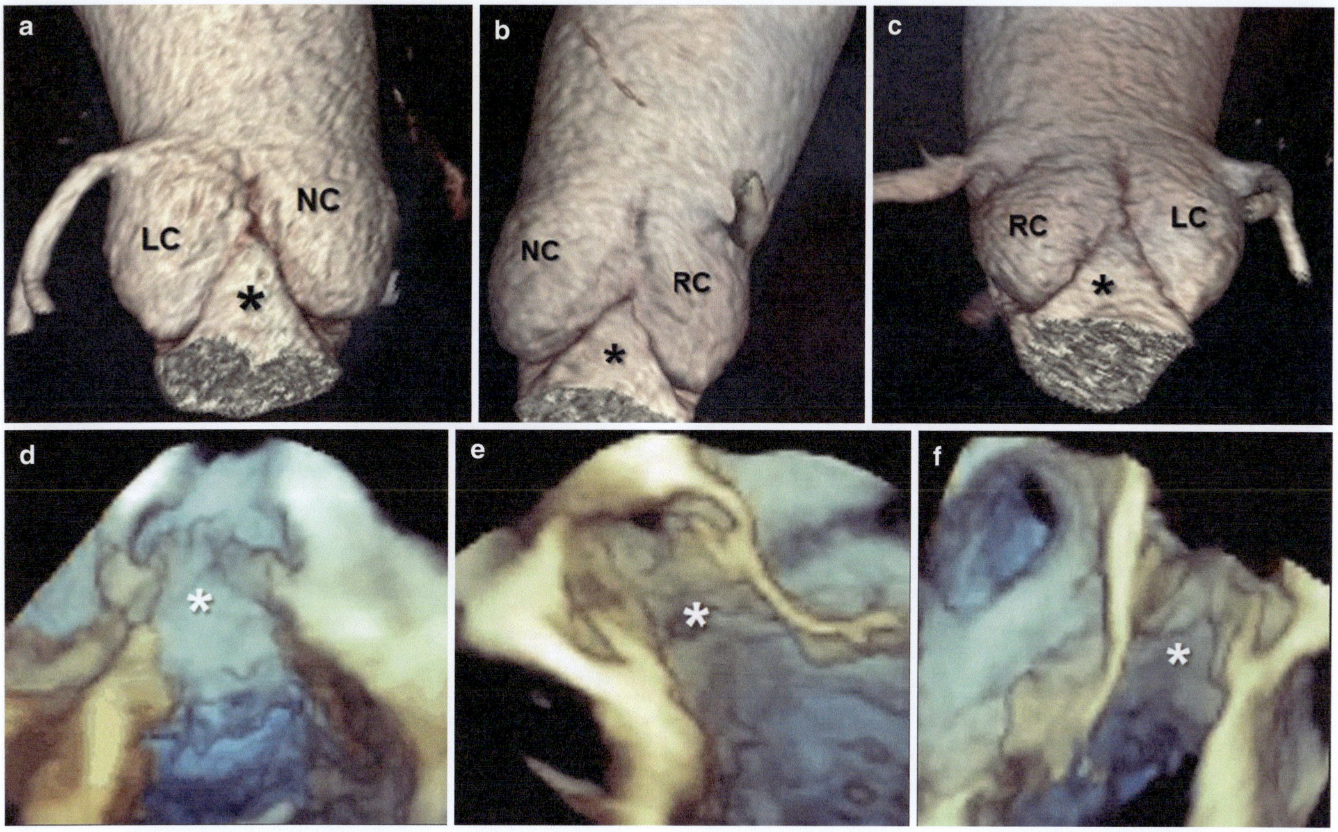

Fig. 11.4 (**a–c**) Electronic cast of the aortic root showing the three interleaflet triangles (asterisks). (**d–f**) 3D TEE longitudinal cross sections of the aortic root. The three interleaflet triangles seen on their ventricular aspect are marked by the asterisks (see text).LC, left coronary; NC, non-coronary; RC, right coronary. Image partially modified from Francesco Faletra et al. in Atlas of non-invasive imaging in cardiac anatomy. Springer-Verlag London, 2020, page 28

pressures. Thus, the interleaflet triangles together with the ventricular surfaces of the semilunar leaflets mark the "hemodynamic" VAJ (Fig. 11.4).

The Sinuses of Valsalva

The sinuses of Valsalva occupy the greater part of the aortic root and consist of three bulges of the aortic root behind the leaflets. They are named according to the origin of the coronary arteries and have different sizes, with the non-coronary sinus being the largest and the left coronary sinus being the smallest. The main function of the sinuses is to preserve the integrity of the aortic leaflets. The most peripheral layers of the flow generated during systole are halted at the STJ and forced back into the space between the leaflets and the sinuses creating eddy currents. These vortexes promote a slow motion of leaflets which approximate each other during late systole, so that the valve is almost closed before forward systolic flow is complete. When blood flow reverses in early diastole, the distance between the valve leaflets is minimal [7]. Therefore, closure of aortic leaflets occurs, at low closing speeds, with minimal hemodynamic stress and in absence of any back-flow leakage (Fig. 11.5).

The elastic capability of the sinuses to distend under pressure, is another relevant characteristic that preserves the leaflets. A cross-section in the middle of the body of the sinuses reveals that, in diastole, the sinuses assume a three-lobed arrangement. This diastolic configuration splits the aortic root into three almost circular subunits formed by the sinus and the corresponding leaflet. The "radius of curvature" of the three subunits is smaller than the aortic root radius in systole and, according to the La Place law, the stress due to diastolic pressure is therefore reduced and shared between the sinuses and the leaflets (Fig. 11.6).

Leaflets

The aortic leaflets represent the "*central piece*" or the "*working component*" of the aortic root. When the leaflets are surgically removed, the aortic valve "de facto" is no longer present. The normal aortic valve has three leaflets with slight differences in size and shape: the non-coronary

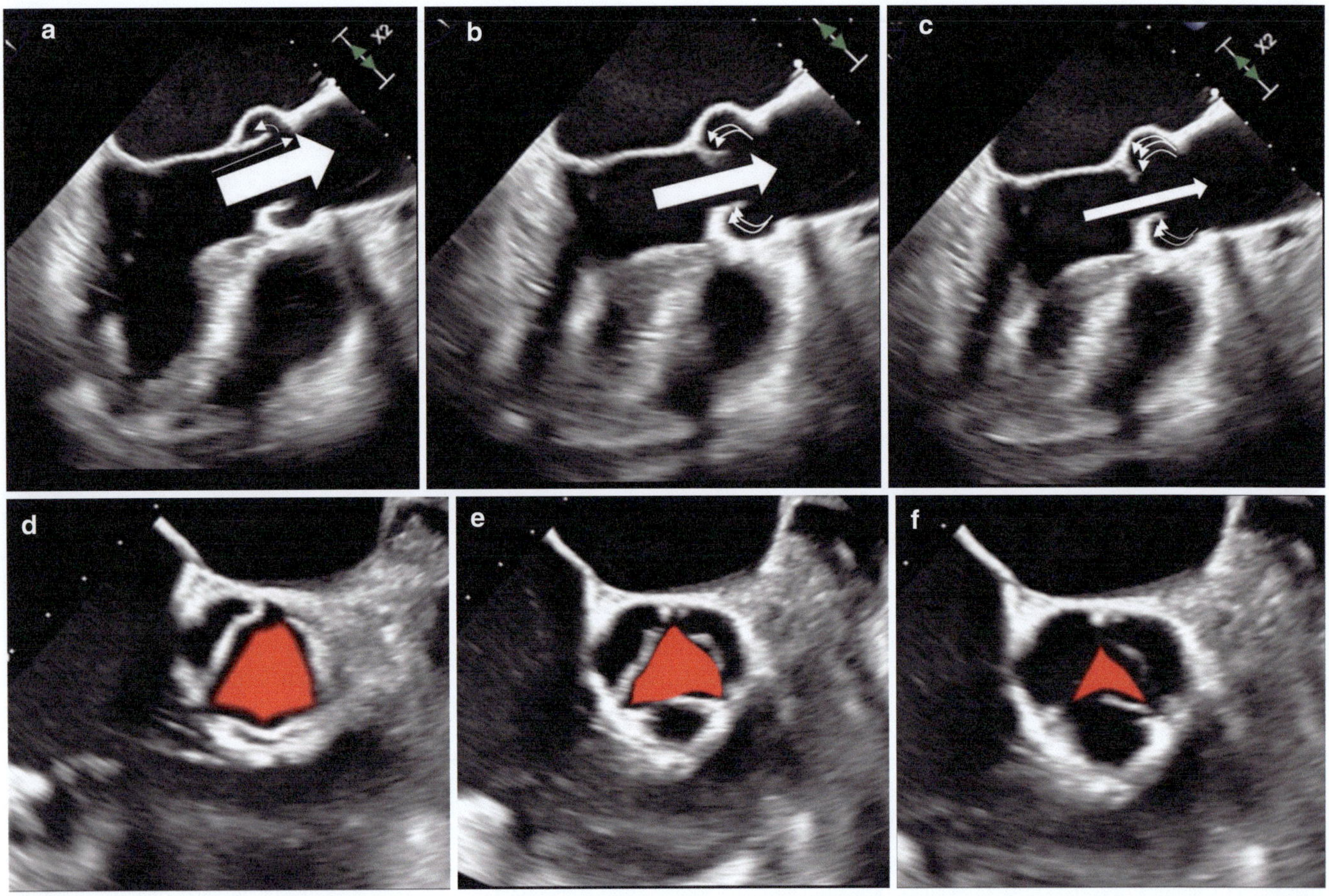

Fig. 11.5 (**a**–**c**) 2D TEE long axis views, showing three time points of the systolic phase (**a**) Early-systole, (**b**) mid-systole and (**c**) end-systole. Please note that as the forward flow through the valve (large arrow) progressively diminishes, the vortexes (curved arrows) approximate the leaflets to each-other (see text). (**d**–**f**) 2D TEE short axis views of the aortic leaflets. The area of the aorta is progressively smaller from early to end-systole. In Contrast, the space between leaflets and sinuses becomes larger and larger due to vortexes (non-represented)

leaflet usually is the largest, and the left coronary leaflet the smallest. Each leaflet has a crescent shape hinge line, a body and an area of apposition known as *lunula* which corresponds to approximately 30% of the leaflet total area. In the middle of the lunula at the free margin (Fig. 11.7), there is a thickened nodule called the *Nodule of Arantius* (see Fig. 12.2, Chap. 12). During diastole, each leaflet, together with the corresponding sinus, takes the appearance of a bird's nest. The insertion line of the leaflet is approximately 1.5 times longer than the length of the free margin, and the height (base-margin) ranges between 12 and 18 mm [3].

Histologically, the leaflets are roughly composed of three layers. These layers are covered, on both sides, by an endothelial layer which acts as a barrier limiting inflammatory cell infiltration and lipid accumulation, and regulates permeability and cell adhesions using paracrine signals. Below the endothelial layer on the aortic side, a layer of collagen fibers is present, with an "undulating" radial arrangement: the fibrosa. During the cardiac cycle, the aortic leaflets change in size. Specifically, their area is about 50% larger in diastole compared to systole. Given its particular collagen fiber arrangement, the fibrosa is therefore "stretched" in diastole and "wrinkled" in systole. On the ventricular side, elastic fibers predominate, and form a layer called the "*ventricularis*". The elastic lamina, stretching in diastole and recoiling in systole, helps the fibrosa to maintain its "corrugated" configuration. Between the fibrosa and ventricularis, there is a layer of loose connective tissue known as the "*spongiosa*". The spongiosa is made up of extracellular matrix (mainly sparse elastin and collagen fibers), complex glycoproteins, a network of nerve fibers and capillaries, and contains an array of different cells types, among which the most representative are the valvular interstitial cells (VICs). Each component of spongiosa confers specific physical properties. *Elastin* allows for recoil after each deformation, and *glycoproteins* provide a "lubricant" characteristic, which reduces mechanical stress. VICs are essential in the processes of regeneration and damage repair. The continuous renewal of all components is one of the secrets of their longevity.

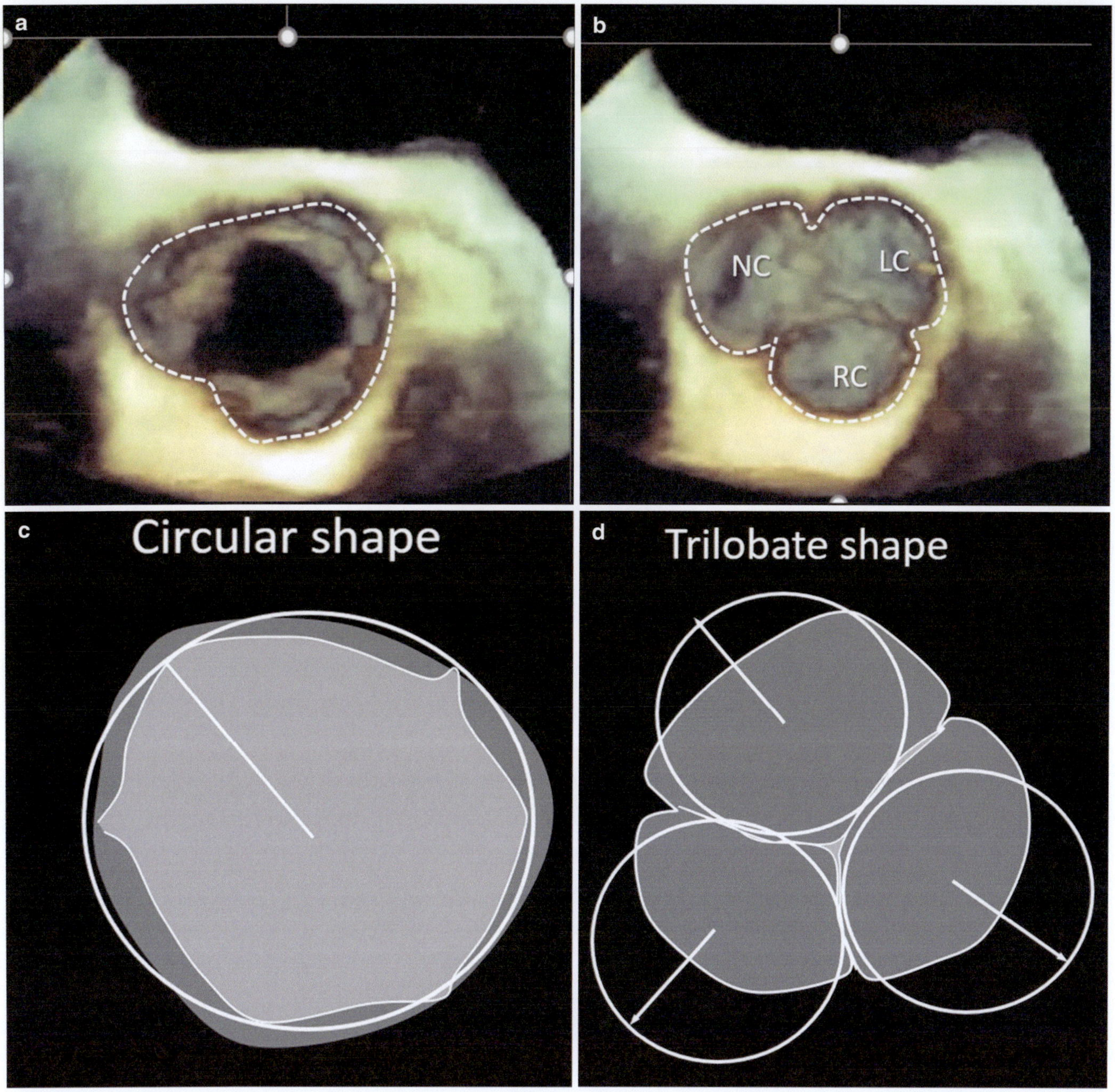

Fig. 11.6 3D TEE cross section in the middle of the aortic sinuses in (**a** and **c**) systole and (**b** and **d**) diastole. From this perspective it is clear that in diastole the sinuses assume a three-lobe arrangement (**d**) resulting in three sub-units with their own radius of curvature (see text)

The Sino-tubular Junction

The sino-tubular junction (STJ) is the most distal part of the aortic root, located between the aortic sinuses and the tubular segment of the ascending aorta. Anatomically, the STJ is made up of circumferentially aligned fibro-elastic lamellae exhibiting a mild waist more pronounced in the proximity to the attachments of the three commissures (Fig. 11.8). In that respect, the STJ is more reminiscent of an "annulus". Because of the strict proximity of STJ to the commissures (the highest points of the crown-shaped annulus), stretching of the STJ (as occurs in aneurysms of the aortic root) results in movement of the commissures away from each other with consequent aortic valve insufficiency. As stated earlier, the STJ plays a role in generating the eddy currents that help in leaflet closure.

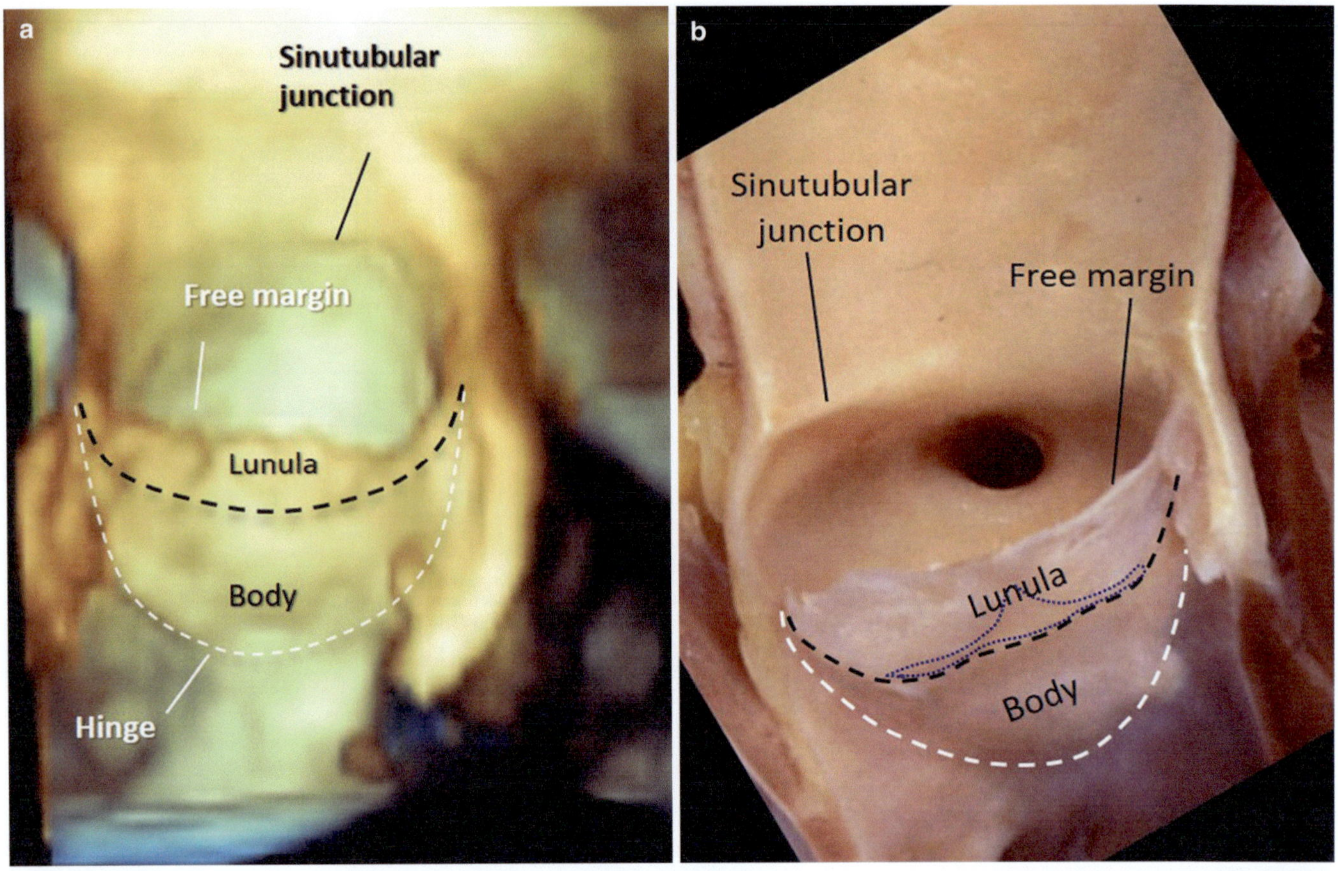

Fig. 11.7 (**a**) 3D TEE images showing the aortic leaflet in "en face" perspective, The black dotted line outlines the inferior border of the lunula, while the white dotted line the hinge line. (**b**) Corresponding anatomic specimen. Image partially modified with permission of Francesco F. Faletra et al. in Atlas of non-invasive imaging in cardiac anatomy. Springer-Verlag, London, 2020, page 30

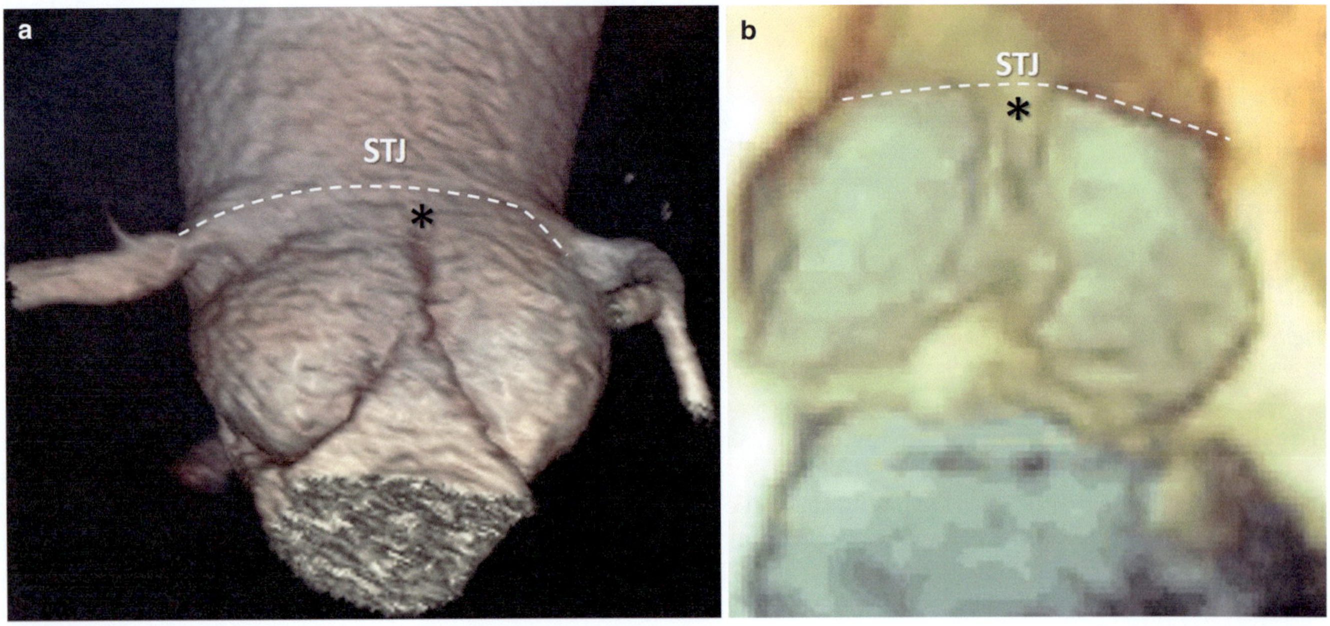

Fig. 11.8 (**a**) CT electronic cast and (**b**) 3D TEE longitudinal cross section showing the close relationship of the sinotubular junction (STJ; dotted line) to the commissure (asterisk) see text for details

References

1. David TE, Feindel CM. An aortic valve-sparing operation for patients with aortic incompetence and aneurysm of the ascending aorta. J Thorac Cardiovasc Surg. 1992;103:617–21.
2. Cribier A, Eltchaninoff H, Bash A, et al. Percutaneous transcatheter implantation of an aortic valve prosthesis for calcific aortic stenosis: First human case description. Circulation. 2002;106:3006–8.
3. Ho SY. Structure and anatomy of the aortic root. Eur J Echocardiogr. 2009;10:i3–i10.
4. Anderson RH. Clinical anatomy of the aortic root. Heart. 2000;84:670–5.
5. Anderson RH, Devine WA, Ho SY, Smith A, McKay R. The myth of the aortic annulus: the anatomy of the subaortic outflow tract. Ann Thorac Surg. 1991;52:640–6.
6. Sutton JP, Ho SY, Anderson RH. The forgotten interleaflet triangles: a review of surgical anatomy of the aortic valve. Ann Thorac Surg. 1995;59:410–27.
7. Pisani G, Scaffa R, Ieropoli O, Dell'Amico EM, Maselli D, Morbiducci U, De Paulis R. Role of the sinuses of valsalva on the opening of the aortic valve. J Thorac Cardiovasc Surg. 2013;145(4):999–1003.

3DE of the Spectrum of Native Aortic Valve and Subvalvular Diseases and Pathological Correlations

12

Jeremy J. Thaden and Joseph F. Maalouf

Introduction

The normal aortic valve (AV) is comprised of three thin leaflets that separate the ascending aorta from the left ventricular cavity during diastole (Fig. 12.1). Each leaflet has a nodule of Arantius that resides centrally along the free margin, at the coaptation point of all three leaflets [1] (Fig. 12.2). The AV leaflets in conjunction with the aortic annulus, the sinuses of Valsalva, the fibrous interleaflet triangles, and the sino-tubular junction comprise the aortic root [1] (see Chap. 11). These structures combine to form a single functional unit.

The AV leaflets are attached at their commissures to the sino-tubular junction in a semilunar fashion thus producing valve cusps and creating interleaflet triangular spaces [1] (Fig. 12.3). The space between the leaflet commissures and the adjacent aortic wall is the sinus of Valsalva (see Chap. 11). The left and right coronary ostia typically arise from the left and right sinuses of Valsalva, respectively [1]. With the rise in recent years of TAVR and surgical AV repair in select patients with aortic regurgitation, there is growing interest in more sophisticated imaging to better visualize, understand, and quantify this complex geometry and the functional interplay of its components. 3D echocardiography provides the ability to image in multiple spatial planes and quantify valvular anatomy and pathology without geometric assumptions, making it well suited for evaluation of the aortic root complex.

3D Echocardiography of the AV: General Considerations

3D echocardiographic (3DE) imaging of the AV presents a number of inherent challenges. Normal AV leaflets are frequently subject to dropout artifact when visualized by 3DE [2] because they are relatively thin and much of the leaflet body is parallel to the ultrasound beam when visualized from the mid-esophagus, creating a suboptimal insonation angle with poor acoustic reflection (Fig. 12.4). Utilization of higher gain settings and 3D smoothing may be helpful to avoid dropout artifact when imaging the AV.

Frequently in diseased states the leaflets are thickened and/or calcified which can improve visualization by 3D echocardiography. However, the presence of severe calcification and shadowing presents unique challenges, particularly when attempting to visualize anterior structures by 3D transesophageal echocardiography (3D TEE).

With currently available 3D TEE systems, adequate frame rate and resolution can typically be obtained with single beat acquisition and narrowed sector widths from the mid-esophageal window. As with other echocardiographic imaging, frequency, gains, focus, and sector size should be optimized prior to acquisition to highlight the subaortic pathology. Gains should be high enough to avoid dropout artifact but not too high as this can amplify acoustic noise and degrade image quality. In subsequent sections we will focus on optimizing 3DE for both qualitative and quantitative assessment of AV pathology.

Supplementary Information The online version of this chapter (https://doi.org/10.1007/978-3-030-72941-7_12) contains supplementary material, which is available to authorized users.

J. J. Thaden (✉)
Assistant Professor of Medicine, Mayo Clinic College of Medicine; Co-Chair for Clinical Practice and Quality, Division of Cardiovascular Ultrasound; Consultant, Department of Cardiovascular Medicine, Mayo Clinic, Rochester, MN, USA
e-mail: Thaden.Jeremy@mayo.edu

J. F. Maalouf
Professor of Medicine, Mayo Clinic College of Medicine; Director, Interventional Echocardiography; Consultant, Department of Cardiovascular Medicine, Mayo Clinic, Rochester, MN, USA
e-mail: maalouf.joseph@mayo.edu

J. F. Maalouf et al. (eds.), *Practical 3D Echocardiography*, https://doi.org/10.1007/978-3-030-72941-7_12

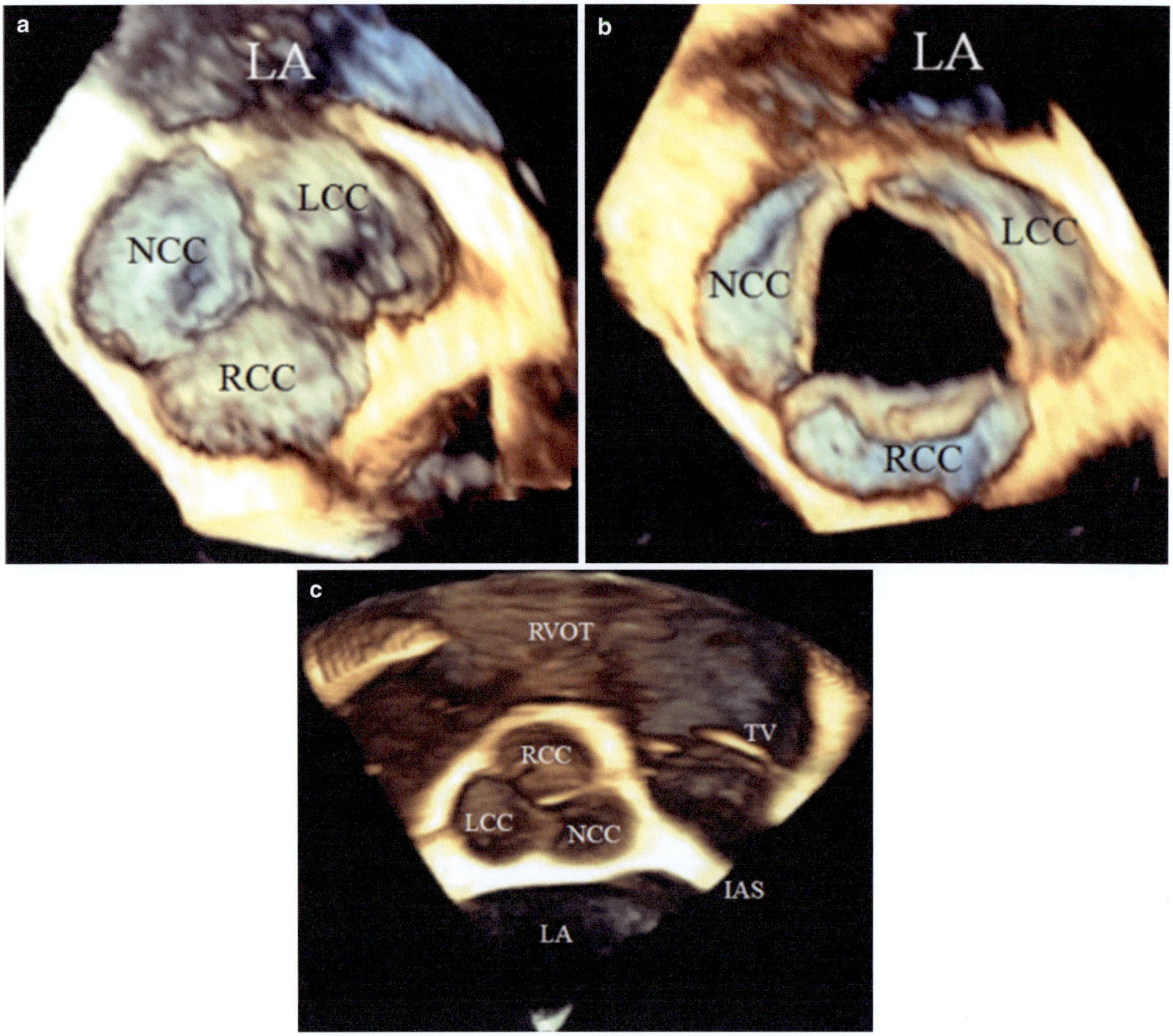

Fig. 12.1 Normal AV. The AV viewed from the perspective of the ascending aorta during diastole (**a**) and systole (**b**). Recommended presentation of the AV is to display the valve from the perspective of the ascending aorta, with the right coronary cusp in the six o'clock position (RCC), the non-coronary cusp at ten o'clock (NCC), and the left coronary cusp at two o'clock (LCC) [2]. (**c**) The AV as viewed by cardiac surgeons intraoperatively. Note that when the AV is viewed intraoperatively via an aortotomy the RCC is at 12 o'clock, the RCC-LCC commissure is at approximately 10 o'clock and the RCC-NCC commissure is at approximately 2 o'clock (Used with permission of Mayo Foundation for Medical Education and Research. All rights reserved). IAS, interatrial septum; LA, left atrium; LCC, left coronary cusp; NCC, non-coronary cusp; RA, right atrium; RCC, right coronary cusp; RVOT, right ventricular outflow tract; TV, tricuspid valve

Spectrum of AV Diseases

Acquired and Congenital AV Stenosis

AV stenosis is among the most common valve disease lesions in economically developed nations [3] and its incidence is suspected to increase as the mean age of the global population increases. Calcific degenerative aortic stenosis most commonly occurs with congenitally normal trileaflet aortic valves (Fig. 12.5), but the process is accelerated in congenitally abnormal unicuspid or bicuspid aortic valves (Figs. 12.6, and 12.7).

Individuals with a unicuspid valve [4] (Fig. 12.7) frequently present at a young age with hemodynamically significant aortic stenosis, but can also present with severe aortic regurgitation or mixed AV disease. Bicuspid valves also have a tendency toward stenosis but typically present

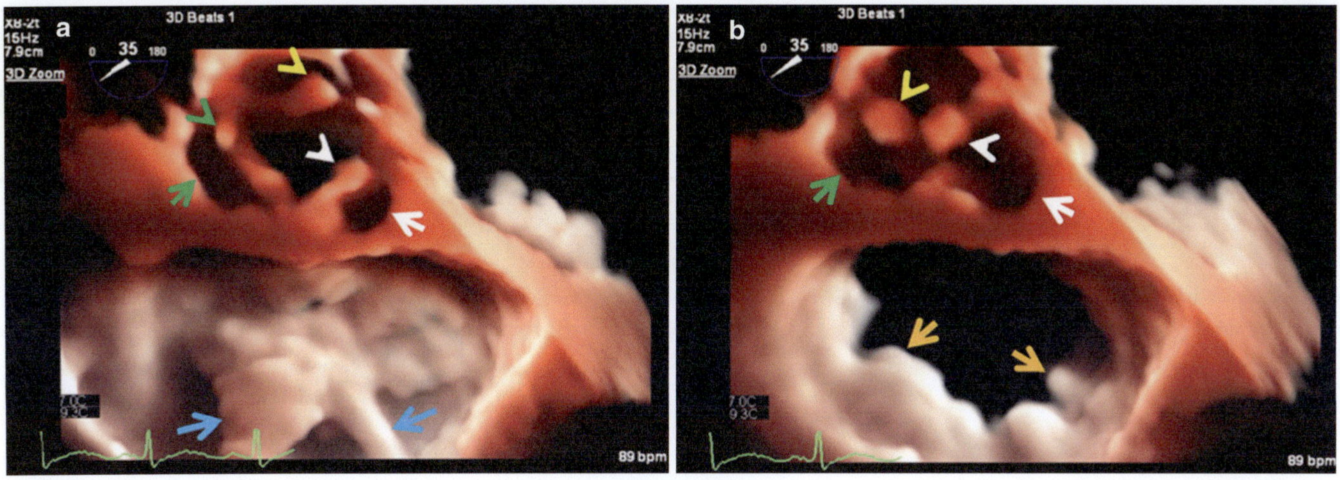

Fig. 12.2 Nodules of Arantius. 3D TEE TrueVue (Philips Healthcare) enface LA views of the mitral and aortic valves in a patient with flail AML A2 segment in both systole (**a**) and diastole (**b**) showing nodules of Arantius (arrow heads) along the free margins of the NCC (white arrow and arrowhead) LCC (green arrow and arrowhead) and RCC (yellow arrow head) and at their coaptation points (**b**). Orange arrows point to PML and blue arrows point to ruptured chordae (Used with permission of Mayo Foundation for Medical Education and Research. All rights reserved). AML, anterior mitral leaflet; LA, left atrium; LCC, left coronary cusp; NCC, noncoronary cusp; PML, posterior mitral leaflet; RCC, right coronary cusp

with significant stenosis later in life and are frequently associated with aortopathy and/or aortic coarctation. Quadricuspid AV is the least common congenital anomaly of the AV with a proposed incidence of only 0.006% [5] (Fig. 12.8). Quadricuspid aortic valves most typically are affected by aortic regurgitation and significant aortic stenosis is much less common.

In economically developed nations, acquired calcific stenosis of a trileaflet valve is more common than calcific stenosis of a congenitally bicuspid or unicuspid valve [6]. Rheumatic aortic stenosis remains an important cause of AV stenosis in countries where rheumatic heart disease remains prevalent (Fig. 12.9).

Echocardiographic imaging for calcific AV disease can be challenging due to the frequent heavy burden of calcification and resultant acoustic shadowing. Because of these limitations, optimal visualization of the entire aortic root may require more than one 3D echocardiographic volumetric dataset by imaging from multiple esophageal positions. The aortic annulus is best imaged at the level of the annular plane (coaxial) or slightly inferior to avoid acoustic shadowing of the anterior portion of the aortic annulus (see later discussion on 3D TEE for assessment of the aortic root pre-TAVR). Conversely, visualization of the tips of the aortic leaflets and the sinuses of Valsalva is typically best from a higher esophageal window because a more inferior window will result in acoustic shadowing of the superior structures. Similarly, direct planimetry of aortic valve area is feasible in many patients and the leaflet tips are often better visualized from a slightly more superior esophageal window. Direct planimetry of the stenotic orifice should be performed using multiplanar reconstruction (MPR) and a dedicated quantitative software package (Fig. 12.10).

Subaortic Stenosis

Subaortic stenosis is the second most common form of left ventricular outflow obstruction, behind valvular stenosis, and it is frequently associated with other congenital cardiac abnormalities. The anatomic cause of subvalvular obstruction is most frequently a thin membrane in the left ventricular outflow tract, but subvalvular narrowing can also be more diffuse and tunnel-like. Subaortic obstruction is typically progressive and can be associated with significant aortic valvular regurgitation.

Subaortic stenosis is frequently well visualized by 3D TEE as a circumferential or near-circumferential fibro-muscular band in the left ventricular outflow tract (Figs. 12.11 and 12.12). Direct visualization by 3D echocardiography, compared to 2D echocardiography, provides a more complete understanding of the circumferential extent of the membrane (Figs. 12.11 and 12.12) and its relationship to the mitral valve and aortic root, which improves pre-surgical planning. 3D echocardiography also allows for direct planimetry of the stenotic orifice using MPR (Fig. 12.13).

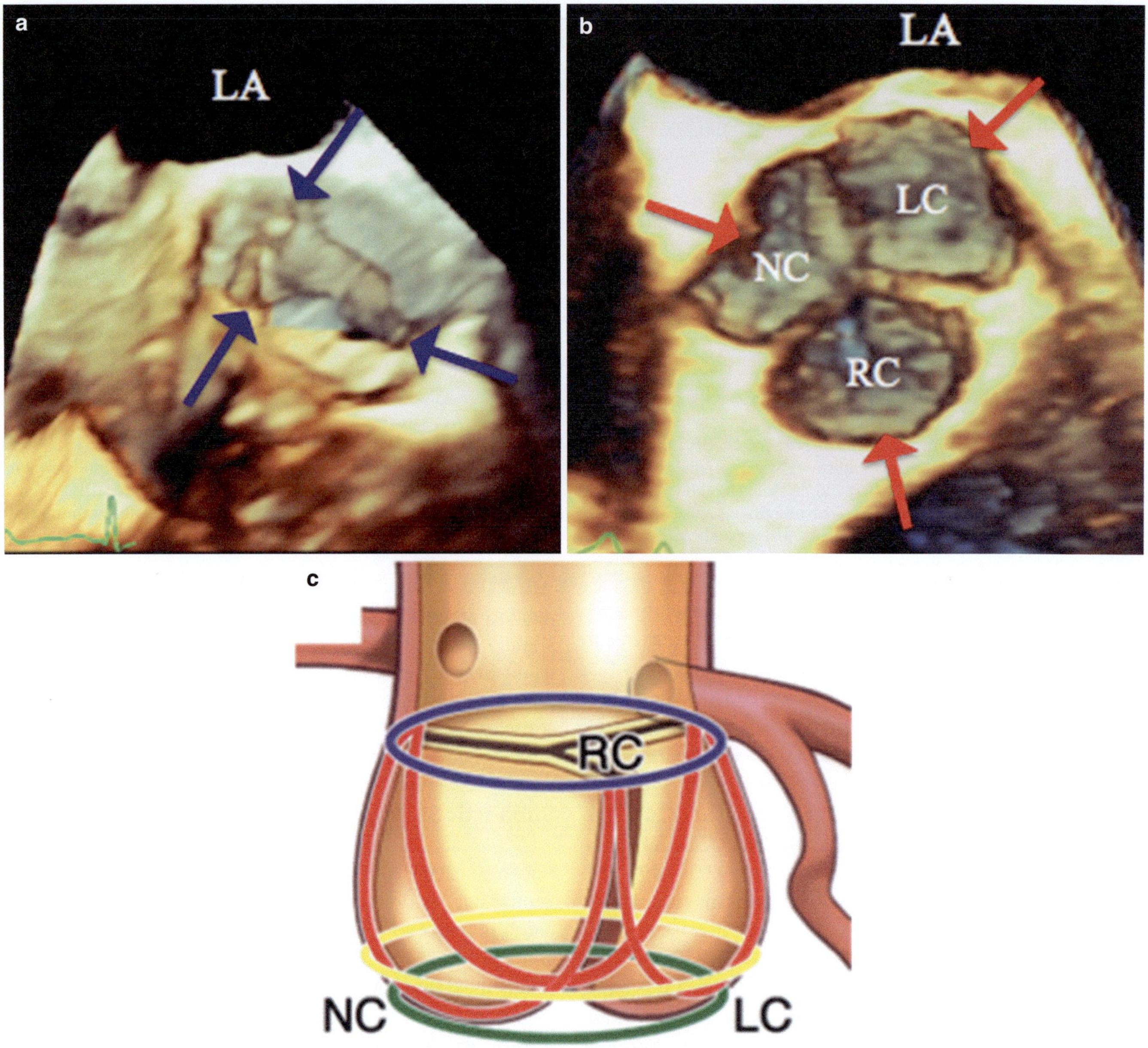

Fig. 12.3 Aortic root anatomy. (**a**) The AV viewed obliquely from the perspective of the ascending aorta shows attachment of the superior margins of the aortic leaflets at the sinotubular junction (blue arrows). (**b**) An en face view of the AV from the ascending aorta during diastole shows the boundaries of the three sinuses of Valsalva (red arrows), including the wall of the aorta, the aortic leaflets, and leaflet coaptation margins which delineate the three sinuses from each other (Images **a** and **b** used with permission of Mayo Foundation for Medical Education and Research. All rights reserved). (**c**) A schematic illustrating the complex anatomy of the aortic root, comprised of the anatomic ventriculo-arterial junction (yellow circle), the sinotubular junction (blue circle), and the crown-like semilunar attachments of the AV leaflets to the aortic wall (red lines). The green circle is the virtual ring formed by joining the basal attachments of the aortic valve leaflets and is the site typically measured for valve sizing prior to TAVR insertion. Jonathon Leipsic, Ronen Gurvitch, Troy M. LaBounty, James K. Min, David Wood, Mark Johnson, Amr M. Ajlan, Namal Wijesinghe and John G. Webb. JACC: Cardiovascular Imaging. Volume 4, Issue 4, April 2011. AV, aortic valve; LA, left atrium; LC, left coronary cusp; NC, non-coronary cusp; RC, right coronary cusp

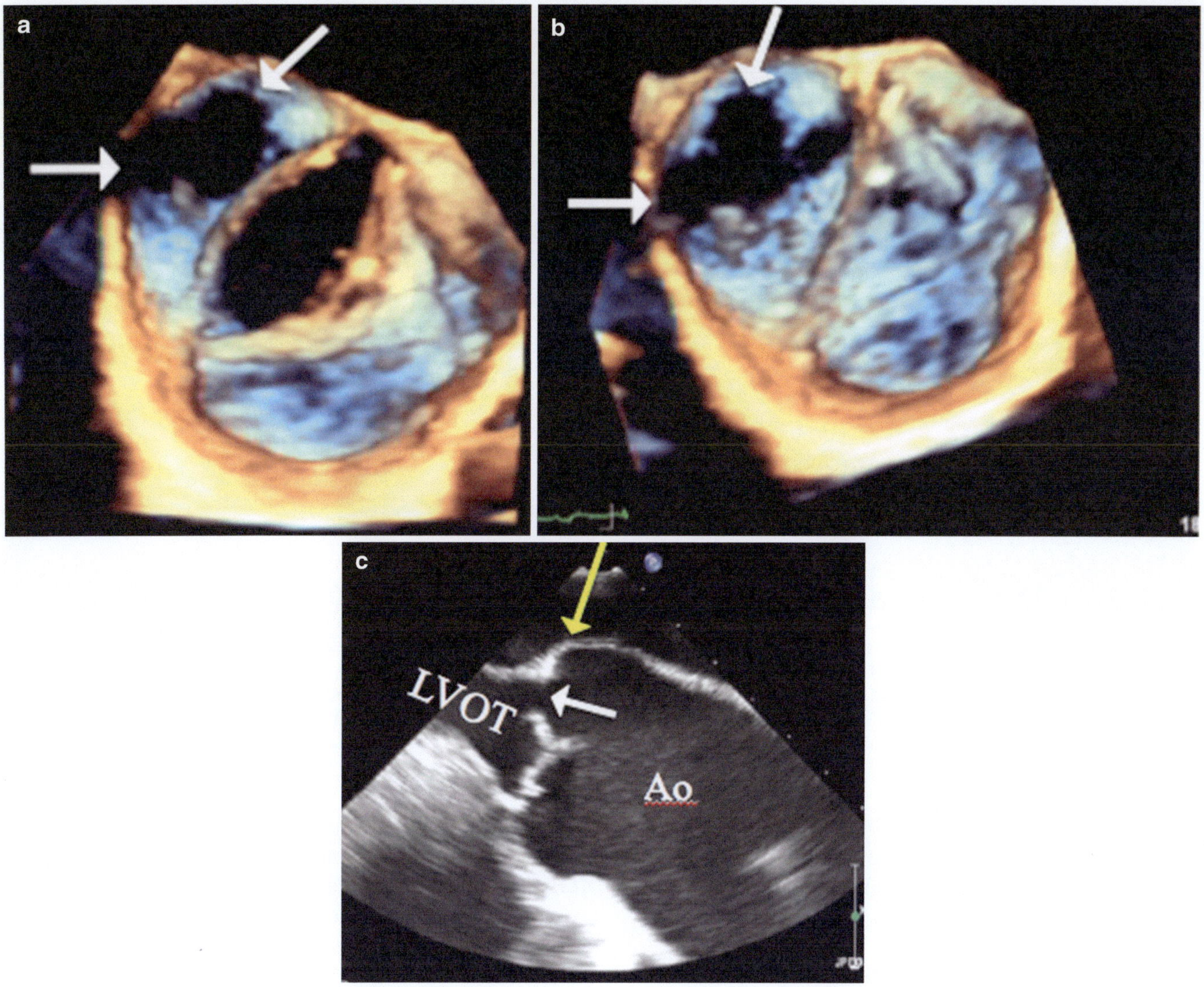

Fig. 12.4 Dropout artifact in a congenitally bicuspid AV. A congenitally bicuspid valve viewed in the conventional orientation during systole (**a**) and diastole (**b**) with fusion of the left and right coronary cusps. The valve is otherwise thin, noncalcified and normally functioning. Note the dropout artifact involving the non-coronary cusp (**a** and **b**, white arrows). Dropout artifact is common because normal AV leaflets are relatively thin and much of the aortic leaflet body is aligned with the ultrasound beam during diastole (**c**, yellow arrow), resulting in a suboptimal insonation angle and poor acoustic reflection (**c**, white arrow). Ao, ascending aorta; AV, aortic valve; LVOT, left ventricular outflow track (Used with permission of Mayo Foundation for Medical Education and Research. All rights reserved)

Supra Valvular Stenosis

Supra-valvular stenosis is the least common form of left ventricular outflow obstruction. It is commonly associated with mutations in the elastin gene which results in a systemic arteriopathy and thickening of the media or intimal layers [7]. Patients typically present within the first two decades of life with a systolic murmur and they may present with symptoms similar to aortic stenosis, including dyspnea, angina, and syncope. Supra-valvular aortic stenosis often occurs as an hourglass shaped stenosis, but the phenotype is variable and can range from a discrete stenosis at the level of the sinotubular junction to diffuse thickening and/or hypoplasia of the ascending aorta, aortic arch, and descending aorta. Because of the

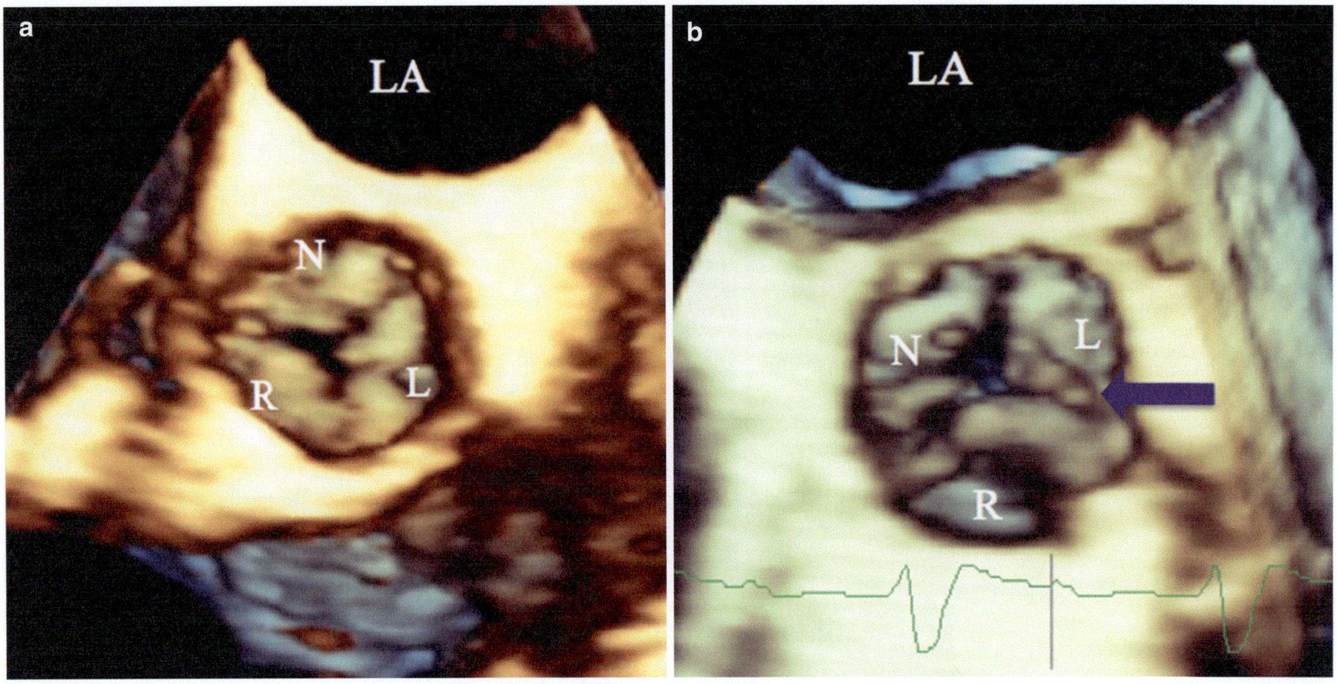

Fig. 12.5 Degenerative/calcific aortic stenosis in a trileaflet AV. (**a**, **b**) Bulky calcification of the body of the aortic leaflets is appreciated when viewed from the perspective of the ascending aorta in patients with degenerative aortic stenosis. Mobile components may be present and in the absence of infection may represent mobile fragments of calcium or in other cases structural valve degeneration, such as torn AV fenestrations (**b**, blue arrow) (Used with permission of Mayo Foundation for Medical Education and Research. All rights reserved). AV, aortic valve; LA, left atrium; L, left coronary cusp; N, non-coronary cusp; R, right coronary cusp

systemic nature of this condition other great vessels are commonly affected, including the mesenteric arteries, the renal arteries, the coronary arteries, and the pulmonary arteries.

Acquired and Congenital Aortic Regurgitation

Aortic regurgitation can result from dilatation of the aortic root or primary pathology related to the AV leaflets themselves. In economically developed countries, the most common causes of aortic regurgitation include dilation of the aortic root, bicuspid AV, and calcific degenerative disease. Rheumatic aortic disease remains an important cause of regurgitation in developing nations.

3D TEE, with surface rendered images and MPR, provides a more detailed understanding of the size and symmetry of the aortic root (Figs. 12.14 and 12.15) which in some cases may aid in understanding the mechanism of aortic regurgitation.

Pre-operative TEE is utilized to determine the feasibility of AV repair. Surgical repair considerations include the etiology of aortic regurgitation (e.g. restricted leaflet mobility, leaflet prolapse, leaflet perforation, annular dilatation, etc.) and specific anatomic measurements including coaptation length (length of leaflet apposition) and effective cusp height (eH, measured from the annulus plane to the tip of leaflet coaptation in diastole). Because the ultrasound beam on 2D imaging of the AV is in an obligatory anteroposterior trajectory, only the eH of the right coronary cusp can be obtained and "off axis" measurements are not possible. With 3D echocardiography, MPR overcomes this limitation by correct alignment of the ultrasound beam with the anatomy of interest thus allowing accurate measurements of the eH of all three cusps (Figs. 12.16, 12.17, 12.18, and 12.19) and their coaptation lengths [8] . 3D TEE with MPR may also help to more precisely visualize prolapse of certain AV segments that are not well seen in available 2D imaging planes. The presence of calcification (whether affecting a cusp or a raphe) is critical to evaluate since optimal repair results occur in valves with minimal or no calcification.

In the future, 3D echocardiography may also improve the quantitation of aortic regurgitation. Direct planimetry of the 3D color Doppler vena contracta (Fig. 12.20) and 3D quantitative Doppler have the potential to more accurately quantify regurgitant orifice area and regurgitant volume to improve risk stratification and patient care [9, 10].

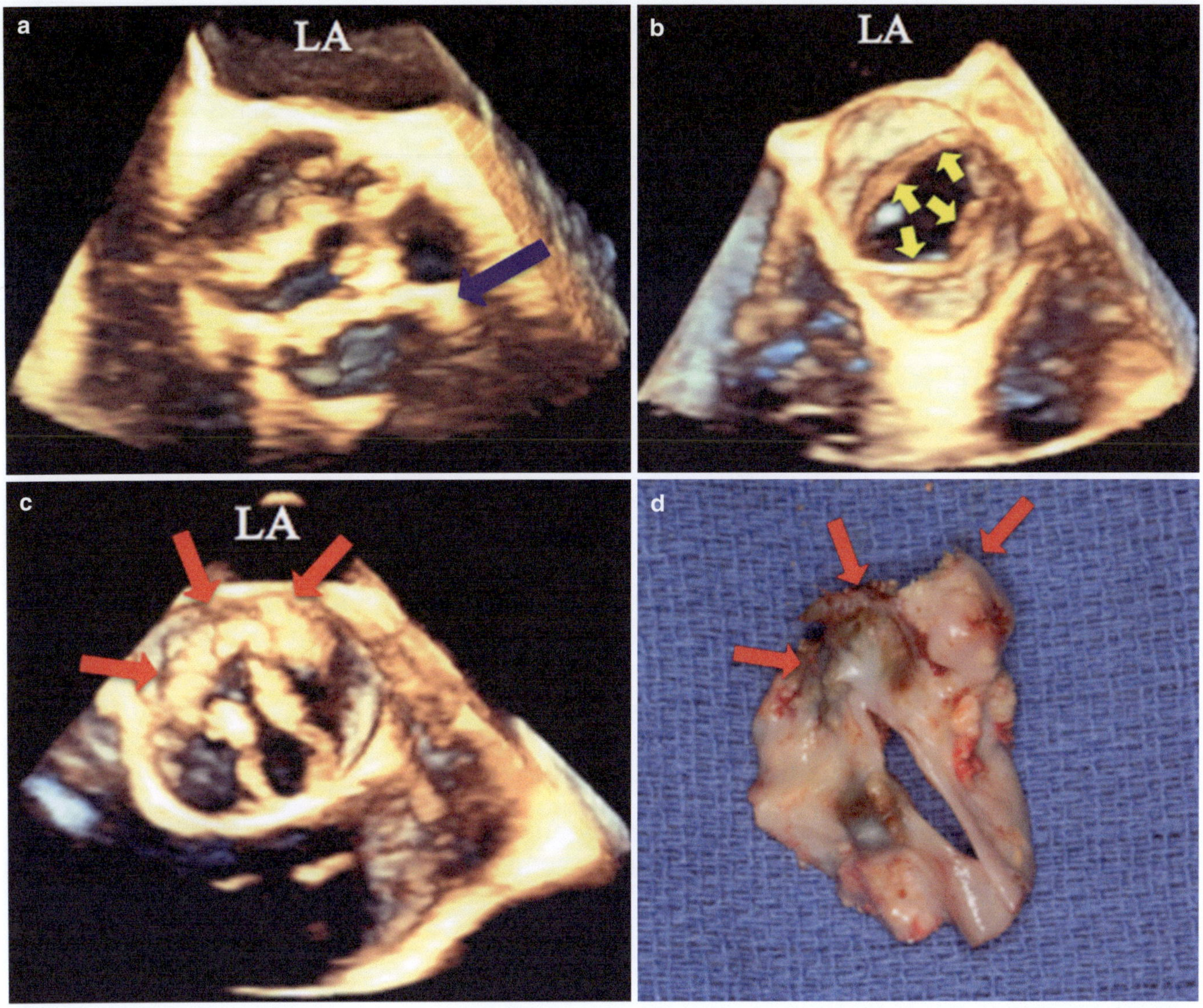

Fig. 12.6 Heterogeneous valve morphology in congenitally bicuspid AV disease. (**a**) Accelerated calcification with progressive AS is commonly present in patients with congenital AS. In this case a heavily calcified raphe is noted on the conjoined left-right coronary cusp (**a**, blue arrow). (**b**) A congenitally bicuspid AV with mild thickening but minimal calcification and relatively preserved leaflet excursion (**b**, yellow arrows). (**c**) A congenitally bicuspid valve with two relatively equal size leaflets and bulky, asymmetric calcification seen posteriorly (**c**, red arrows) along with leaflet thickening resulting in AS. (**d**) The pathological correlate to Panel **C** following surgical excision showing asymmetric calcification (**d**, red arrows) (Used with permission of Mayo Foundation for Medical Education and Research. All rights reserved). AS, aortic stenosis; AV, aortic valve; LA, left atrium

AV Endocarditis

The AV is involved in close to 40% of patients with infective endocarditis. Depending on the organism involved and host factors, clinical presentation may vary between subacute with symptoms of low-grade infection or acute with severe febrile illness rapidly progressing to congestive heart failure and potentially complicated by systemic embolism, paravalvular extension of infection, or complete heart block. Although echocardiography cannot make a pathologic diagnosis, echocardiographic findings consistent with a vegetation are included as a major criteria for the clinical diagnosis of infective endocarditis.

Vegetations involving the AV are most commonly attached to the ventricular aspect of the valve, are frequently irregularly shaped, and they typically move with the AV, but have their own independent oscillatory motion. Additional

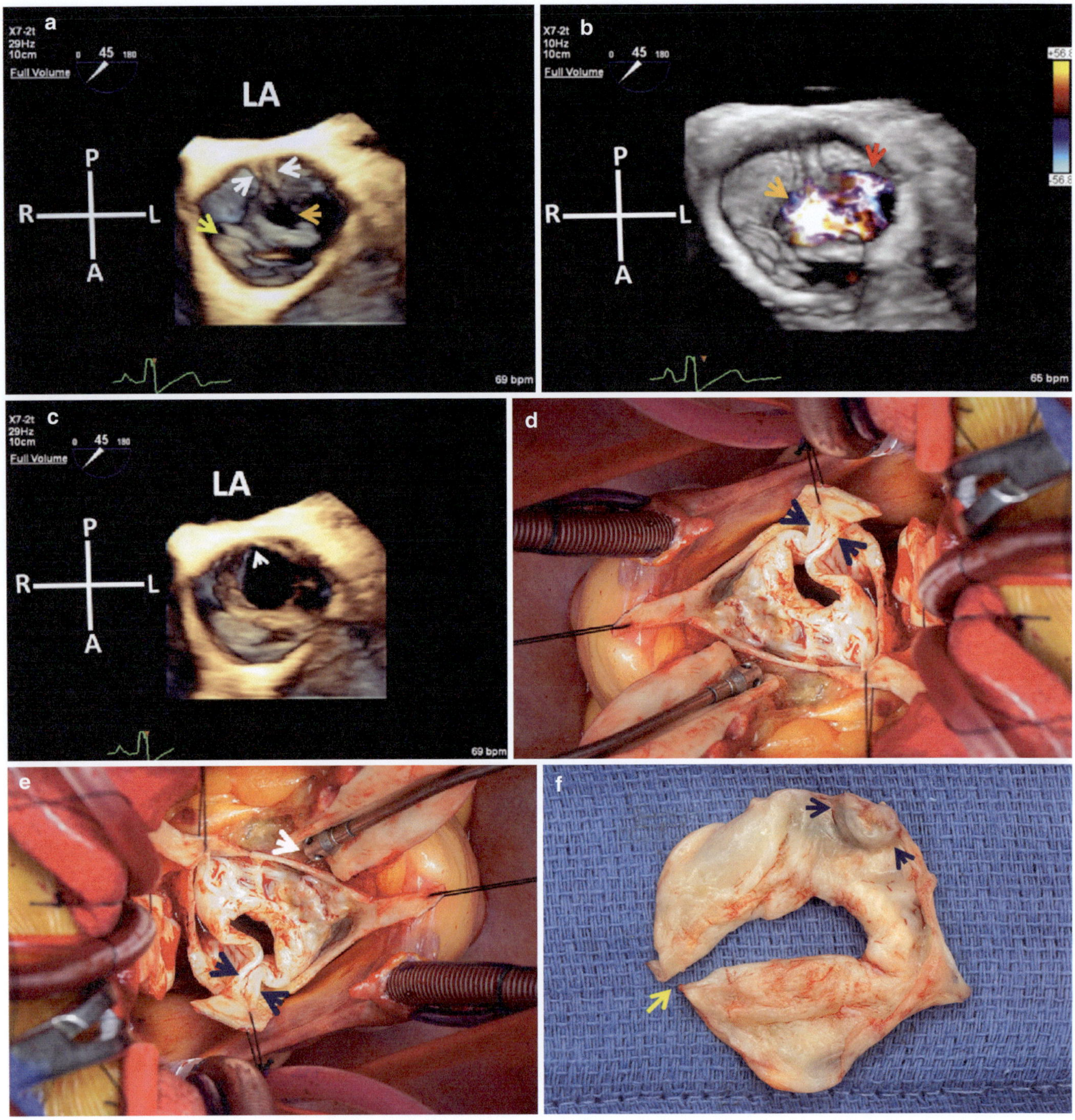

Fig. 12.7 54 year old man with unicuspid AV. 3D TEE Enface views of AV from aortic perspective in diastole (**a**, **b**) and systole (**c**) showing a single thick commissure (white arrows) and a calcified ridge (yellow arrow). There is central malcoaptation in diastole (orange arrow) with severe regurgitation on CFD (**b**) that is both central (orange arrow) and cusp related (red arrow). Intraoperative view of the valve oriented to match the 3D view (**d**) and as viewed by the surgeon (**e**) shows the thickened commissure (dark blue arrows), white arrow points to position of RCA ostium). The explanted valve in (**f**) shows site of commissure (yellow arrow) and calcification (dark blue arrows) seen on 3D (Used with permission of Mayo Foundation for Medical Education and Research. All rights reserved). A, anterior; AV, aortic valve; CFD, color flow Doppler; L, left; LA, left atrium; P, posterior; R, right; RCA, right coronary artery

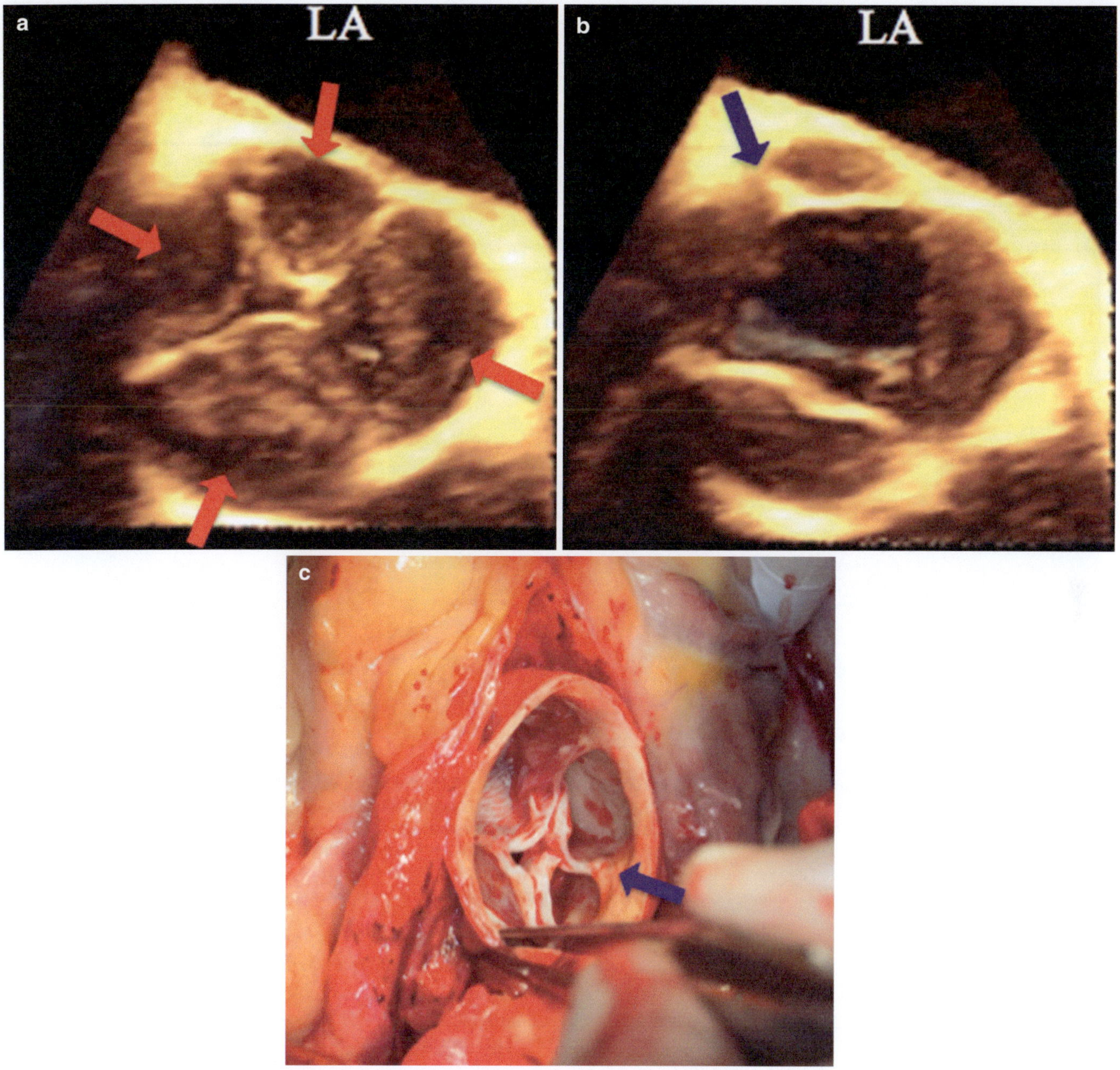

Fig. 12.8 Quadricuspid AV in a patient with severe aortic regurgitation. TEE prior to AV replacement for severe aortic regurgitation reveals a quadricuspid AV with four clearly defined leaflets (**a**, red arrows). 3D images examined during systole show partial fusion of the cusp in the non-coronary position (**b**, blue arrow) and this is confirmed on gross inspection of the valve at the time of operation (**c**, blue arrow) (Used with permission of Mayo Foundation for Medical Education and Research. All rights reserved). AV, aortic valve; LA, left atrium

findings which are not necessary for the diagnosis, but are supportive include destruction of the AV leaflets, cusp perforation, evidence of perivalvular extension or abscess formation, and pseudoaneurysm formation.

3D TEE is often helpful to clarify the location and number of vegetations and also provides a more comprehensive understanding of cusp involvement and valve destruction (Figs. 12.21, 12.22, and 12.23; see also Chap. 17).

In the setting of AV endocarditis the leaflets are often thickened which aids in visualization of the valve by 3D TEE by reducing dropout artifact. However, 3D color Doppler imaging is necessary to confirm flow through observed cusp defects, thus differentiating true perforations from dropout artifact (Figs. 12.21 and 12.23). 3D TEE can also be helpful to better characterize complex perivalvular extension and pseudoaneurysm and more precisely localize mobile vegeta-

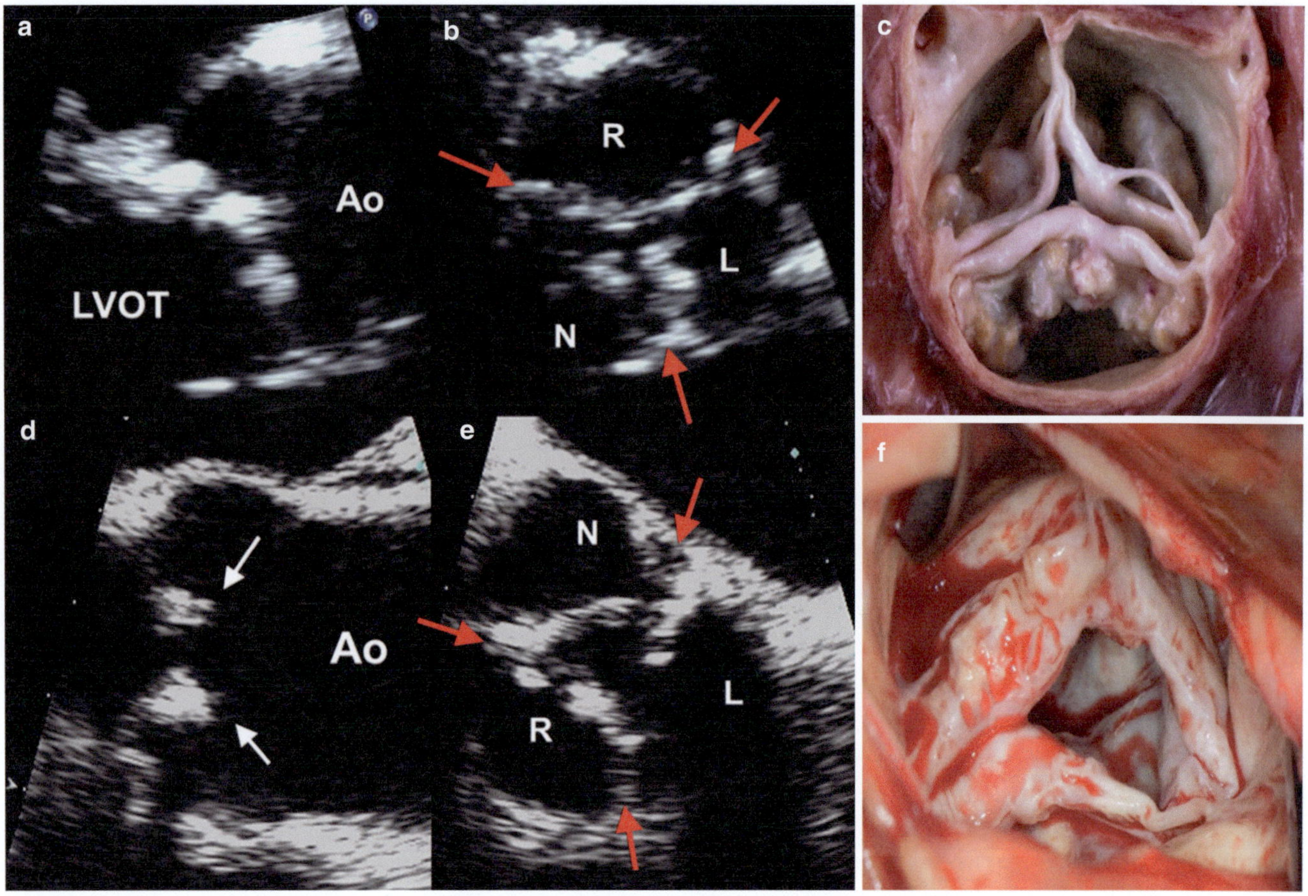

Fig. 12.9 Typical echocardiographic and pathologic findings for degenerative and rheumatic aortic stenosis. Panels **a**–**c** show typical features of calcific or degenerative AV stenosis, characterized by bulky calcification of the body of the aortic leaflets and relative sparing of the AV commissures (**b**, red arrows). Panel **c** is the pathologic correlate for panels **a** and **b**. Panels **d**–**f** show typical features of rheumatic aortic stenosis, which typically involves thickening of the aortic leaflet tips (**d**, white arrows) and commissural fusion (**e**, red arrows). Panel **f** is the pathologic correlate for Panels **d** and **e** (Used with permission of Mayo Foundation for Medical Education and Research. All rights reserved). Ao, ascending aorta; AV, aortic valve; L, left coronary cusp; LVOT, left ventricular outflow track; N, non-coronary cusp; R, right coronary cusp

tions and their proximity to critical structures such as the coronary artery ostia.

Tumors and Masses Involving the AV (See Also Chap. 26)

The two most common AV masses encountered in routine clinical practice are papillary fibroelastoma and Lambl's excrescence (Figs. 12.24 and 12.25). Additional considerations in the appropriate clinical scenario include infective endocarditis (discussed above) and nonbacterial thrombotic endocarditis. 3D TEE provides a robust characterization of the size and morphology of AV masses (Figs. 12.24 and 12.25). Particularly when there are multiple small masses, 3D TEE can often better delineate their location and number which in some cases can help narrow the differential diagnosis.

The aortic annulus and valve leaflets are dynamic structures, which require adequate frame rates for optimal visualization. Accordingly, it is important to optimize image settings to maximize frame rate for 3D TEE prior to image acquisition. In clinical practice this is most easily achieved by narrowing the sector size, acquiring the dataset in a zoomed view, and/or performing a multi-beat acquisition. As discussed above, there is often difficulty with dropout artifact in the body of the aortic leaflets, but frequently AV masses are directed more perpendicular to the ultrasound beam (when viewed from the mid-esophagus) and therefore, dropout artifact is not typically a major limitation when visualizing these masses.

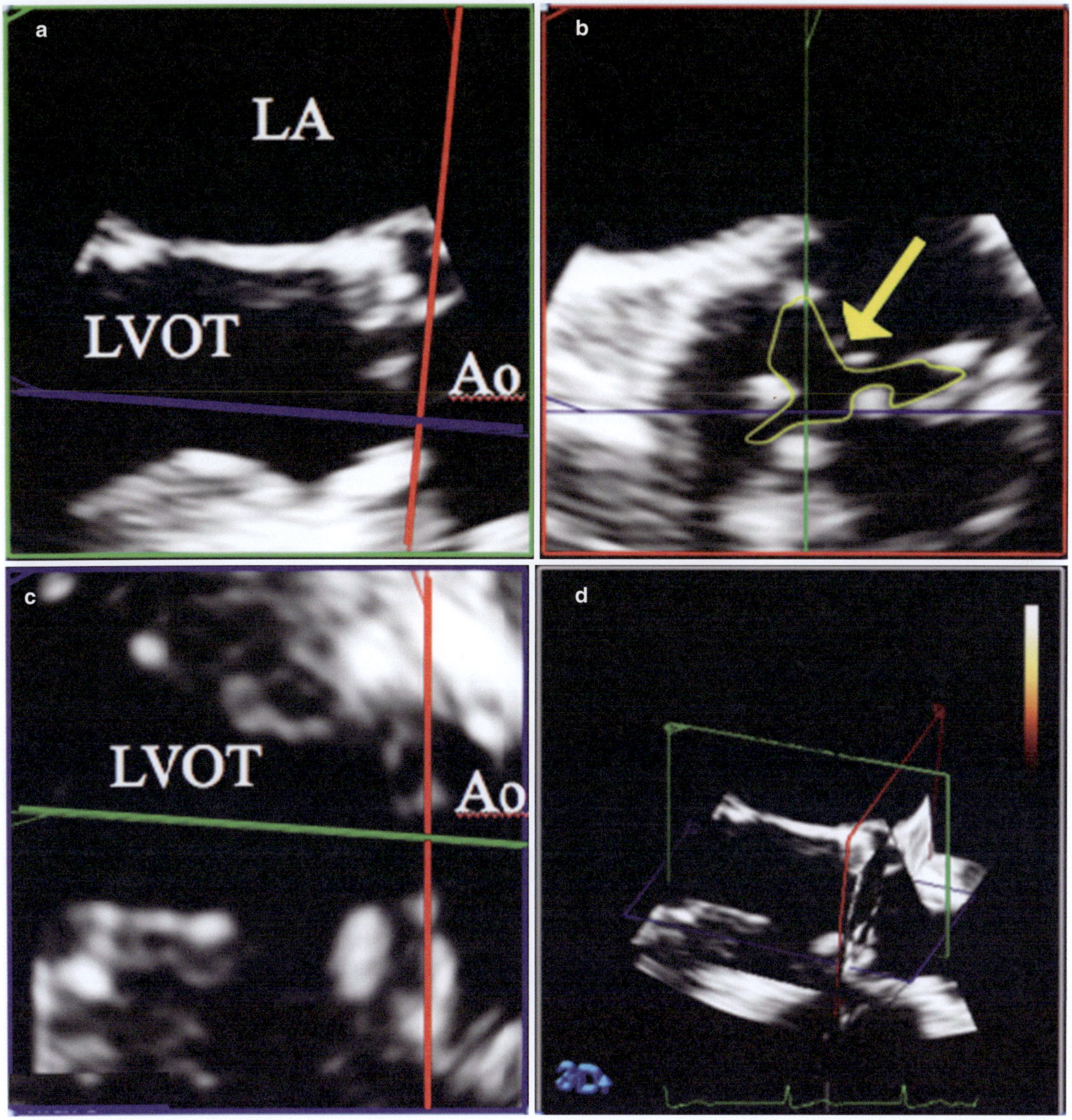

Fig. 12.10 Direct planimetry of aortic valve area by MPR. A 3D volumetric dataset of the aortic root is opened in the MPR software package and a mid-systolic frame is selected. An en face view of the stenotic orifice for direct planimetry (yellow arrow, **b**) is achieved by aligning the red plane in the two corresponding long axis views of the left ventricular outflow tract and aortic root (red lines, **a** and **c**) (Used with permission of Mayo Foundation for Medical Education and Research. All rights reserved). Abbreviations: Ao, ascending aorta; LA, left atrium; LVOT, left ventricular outflow tract; MPR, multiplanar reconstruction

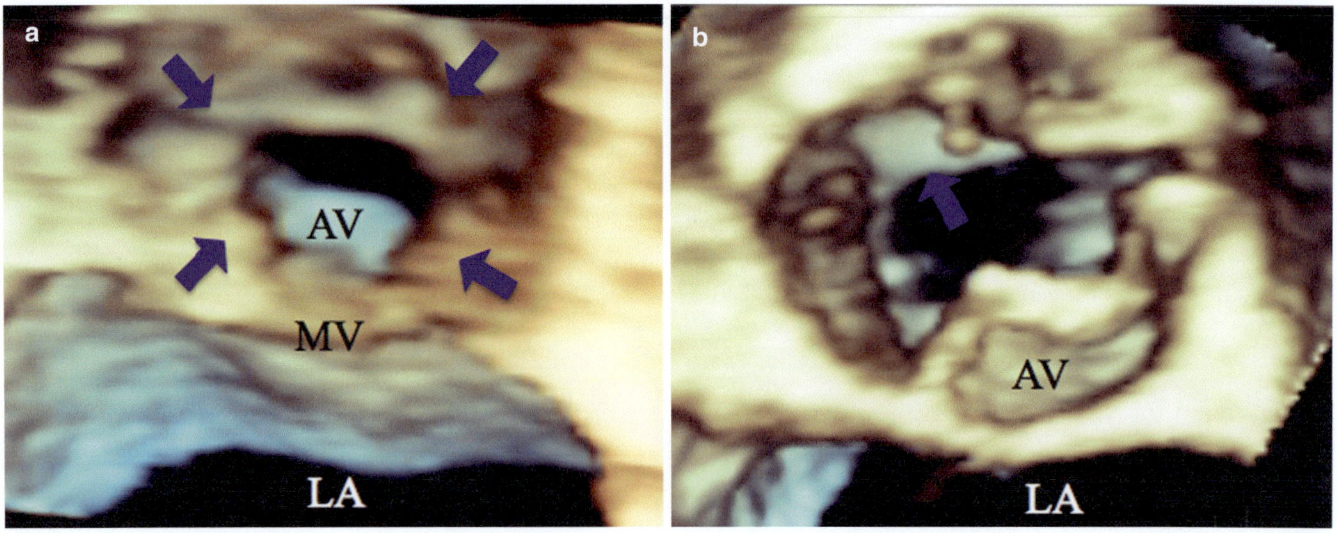

Fig. 12.11 Subaortic membrane visualization by 3D echocardiography. A thin, near-circumferential subaortic membrane (**a** and **b**, blue arrows) is seen from the perspective of the left ventricular outflow tract (**a**) and the ascending aorta as viewed through the AV during systole (**b**, blue arrow) (Used with permission of Mayo Foundation for Medical Education and Research. All rights reserved). AV, aortic valve; LA, left atrium; MV, mitral valve and mitral-aortic continuity

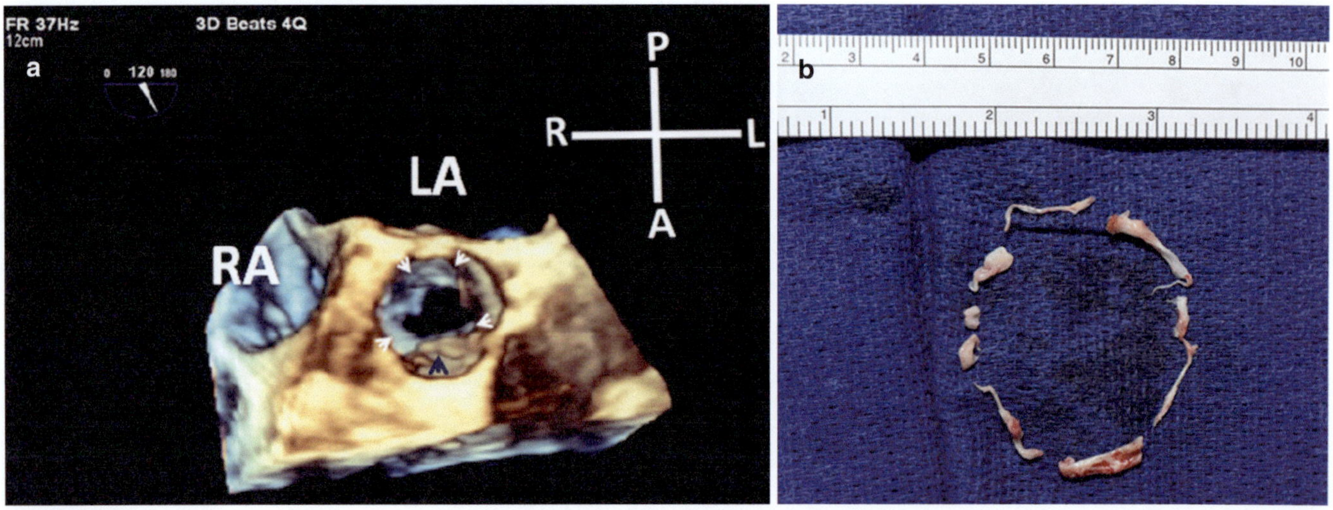

Fig. 12.12 (**a**) Another subaortic membrane (white arrows) as viewed from ascending aorta after cropping off most of the AV (dark blue arrow). Note the non-uniform circumferential extent of the membrane. (**b**) Intraop photo of the resected membrane (Used with permission of Mayo Foundation for Medical Education and Research. All rights reserved). A, anterior; AV, aortic valve; L, left; LA, left atrium; P, posterior; R, right; RA, right atrium

3D TEE for Assessment of the Aortic Root Pre-TAVR

Under-sizing of the aortic annulus prior to transcatheter AV insertion is a risk factor for significant paravalvular regurgitation post-procedure [11–13]. Previous studies have demonstrated that the aortic annulus is not typically circular, but elliptical and can be irregularly shaped (Fig. 12.26).

As such, 3D assessment of the aortic annulus has been shown to be superior to 2D measurement of the aortic annulus and 3D TEE has been shown to be equivalent to CT in experienced hands [12]. 3D TEE can be used to accurately measure aortic annular area and circumference, height to the coronary ostia, sinus of Valsalva dimensions, and sinotubular junction diameter.

Obtaining a high quality 3D volumetric data set is the first step for accurate assessment and quantitation of the aortic root. The 3D dataset should be obtained from the mid-esophageal window at a level that is coaxial or slightly inferior (caudal) to the plane of the aortic root. If the dataset is

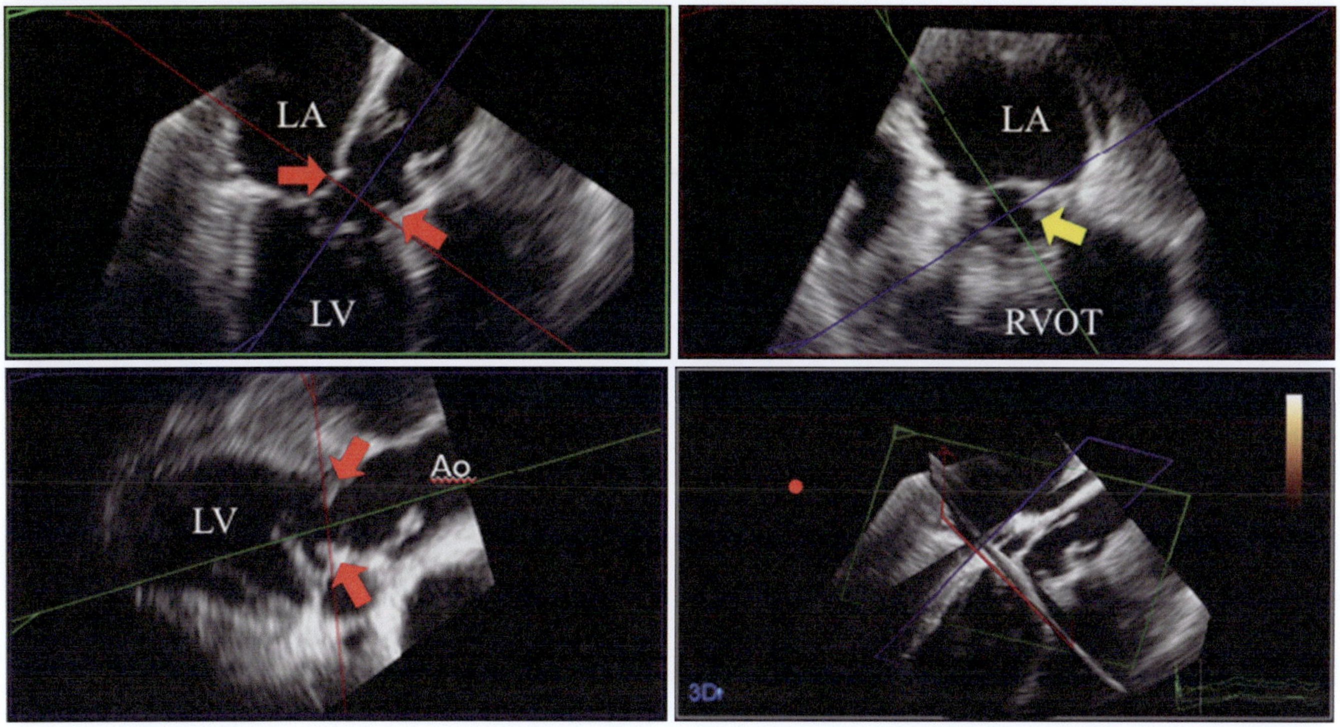

Fig. 12.13 Direct planimetry of subaortic stenosis by MPR. A short axis view of a subaortic membrane is created by aligning with the plane of the membrane in a double-oblique technique using two orthogonal views of the left ventricular outflow tract (upper and lower left panels, red arrows). Planimetry of the stenotic orifice can be performed in the short axis image (upper right panel, yellow arrow) (Used with permission of Mayo Foundation for Medical Education and Research. All rights reserved). Ao, ascending aorta; LA, left atrium; LV, left ventricle; MPR, multiplanar reconstruction; RVOT, right ventricular outflow tract

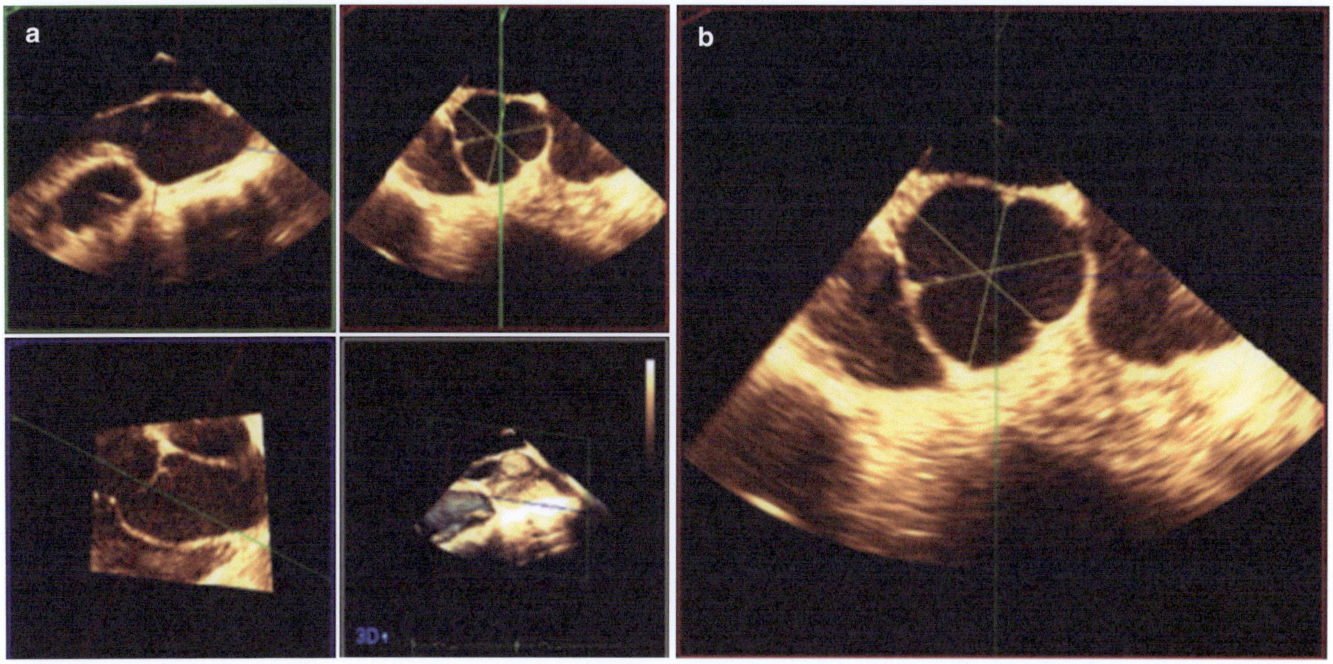

Fig. 12.14 Aortic root assessment by 3D TEE with MPR in a patient with Marfan syndrome and typical aortic root pathologic findings. There is symmetric enlargement of the sinuses of Valsalva with effacement of the sino-tubular junction and relatively early tapering of the ascending aorta to normal diameter. MPR (**a**) allows coplanar alignment with the sinuses of Valsalva and aortic root measurements (**b**) similar to cardiac CT or MRI (Used with permission of Mayo Foundation for Medical Education and Research. All rights reserved). MPR, multiplanar reconstruction

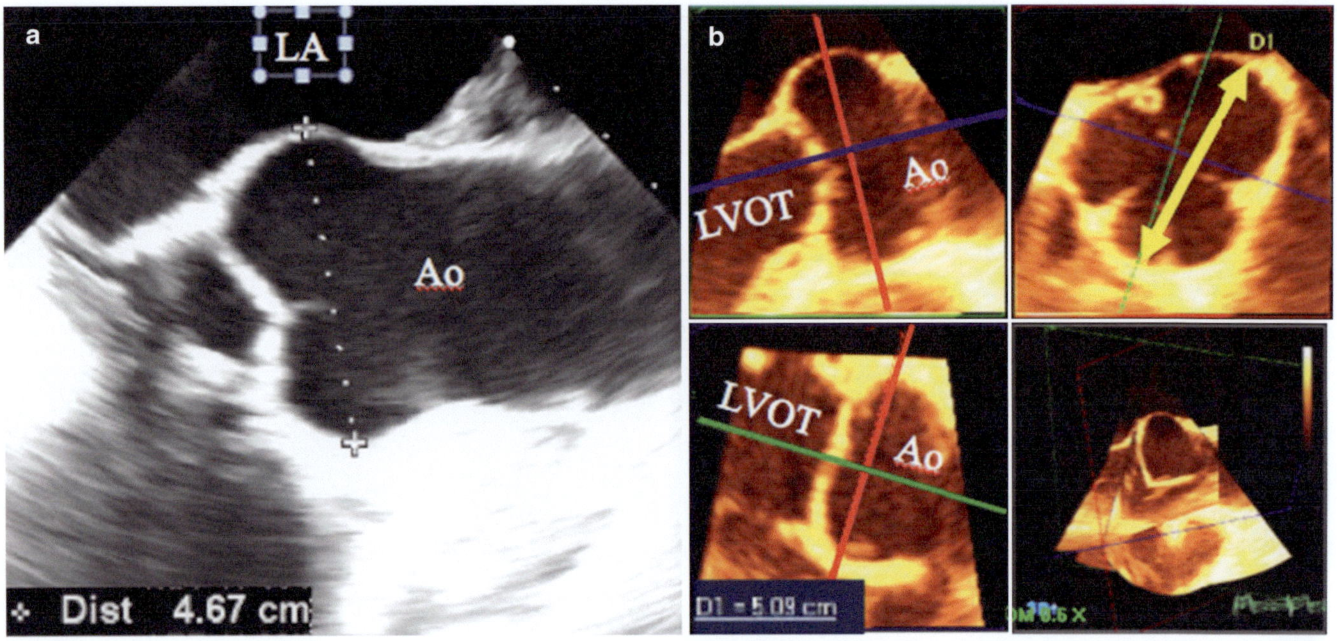

Fig. 12.15 3D TEE for asymmetric sinus of Valsalva enlargement. The sinus of Valsalva diameter measured by 2D TEE from a conventional long axis view is 4.7 cm (**a**). Using a 3D TEE dataset and MPR (**b**), the imaging plane is aligned with the sinuses of Valsalva in two long axis views of the aortic root (red lines, left upper and lower panels) which provides a short axis view of the sinuses and demonstrates asymmetric enlargement of left sinus of Valsalva (**b**, right upper panel) which was not as well appreciated on available 2D imaging planes. By 3D TEE (**b**), the maximum sinus of Valsalva diameter measures 5.1 cm between the left and right coronary sinuses of Valsalva (yellow arrow, right upper panel) (Used with permission of Mayo Foundation for Medical Education and Research. All rights reserved). Ao, aorta; LA, left atrium; LVOT, left ventricular outflow track; MPR, multiplanar reconstruction

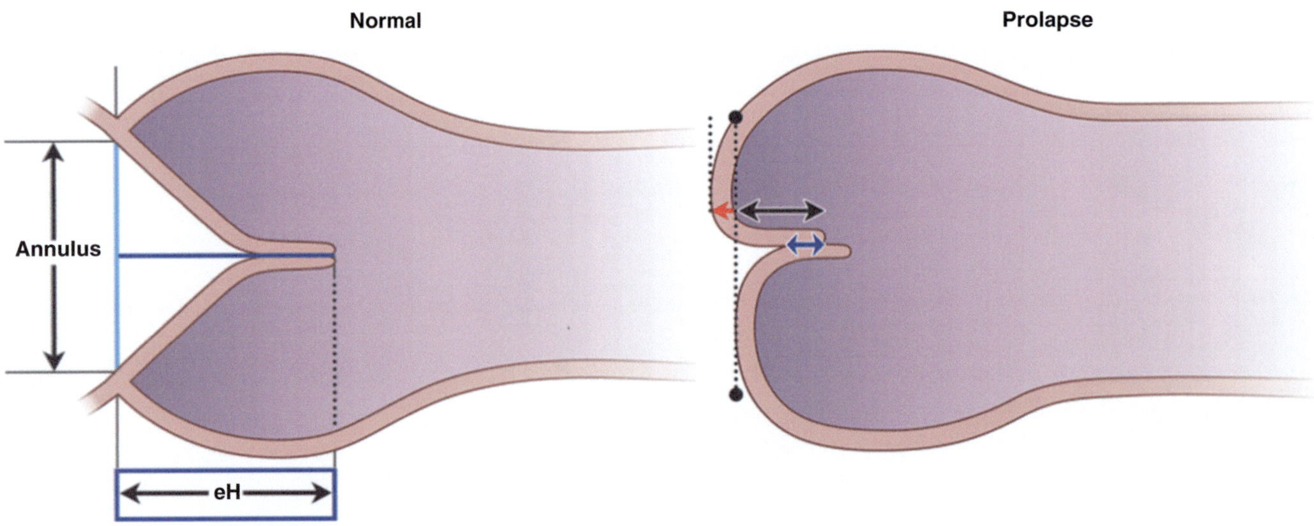

Fig. 12.16 Schematic diagram of normal aortic leaflet effective height (eH) on the left and AV prolapse on the right with reduced eH due to valve prolapse (black double arrow) and decreased coaptation length (blue double arrow). Adapted from le Polain de Waroux JB, Pouleur AC, Robert A et al. Mechanisms of recurrent aortic regurgitation after AV repair: predictive value of intraoperative transesophageal echocardiography. JACC Cardiovasc Imaging 2009;2:931–9 [8]. AV, aortic valve; eH, effective height

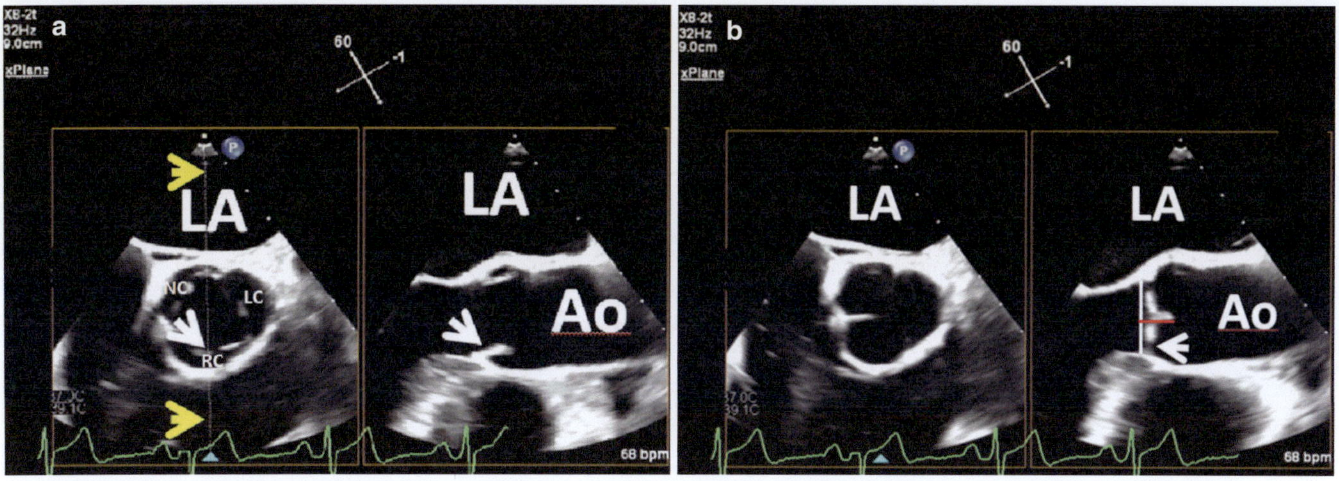

Fig. 12.17 x-Plane of AV in systole (**a**) and diastole (**b**). The tilt cursor (**a**, yellow arrows) cuts through the NC close to the commissure that separates it from the LC, and bisects the body of the RC (white arrow). The corresponding image in the long axis of the ascending aorta (Ao) shows the fully open RC (white arrow). **b**, The RC (white arrow) eH (solid red line) is measured from plane of aortic valve annulus (solid white line) (Used with permission of Mayo Foundation for Medical Education and Research. All rights reserved). Ao, ascending aorta; AV, aortic valve; LA, left atrium; LC, left coronary cusp; NC, non-coronary cusp; RC, right coronary cusp

acquired from a higher esophageal window the calcified valve can cause acoustic shadowing of the anterior aortic annulus which makes measurement challenging (Fig. 12.27). Ideally, one should avoid a multi-beat acquisition for annular sizing as unrecognized stitch artifact could render measurements inaccurate. It is therefore important to narrow the sector size for single beat (live 3D) full volume acquisition or if the dataset is acquired in a zoomed mode to achieve adequate frame rate; in general, 10 frames/s provide adequate systolic frames for analysis.

Measurement of the aortic annulus area and circumference are most accurately performed using MPR on the previously acquired dataset. Recently, some vendors have developed automated software to measure the aortic annulus while other systems require manual measurement and both methods have been shown to correlate well with cardiac CT [12–14] (Fig. 12.28). Even with automated measurements, care must be taken to confirm the accuracy of the measurement and manually adjust as necessary.

Although the details of manual measurement vary slightly according to the vendor software used, the principles necessary to produce accurate and reproducible results are similar. Here is our recommendation for manual planimetry of the aortic annulus:

1. Obtain a high quality, single beat 3D volumetric dataset of the aortic root, including the left ventricular outflow tract to the sino-tubular junction with careful attention to avoid acoustic shadowing of the anterior aortic annulus.
2. Open the appropriate software package with MPR and quantitative measurement capability.
3. Optimize gains and magnify/zoom on the aortic root if necessary.
4. Identify a systolic frame (preferably mid-systole) where the complete circumference of the aortic annulus is well visualized.
5. Designate the MPR plane which will be used for the aortic annulus measurement and align that plane so that it is roughly coplanar with the aortic annulus.
6. Rotate the designated plane axially to make fine adjustments in the position by aligning this plane with the nadir (most inferior position) of each of the 3 aortic cusps.
7. Use direct planimetry to measure aortic annular area and circumference.

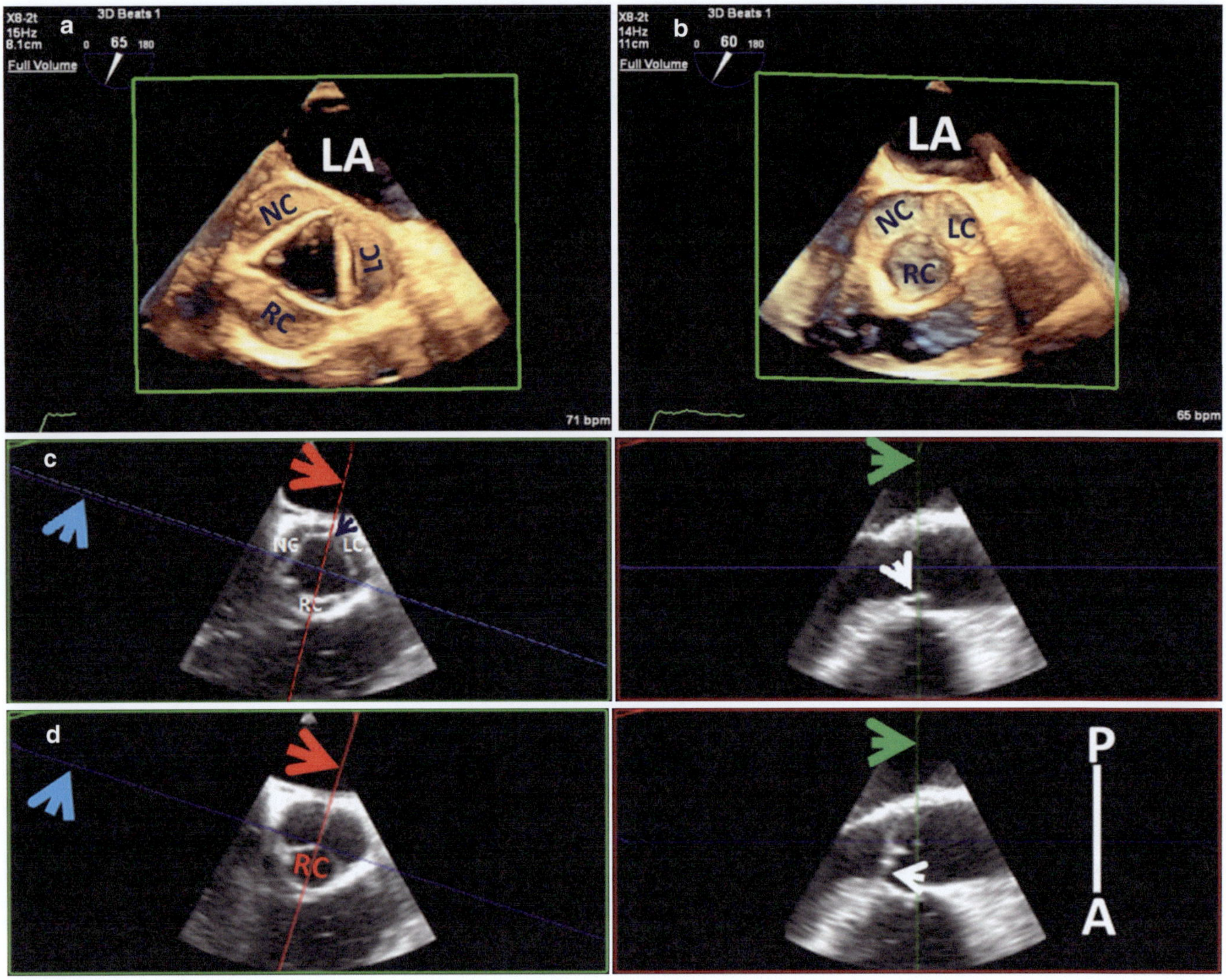

Fig. 12.18 Live single beat FV AV in systole (**a**) and diastole (**b**). MPR AV (**c**, **d**) shows the red plane (red line and arrow) bisecting the body of the RC and through the interleaflet trigone between the non and left coronary cusps (dark blue arrow) in both systole (**c**, left) and diastole (**d**, left) with corresponding images of the RC (white arrows) in the orthogonal 2D long-axis AV and ascending aorta planes (**c** and D, right). Blue and green arrows point to the orthogonal blue and green planes (Used with permission of Mayo Foundation for Medical Education and Research. All rights reserved). A, anterior; AV, aortic valve; FV, Full Volume; LA, left atrium; LC, left coronary cusp; MPR, multiplanar reconstruction; NC, non-coronary cusp; P, posterior; RC, right coronary cusp

8. Rotate the designated plane axially again, using the orthogonal (long axis) views of the aortic annulus to confirm the accuracy of the aortic annular points.

Additional measurements including aortic annular minimum and maximum diameter, distance to the coronary ostia, sinus of Valsalva diameter, and sino-tubular junction diameter are highly feasible and best done within an MPR package. In our experience we have found that this technique is highly feasible and reproducible in the majority of patients when done by an experienced operator. Poor feasibility is occasionally seen in patients with poor acoustic windows and poor echocardiographic image quality or in those with heavy calcification of the subvalvular left ventricular outflow tract, particularly if it involves the aorto-mitral continuity as this can cause acoustic shadowing of the aortic annulus.

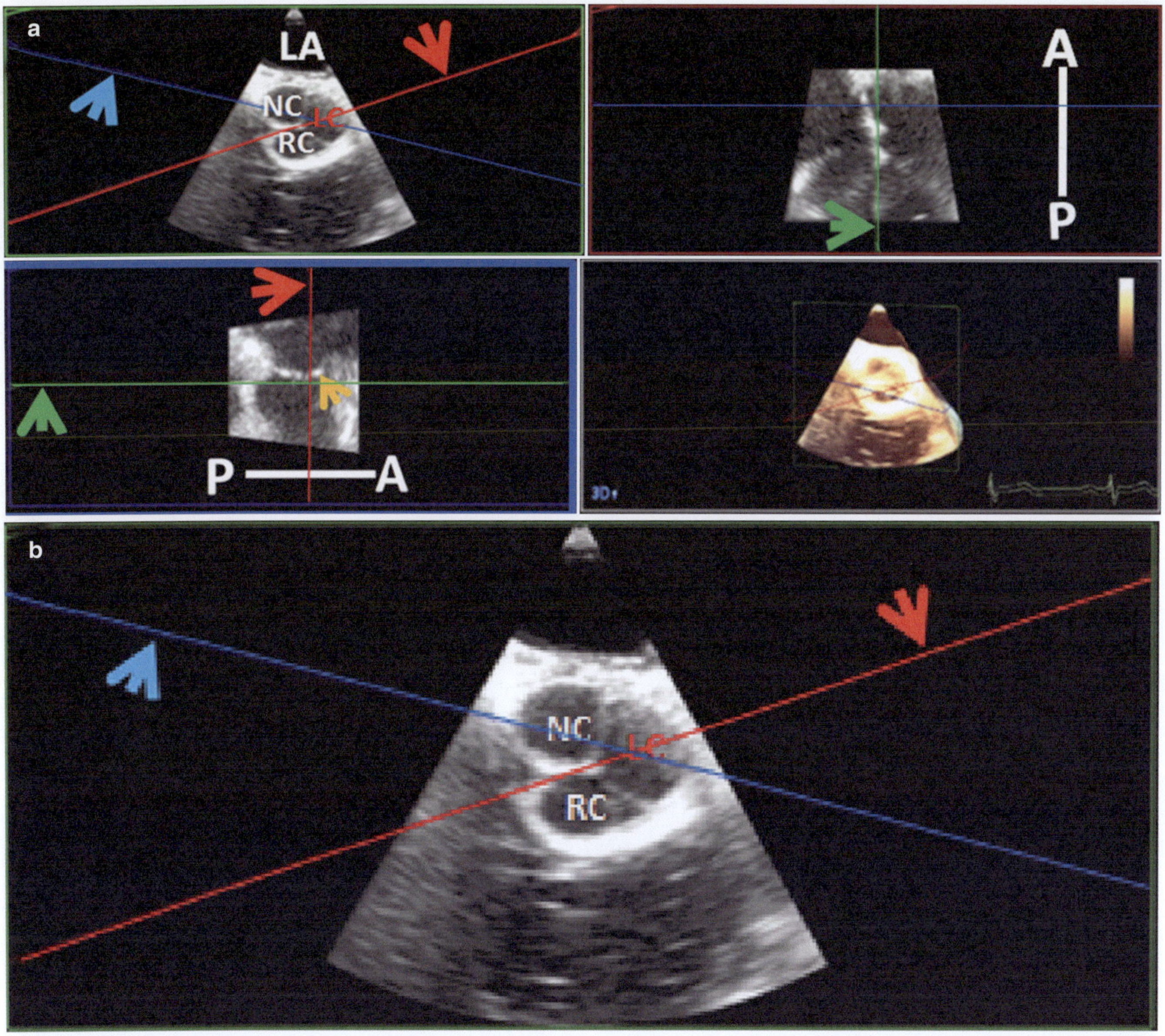

Fig. 12.19 Effective height non-coronary and left coronary cusps. Using the same approach as shown in Fig. 12.18. eH measurements for both left (**a–c**) and non-coronary (**d–f**) cusps can be obtained. (**a**) MPR of AV with focus on ***left coronary cusp***. Red plane (red arrow, upper left) is directed through middle of body of the left coronary cusp and through the interleaflet trigone separating the right and non-coronary cusps (**a**, **b**). Left cusp (orange arrow) is identified by intersection of red plane (red line and arrow) with AV in the blue transverse plane (blue box, left lower quadrant **a** and **c**) allowing measurement of eH (orange line, **c**) from plane of aortic annulus (white line, **c**). (**d**) MPR of AV with focus on ***non-coronary cusp***. Red plane (red arrow, upper left) is directed through middle of body of the non-coronary cusp and through the interleaflet trigone separating the right and left coronary cusps (**d**, **e**). Non-coronary cusp (yellow arrow) is identified by intersection of red plane (red line and arrow) with AV in the blue transverse plane (blue box, left lower quadrant **d** and **f**) allowing measurement of eH (dashed orange line, **f**) from plane of aortic annulus (white line, **f**). The antero-posterior trajectory of the green plane (green line and arrows) is determined from the long-axis 2D view of the AV and ascending aorta in the red box in right upper quadrants of **a** and **d**. Note that the non-coronary cusp is posterior to the left coronary cusp. Also note that the blue plane (blue lines and arrows) cuts across the left and non-coronary cusps only (). A, anterior; AV, aortic valve; eH, effective height; LA, left atrium; LC, left coronary cusp; MPR, multiplanar reconstruction; NC, non-coronary cusp; P, posterior; RC, right coronary cusp

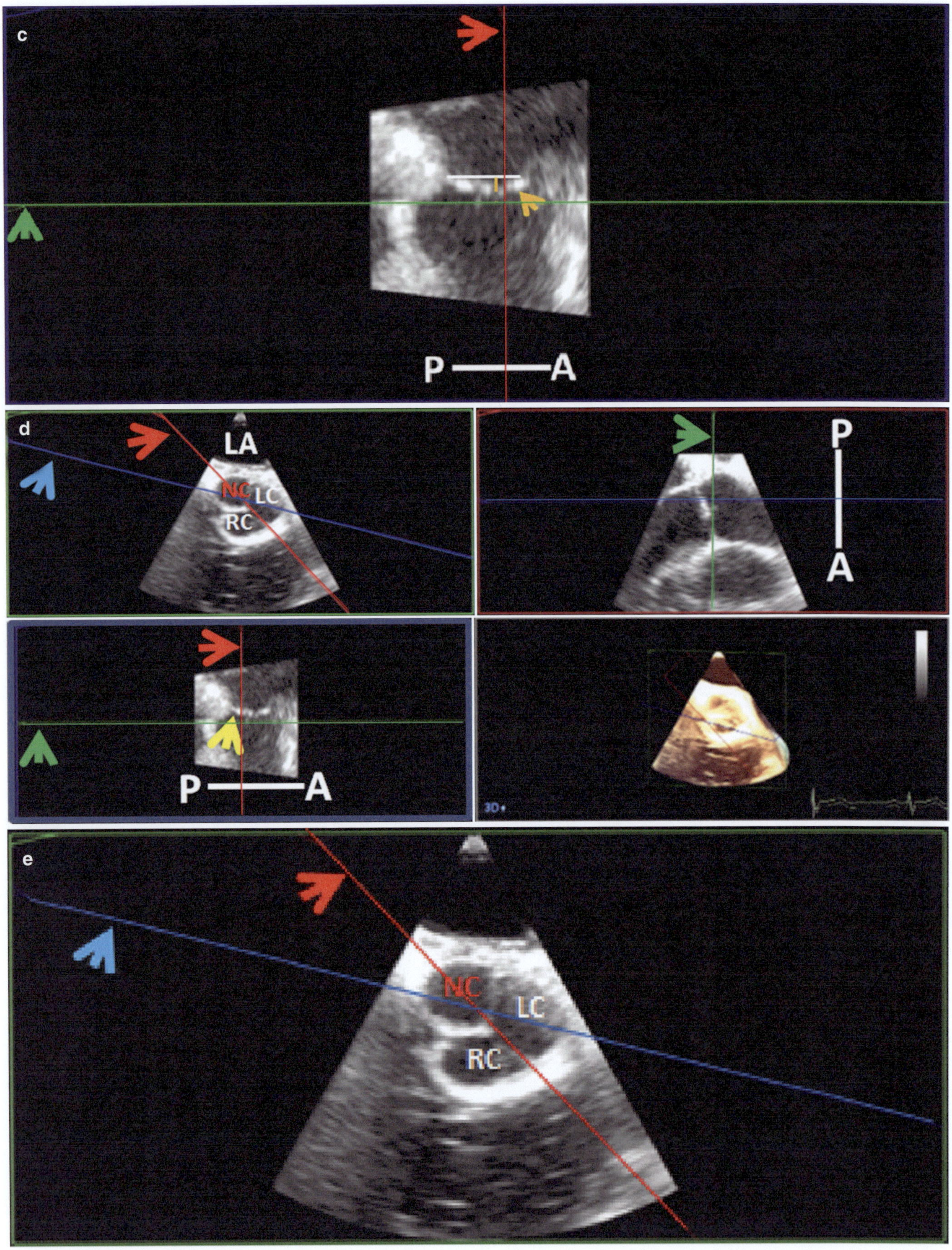

Fig. 12.19 (continued)

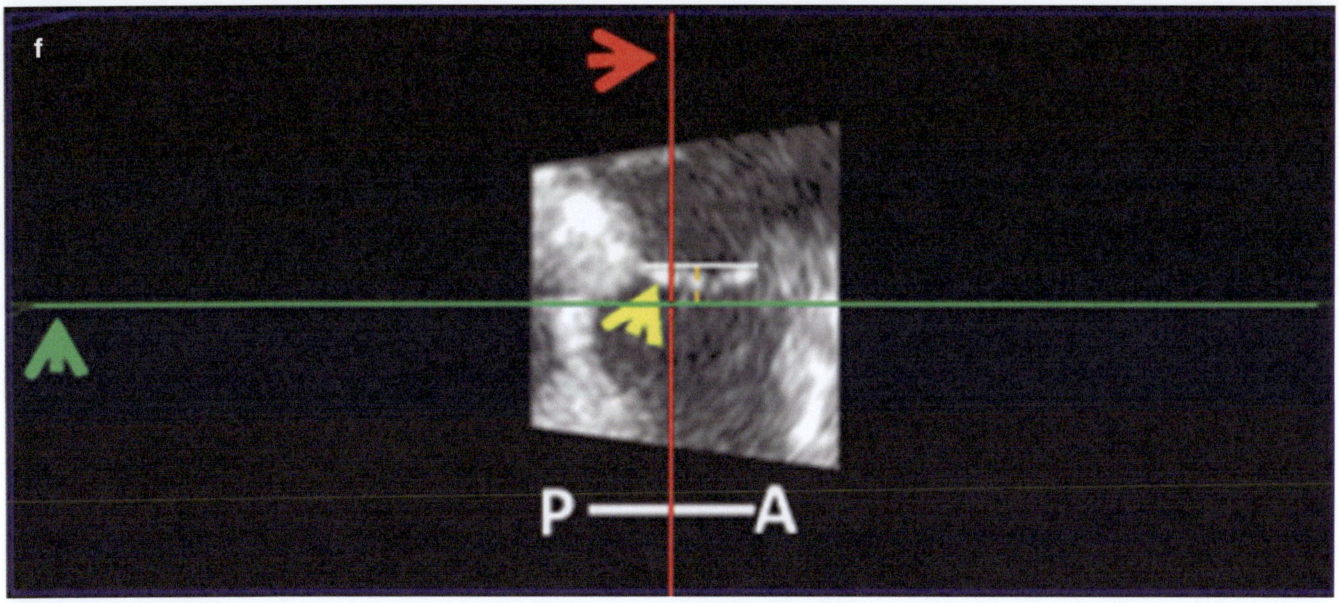

Fig. 12.19 (continued)

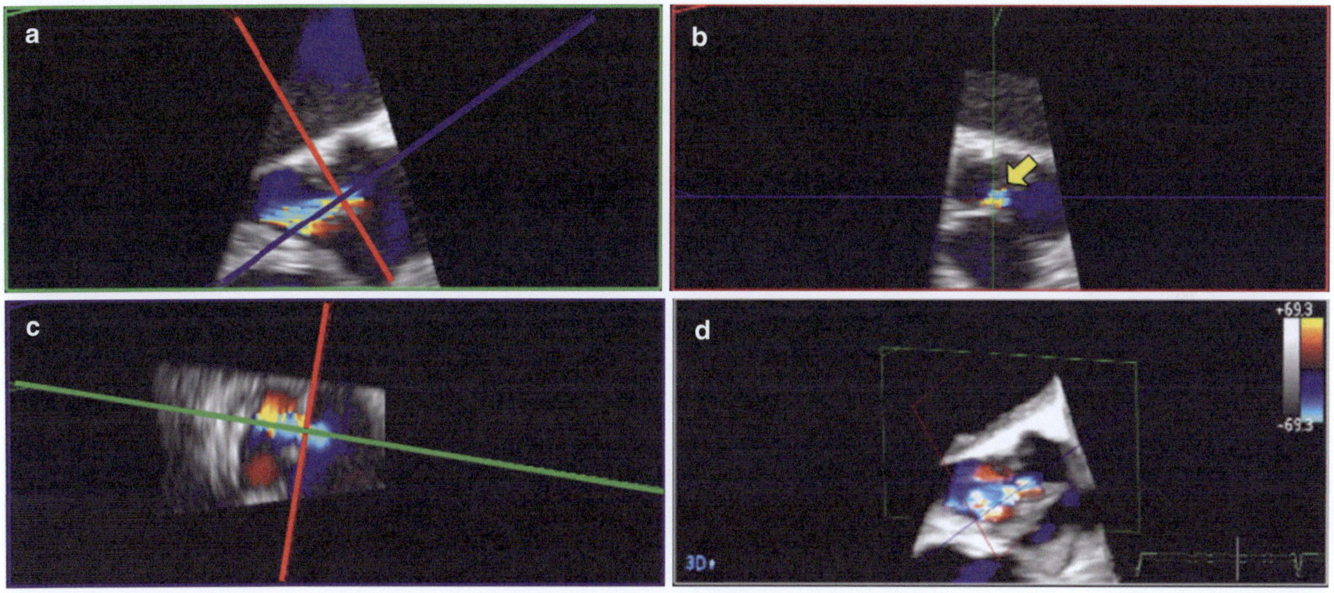

Fig. 12.20 3D color Doppler vena contracta area for aortic regurgitation. Three orthogonal views of an AV regurgitant jet are shown (**a**–**c**). By aligning the red plane in 2 orthogonal views of the vena contracta (**a** and **c**, red lines), a short axis view of the vena contracta area is created (**b**, yellow arrow) for direct planimetry. A cropped version of the 3D color Doppler volumetric dataset is shown in **d** (Used with permission of Mayo Foundation for Medical Education and Research. All rights reserved)

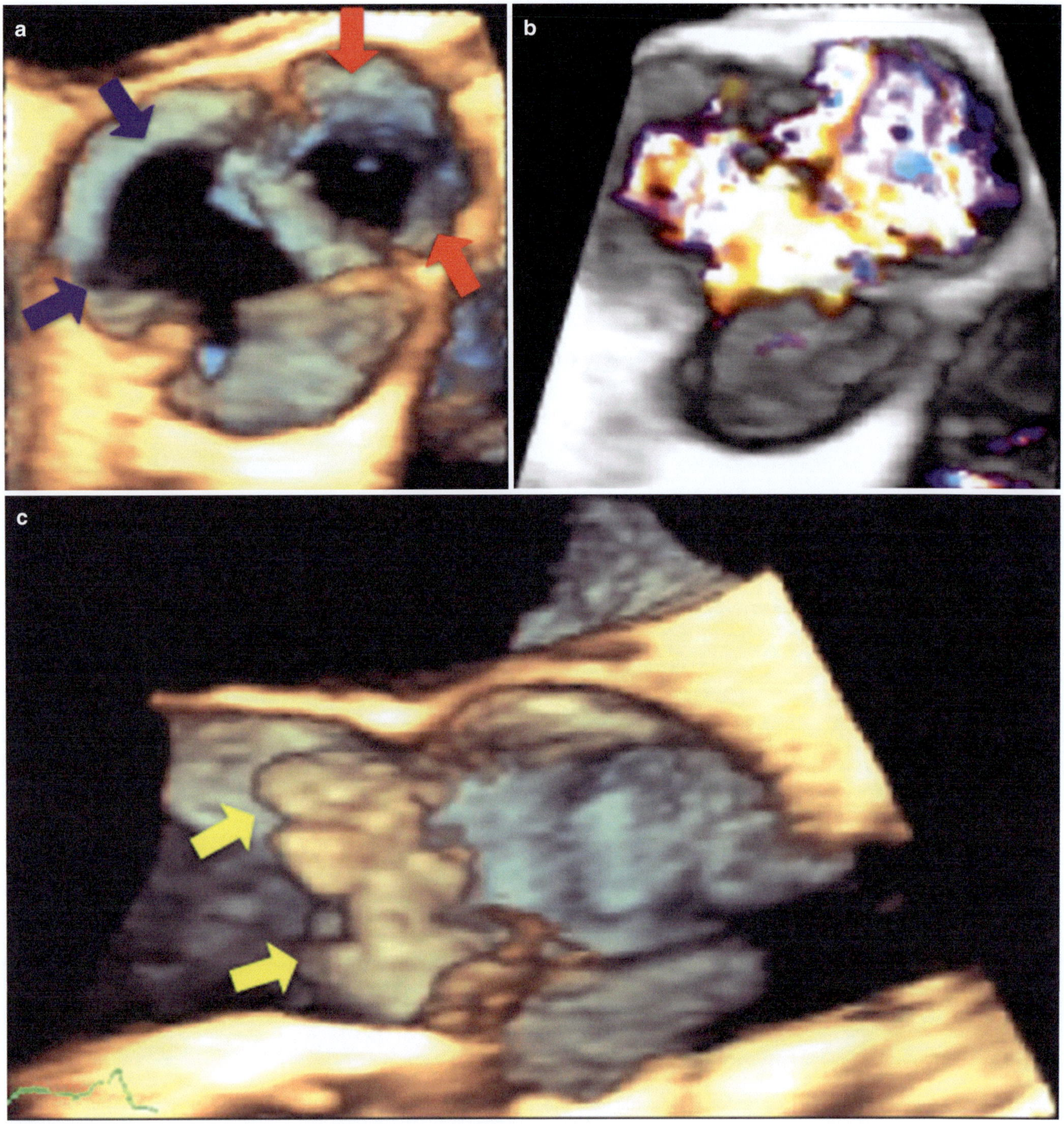

Fig. 12.21 AV endocarditis with severe valve destruction. A patient with acute bacterial endocarditis related to *Corynebacterium pseudodiphtheriticum* with extensive AV destruction. Viewed from the ascending aorta (**a**), there is very little remaining non-coronary cusp tissue (blue arrows, **a**) and there is a large perforation in the left coronary. cusp (red arrows, **a**) with severe regurgitation confirmed by 3D color Doppler imaging (**b**). The large vegetations adherent to the left coronary cusp are seen in cross section of the LVOT and aortic root (yellow arrows, **c**) (Used with permission of Mayo Foundation for Medical Education and Research. All rights reserved). AV, aortic valve; LVOT, left ventricular outflow tract

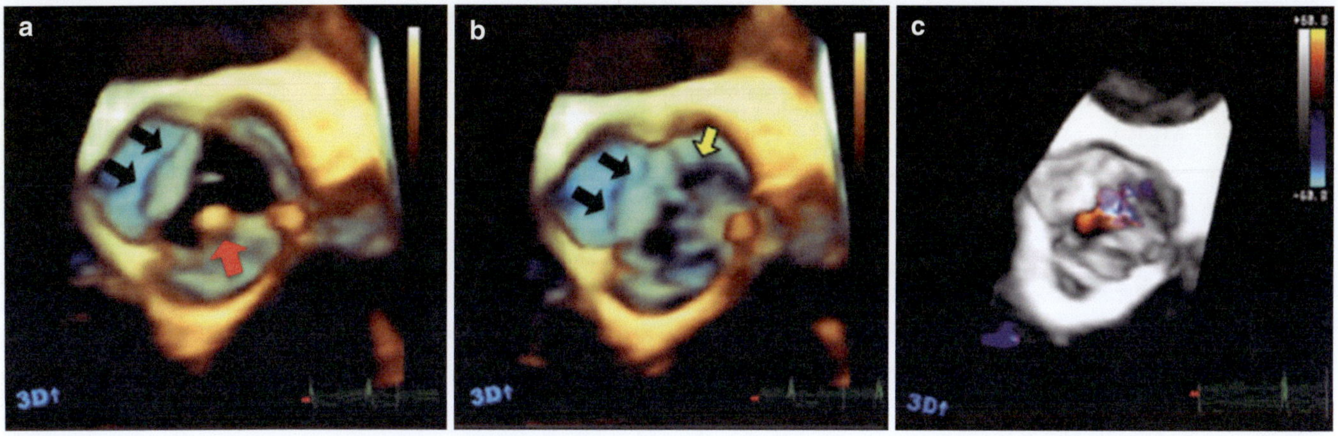

Fig. 12.22 AV endocarditis. A patient with AV endocarditis caused by *Enterococcus faecalis* viewed in systole (**a**), diastole (**b**), and diastole with 3D color Doppler to evaluate for valvular regurgitation (**c**). Note the thickened leaflets, in particular the free margin of the non-coronary cusp (black arrows, **a**, **b**) and the AV vegetation attached to the right coronary cusp (red arrow, **a**). The left and portions of the right coronary cusp have a "moth-eaten" appearance due to leaflet destruction related to the endocarditis (yellow arrow, **b**). Color flow Doppler confirms regurgitation through these defects (**c**) (Used with permission of Mayo Foundation for Medical Education and Research. All rights reserved). AV, aortic valve

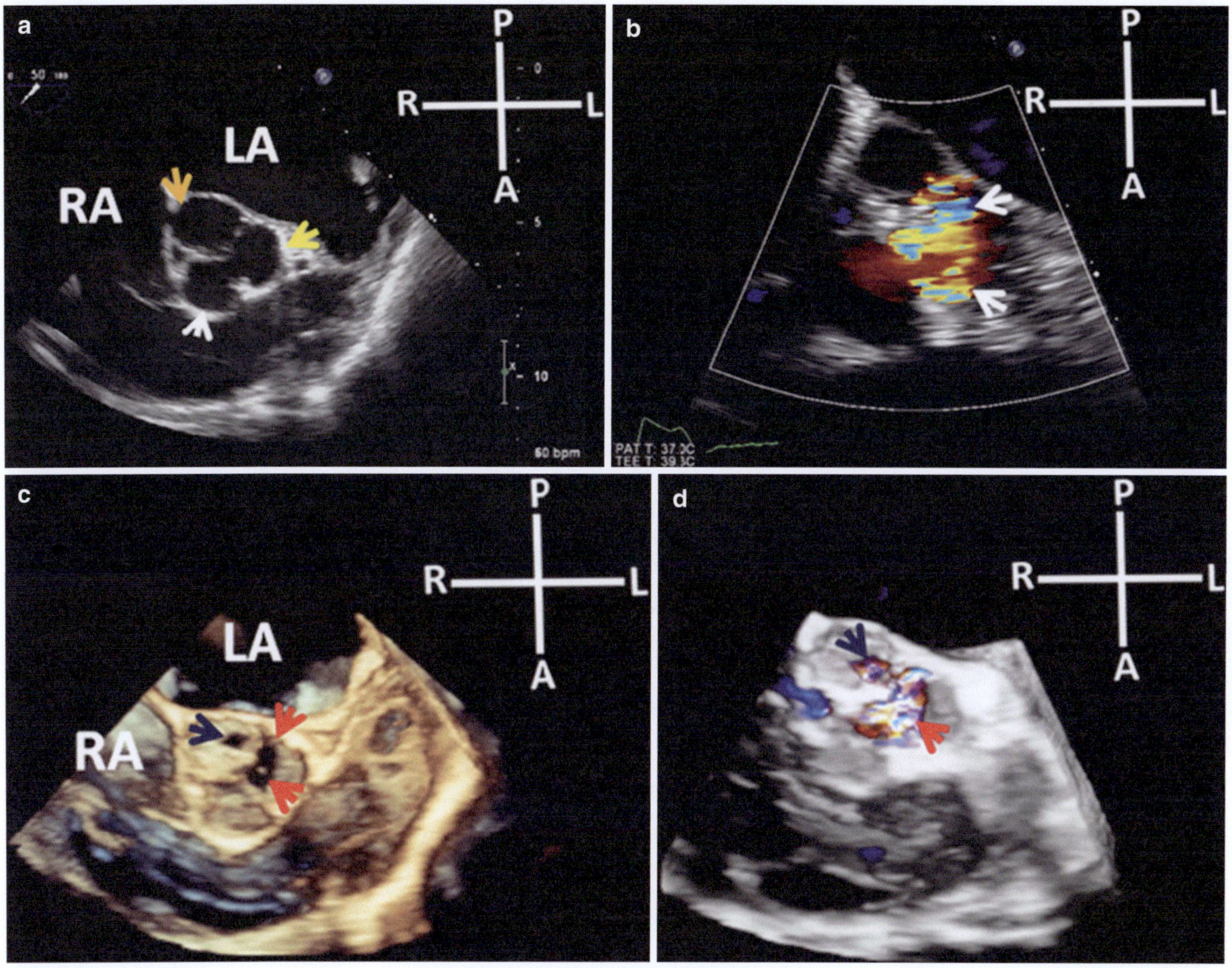

Fig. 12.23 Post AV endocarditis. **Top panel**: 2D TEE short-axis AV (**a**) not showing any apparent pathology . white, yellow, and orange arrows point to the RCC, LCC, and NCC respectively. Significant AR (white arrows) seen on color flow Doppler (**b**). (**c**) Live 3D of the same view shown in **a**. The added depth provided by 3D unmasks extensive destruction of the LCC (red arrows) and a perforation in the NCC (dark blue arrow). These findings are confirmed on 3D color Doppler imaging (**d**) that shows regurgitant flow through the observed defects (Used with permission of Mayo Foundation for Medical Education and Research. All rights reserved). A, anterior; AV, aortic valve; L, left; LA, left atrium; LCC, left coronary cusp; NCC, non coronary cusp; P, posterior; R, right; RA, right atrium; RCC, right coronary cusp

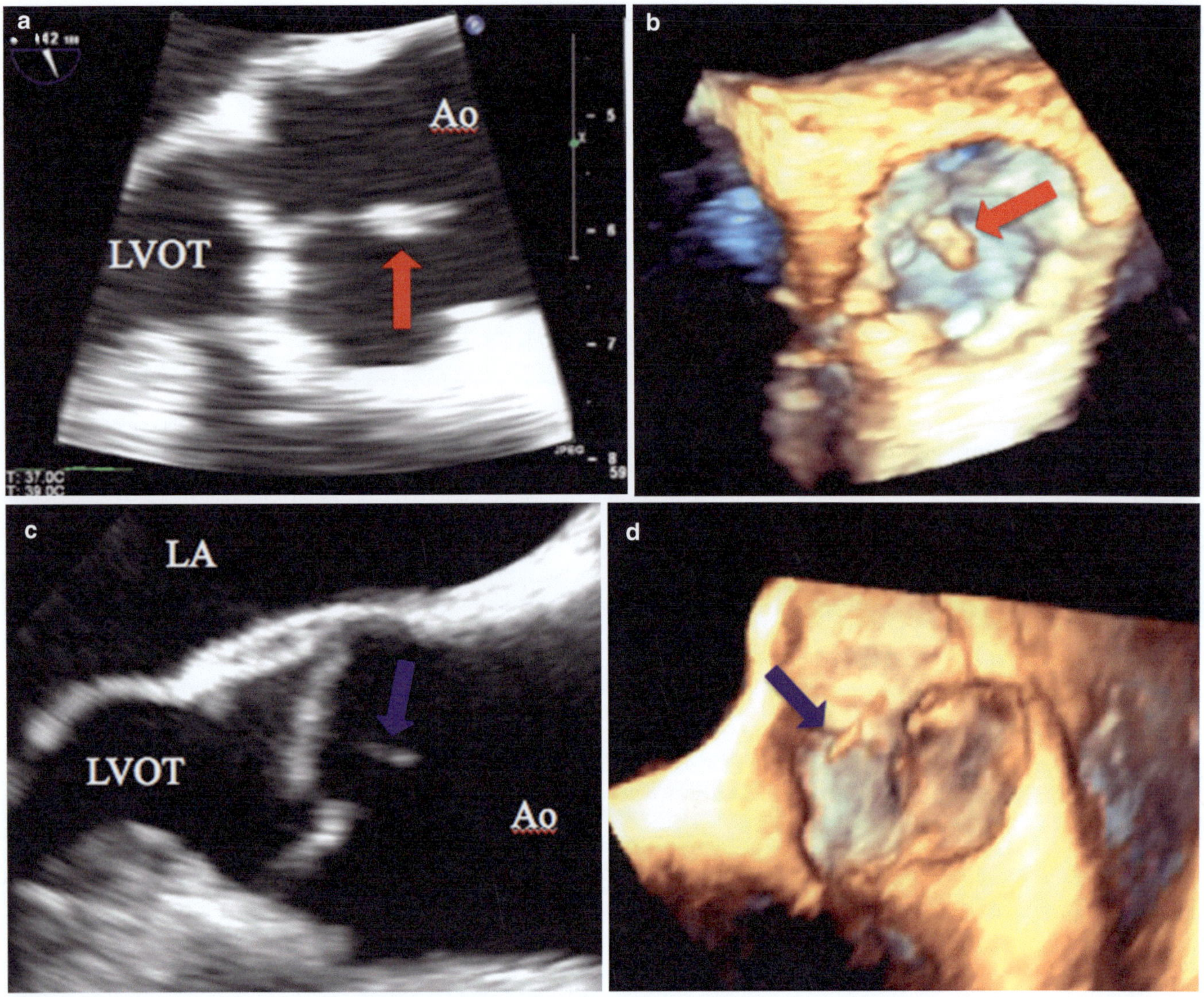

Fig. 12.24 3D TEE of AV masses. (**a**, **b**) A small papillary fibroelastoma is seen attached to the non-coronary cusp of the AV by 2D (**a**, red arrow) and 3D TEE (**b**, red arrow). Papillary fibroelastomas are most commonly attached to the aortic surface of the valve and typically have a "pom-pom" appearance by echocardiography with a short stalk and multiple small fronds of varying length. (**c**, **d**) A Lambl's excrescence is seen on the AV by 2D (**c**, blue arrow) and 3D (**d**, blue arrow) echocardiography. Lambl's excrescence are commonly seen as small, linear mobile echo-densities adherent to the AV (Used with permission of Mayo Foundation for Medical Education and Research. All rights reserved). Ao, ascending aorta; LA, left atrium; LVOT, left ventricular outflow track

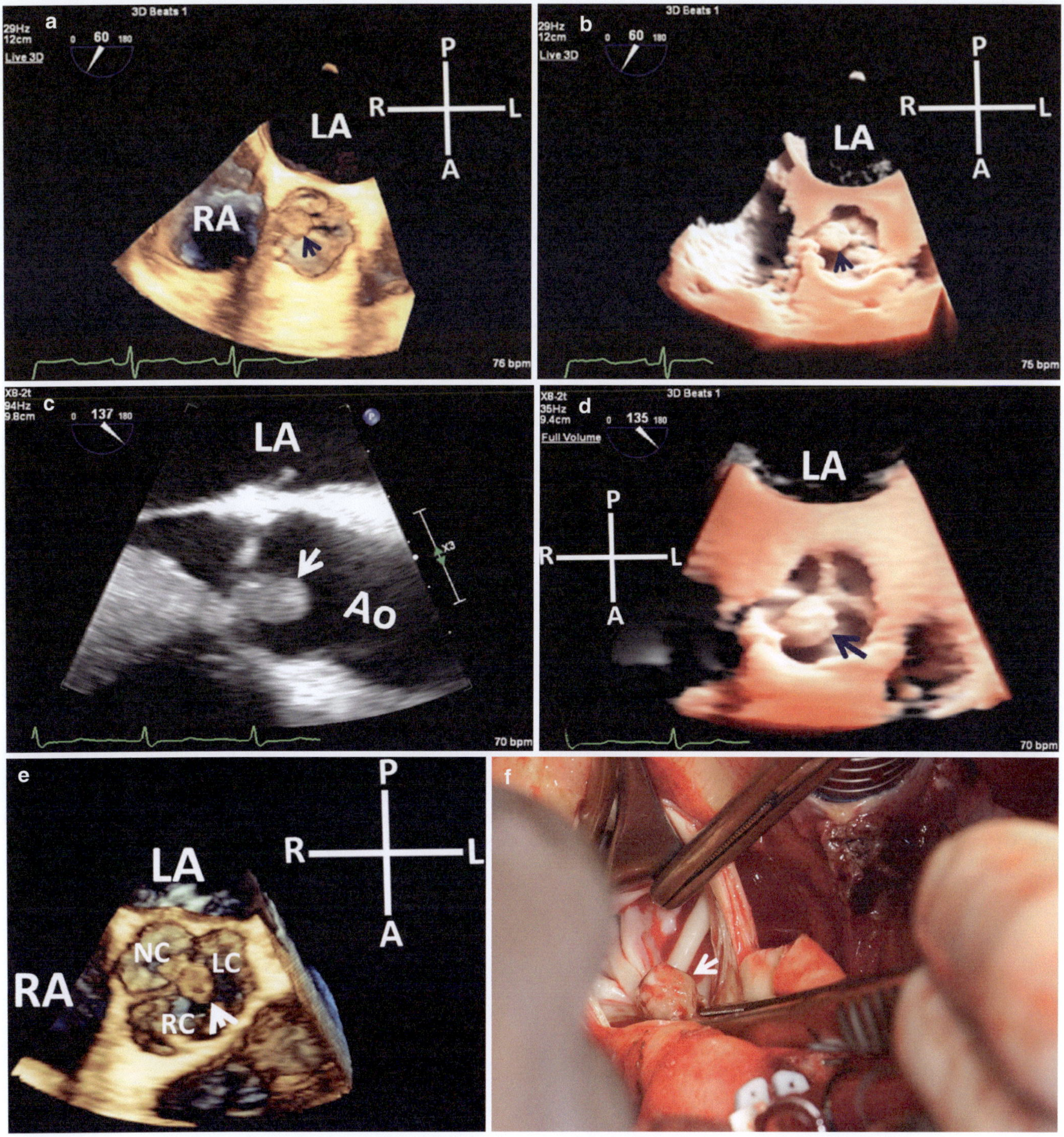

Fig. 12.25 3D TEE of AV masses. Top panel: Papillary fibroelastoma in NC using standard 3D vision (**a**, arrow), and after adding a virtual light source (**b**, TrueVue; Philips Healthcare, arrow). Note the smooth and well-rounded appearance. (**c**, **d**) 2D long-axis AV view of another RC Papillary fibroelastoma (**c**, white arrow) and corresponding 3D short-axis view in TrueVue (**d**, dark blue arrow). (**e**) Ruptured papillary muscle prolapsing through the AV (**e**, arrow) simulating an AV mass, and intraoperative appearance (**f**, arrow) (Images **a**, **c**, **d**, **e**, and **f** used with permission of Mayo Foundation for Medical Education and Research.) A, anterior; Ao, ascending aorta; AV, aortic valve; P, posterior; L, left; LA, left atrium; LC, left coronary cusp; NC, non coronary cusp; R, right; RA, right atrium; RC, right coronary cusp

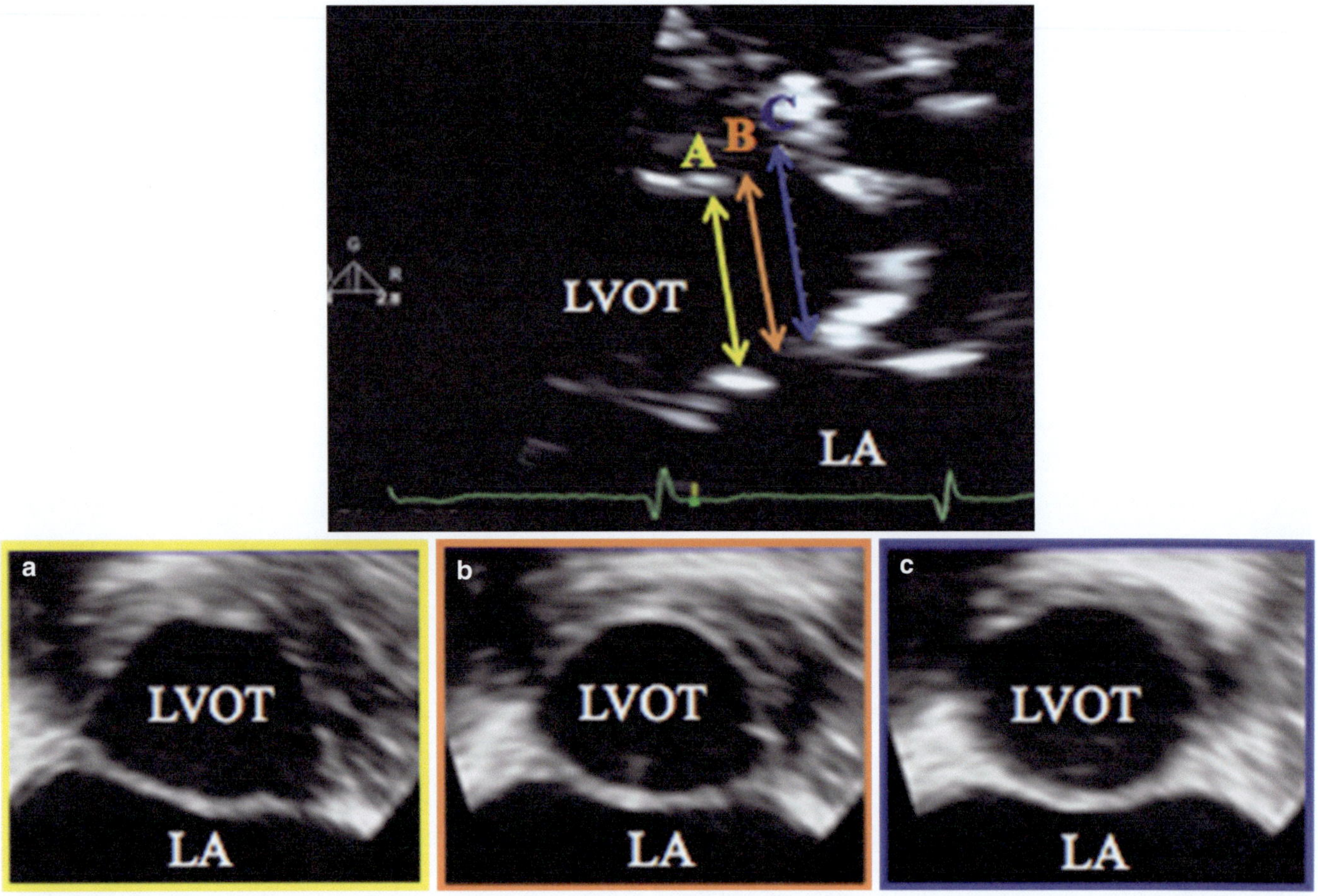

Fig. 12.26 Elliptical shape of the aortic annulus and left ventricular outflow tract. A 2D long axis view of the left ventricular outflow tract is shown in the upper panel and multiple corresponding tomographic slices of the outflow tract derived from a 3D TEE dataset are shown in **a**–**c**. Typically, the left ventricular outflow tract becomes progressively more elliptical and irregularly shaped when moving from the aortic annulus (**c**) toward the left ventricle (**a**, **b**). Even at the level of the aortic annulus the aortic root is elliptical (**c**), highlighting the challenge of properly sizing the aortic annulus by a single 2D linear dimension (Used with permission of Mayo Foundation for Medical Education and Research. All rights reserved). LA, left atrium; LVOT, left ventricular outflow tract

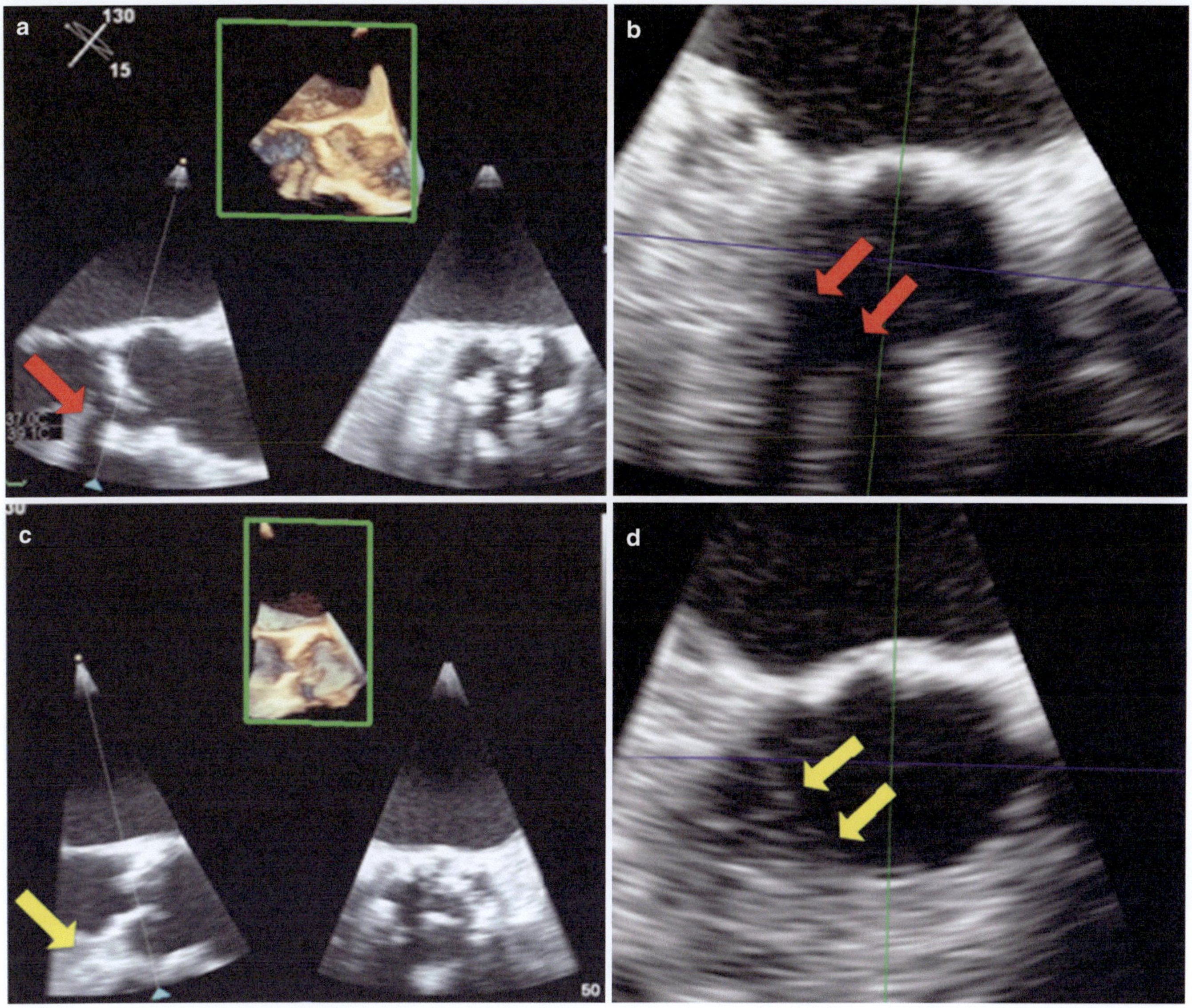

Fig. 12.27 Optimizing 3D TEE acquisition for aortic annulus measurement: avoiding acoustic shadowing. 3D TEE full volume acquisitions are shown in the same patient from two different positions in the esophagus. Panels **a** and **b** are from a superior esophageal window. Bulky calcification of the AV leaflets results in acoustic shadowing of the anterior aortic annulus and left ventricular outflow tract (**a**, red arrow). In panel **b** a short axis view demonstrates the acoustic shadowing (red arrows) which makes precise measurement more challenging. Panels **c** and **d** show a 3D acquisition in the same patient from a more inferior esophageal transducer position, thus avoiding the calcium on the AV leaflets and resolving the acoustic shadowing (**c**, yellow arrow). Panel **d** shows the aortic annulus in short axis view and improved visualization of the anterior border (yellow arrows) from the more inferior transducer position which improves the confidence in the measurement (Used with permission of Mayo Foundation for Medical Education and Research. All rights reserved)

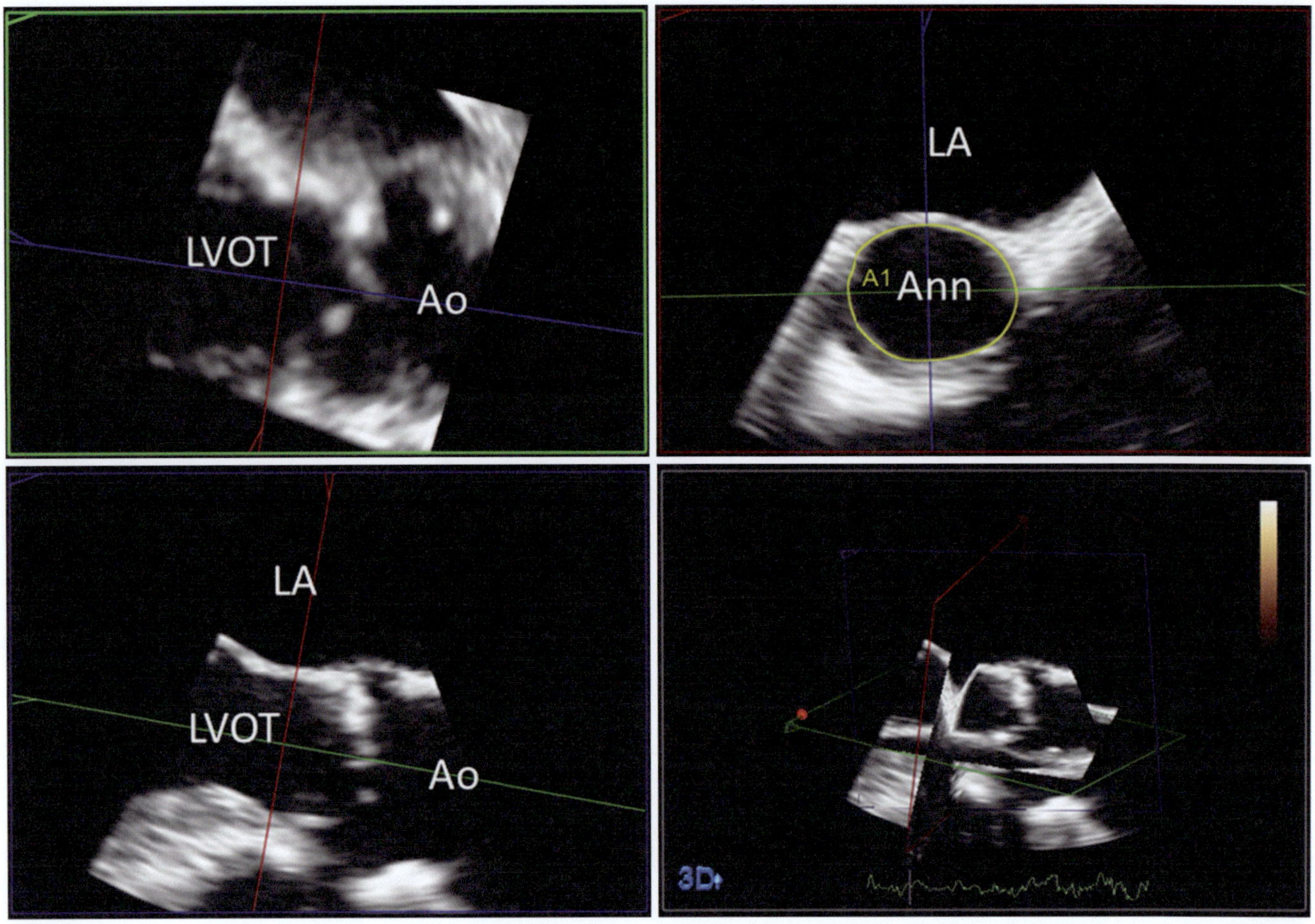

Fig. 12.28 MPR for aortic annulus measurement. Three orthogonal planes bisecting the aortic root are shown. The plane of the aortic annulus is shown in two orthogonal long axis views in the upper left and lower left panels. Direct planimetry of the annulus is then performed to obtain annular area and perimeter for transcatheter AV sizing (upper right panel) (Used with permission of Mayo Foundation for Medical Education and Research. All rights reserved). *Ann*, aortic annulus; *Ao*, ascending aorta; AV, aortic valve; LA, left atrium; LVOT, left ventricular outflow tract

References

1. Malouf JF, Maleszewski JJ, Tajik AJ, Seward JB. Section 2: Foundations of cardiovascular medicine, Chapter 4: Functional anatomy of the heart. In: Fuster V, Harrington RA, Narula J, Eapen ZJ, editors. Hurst the heart. 14th ed. New York: McGraw Hill; 2017.
2. Lang RM, Badano LP, Tsang W, et al. EAE/ASE recommendations for image acquisition and display using three-dimensional echocardiography. J Am Soc Echocardiogr. 2012;25:3–46.
3. Nkomo VT, Gardin JM, Skelton TN, Gottdiener JS, Scott CG, Enriquez-Sarano M. Burden of valvular heart diseases: a population-based study. Lancet. 2006;368:1005–11.
4. Slostad BD, Witt CM, O'Leary PW, Maleszewski JJ, Scott CG, Dearani JA, Pellikka PA. Unicuspid aortic valve: demographics, comorbidities, echocardiographic features, and long-term outcomes. Circulation. 2019;140:1853–5.
5. Tsang MY, Abudiab MM, Ammash NM, et al. Quadricuspid aortic valve: characteristics, associated structural cardiovascular abnormalities, and clinical outcomes. Circulation. 2016;133:312–9.
6. Iung B, Baron G, Butchart EG, et al. A prospective survey of patients with valvular heart disease in Europe: The Euro Heart Survey on Valvular Heart Disease. Eur Heart J. 2003;24:1231–43.
7. Merla G, Brunetti-Pierri N, Piccolo P, Micale L, Loviglio MN. Supravalvular aortic stenosis: elastin arteriopathy. Circ Cardiovasc Genet. 2012;5:692–6.
8. le Polain de Waroux JB, Pouleur AC, Robert A, et al. Mechanisms of recurrent aortic regurgitation after aortic valve repair: predictive value of intraoperative transesophageal echocardiography. JACC Cardiovasc Imaging. 2009;2:931–9.
9. Choi J, Hong GR, Kim M, et al. Automatic quantification of aortic regurgitation using 3D full volume color Doppler echocardiography: a validation study with cardiac magnetic resonance imaging. Int J Cardiovasc Imaging. 2015;31:1379–89.
10. Perez de Isla L, Zamorano J, Fernandez-Golfin C, et al. 3D color-Doppler echocardiography and chronic aortic regurgitation: a novel approach for severity assessment. Int J Cardiol. 2013;166:640–5.
11. Jilaihawi H, Kashif M, Fontana G, et al. Cross-sectional computed tomographic assessment improves accuracy of aortic annular sizing for transcatheter aortic valve replacement and reduces the incidence of paravalvular aortic regurgitation. J Am Coll Cardiol. 2012;59:1275–86.

12. Khalique OK, Kodali SK, Paradis JM, et al. Aortic annular sizing using a novel 3-dimensional echocardiographic method: use and comparison with cardiac computed tomography. Circ Cardiovasc Imaging. 2014;7:155–63.
13. Willson AB, Webb JG, Labounty TM, et al. 3-dimensional aortic annular assessment by multidetector computed tomography predicts moderate or severe paravalvular regurgitation after transcatheter aortic valve replacement: a multicenter retrospective analysis. J Am Coll Cardiol. 2012;59:1287–94.
14. Calleja A, Thavendiranathan P, Ionasec RI, et al. Automated quantitative 3-dimensional modeling of the aortic valve and root by 3-dimensional transesophageal echocardiography in normals, aortic regurgitation, and aortic stenosis: comparison to computed tomography in normals and clinical implications. Circ Cardiovasc Imaging. 2013;6:99–108.

13

Correlation of 3DE with CT and MRI in the Diagnosis and Assessment of Valvular Heart Disease and New Trends

Prajwal Reddy, Htin Aung, Nandan S. Anavekar, and Thomas A. Foley

Echocardiography remains the first line assessment in the clinical evaluation of VHD [1, 2]. Well established guidelines exist for severity, ventricular function, and chamber enlargement primarily relying on echocardiographic data [3, 4]. Cardiac CT and Cardiac MR (CMR) are increasingly used as adjunct tests in the multi-modality evaluation of VHD. The role of CT specifically has expanded with the advances in percutaneous interventional therapies and provides valuable information for pre-procedural planning including anatomic sizing, feasibility of percutaneous procedures, functional assessment of severity and mechanism [5].

In mitral valve prolapse, identification of prolapsed and flail segments can be difficult to visualize via echocardiography. Pre-operative assessment with CT can be used in predicting suitability for repair before surgery with leaflet thickening and calcification as predictors of valve replacement (Figs. 13.1, 13.2, 13.3) [6].

In low risk patients with mitral valve prolapse and regurgitation necessitating surgery, CT can provide the coronary evaluation avoiding the need for pre-operative invasive coronary angiography (Fig. 13.4).

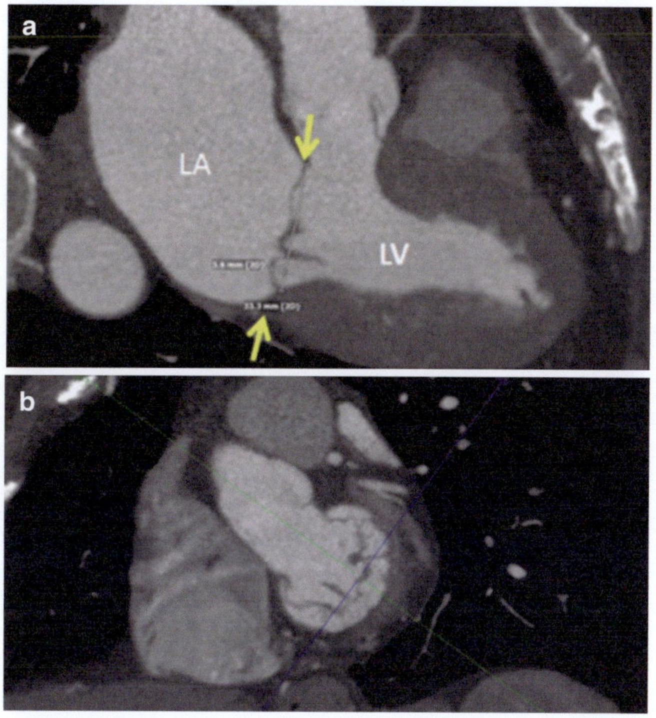

Fig. 13.1 Multi-planar reconstruction in cardiac computed tomography for assessment of mitral valve prolapse. (**a**): Diagnostic image of mitral valve leaflet prolapse (arrows) in the three-chamber view. (**b**): The corresponding short axis view. Used with permission of Mayo Foundation for Medical Education and Research. All rights reserved. LA, left atrium; LV, left ventricle

P. Reddy · H. Aung
Cardiovascular Disease, Mayo Clinic, Rochester, MN, USA
e-mail: reddy.prajwal@mayo.edu; aung.htin@mayo.edu

N. S. Anavekar
Professor of Medicine, Mayo Clinic College of Medicine; Consultant, Department of Cardiovascular Medicine, Mayo Clinic, Rochester, MN, USA
e-mail: Anavekar.Nandan@mayo.edu

T. A. Foley (✉)
Assistant Professor of Radiology, Mayo Clinic College of Medicine; Consultant, Division of Cardiovascular Radiology, Department of Radiology, Mayo Clinic, Rochester, MN, USA
e-mail: Foley.Thomas@mayo.edu

J. F. Maalouf et al. (eds.), *Practical 3D Echocardiography*, https://doi.org/10.1007/978-3-030-72941-7_13

CT plays a vital role in percutaneous valve therapies, such as annular measurements which are highly reproducible and are used for transcatheter heart valve sizing [7]. Moreover, CT offers assessment of vascular access sites and evaluation of the coronary arteries (Figs. 13.5 and 13.6) [8]. Similarly, CT offers a wealth of information with the advent of percutaneous mitral valve replacement. Cross sectional imaging aids in determining: mitral annular size and geometry; the characterization of the landing zone, specifically assessing mitral annular calcification; prediction of left ventricular outflow tract (LVOT) or coronary obstruction risk; predicting fluoroscopic angles that are coplanar with the mitral annulus, and access planning (Figs. 13.7, 13.8, and 13.9) [5, 6]. Cardiac CT has also cemented a role in pre-procedural assessment for transcatheter aortic valve replacements (TAVR). Figures 13.10, 13.11, 13.12, and 13.13 highlight the typical imaging protocol prior to TAVR.

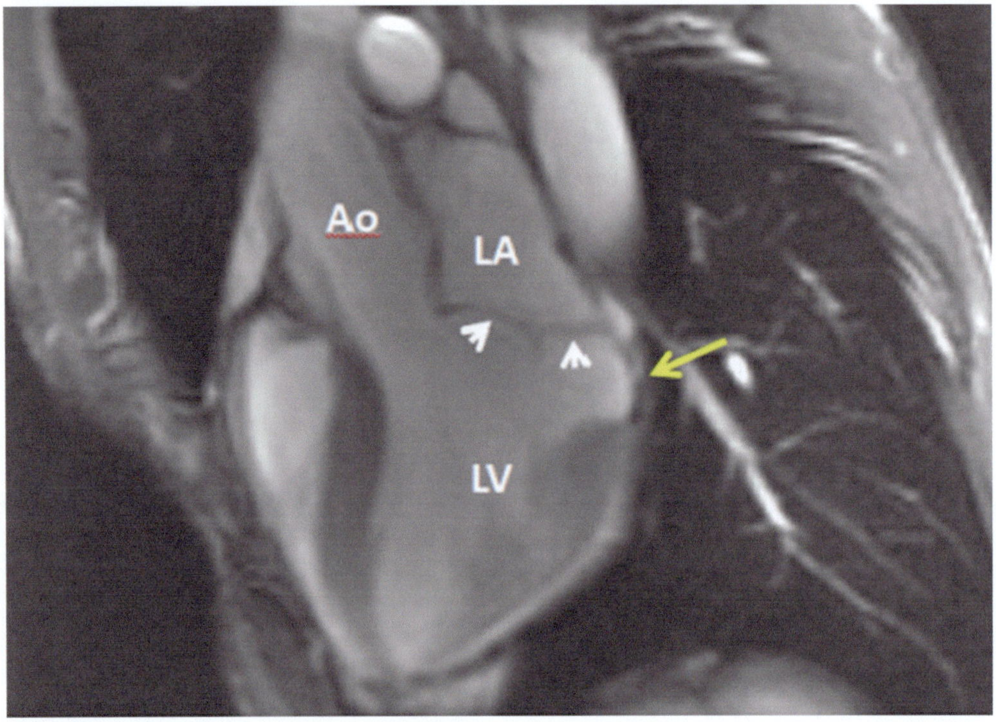

Fig. 13.2 Cardiac magnetic resonance image of the heart in the three-chamber view. The steady-state free precession images demonstrate severe mitral valve leaflet prolapse (white arrow heads) and mitral annular disjunction (yellow arrow). Used with permission of Mayo Foundation for Medical Education and Research. All rights reserved. Ao, ascending aorta; LA, left atrium; LV, left ventricle

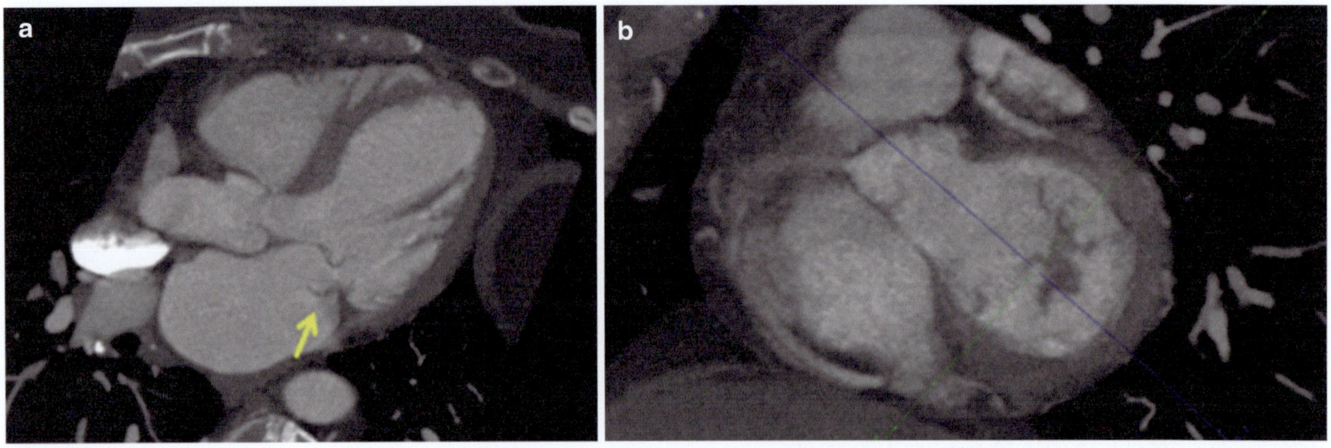

Fig. 13.3 (**a** and **b**): Multi-planar reconstruction in cardiac computed tomography demonstrates the flail middle (P2) segment (**a**, arrow) of the posterior leaflet of the mitral valve and corresponding short-axis view (**b**). Used with permission of Mayo Foundation for Medical Education and Research. All rights reserved

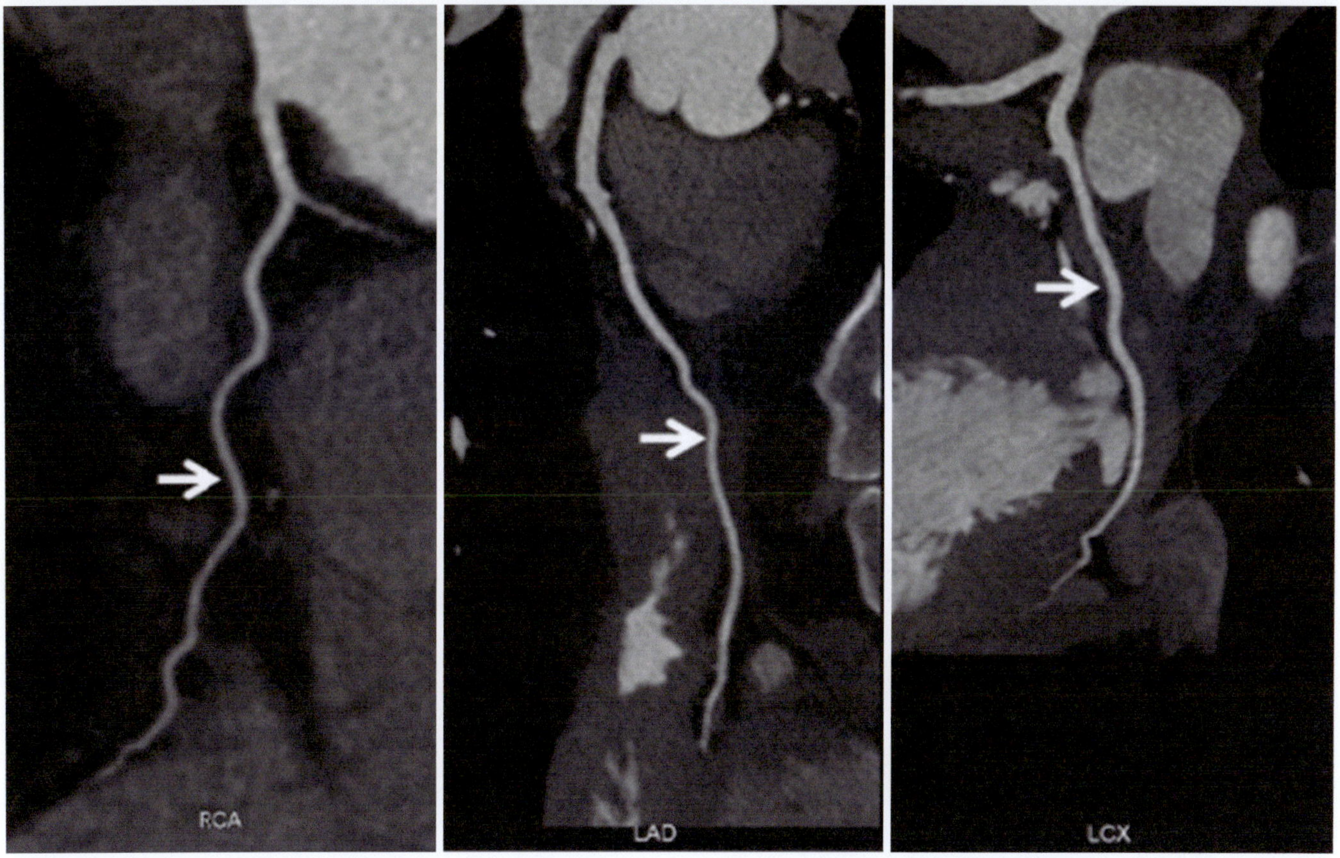

Fig. 13.4 Curve planar reformatted images demonstrating coronary artery anatomy (arrows). Used with permission of Mayo Foundation for Medical Education and Research.

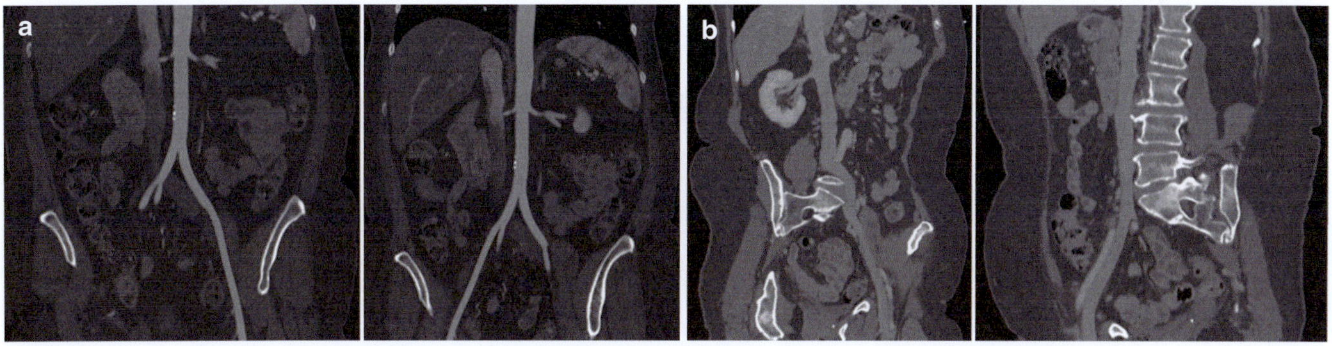

Fig. 13.5 (**a**): CT angiography of the abdomen and pelvis with curved planar reformatted images of the aorto-iliac arteries. (**b**): Delayed-phase CT angiography of the abdomen and pelvis with curved planar reformatted images of the iliac veins and the inferior vena cava. Used with permission of Mayo Foundation for Medical Education and Research.

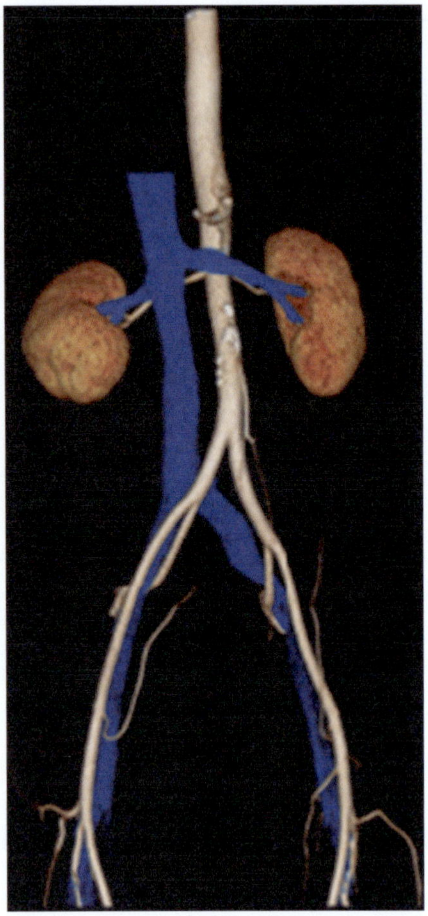

Fig. 13.6 Three-dimensional volume tracing of the abdominal aorta and the iliofemoral arteries along with the iliofemoral veins in the inferior vena cava. Used with permission of Mayo Foundation for Medical Education and Research. All rights reserved

Echocardiography offers a real-time hemodynamic assessment of severity; however suboptimal echocardiographic views can lead to discrepant severity parameters. Multiple VHD guidelines have suggested the use of CMR in these situations [3, 4]. The reproducibility of ventricular volumes, measurement of regurgitant volumes, and assessment of myocardial fibrosis has the potential to amend our current guidelines for intervention [9]. Moreover, cardiac MRI offers a more accurate evaluation of right ventricular systolic function and size which often is difficult to assess with 2D transthoracic echocardiograms. Accurate RV assessment could be instrumental as guidelines and interventions target the tricuspid valve. More investigation is needed to validate specific CMR thresholds of mitral regurgitation severity and ventricular dimensions in both primary and secondary MR with outcome data [3–5]. Multi-modality imaging offers the hope of harnessing the strengths of each imaging modality in identifying optimal time for valve intervention.

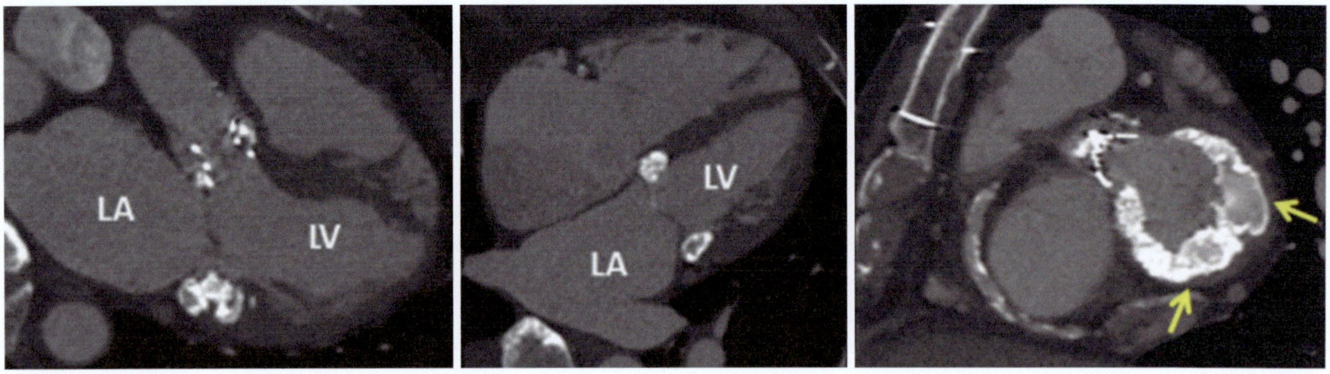

Fig. 13.7 Multi-planar reconstruction in cardiac computed tomography demonstrating severe mitral annular calcification (arrows). Used with permission of Mayo Foundation for Medical Education and Research. All rights reserved. LA, left atrium; LV, left ventricle

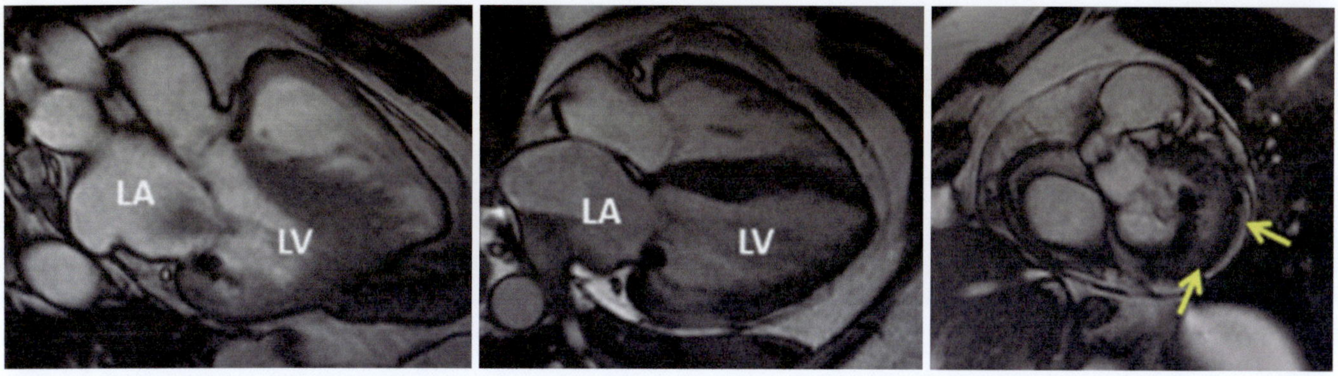

Fig. 13.8 Cardiac magnetic resonance images of the heart in the three-chamber, four-chamber, and short-axis views. The steady-state free precession images demonstrate severe mitral annular calcifications (arrows). Used with permission of Mayo Foundation for Medical Education and Research. All rights reserved. LA, left atrium; LV, left ventricle

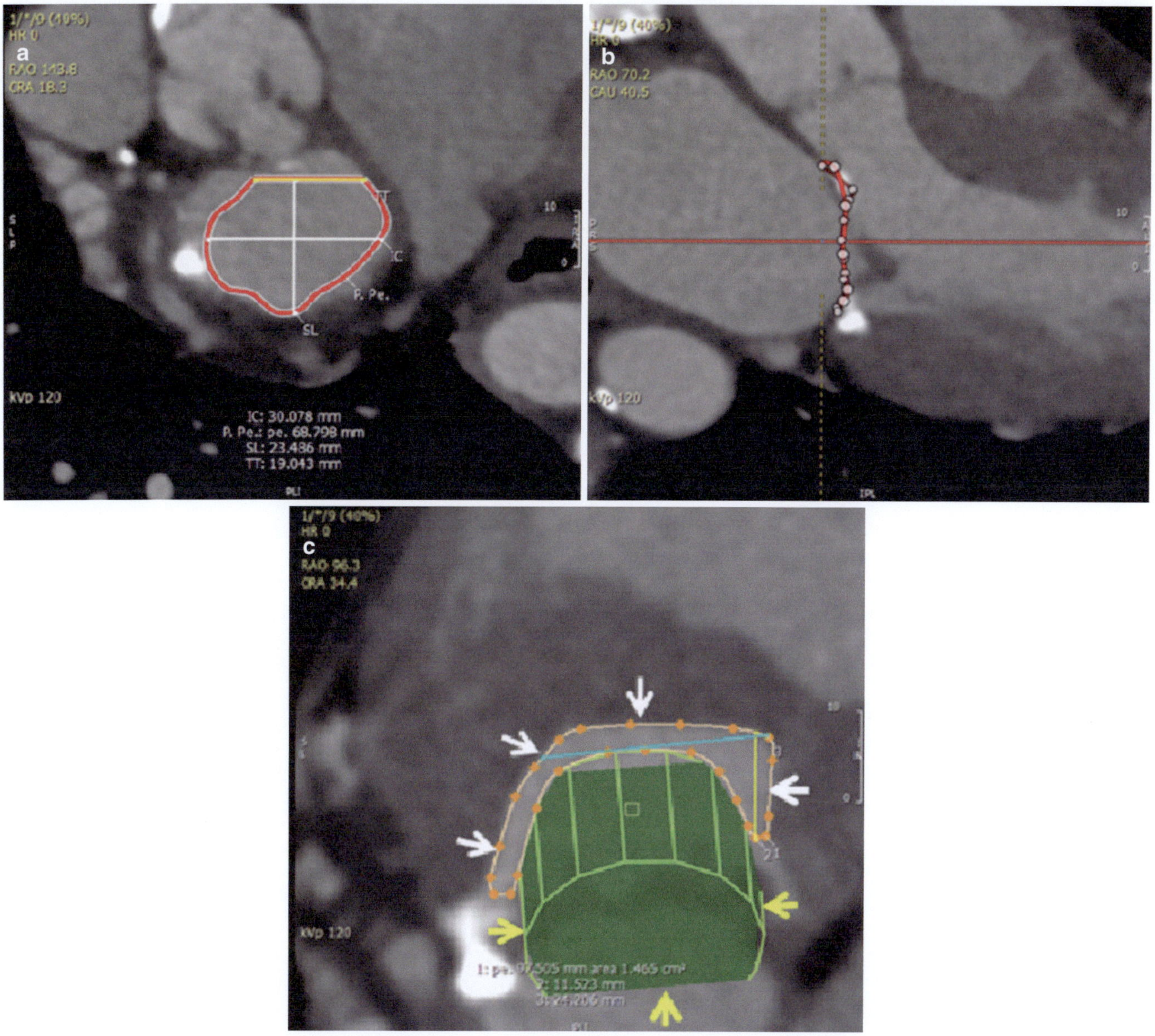

Fig. 13.9 Multiplanar cardiac computed tomography for mitral valve sizing prior to transcatheter mitral valve replacement. Proprietary software utilized for the measurement of mitral valve annular area (**a** and **b**) along with measurement of the neo-left ventricular outflow tract (**c**, white arrows) following placement of a virtual valve (yellow arrows). The measurements are performed in systolic and diastolic phases. Used with permission of Mayo Foundation for Medical Education and Research. All rights reserved

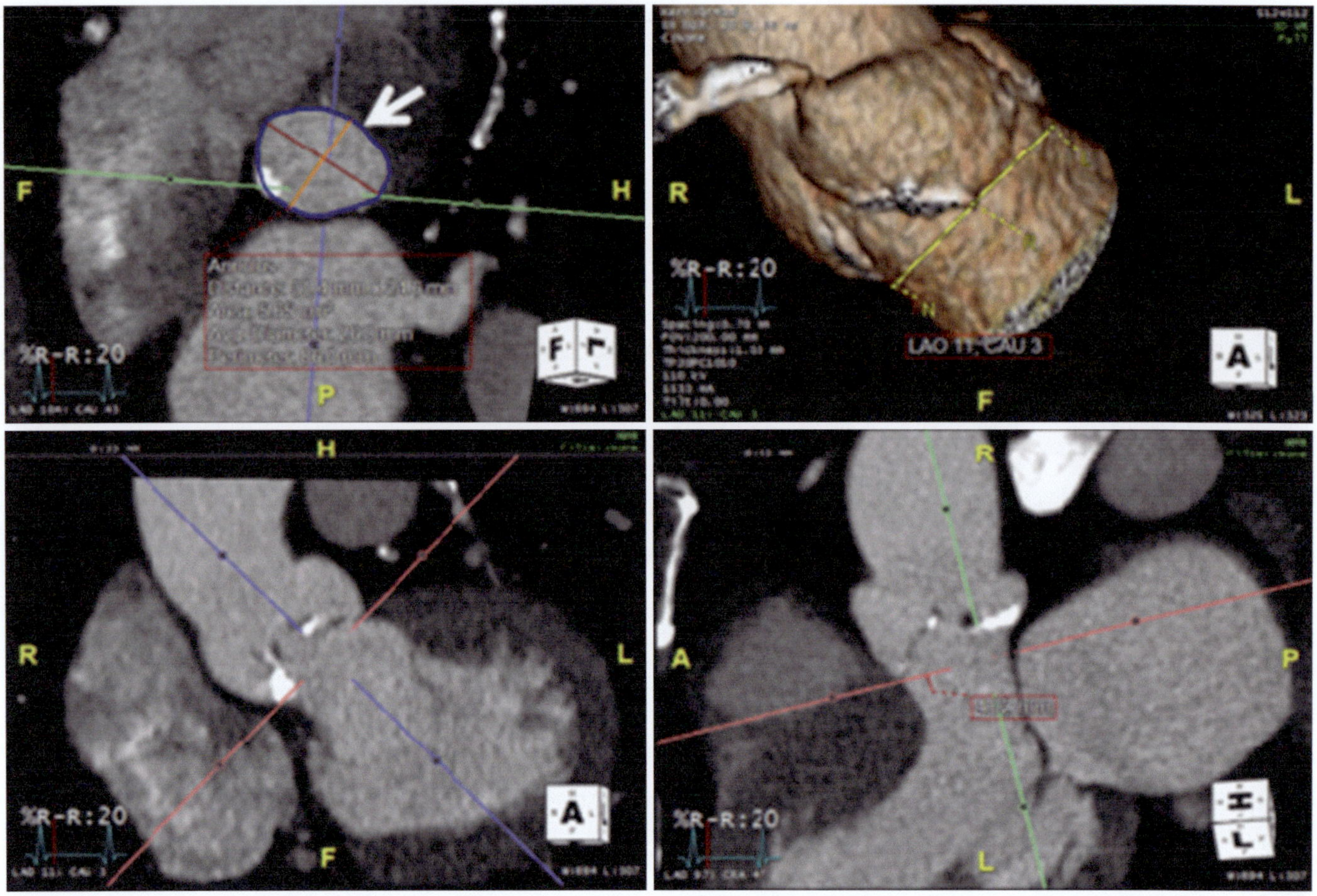

Fig. 13.10 Multiplanar cardiac computed tomography of the heart for planning transcatheter aortic valve replacement. Best systolic phase is obtained when the aortic valve is at its greatest area. The aortic valve annular area (arrow) is measured at the lowest points of the coronary cusps. Used with permission of Mayo Foundation for Medical Education and Research.

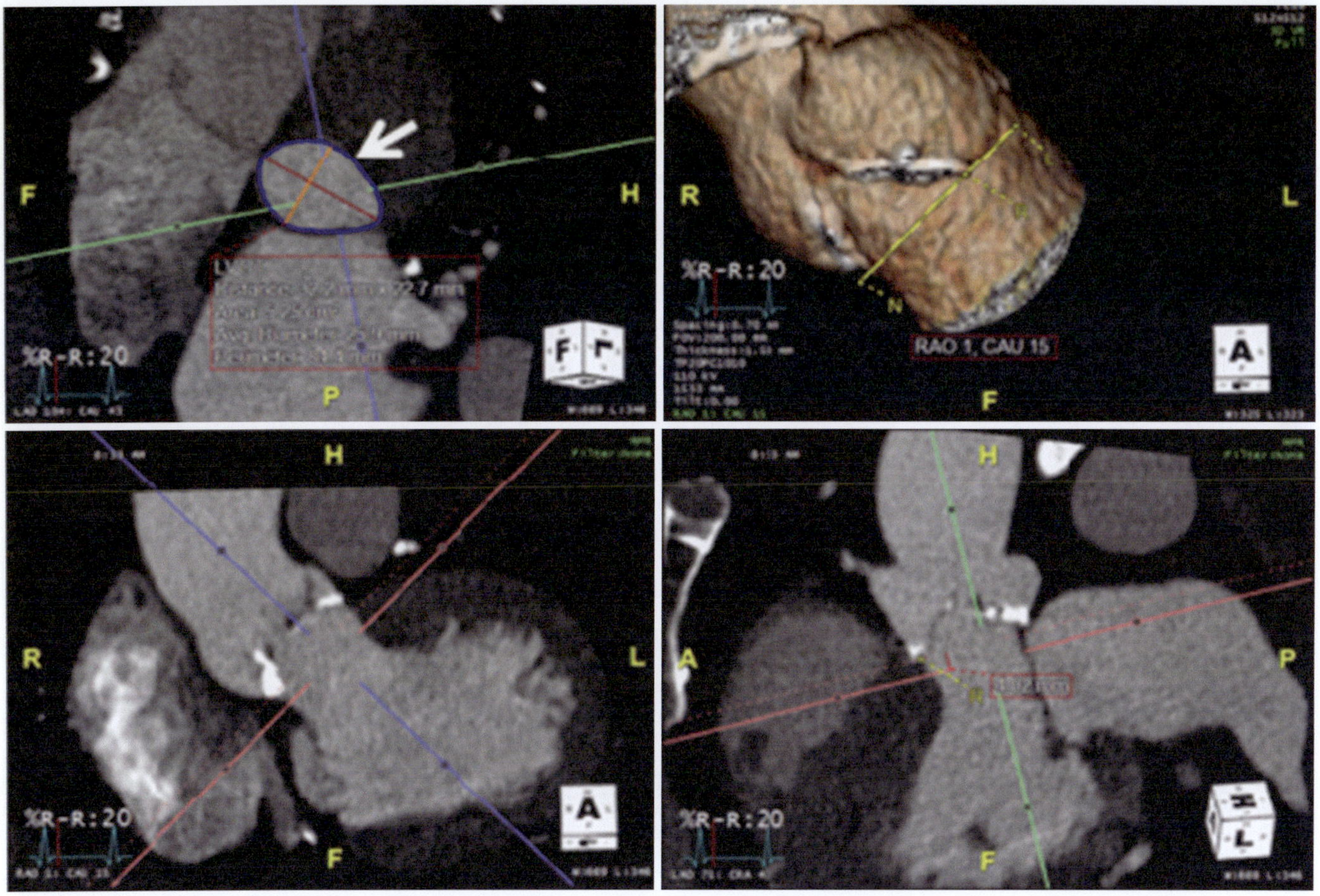

Fig. 13.11 Four millimeters below the aortic valve annulus, the left ventricular outflow tract area (arrow) is measured. Used with permission of Mayo Foundation for Medical Education and Research.

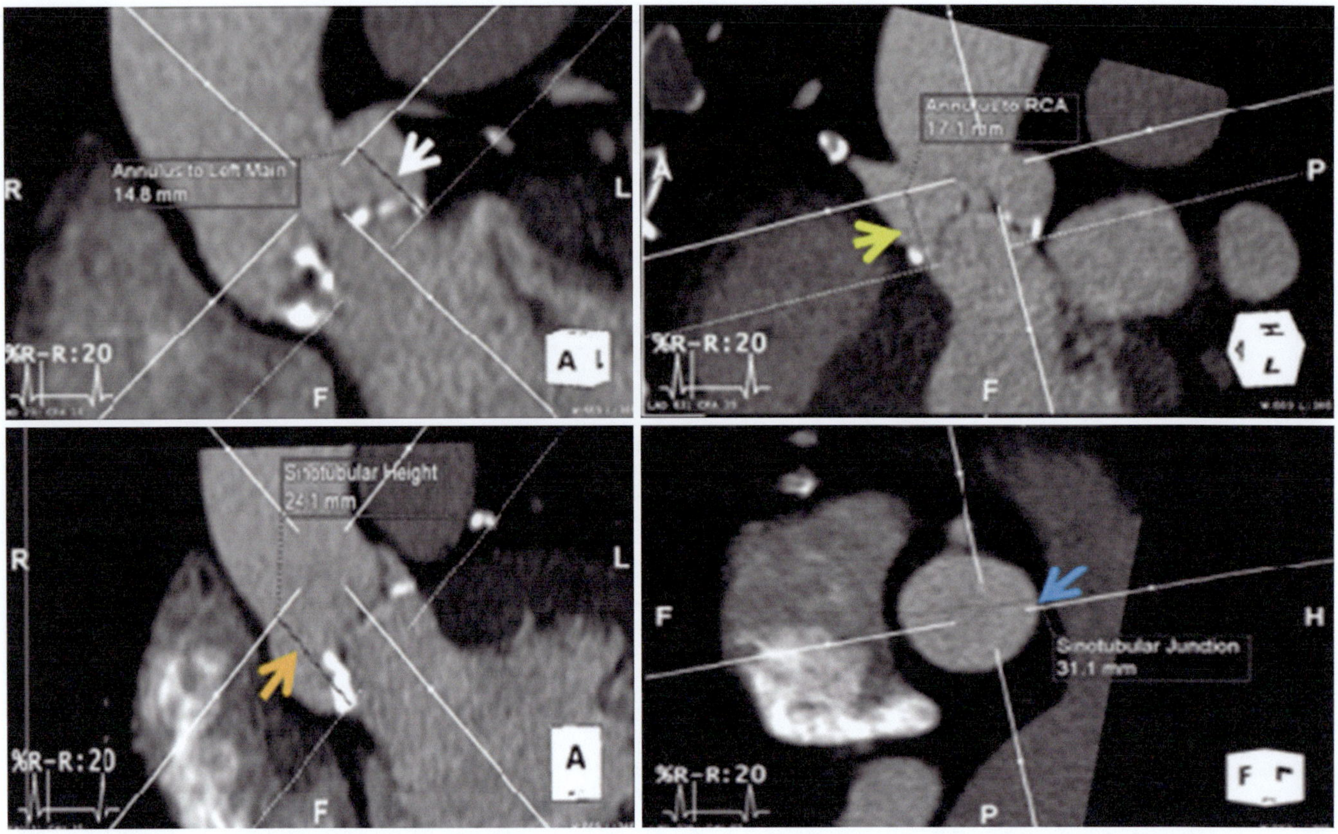

Fig. 13.12 Following measurements of the aortic valve annular and the left ventricular outflow tract areas, the heights of the left main coronary artery (white arrow) and the right coronary artery (yellow arrow) are measured from the level of the aortic valve annulus. The sinotubular junction height (orange arrow) as well as the diameter of the sinotubular junction (blue arrow) are also measured. Used with permission of Mayo Foundation for Medical Education and Research.

Fig. 13.13 Typical report format for the measurements that are performed for a cardiac computed tomography protocol in planning transcatheter aortic valve replacement for the cardiac portion. Similar to the mitral valve prolapse protocol, an abdomen/pelvis CT angiogram is also performed concomitantly. However, a delayed phase is not necessary for the pre-TAVR protocol, but measurements of the abdominal aorta and the iliofemoral arterial diameters are performed. Used with permission of Mayo Foundation for Medical Education and Research. All rights reserved

Aortic Valve Planes	
Aortic Valve Plane N-R-L	LAO 6, CAU 17
Aortic Valve Plane at LAO 0	LAO 1, CAU 26
Aortic Valve Plane at LAO 10	LAO 10, CAU 11
Aortic Valve Plane at RAO 10	RAO 10, CAU 39
Measurements	**Diameter Units (mm)**
Aortic Root	
a = Distance from annulus to left main coronary	12.1
b = Distance from annulus to RCA	14.0
c Sinuses of Valsalva	
c1 = Right coronary sinus to left-non commissure.	31.5
c2 = Left coronary sinus to right-non commissure.	33.9
c3 = Noncoronary sinus to right-left commissure.	35.4
c4= Right coronary sinus to left coronary sinus.	33.0
c5 = Left coronary sinus to non-coronary sinus.	38.4
c6 = Non-coronary sinus to right coronary sinus.	36.7
Annulus Distance	30.8 × 20.7
LVOT Distance	33.1 × 23.9
d = Sinotubular junction	29.0
e = Aortic annulus to innominate	100

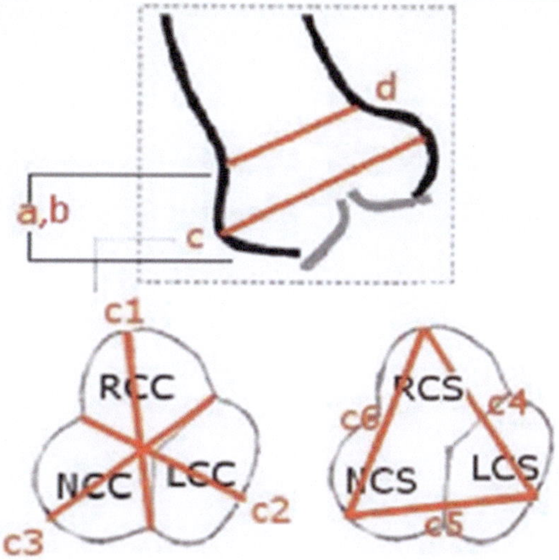

References

1. Iung B, Vahanian A. Epidemiology of valvular heart disease in the adult. Nat Rev Cardiol. 2011;8(3):162–72.
2. Iung B, Vahanian A. Epidemiology of acquired valvular heart disease. Can J Cardiol. 2014;30(9):962–70.
3. Nishimura RA, et al. 2014 AHA/ACC guideline for the Management of Patients with Valvular Heart Disease: a report of the American College of Cardiology/American Heart Association task force on practice guidelines. Circulation. 2014;129(23):e521–643.
4. Baumgartner H, et al. 2017 ESC/EACTS guidelines for the management of valvular heart disease. Eur Heart J. 2017;38(36):2739–91.
5. Naoum C, et al. Cardiac computed tomography and magnetic resonance imaging in the evaluation of mitral and tricuspid valve disease: implications for transcatheter interventions. Circ Cardiovasc Imaging. 2017;10(3):e005331.
6. Suh YJ, et al. Utility of cardiac CT for preoperative evaluation of mitral regurgitation: morphological evaluation of mitral valve and prediction of valve replacement. Korean J Radiol. 2019;20(3):352–63.
7. Liu Q, Hahn RT. The role of multimodality imaging in Transcatheter aortic valve replacement. Curr Cardiol Rep. 2019;21(8):84.
8. Nguyen G, Leipsic J. Cardiac computed tomography and computed tomography angiography in the evaluation of patients prior to transcatheter aortic valve implantation. Curr Opin Cardiol. 2013;28(5):497–504.
9. Park SJ, et al. Assessment of myocardial fibrosis using multimodality imaging in severe aortic stenosis: comparison with histologic fibrosis. JACC Cardiovasc Imaging. 2019;12(1):109–19.

3DE Appearance of the Different Types of Normal Mechanical and Biological Valves

14

Sushil Allen Luis and Joseph F. Maalouf

Introduction

Cardiac valve prostheses should be carefully assessed by both 2D and 3D echocardiography for evaluation of prosthetic valve function [1]. A clear appreciation of normal prosthesis morphology and occluder mechanism of different prosthesis types (Fig. 14.1) is a prerequisite for the evaluation of prosthetic valve dysfunction. As will be illustrated in this chapter, 3D transesophageal echocardiography (3D TEE) adds incremental value to valve prosthesis assessment by 2D echocardiography (2DE) alone, particularly for mitral prostheses analogous to imaging of the native mitral valve. By providing a panoramic view of the valve prosthesis and surrounding bed, from a single imaging window, prosthesis morphology including subtle findings that cannot be seen on 2DE, and prosthesis occluder mechanism including spatial orientation can be better appreciated. A comprehensive understanding of normal prosthetic valve anatomy and function, in conjunction with their 3D TEE appearances, is therefore, essential to understand and identify pathologic states. Heart valve prostheses can be classified into mechanical (bileaflet, tilting disk, and ball-and-cage), surgical biologic valves (stented, unstented or homografts), and transcathter bioprosthetic valves. For patients who undergo, mitral valve repair, the annuloplasty band or ring can also be readily appreciated on 3D echocardiography.

With 3D TEE, the sewing ring of surgical mitral prostheses can be readily imaged and normal occluder mechanism ascertained (Figs. 14.2 and 14.3). All mechanical prostheses have built in mild regurgitation (commonly referred to as washing or closing jets) to minimize the risk of valve thrombosis. And, each mechanical prosthesis type has its own distinctive built in regurgitation appearance that is readily appreciated on 3DE and serves as the prosthesis type fingerprint. *Mild prosthetic regurgitation can be observed with some bioprostheses.*

Mechanical Heart Valves

Bileaflet Valves

Bileaflet mechanical valves are currently the most commonly implanted heart valve prostheses, with the best hemodynamic performance of all cardiac valve prostheses available. Bileaflet prostheses consist of two semicircular disc occluders each attached to a rigid circular annular ring by two small hinges (Fig. 14.1). Valve leaflets open to an angle of 75–90° relative to the annular plane, with a smaller slit like central orifice and two larger semicircular orifices (Fig. 14.2). Normal built-in regurgitation consists of a small central jet (from regurgitation between the two occluder disc leaflets) and two or more small peripheral jets (from regurgitation that occurs between the occluder disc leaflets and adjacent sewing ring). Additional trivial regurgitation can occur at the hinges of the occluders. They are all referred to as washing or closing jets (Fig. 14.2).

Bileaflet prostheses vary according to placement of the prosthesis within or above the native valve annulus. Intra-annular valves include the St. Jude standard and Carbomedics standard valves, and supra-annular valves

Supplementary Information The online version of this chapter (https://doi.org/10.1007/978-3-030-72941-7_14) contains supplementary material, which is available to authorized users.

S. A. Luis (✉)
Associate Professor of Medicine, Mayo Clinic College of Medicine; Consultant, Department of Cardiovascular Medicine, Mayo Clinic, Rochester, MN, USA
e-mail: Luis.S@mayo.edu

J. F. Maalouf
Professor of Medicine, Mayo Clinic College of Medicine; Director, Interventional Echocardiography; Consultant, Department of Cardiovascular Medicine, Mayo Clinic, Rochester, MN, USA
e-mail: maalouf.joseph@mayo.edu

J. F. Maalouf et al. (eds.), *Practical 3D Echocardiography*, https://doi.org/10.1007/978-3-030-72941-7_14

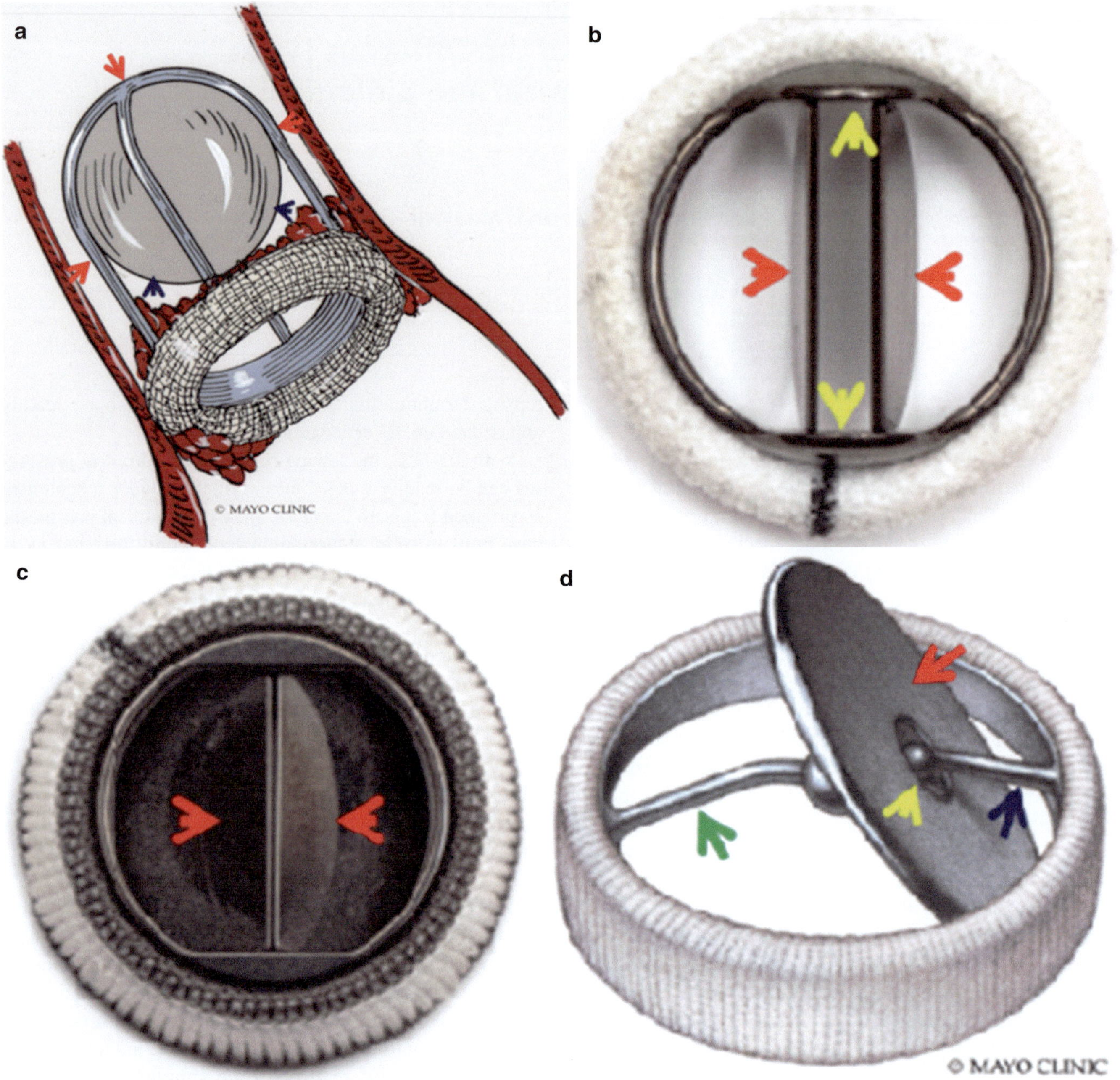

Fig. 14.1 (**a**) Schematic diagram of Starr-Edwards caged-ball. The silastic ball occluder (dark blue arrows) is contained within cage metal struts (red arrows). (**b**, **c**) Mechanical bileaflet prosthesis in open (**b**) and closed (**c**) positions. Red arrows point to the two occluder leaflets and yellow arrows point to prosthesis hinges. (**d**, **e**) Medtronic-Hall single tilting disc prosthesis. Schematic diagram (**d**) and actual prosthesis (**e**). Green arrows point to sigmoid shaped central strut, light blue arrows point to two small inlet struts, and dark blue arrow points to a smaller outlet stop strut. Yellow arrow points to central occluder pivot hole. Red arrow points to disc occluder in schematic and to smaller outlet stop strut in the actual prosthesis. Used with permission of Mayo Foundation for Medical Education and Research. All rights reserved

e

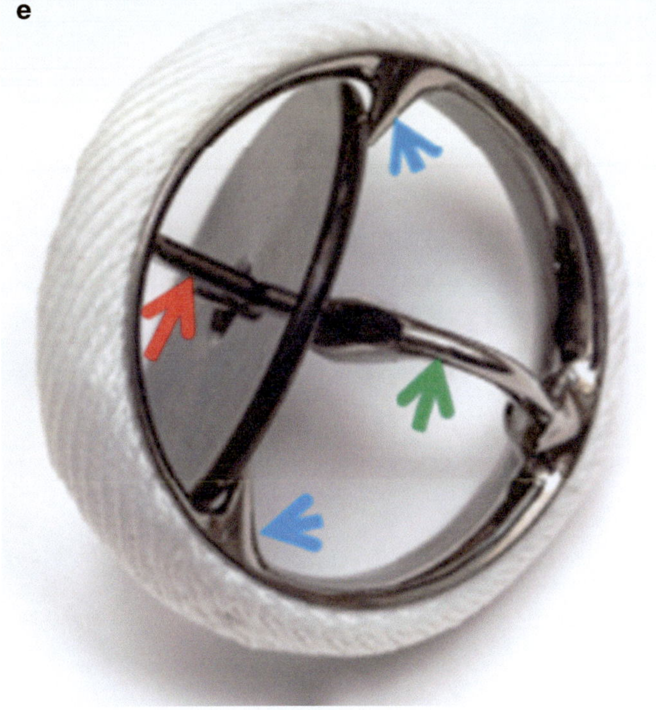

Fig. 14.1 (continued)

include the Carbomedics Top Hat and St. Jude HP valves. Supra-annular prostheses are typically associated with a larger effective orifice area and superior hemodynamic performance when compared to intra-annular prostheses *For mechanical bileaflet mitral valve prostheses, the leaflet pivots including hinge mechanism and coaptation surface project above the plane of the sewing ring (SR) for standard St.Jude valves (Fig. 14.3), but are within the SR plane for standard Carbomedics valves. The added depth associated with 3D imaging compared with 2D imaging facilitates viewing of the leaflets of aortic mechanical prostheses (Fig. 14.4). Blurring or amplification artifacts can cause sewing ring stitches to appear thicker than they actually are, and metallic prosthesis components such as occluders and hinges are subject to blooming artifacts (Figs. 14.2* and *14.5, see Chap. 3).*

The two hinge pivots of mechanical mitral bileaflet prostheses can have one of two spatial orientations that can be readily recognized on 3D TEE: Either parallel to the line connecting the two native mitral commissures (referred to as anatomic) or perpendicular to it (referred to as antianatomic, Figs. 14.2 and 14.6). The anatomic orientation has been associated with asymmetric leaflet motion whereas the anti-anatomic orientation has been associated with symmetric leaflet motion and better intracardiac flow dynamics [2, 3], but data are limited.

Tilting-Disc Valves

Tilting disc valves include the Bjork-Shiley and Medtronic Hall valves. Although no longer implanted in clinical practice they may be seen not infrequently in patients with prior valve replacements. These valves consist of a single circular disc which pivots over a central strut. The disc typically opens to 60–80° relative to the annular plane, resulting in a larger and smaller orifice. Both tilting disc valve types have multiple small jets of regurgitation arising from within the sewing ring. Additionally, the Medtronic Hall valve also has a larger jet of regurgitation arising from a central hole in the occluder disc (Fig. 14.7).

Ball-Cage Valves

The prototype for ball-cage valves is the Starr Edwards valve, which is no longer available for implantation but is still encountered in clinical practice. This type of valve prostheses consists of a silastic ball within a cage made up of two perpendicular arches (see Fig. 14.1). When, in the mitral position (Fig. 14.8), the prosthesis opens in diastole with movement of the ball towards the left ventricle allowing flow from left atrium to left ventricle. In early systole, left ventricular contraction results in atrial displacement of the ball closing the valve. This atrial displacement of the ball results in displacement or regurgitation of a small amount of blood within the cage into the left atrium.

Bioprosthetic Valves

Stented Bioprostheses

Stented bioprostheses consist of a circular annular ring onto which three leaflets are attached, with three struts extending into the outflow portion of the prostheses (Fig. 14.9). These bioprostheses leaflets are made up of porcine valvular tissue or bovine pericardium. Prosthetic regurgitation is not typical, although trivial or mild central jets may be seen (Fig. 14.9).

Stentless Bioprostheses

Stentless bioprostheses may be seen in the aortic position and were designed to provide superior hemodynamics when compared to stented bioprostheses. These bioprostheses may be made from porcine aortic valve or bovine pericardium. Prosthetic regurgitation is not typical, although trivial central jets may be seen.

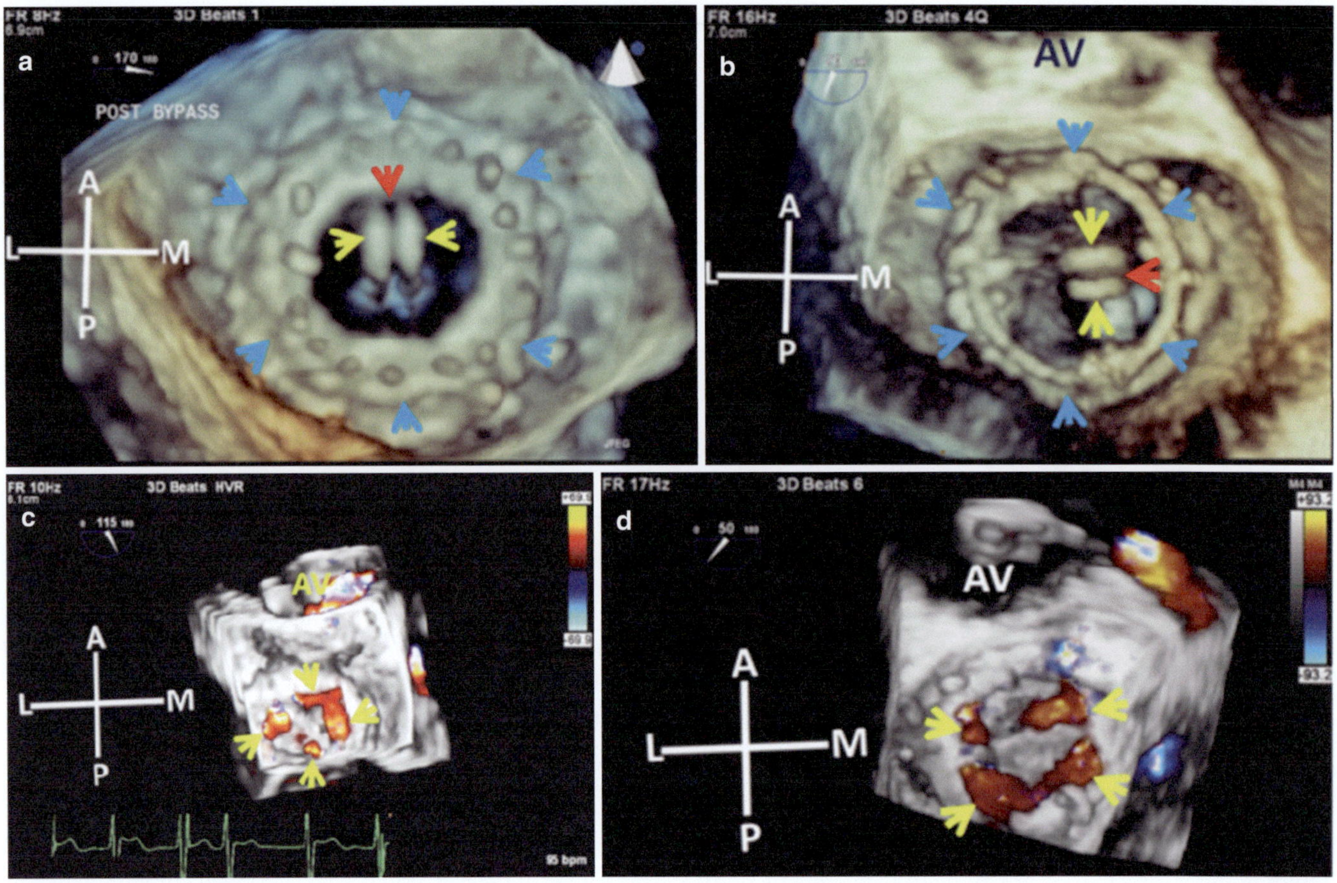

Fig. 14.2 (**a**, **b**) 3D TEE enface LA views of two mechanical bileaflet mitral prostheses. The two occluder leaflets (yellow arrows) and sewing ring (blue arrows) are well seen. The orientation of the occluder leaflets is *antianatomic* (**a**) and *anatomic* (**b**). Note the parallel alignment of the occluder leaflets in both prostheses, the slit like central orifice (red arrows) and adjacent two larger semicircular orifices. Also note that the occluder leaflets appear thick due to blooming artifacts. (**c**, **d**) Typical washing jets of a mechanical bileaflet prosthesis (arrows). Used with permission of Mayo Foundation for Medical Education and Research. All rights reserved. A, anterior; AV, aortic valve; L, lateral; M, medial; P, posterior

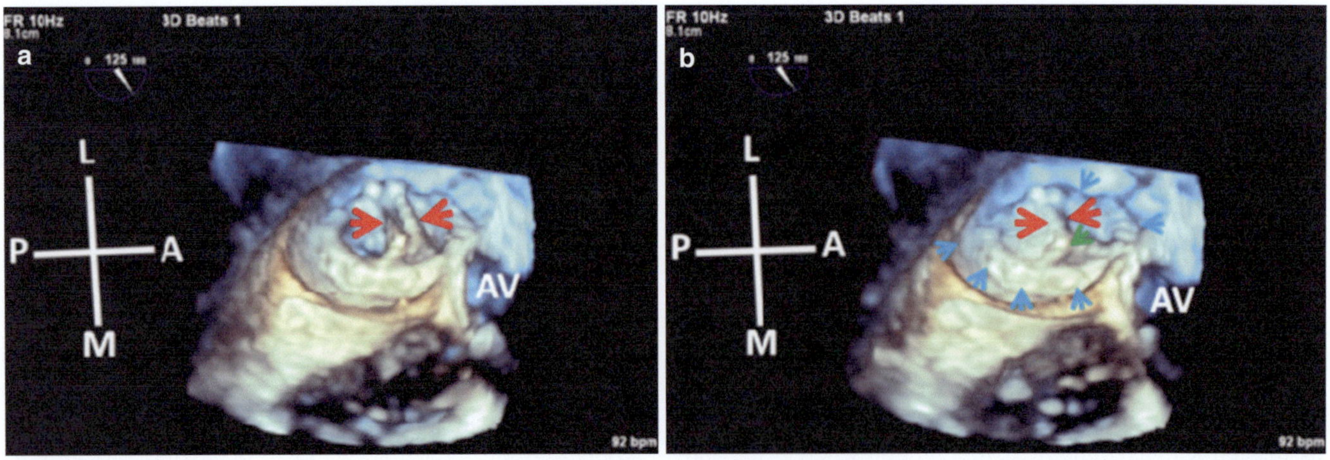

Fig. 14.3 3D TEE enface LA views of a St.Jude mechanical bileaflet mitral prosthesis with the valve open (**a**) and closed (**b**). The occluder leaflets (red arrows) have an anatomic orientation. Note that the closed leaflet coaptation surface (**b**, red arrows) is above plane of the SR (blue arrows). The green arrow points to the medial hinge. Used with permission of Mayo Foundation for Medical Education and Research. All rights reserved. A, anterior; AV, aortic valve; L, lateral; LA, left atrial; M, medial; P, posterior; SR, sewing ring

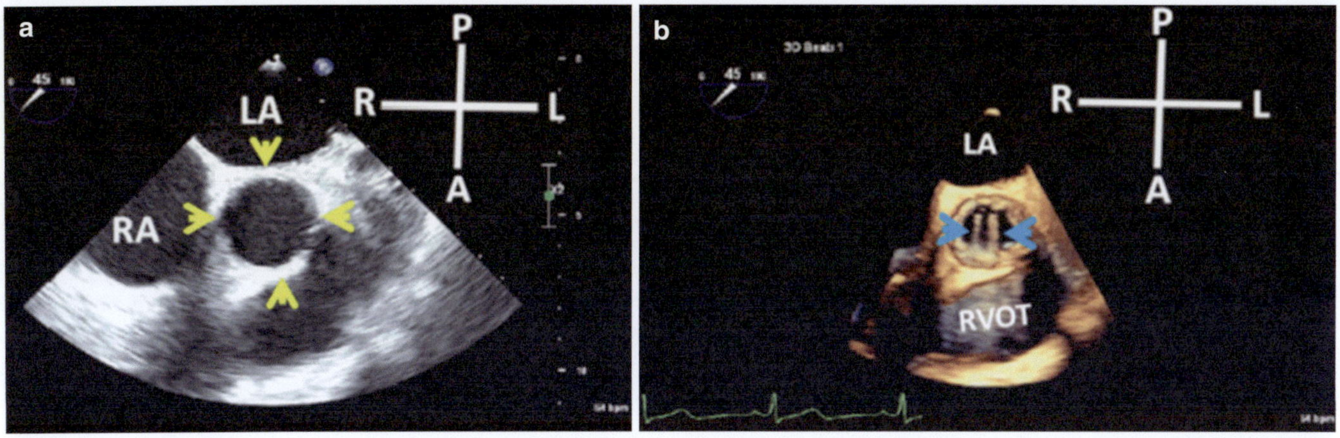

Fig. 14.4 (**a**) 2D TEE mid-esophageal short-axis aortic valve view (yellow arrows) in a patient with a mechanical bileaflet prosthesis. The prosthesis leaflets are not seen. (**b**) By turning on 3D imaging, the prosthesis leaflets (blue arrows) are now well seen in the open position because of the added depth provided by 3D. Used with permission of Mayo Foundation for Medical Education and Research. All rights reserved. A, anterior; L, left; LA, left atrium; P, posterior; R, right; RA, right atrium; RVOT, right ventricular outflow tract

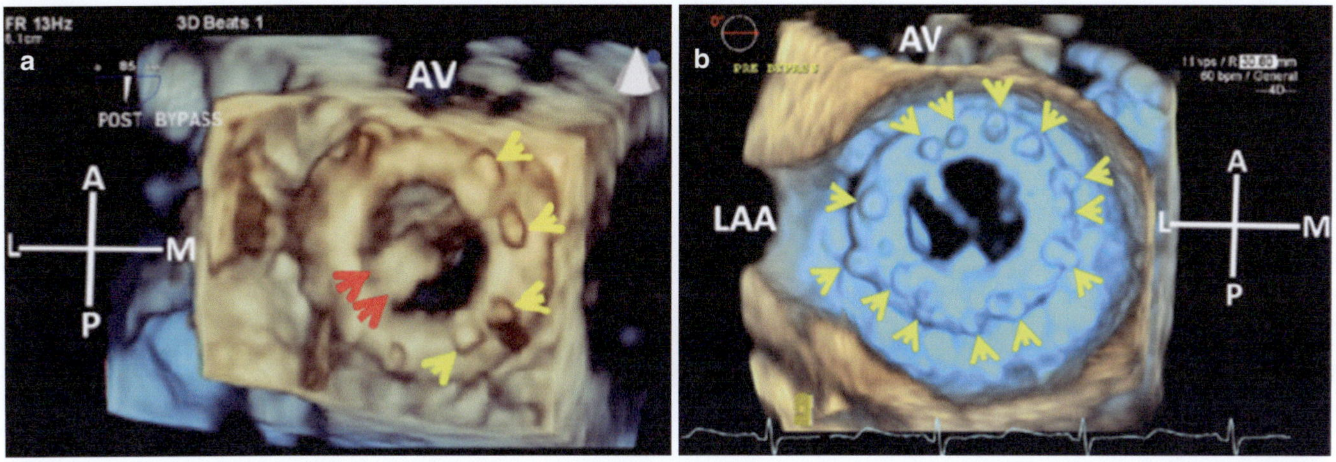

Fig. 14.5 3D TEE enface LA views of a mechanical mitral bileaflet prosthesis (**a**) and mitral bioprosthesis (**b**). Note the asymmetrical distribution of the SR sutures/stitches (yellow arrows) which appear thick due to blurring or amplification artifacts. The posterior component of the bileaflet occluder leaflets (red arrows) also appear thick due to blooming artifact. Used with permission of Mayo Foundation for Medical Education and Research. All rights reserved. A, anterior; AV, aortic valve; L, lateral; LA, left atrium; LAA, left atrial appendage; M, medial; P, posterior; SR, sewing ring

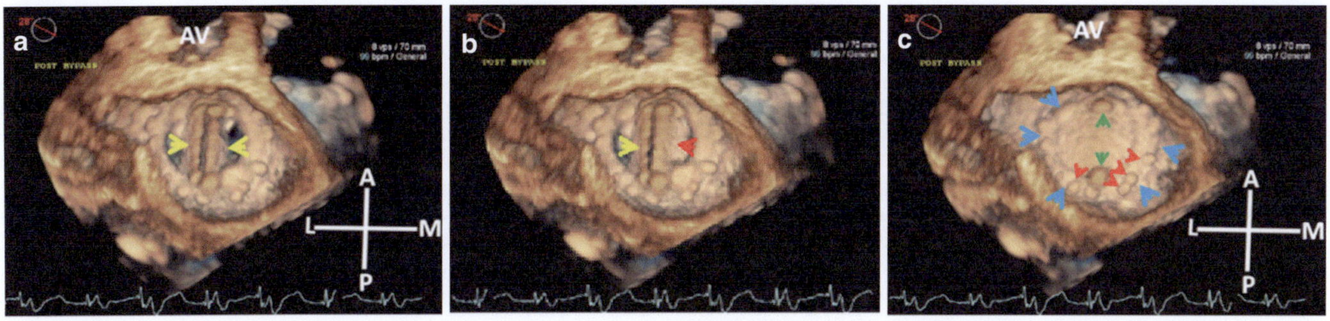

Fig. 14.6 3D TEE enface LA views of St. Jude mitral prosthesis during different phases of the cardiac cycle. (**a**) Mid diastole, (**b**) late diastole and (**c**) systole. Note the antianatomic orientation of the prosthesis leaflets (arrows in **a** and **b**) and asymmetric closure of the prosthesis leaflets in **b**. Blue arrows point to SR and green arrows to anterior and posterior hinges. Red arrow heads in **c** point to suture material. Used with permission of Mayo Foundation for Medical Education and Research. All rights reserved. A, anterior; AV, aortic valve; L, lateral; LA, left atrium; M, medial; P, posterior; SR, sewing ring

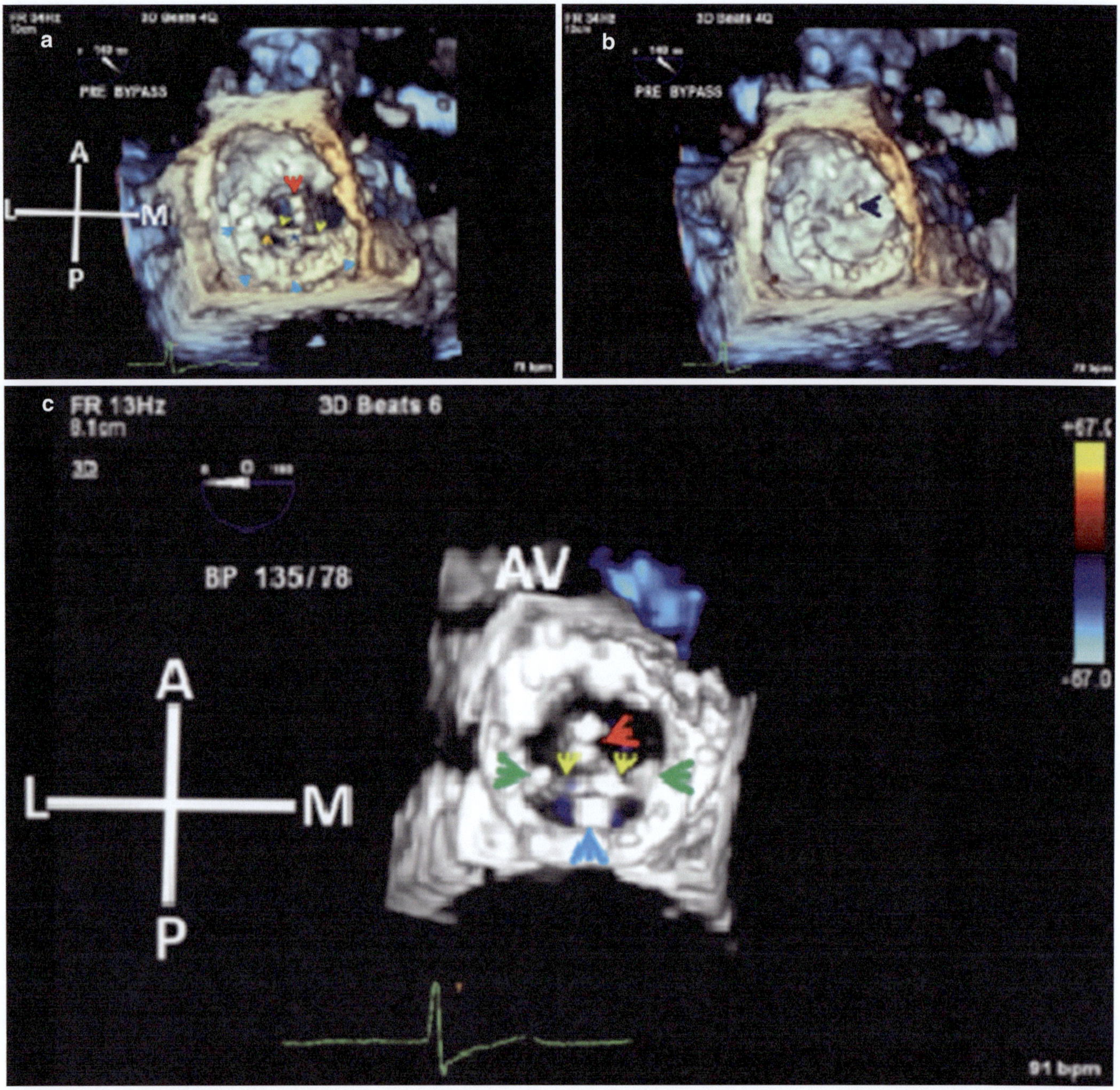

Fig. 14.7 3D TEE of MH tilting disc prosthesis in the mitral position. (**a**) Diastolic and (**b**) systolic frames. Yellow arrows point to circular disc occluder and red arrow points to sigmoid shaped central strut. Orange arrow points to one of two small inlet struts. The central hole can also be seen (blue star in diastole, and dark blue arrow in systole). (**c**) Enlarged color suppress view of the MH tilting disc in diastole. Note the central strut (red arrow), the smaller stop strut (blue arrow) and two inflow struts (green arrows) that flank the disc occluder (yellow arrows). Also note the two large orifices anteriorly and two small orifices posteriorly. (**d**, **e**) Same images in diastole but tilted with color suppress (**d**) and color Doppler on showing diastolic flow (**e**). (**f**, **g**) Systolic frames from two different MH tilting disc prostheses. Central prosthesis regurgitation (blue and red arrows) characteristic of MH tilting disc prosthesis can be seen. There is also posterior periprosthetic regurgitation (yellow arrow) associated with the MH prosthesis in **g**. (**h**, **i**) Systolic frames of a MH tilting disc prosthesis in the aortic position. The disc occluder (red arrows) is seen in early (**h**) and late (**i**) systole. Light blue arrows point to prosthesis SR in **a** and **h**. Used with permission of Mayo Foundation for Medical Education and Research. A, anterior; AV, aortic valve; L, lateral; LA, left atrium; M, medial; MH, Medtronic-Hall; P, posterior; SR, sewing ring

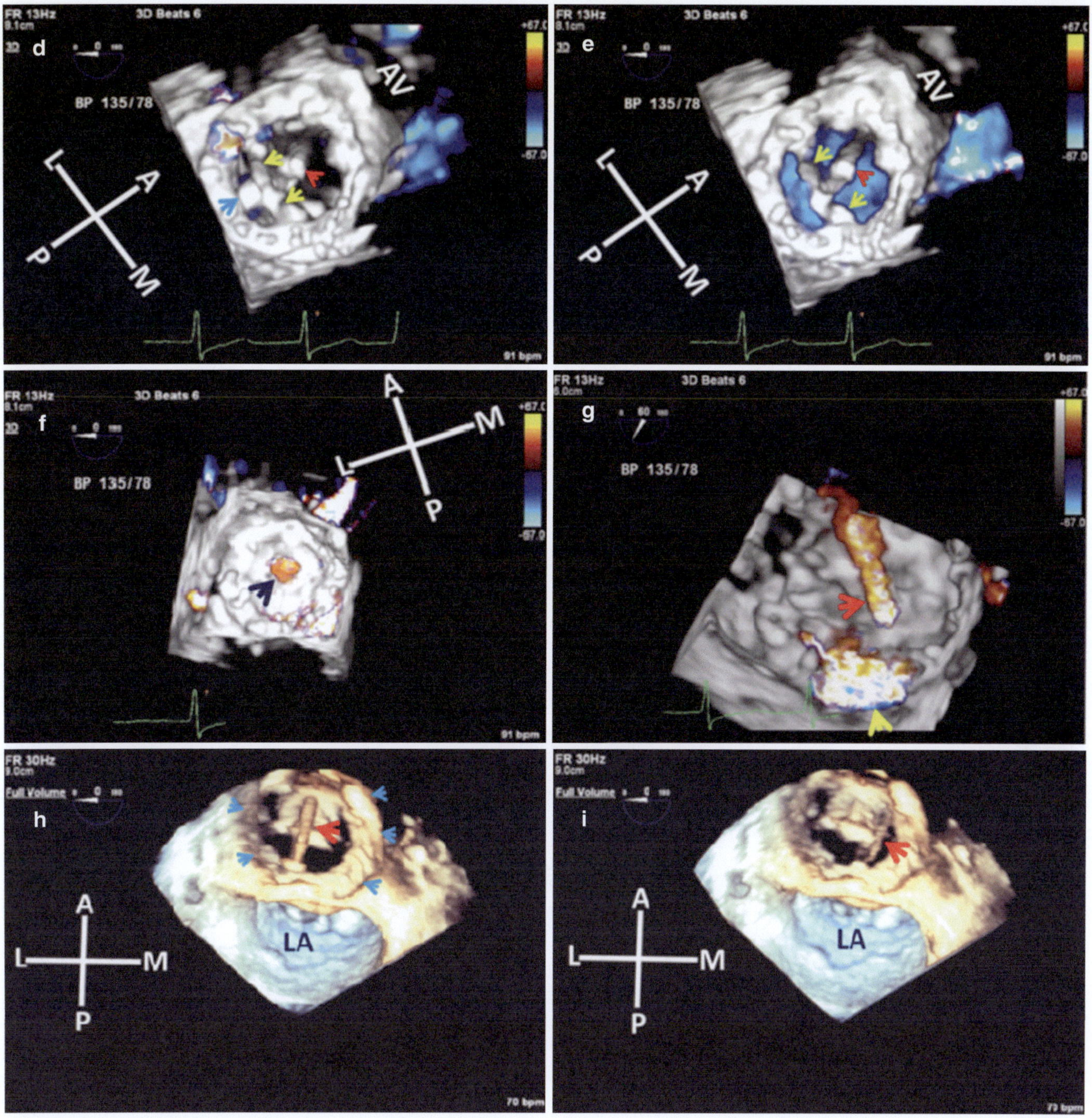

Fig. 14.7 (continued)

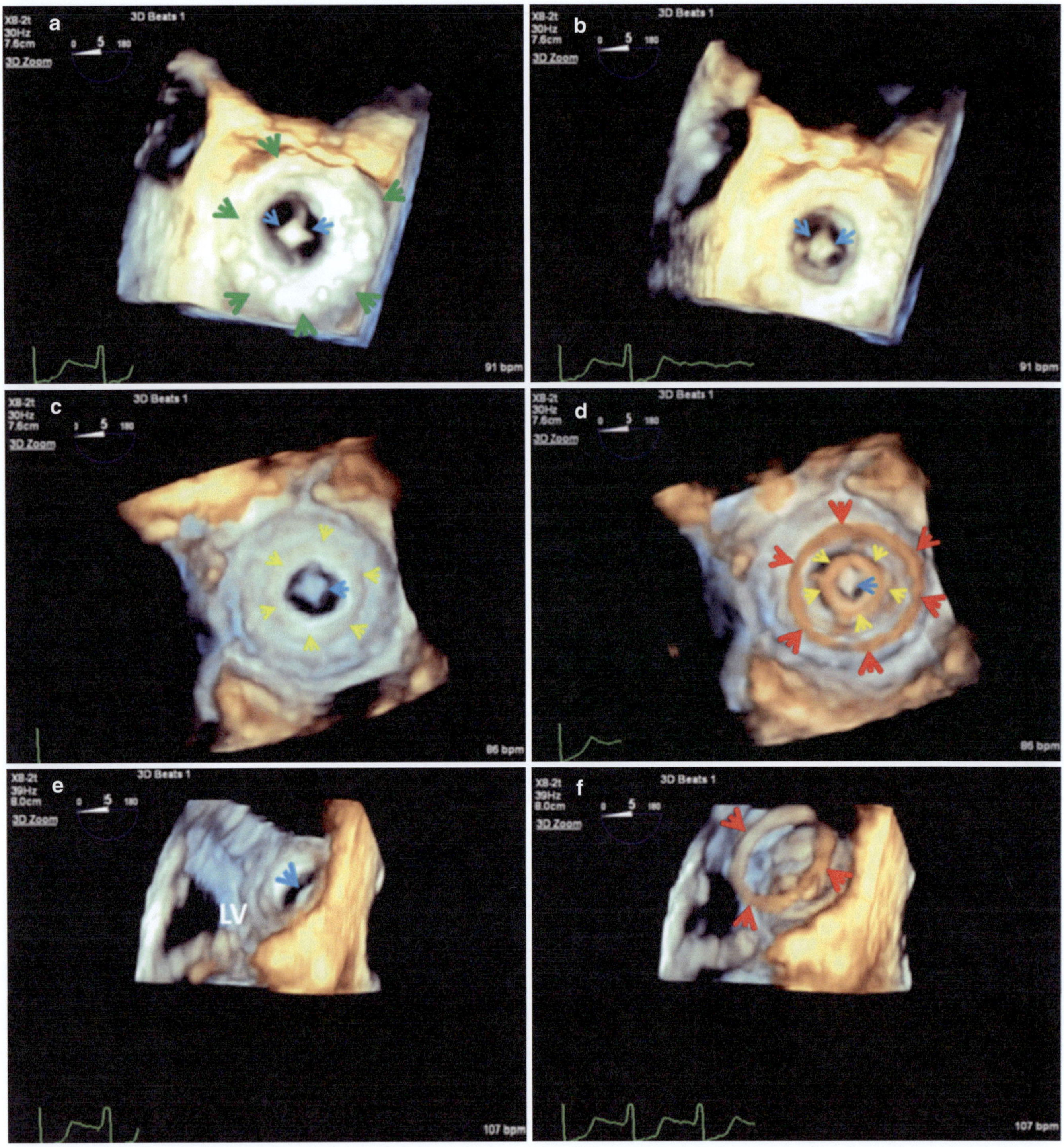

Fig. 14.8 3D TEE of Starr Edwards caged ball mitral valve prosthesis. (**a**, **b**) enface LA views in late systole (**a**) and diastole (**b**). The ball occluder can be seen (light blue arrows); green arrows point to SR. (**c**, **d**) Enface LV views of the same prosthesis. Note the circular motion artifact (red arrows) created by the ball occluder (light blue arrows) as it moves down the cage. The yellow arrows point to the SR. (**e**, **f**) Same LV views with the image tilted sideways in order to appreciate the spatial relationship of the ball valve motion artifact (red arrows) to the closed ball-valve prosthesis (blue arrow, **e**). Used with permission of Mayo Foundation for Medical Education and Research. All rights reserved. LA, left atrium, LV, left ventricle; SR, sewing ring

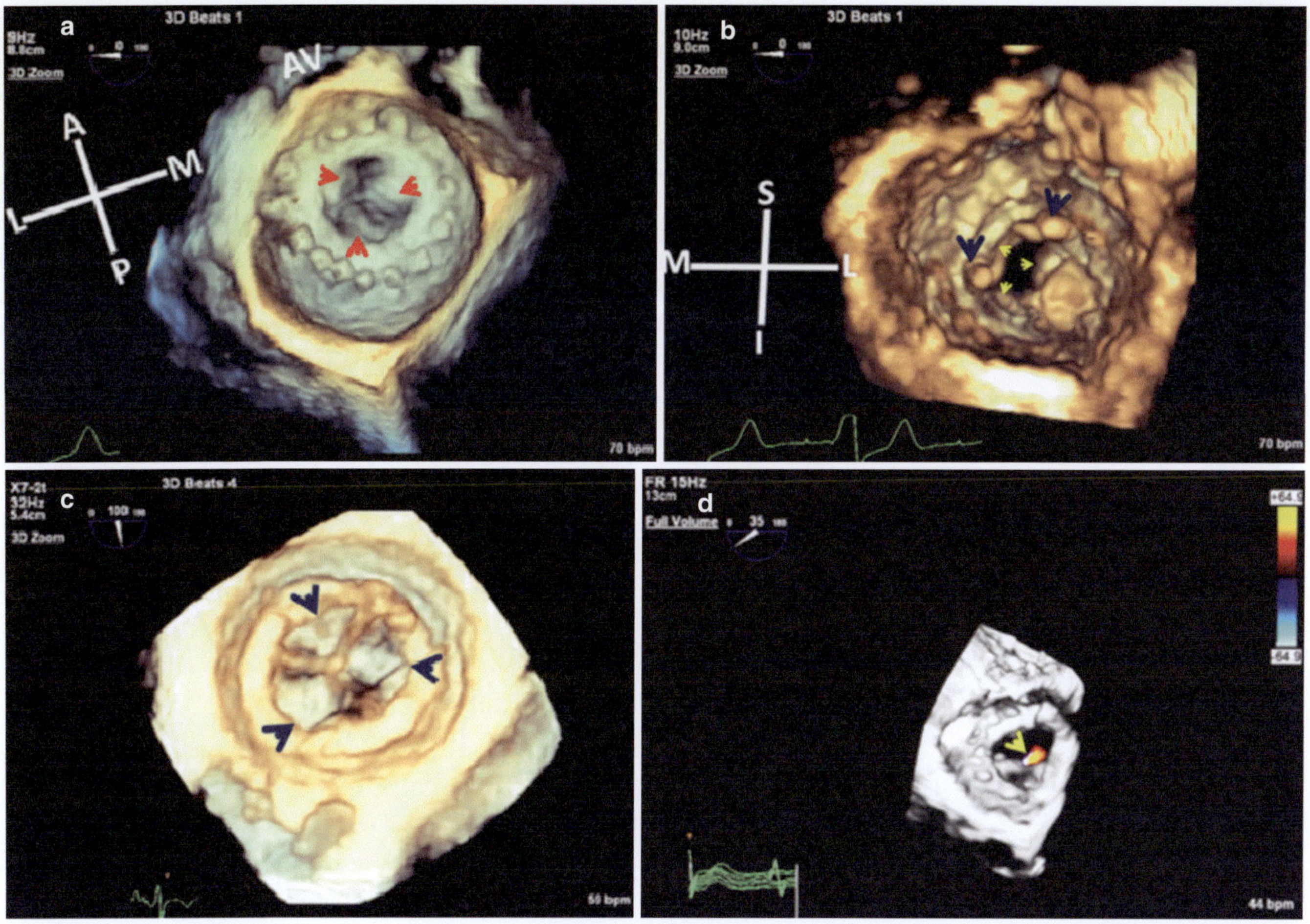

Fig. 14.9 **Top panel**: 3D TEE enface LA (**a**) and LV (**b**) views of a mitral bioprosthesis (27 mmCE Perimount Magna Ease) showing the three bioprosthesis cusps (red arrows in **a** and yellow arrows in **b**). Note the two prosthesis struts (dark blue arrows). **Bottom panel**: (**c**) LA view of another mitral bioprosthesis (33 mm Hancok II) showing the symmetrical trileaflet prosthesis anatomy (arrows). (**d**) Mild central bioprosthesis regurgitation (arrow) on CFD. Used with permission of Mayo Foundation for Medical Education and Research. All rights reserved. A, anterior; AV, aortic valve; CFD, color flow Doppler; I, inferior; L, lateral; LA, left atrial; LV, left ventricular; M, medial; P, posterior; R, right; S, superior

Sutureless Bioprostheses

Sutureless bioprostheses may be placed in the aortic valve position, using conventional surgical techniques, including cardiopulmonary bypass. The Perceval sutureless aortic bioprosthesis (Fig. 14.10) is a bovine pericardial prosthesis placed on a stent consisting of two rings and nine vertical struts. The stent both supports the valve and holds it in place without the need for surgical sutures.

Transcatheter Valves

The most commonly used transcathter aortic valves are the Medtronic CoreValve and Edwards Sapien prostheses. The Medtronic CoreValve (Fig. 14.11) is a supra-annular, porcine bioprosthesis with a self-expanding Nitinol stent frame. This prosthesis is longer than the Edwards Sapien prosthesis, with the distal portion of the prosthesis positioned at the sinotubular junction. The Edwards Sapien prosthesis is an

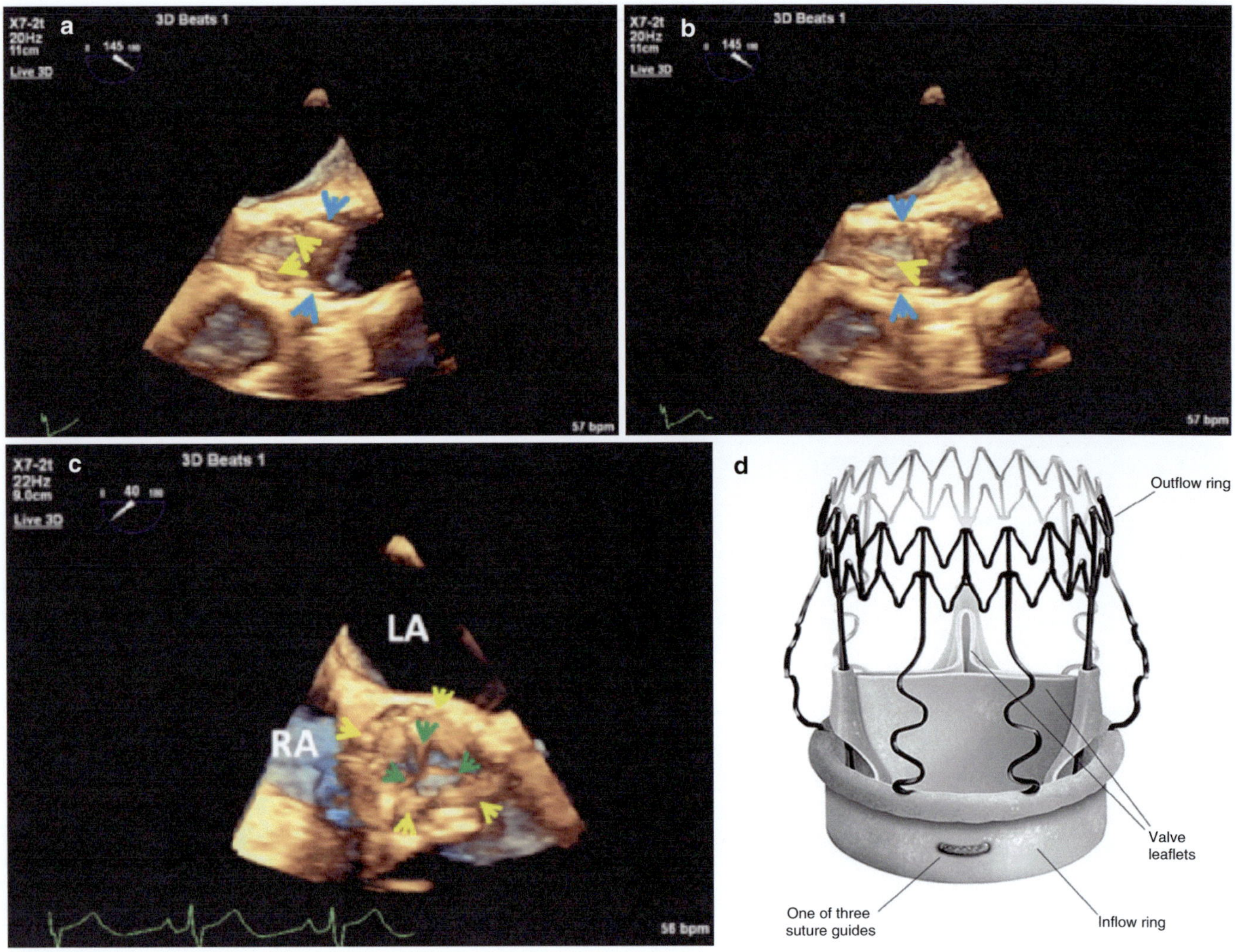

Fig. 14.10 3D TEE views of a Perceval sutureless valve. **Top panel**: Perceval sutureless aortic valve in systole (**a**) and diastole (**b**). Yellow arrows point to Perceval valve leaflets. Blue arrows point to valve stents. **Bottom panel**: (**c**) Perceval sutureless valve seen enface from aortic perspective. Green arrows point to Perceval valve leaflets and yellow arrows to circular ring. Images **a**–**c** are Used with permission of Mayo Foundation for Medical Education and Research. All rights reserved. (**d**) Perceval valve (courtesy of LivaNova PLC). LA, left atrium; RA, right atrium

intra-annular, bovine pericardial valve prosthesis with a balloon-expandable cobalt-chromium stent frame. In addition to treating native aortic valve stenosis, the Edwards Sapien valve prosthesis is also licensed by the FDA for valve-in-valve implantation for the treatment of bioprosthesis degeneration (Fig. 14.12). The Edwards Sapien transcatheter heart valve has also been used for valve-in complete mitral ring implantation (Fig. 14.13)

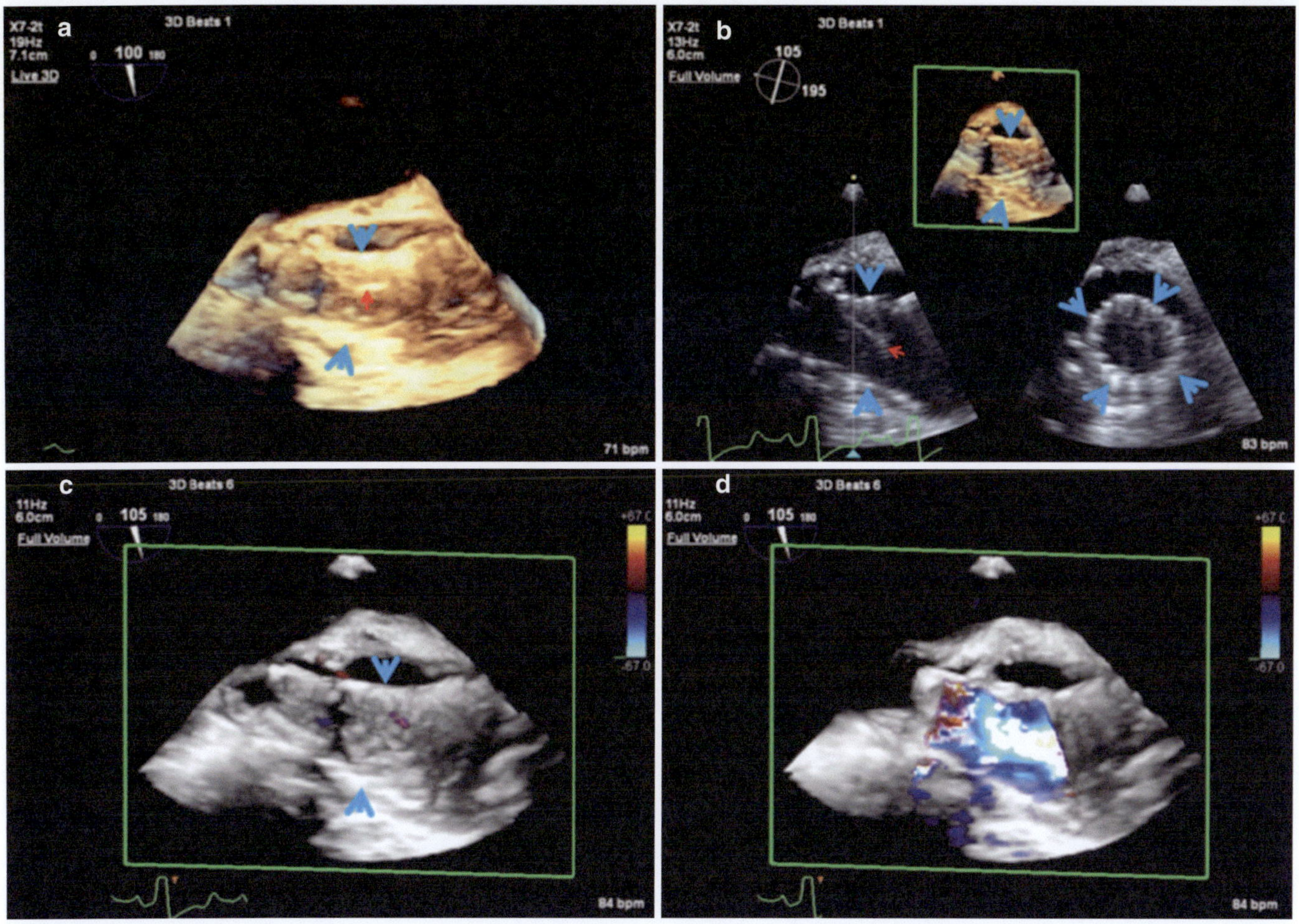

Fig. 14.11 3D TEE views of a fully deployed transcatheter CoreValve in the aortic position. (**a**, **b**) Fully expanded CoreValve. The stents (blue arrows) and leaflets (red arrows) can be seen. Note the circular shape at the waist of this THV site of leaflet insertion. (**c**, **d**) 3D CFD of the prosthesis in diastole (**c**) and systole (**d**). Note that there is no evidence of periprosthetic regurgitation. Used with permission of Mayo Foundation for Medical Education and Research. All rights reserved. CFD, color flow Doppler; THV, transcatheter heart valve

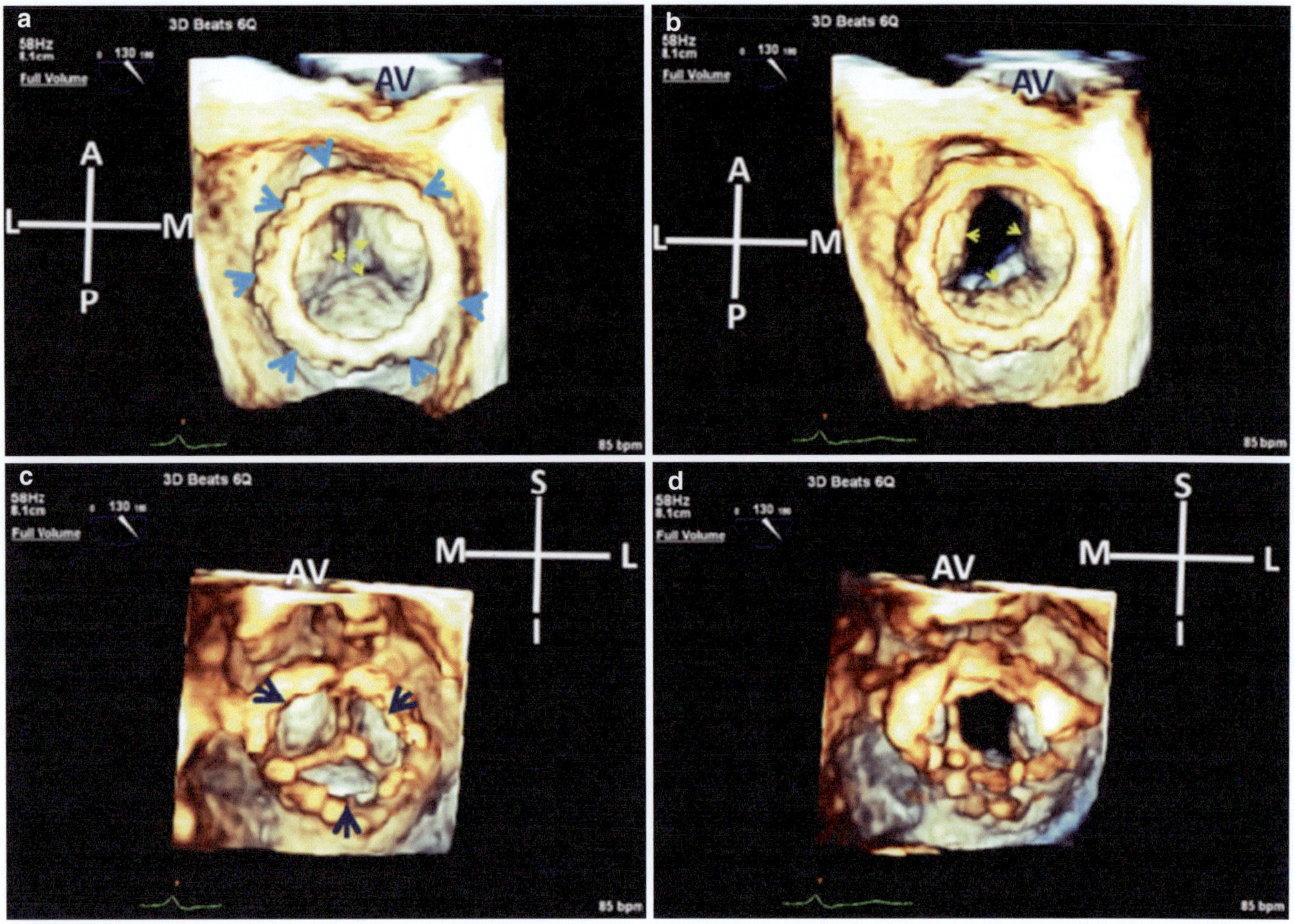

Fig. 14.12 3D TEE of Sapien S3 mitral valve-in-valve implantation. **Top panel**: Enface LA views in systole (**a**) and diastole (**b**). Yellow arrows point to the THV cusps and blue arrows to the THV stent. **Bottom panel**: Enface LV views in systole (**c**) and diastole (**d**). Dark blue arrows point to the three THV cusps. Used with permission of Mayo Foundation for Medical Education and Research. All rights reserved. A, anterior; AV, aortic valve; I, inferior; L, lateral; LA, left atrium; LV, left ventricle; M, medial; S, superior; THV, transcatheter heart valve

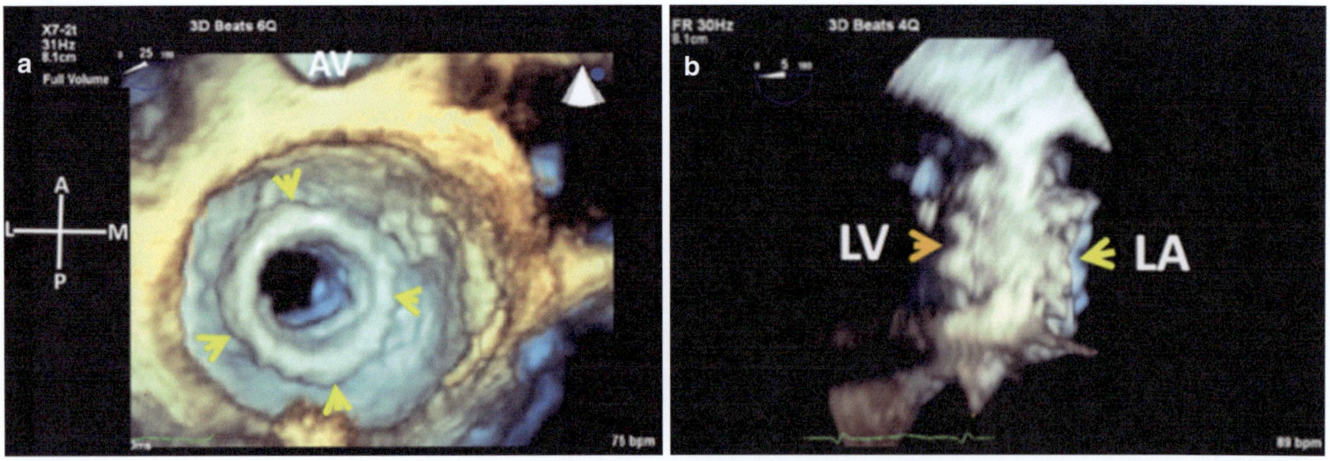

Fig. 14.13 3D TEE LA view of valve-in complete ring implantation of a Sapien THV. (**a**) The height of the THV stent framework (arrows) within the LA can be appreciated. (**b**) Same THV viewed sideways showing the atrial (yellow arrow) and ventricular (orange arrow) stent components. Used with permission of Mayo Foundation for Medical Education and Research. All rights reserved. A, anterior; AV, aortic valve; L, lateral; LA, left atrium; LV, left ventricle; M, medial; P, posterior; THV, transcatheter heart valve

References

1. Zoghbi WA, et al. Recommendations for evaluation of prosthetic valves with echocardiography and Doppler ultrasound. J Am Soc Echocardiogr. 2009;22(9):975–1014.
2. Mächler H, Perthel M, Reiter G, Reiter U, Zink M, Bergmann P, Waltensdorfer A, Laas J. Influence of bileaflet prosthetic mitral valve orientation on left ventricular flow—an experimental in vivo magnetic resonance imaging study. Eur J Cardiothorac Surg. 2004;26(4):747–53.
3. Deng Y, Belfar A, Powell T. Early prosthetic valve malfunction leading to cardiogenic shock and emergency redo mitral valve replacement. J Cardiothorac Vasc Anesth. 2019;33:2866–9.

15 3DE Assessment of the Pathological Spectrum of Mitral Prosthesis and Sewing Ring Dysfunction: Incremental Value over 2DE

Sushil Allen Luis and Joseph F. Maalouf

Introduction

Prosthetic valve dysfunction covers a wide spectrum that includes prosthesis thrombosis, pannus tissue ingrowth (an overgrowth of fibrous tissue from sewing ring (SR) into the valve orifice), and prosthesis dehiscence [1]. Bioprosthetic valve cusps are prone to degeneration which can result in prosthesis regurgitation due to cusp prolapse, avulsion or perforation, or prosthesis stenosis due to cusp calcification, thrombosis, or both [1]. Mechanical prostheses are more prone to thrombosis [1]. Three-dimensional echocardiography (3DE) and in particular 3D TEE is invaluable for determining the mechanism of mitral prosthesis dysfunction and in localizing the site of thrombus formation and SR dehiscence [1]. 3DE also provides the opportunity to visualize the entire mitral valve prosthesis, and post mitral valve repair annuloplasty bands or rings, together with their surrounding bed, in a single view, and in real time. This enhances understanding the location and relationships of abnormalities to normal structures.

Supplementary Information The online version of this chapter (https://doi.org/10.1007/978-3-030-72941-7_15) contains supplementary material, which is available to authorized users.

S. A. Luis (✉)
Associate Professor of Medicine, Mayo Clinic College of Medicine; Consultant, Department of Cardiovascular Medicine, Mayo Clinic, Rochester, MN, USA
e-mail: Luis.S@mayo.edu

J. F. Maalouf
Professor of Medicine, Mayo Clinic College of Medicine; Director, Interventional Echocardiography; Consultant, Department of Cardiovascular Medicine, Mayo Clinic, Rochester, MN, USA
e-mail: maalouf.joseph@mayo.edu

Prosthetic Valve Dehiscence

Periprosthetic leak (PPL; also known as paravalve leak) is a complication associated with the implantation of a prosthetic heart valve , and refers to regurgitation between two cardiac chambers that skirts the valve prosthesis [1]. Surgical PPL is due to incomplete seal between the implanted prosthesis (mechanical or biologic) sewing ring (SR) and native annulus either because of annular calcification that precludes adequate suturing of the SR to the annulus or breakdown of SR sutures, frequently due to endocarditis, leading to detachment or dehiscence of the prosthesis from its annulus (Fig. 15.1) . With transcatheter valve-in-valve implantation, PPL is due to incomplete seal of the stented transcatheter valve and native mitral annulus or bioprosthesis SR (Fig. 15.2). Mitral PPL results in abnormal systolic flow from the left ventricle to the left atrium through the periprosthetic defect.

Although the PPL may be severe and cause heart failure, it may be clinically significant even in the absence of severe regurgitation because of hemolysis

Anatomic Defect Localization

Successful percutaneous PPL closure (see Chap. 30) is dependent on determining the circumferential extent, number and location of periprosthetic defects, and accurate characterization of PPL anatomic pathology. As with assessment of the native mitral valve, TEE is particularly well suited for evaluating mitral periprosthetic leaks. With 2D TEE, the site of PPL and circumferential extent is determined by careful systematic scanning of the entire prosthesis sewing ring in multiple imaging views from different acoustic windows. Nonetheless, a PPL defect may be missed (Figs. 15.3 and 15.4) or its circumferential extent may not be fully appreciated even when the TEE is performed by an experienced operator (Fig. 15.5). With 3D TEE, the entire mitral valve prosthesis and its bed can be imaged from a single acoustic

J. F. Maalouf et al. (eds.), *Practical 3D Echocardiography*, https://doi.org/10.1007/978-3-030-72941-7_15

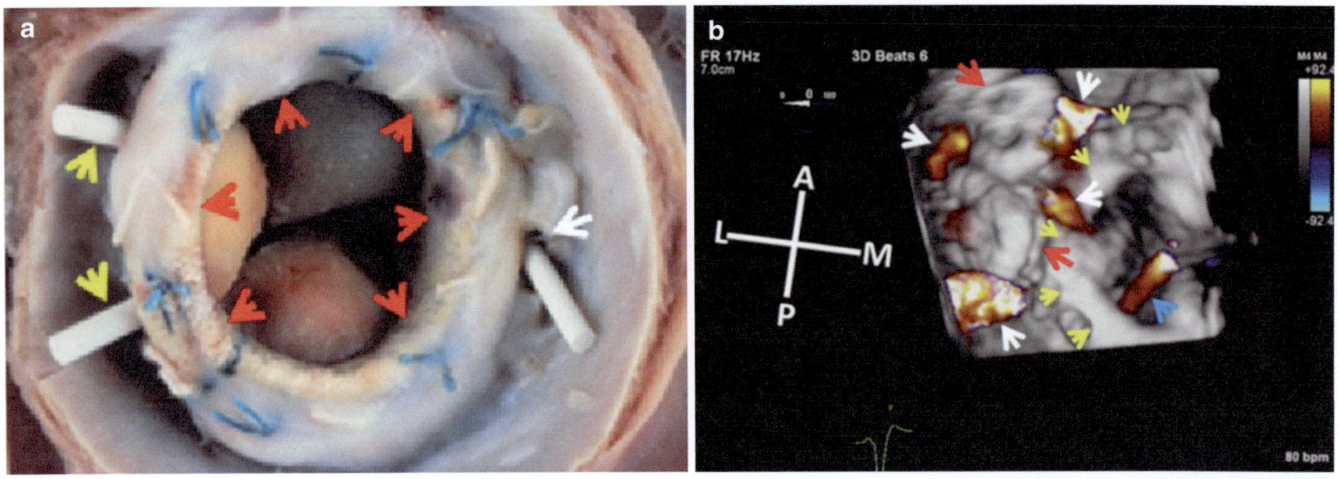

Fig. 15.1 (**a**) Pathology of mitral PPL, courtesy of Dr. William Edwards (Mayo Clinic), showing three periprosthetic defects. Two (yellow arrows) can be seen at underbelly of the SR (red arrows), and the third (white arrow) is in the atrial bed adjacent to the SR. (**b**) 3D TEE enface LA CFD post PPL closure with two AVP devices (red arrows) showing persistent PPL (white arrows) around the deployed AVP devices. Yellow arrows point to bioprosthesis SR and blue arrow points to mild central prosthesis regurgitation. Used with permission of Mayo Foundation for Medical Education and Research. All rights reserved. A, anterior; AVP, Amplatzer Vascular Plug; CFD, color flow Doppler; L, lateral; LA, left atrium; M, medial; P, posterior; PPL, periprosthetic leak; SR, sewing ring

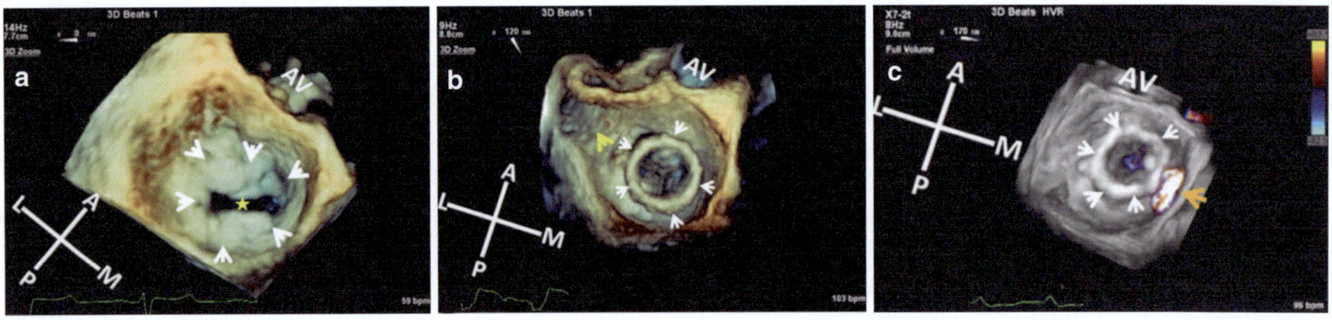

Fig. 15.2 Live 3D TEE enface LA views of MV and PPL following valve-in-valve implantation of a Sapien THV. (**a**) Severe MAC (white arrows) with secondary severe narrowing of MV orifice (star). (**b**, **c**) Sapien THV showing a medial PPL (orange arrow) on CFD. White arrows point to THV stent frame and yellow arrow points to LAA. Used with permission of Mayo Foundation for Medical Education and Research. All rights reserved. A, anterior; AV, aortic valve; CFD, color flow Doppler; L, lateral; LA, left atrium; LAA, left atrial appendage; M, medial; MAC, mitral annular calcification; MV, mitral valve; P, posterior; PPL, periprosthetic leak; THV, transcatheter heart valve

window, thus obviating the often extensive TEE probe manipulation needed to obtain diagnostic 2D images. Moreover, 3D TEE also provides an intuitive en face "surgeon's view" of the mitral valve prosthesis and surrounding anatomy that is readily recognizable by interventional cardiologists with no or limited experience in echocardiography (Figs. 15.4 and 15.5).

Accurate localization of a mitral PPL is a prerequisite for guiding percutaneous closure of the defect. This can be readily achieved with 3D TEE through use of a simple triangulation method [2] that is based on standard spatial coordinates and three fixed anatomic land marks (the anteriorly located aortic valve, the anterolaterally located left atrial appendage, and the medially located atrial septum (Fig. 15.6)

3D TEE also provides crucial information regarding defect (s) shape (most mitral paravalvular defects are crescentic or oblong rather than being cylindrical holes), and size (Figs. 15.6, 15.7, and 15.8).

When there is suspicion of a periprosthetic defect on 3D TEE, great care must be taken to avoid creation of drop out artifacts due to excessive tissue cropping or low gain settings (see Chap. 3). False periprosthetic defects due to drop out artifacts can also be produced by acoustic shadowing caused by prosthetic material or calcification (see Fig. 3.8, Chap. 3). Demonstration of flow through any observed defect using color Doppler is therefore, a must to confirm its true nature (see Fig. 3.8, Chap. 3). *A periprosthetic defect may not be identified by 3D imaging alone without use of 3D color flow Doppler (Fig. 15.9) particularly when located at underbelly*

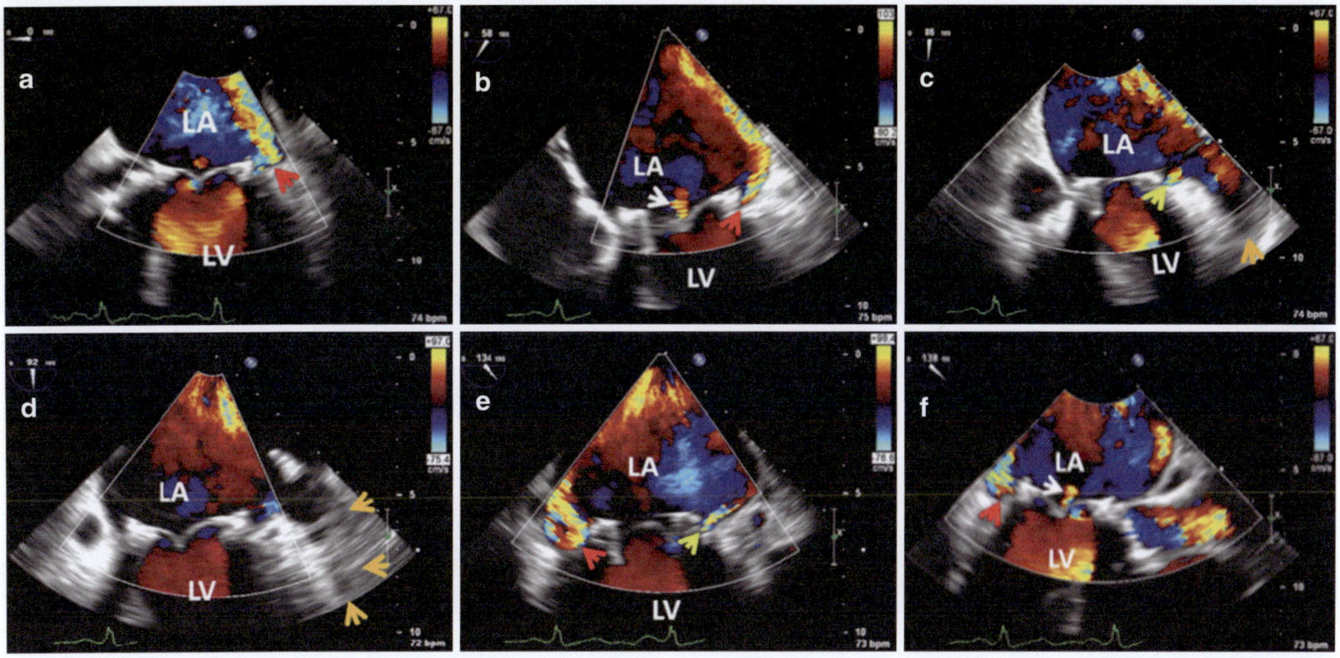

Fig. 15.3 (a–f) 2D TEE CFD of mitral PPL: With the TEE probe in the mid esophagus, the SR is scanned from horizontal (0°; medial to lateral) to long-axis aorta (138° anterior to posterior) planes. A large postero-lateral defect (red arrows) and a small anterolateral PPL (yellow arrows) adjacent to the LAA (orange arrows) are seen. White arrows point to trivial prosthesis regurgitation. Used with permission of Mayo Foundation for Medical Education and Research. All rights reserved. CFD, color flow Doppler; LA, left atrium; LAA, left atrial appendage; LV, left ventricle; PPL, periprosthetic leak; SR, sewing ring

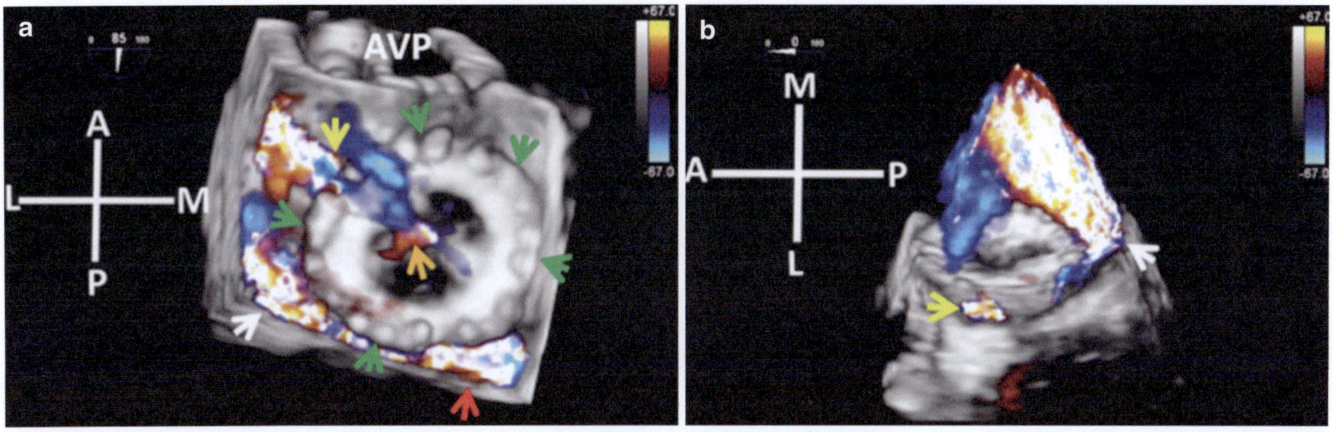

Fig. 15.4 (a, b) 3D CFD enface LA view of MV bioprosthesis from same patient as in Fig. 15.3 shows three PPL sites, a large posterolateral leak (white arrows), a smaller postero-medial leak (red arrow) and a tiny antero-lateral leak (yellow arrows) facing ostium of the LAA. Green arrows point to prosthesis SR, and orange arrow points to trivial central prosthesis regurgitation. Used with permission of Mayo Foundation for Medical Education and Research. All rights reserved. A, anterior; AVP, aortic valve prosthesis; CFD, color flow Doppler; L, lateral; LA, left atrium; LAA, left atrial appendage; M, medial; MV, mitral valve; P, posterior; PPL, periprosthetic leak; SR, sewing ring

of the SR or in very close proximity to it (see Fig. 30.5, Chap. 30), or if adjacent to the leaflet hinges of a mechanical prosthesis (Fig. 15.9).

In patients undergoing surgical mitral valve (MV) repair and insertion of an annuloplasty band or ring, suture breakdown can cause separation of the annuloplasty band or ring from the underlying annulus (Figs. 15.10 and 15.11). In contrast to PPL associated with surgical mitral prostheses, annuloplasty dehiscence associated with MV repair rarely disrupts the attachment between the mitral valve leaflets and native annulus. The resultant regurgitant systolic flow therefore, is usually due to the underlying mitral valve pathology and is caused by loss of annular band/ring support, hence, not amenable to treatment by percutaneous closure of the dehiscence with a vascular plug. *The posterior segment of annuloplasty bands/rings is more susceptible to dehiscence because the*

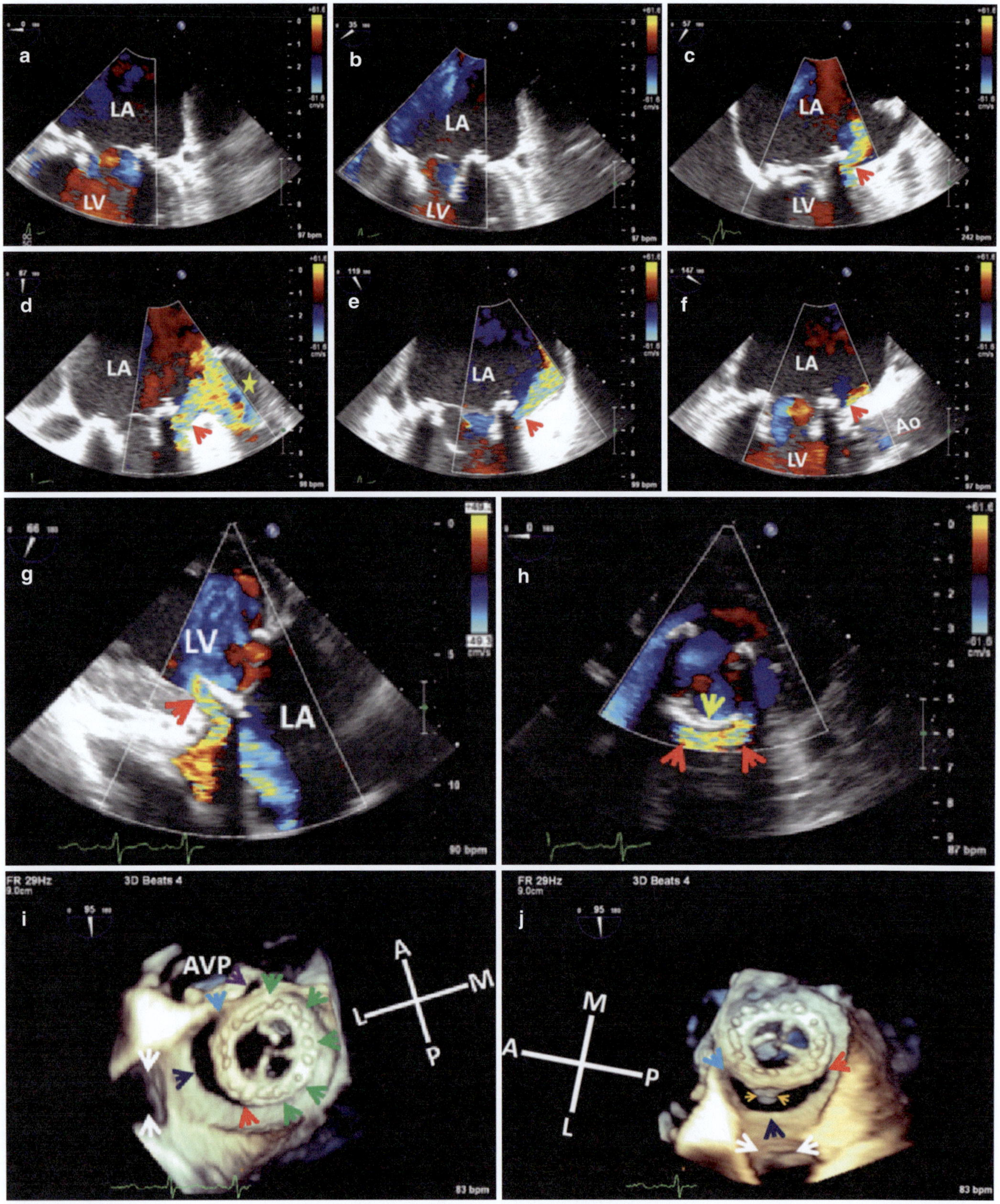
a
LA
LV
b
LA
LV
c
LA
LV
d
LA
e
LA
f
LA
Ao
LV
g
LV
LA
h
FR 29Hz
9.0cm
3D Beats 4
i
AVP
A
M
L
P
j
M
A
P
L
83 bpm

Fig. 15.5 (**a**–**f**) 2D TEE CFD images of a mitral bioprosthesis from the mid esophagus with the SR carefully scanned from horizontal 0° to long-axis aorta at 147°. There is a severe anterolateral leak (red arrows) with the regurgitation directed towards the LAA (star). (**g**, **h**) TG CFD of the PPL(red arrows). Note that the short-axis view (**h**) is best suited to assess the circumferential extent of the PPL, but is not always feasible. Yellow arrow points to prosthesis SR. (**i**, **j**) Multibeat 3D TEE enface views of the mitral bioprosthesis. There is a very large SR dehiscence (dark blue arrows) adjacent to LAA ostium (white arrows) that spans nearly a third of the SR circumference from anterior (light blue arrow) to posterior (red arrow). The extent of SR dehiscence makes it unsuitable for percutaneous closure. Green arrows point to prosthesis SR. Note that one of the bioprosthesis struts (**j**, orange arrows) can be seen projecting into the LV opposite the LAA. Used with permission of Mayo Foundation for Medical Education and Research. All rights reserved. A, anterior; Ao, ascending aorta; AVP, aortic valve prosthesis; CFD, color flow Doppler; L, lateral; LA, left atrium; LAA, left atrial appendage; LV, left ventricle; M, medial; MV, mitral valve; P, posterior; PPL, periprosthetic leak; SR, sewing ring; TG, transgastric

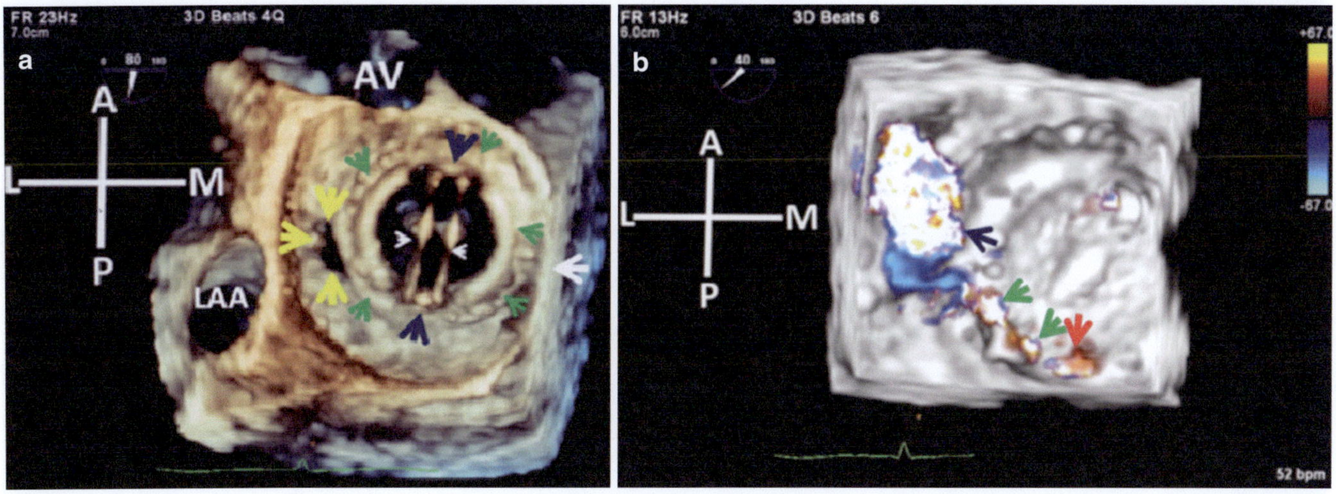

Fig. 15.6 (**a**) Triangulation method used to localize mitral PPL on 3D TEE. The location of a periprosthetic defect (yellow arrows) is reported in relation to three fixed anatomic landmarks: anterior AV, anterolateral LAA, and medial atrial septum (white arrow). Note the crescent shape of the periprosthetic defect. The hinges of mechanical bileaflet prostheses (dark blue arrows) can also serve as fluoroscopic beacons to location of the PPL. Green arrows point to prosthesis SR. The periprostheic defect can be measured using MPR. Note that measurements can also be obtained using on line calipers but the accuracy of such measurements has not been validated clinically. (**b**) Multibeat 3D CFD showing flow through the periprosthetic defect (dark blue arrow). Green arrows point to built in trivial regurgitation associated with the posterior occluder hinge and red arrow points to built in trivial regurgitation associated with the prosthesis leaflet occluder. Used with permission of Mayo Foundation for Medical Education and Research. All rights reserved. A, anterior; AV, aortic valve; CFD, color flow Doppler; L, lateral; LA, left atrium; LAA, left atrial appendage; M, medial; MPR, multiplanar reconstruction; MV, mitral valve; P, posterior; PPL, periprosthetic leak; SR, sewing ring

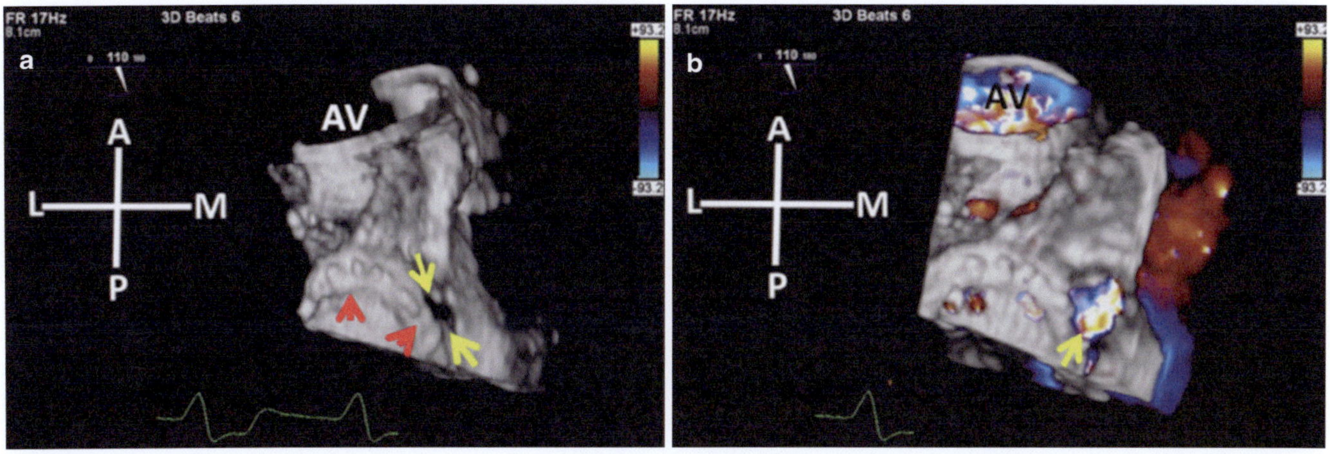

Fig. 15.7 (**a**, **b**) Enface 3D TEE LA view of an anteromedial PPL with regurgitant flow on CFD (yellow arrows) in a patient who also underwent a composite aortic valved conduit (AV). The use of color filter (see Chap. 3, Fig. 3.5) can be very helpful in optimizing the image by bringing out the origin of the regurgitant jet. Red arrows point to anterior prosthesis SR. Used with permission of Mayo Foundation for Medical Education and Research. All rights reserved. A, anterior; CFD, color flow Doppler; L, lateral; LA, left atrium; M, medial; P, posterior; PPL, periprosthetic leak; SR, sewing ring

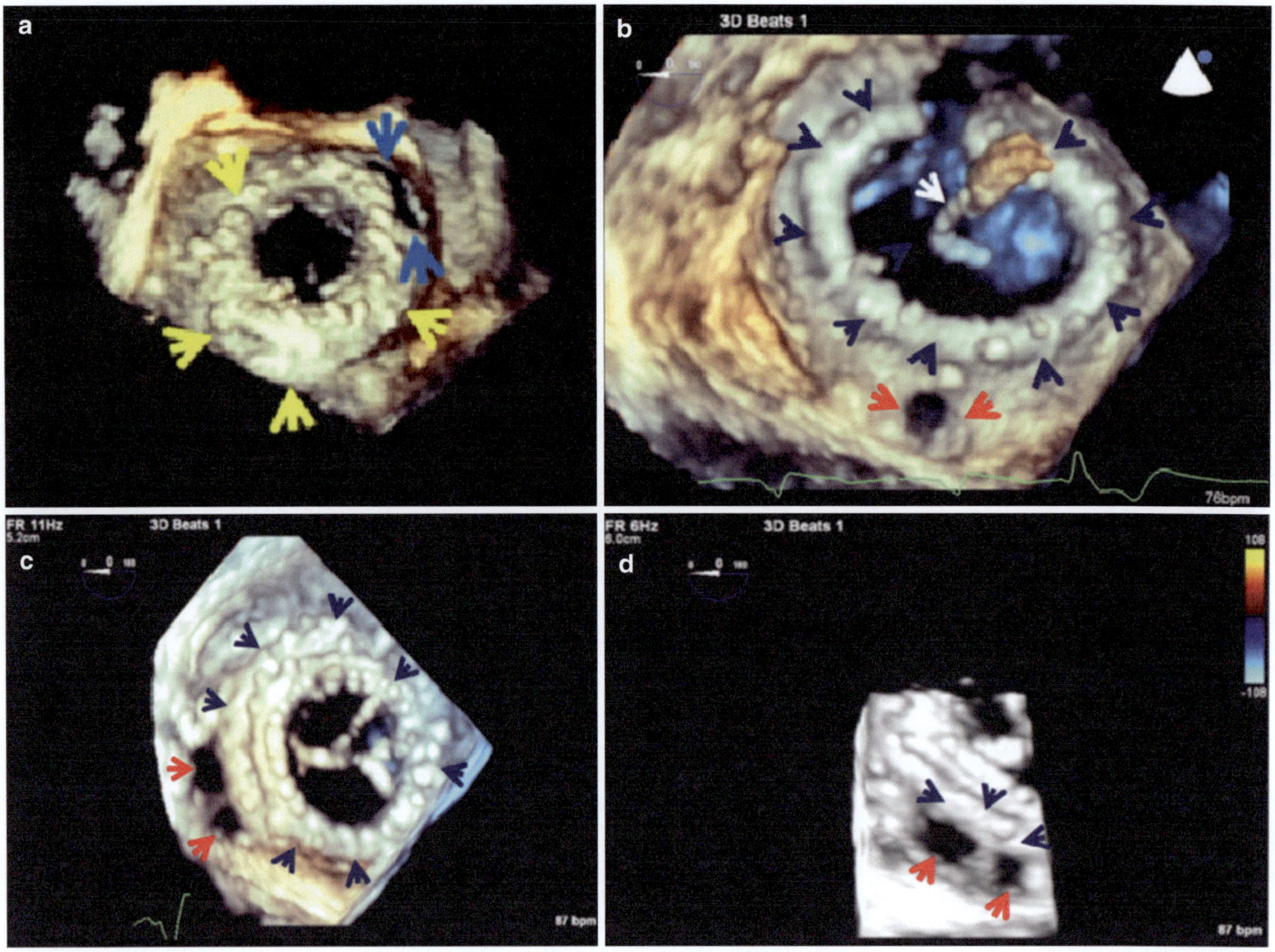

Fig. 15.8 Various periprosthetic defect shapes as seen on 3D TEE. **Top panel**: (**a**) Irregular crescent shaped periprostheic defect (blue arrows); yellow arrows point to prosthesis SR. (**b**) Single circular periprosthetic defect (red arrows) in a patient who underwent MV repair with insertion of a complete annuloplasty ring (dark blue arrows). White arrow points to a wire in MV orifice. **Bottom panel**: (**c**, **d**) Two adjacent and round periprosthetic defects separated by small amount of tissue (red arrows). Dark blue arrows point to prosthesis SR. Used with permission of Mayo Foundation for Medical Education and Research. All rights reserved. MV, mitral valve; SR, sewing ring

posterior mitral annulus is located deeper in the surgical field thus limiting surgical exposure which may also inadvertently result in a periannular defect (Fig. 15.12). Annular calcification, when present, usually involves the posterior mitral annulus and prevents effective suture placement. Moreover, because the left circumflex coronary artery runs posteriorly, surgeons intentionally avoid deep placement of sutures.

There is no gold standard for determining severity of mitral PPL and integration of multiple echocardiographic parameters is thus required. In some circumstances the regurgitant orifice area can also be measured by planimetry using multiplanar reconstruction of the 3D color Doppler data set (Fig. 15.13), but care must be taken during image acquisition to avoid acoustic shadowing from the prosthesis sewing ring.

Prosthetic Valve Dysfunction and Thrombosis

Aside from PPL, prosthesis thrombosis (Fig. 15.14) and pannus ingrowth account for the vast majority of non-infectious causes of prosthetic valve dysfunction [1, 3, 4]. Both thrombus and pannus tissue overgrowth can present as masses on the sewing ring or adjacent to it and can cause prosthesis obstruction [1, 3, 4]. Differentiation of thrombus from pan-

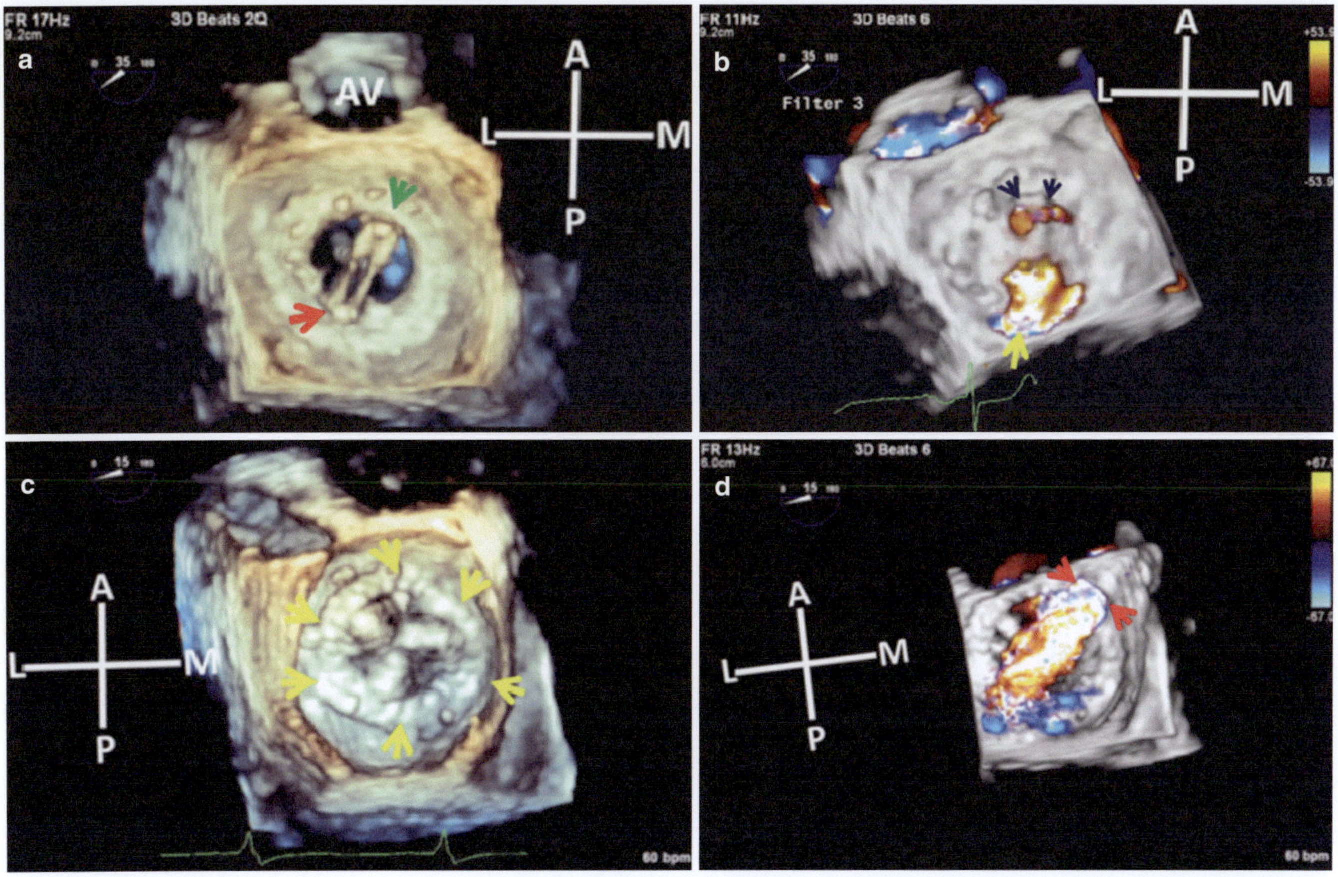

Fig. 15.9 **Top panel**: 3D TEE enface LA views of a mechanical mitral bileaflet prosthesis with PPL adjacent to posterior hinge (**a**, red arrow) but only seen on CFD (**b**, yellow arrow). The two small MR jets anteriorly (dark blue arrows) are normal built in regurgitation. Green arrow points to anterior hinge. **Bottom panel**: (**c**, **d**) 3D TEE LA view of antero-medial mitral bioprosthesis PPL that is only apparent on CFD (red arrows). Yellow arrows point to prosthesis SR. Used with permission of Mayo Foundation for Medical Education and Research. All rights reserved. A, anterior; AV, aortic valve; CFD, color flow Doppler; L, lateral; LA, left atrium; M, medial; MR, mitral regurgitation; P, posterior; PPL, periprosthetic leak; SR, sewing ring

nus overgrowth can be very challenging or not possible despite integration of clinical and multimodality imaging including fluoroscopy, and both thrombus and pannus tissue may coexist [1, 3, 4]. Moreover, neither mass mobility or size can reliably differentiate thrombus from pannus [3, 4]. However, mechanical prosthesis obstruction due to thrombus is associated with a mass on TEE and restriction to occluder leaflet mobility in nearly all patients [3]. In contrast, when the obstruction is caused by pannus tissue, there may be no restriction to prosthesis leaflet mobility, and a mass is not seen on TEE in the majority of cases [3]. Therefore, if mechanical prosthesis obstruction is associated with normal prosthesis occluder mobility, thrombus is highly unlikely as the cause of obstruction and pannus ingrowth is the likely underlying mechanism. However, if there is restriction to prosthesis occluder function, either pannus or thrombus can be the underlying cause. Thrombosis is a more common cause of mechanical mitral prosthesis dysfunction than pannus ingrowth, however. Bioprosthesis degeneration can be in the form of stenosis (Fig. 15.14), regurgitation or both [5]. Post MV repair sewing ring thrombosis is rare but has been reported (Fig. 15.14).

In patients undergoing mitral valve replacement with a mechanical valve, 3D TEE can be very useful for verifying normal occluder function on coming off bypass (Fig. 15.15). This is important because mechanical prosthesis occluder malfunction may not become clinically apparent until after surgery.

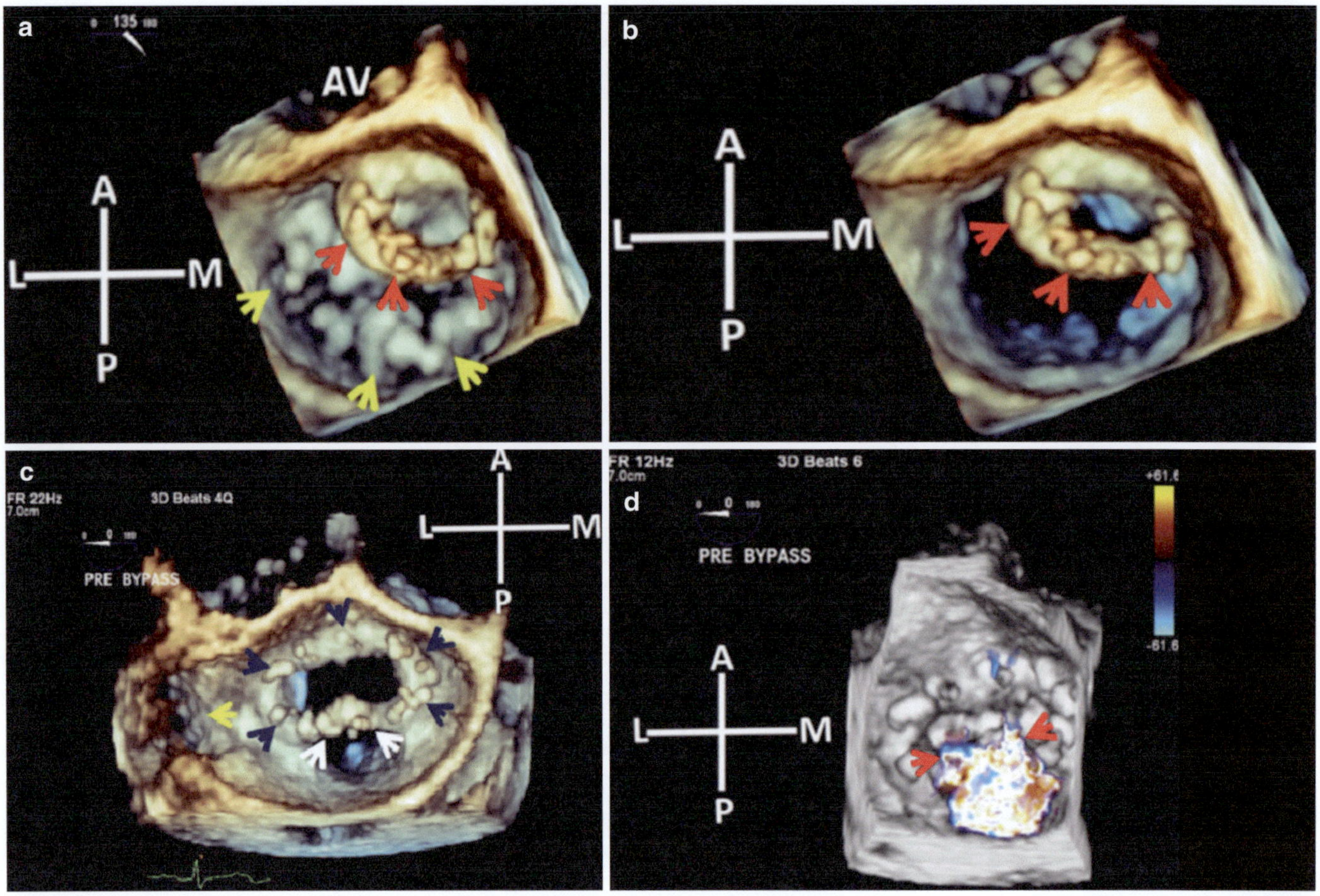

Fig. 15.10 3D TEE Enface LA views in two patients status post-surgical mitral valve repair and insertion of complete annuloplasty rings. **Top panel**: first patient: Systole (**a**) and diastole (**b**). There is complete dehiscence of the annuloplasty ring posteriorly (red arrows). Yellow arrows point to PML. **Bottom panel**: second patient (**c**) Partial dehiscence of posterior annuloplasty ring (white arrows) adjacent to P2 segment of PML. Dark blue arrows point to annuloplasty ring and yellow arrow points to LAA. (**d**) Mitral regurgitation (red arrows) secondary to partial annuloplasty dehiscence. Annuloplasty dehiscence has a predilection for the posterior annulus and is more common with complete rings. Used with permission of Mayo Foundation for Medical Education and Research. All rights reserved. A, anterior; AV, aortic valve; L, lateral; LA, left atrium; LAA, left atrial appendage; M, medial; P, posterior; PML, posterior mitral leaflet

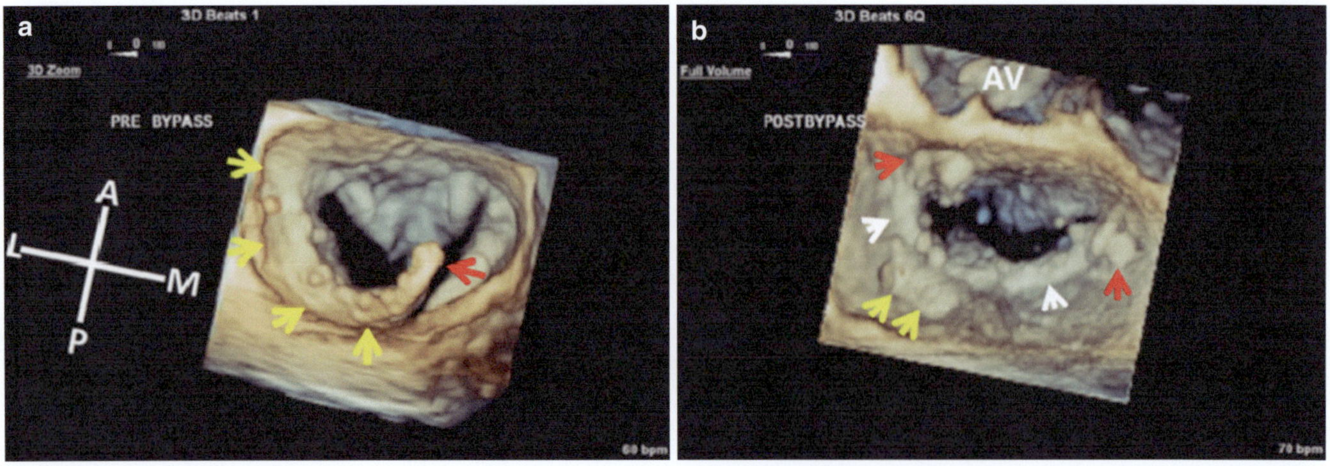

Fig. 15.11 3D TEE enface LA views of posterior annuloplasty bands following surgical MV repair. (**a**) Medial dehiscence of annuloplasty band (red arrow). Yellow arrows point to rest of the band. (**b**) Following placement of a new annuloplasty band (white arrows). Note the reinforcing sutures that were placed at the two trigones (red arrows) posterior to P2 (yellow arrows). The sutures appear thick due to blurring artifacts (see Chap. 3). Used with permission of Mayo Foundation for Medical Education and Research. All rights reserved. A, anterior; AV, aortic valve; L, lateral; LA, left atrium; M, medial; MV, mitral valve; P, posterior

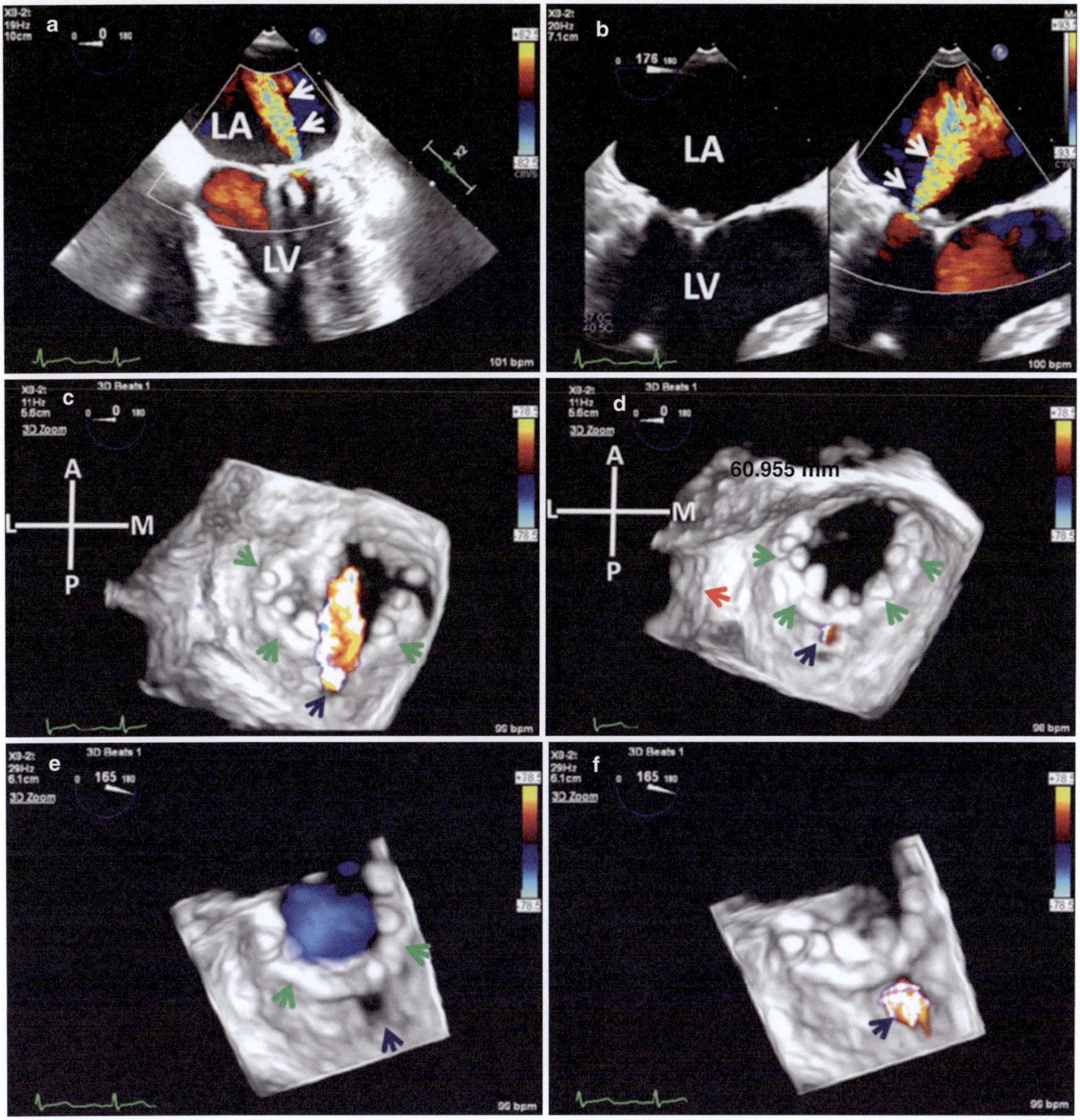

Fig. 15.12 Periannular regurgitation in a patient following surgical MV repair with insertion of posterior annuloplasty band. **Top panel**: (**a**, **b**) 2D TEE shows MR (white arrows) but the origin of the MR jet is not seen. **Middle panel**: 3D TEE enface LA views of the MV and posterior annuloplasty band in late systole (**c**) and end systole (**d**) showing the MR jet (dark blue arrows) originating from a circular defect in the LA bed adjacent to the annuloplasty band posteriorly. There is otherwise, no evidence of dehiscence of the annuloplasty band. **Bottom panel**: (**e**, **f**) Focused 3D images of the circular periannular defect (dark blue arrows) with regurgitant flow through it in systole. Green arrows (**c**, **d**, **e**) point to annuloplasty band and red arrow to ostium of LAA. Used with permission of Mayo Foundation for Medical Education and Research. All rights reserved. A, anterior; AV, aortic valve; L, lateral; LA, left atrium; LAA, left atrial appendage; LV, left ventricle; M, medial; MR, mitral regurgitation; MV, mitral valve; P, posterior

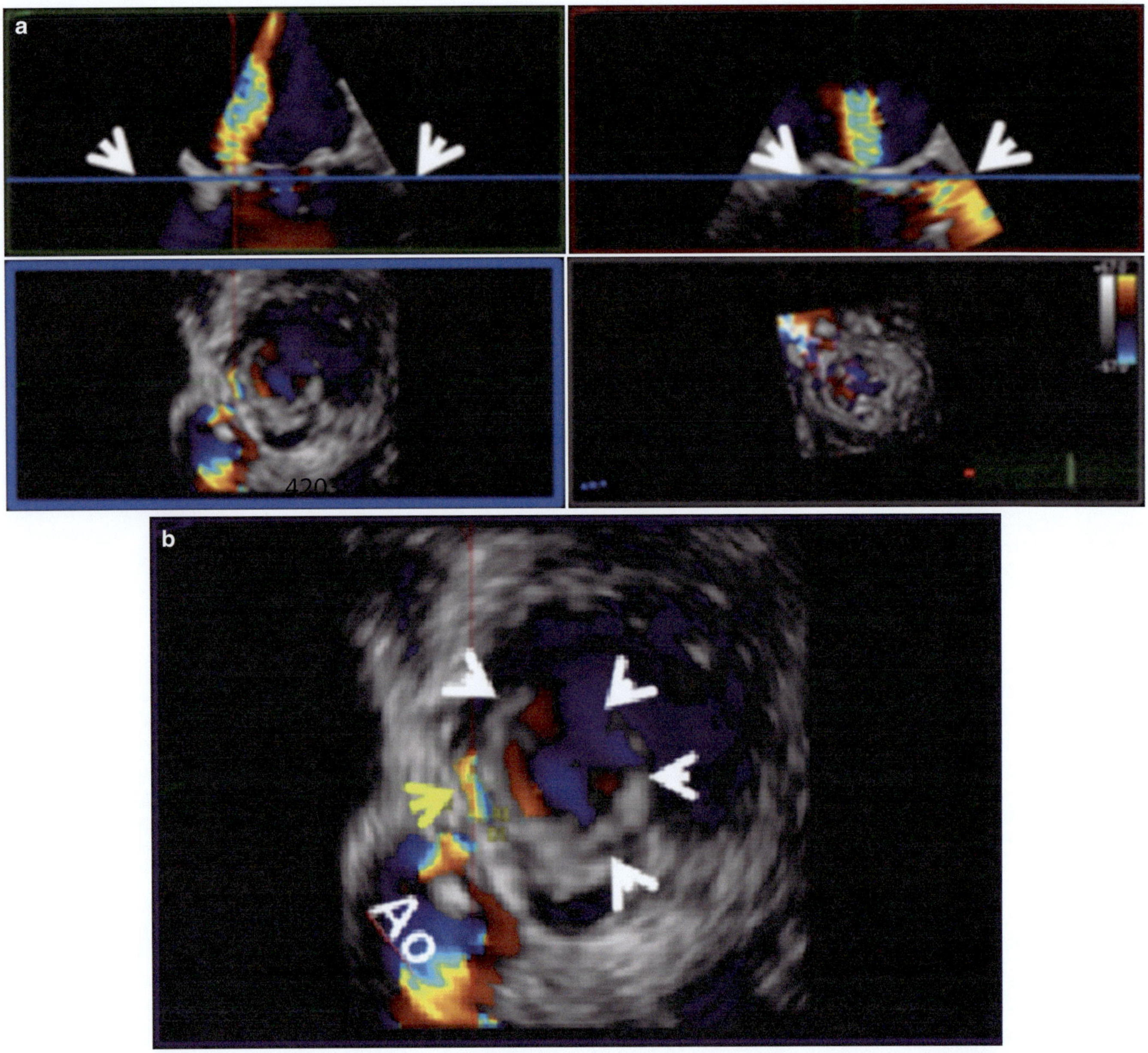

Fig. 15.13 (**a**) MPR of anterior mitral PPL. Transverse plane (blue line, arrows) at site of origin of PPL in two orthogonal planes [coronal or frontal (green), and sagittal or vertical (red)] produces a slit like color flow Doppler defect, which represents the VC of the mitral PPL, in the transverse plane (Blue rectangle, left lower quadrant). (**b**) Enlarged image of the transverse plane showing the slit like PPL VC (yellow arrow) that can be planimetered. White arrows point to prosthesis SR. Used with permission of Mayo Foundation for Medical Education and Research. All rights reserved. Ao, ascending aorta; MPR, multiplanar reconstruction; PPL, periprosthetic leak; SR, sewing ring; VC, vena contracta

Fig. 15.14 **Top panel**: (**a**, **b**) 3D TEE enface LA (**a**) and LV (**b**) views of degenerated bioprosthesis stenosis. Note the very narrowed prosthesis orifice (red arrows). Green arrows point to prosthesis SR in the LA and yellow arrows point to the three prosthesis struts in the LV. (**c**) 3D TEE of a prosthetic valve with small thrombus (red arrow) projecting into the orifice of the prosthesis from the SR anteriorly (dark blue arrows). (**d**) Intraoperative photograph of the thrombus (arrow). (**e**) Large amount of thrombus (dark blue arrows) on annuloplasty band (green arrows) 2 years after successful surgical MV repair. (**f**) 3D TEE enface LV view of bioprosthesis thrombosis (dark blue arrows) with secondary severe bioprosthesis stenosis (green arrow). **Bottom panel**: Explanted thrombosed bioprosthesis. (**g**) Bioprosthesis leaflets (white arrows) as seen from LA. No thrombus is seen. (**h**) LV view of same prosthesis showing extensive thrombus involving the ventricular surface of all three cusps (yellow arrows). White arrows point to bioprosthesis struts. Used with permission of Mayo Foundation for Medical Education and Research. All rights reserved. A, anterior; AV, aortic valve; I, inferior; L, lateral; LA, left atrium; LAA, left atrial appendage; LV, left ventricle; M, medial; MV, mitral valve; P, posterior; S, superior; SR, sewing ring

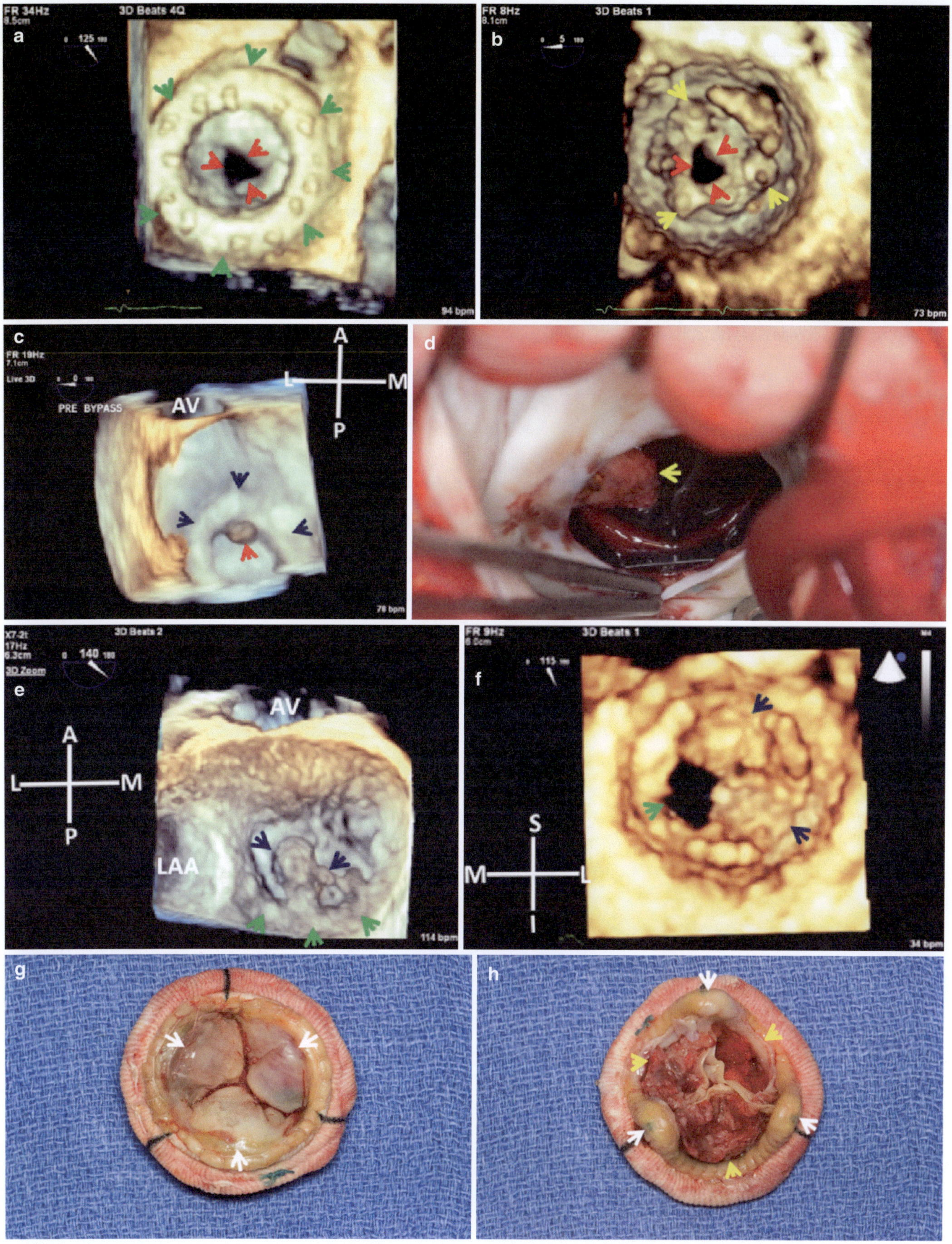
a
FR 34Hz
8.5cm
3D Beats 4Q
125
94 bpm
b
FR 8Hz
8.1cm
3D Beats 1
73 bpm
c
FR 19Hz
7.1cm
Live 3D
PRE BYPASS
AV
A
L
M
P
78 bpm
d
e
X7-2t
17Hz
6.3cm
3D Zoom
3D Beats 2
140
AV
A
L
M
P
LAA
114 bpm
f
FR 9Hz
3D Beats 1
115
S
M
L
I
34 bpm
g
h

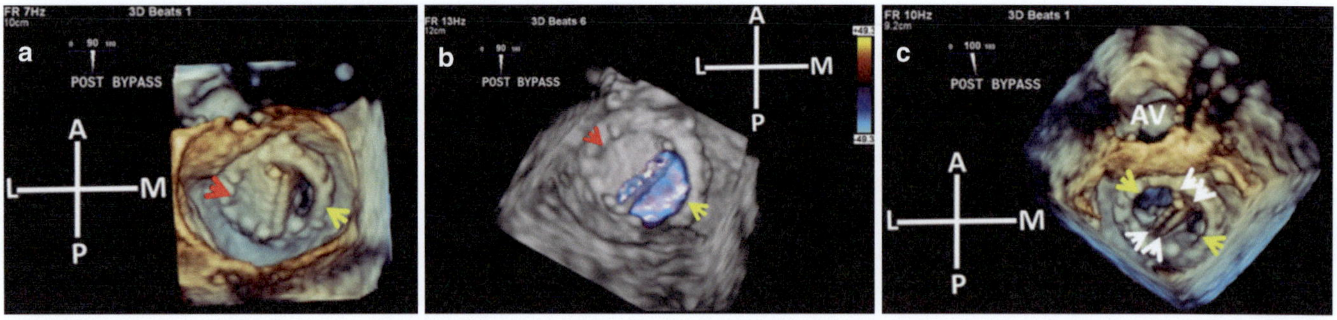

Fig. 15.15 Intraoperative post pump 3D TEE enface LA views of a mechanical bileaflet prosthesis implanted in the mitral position. (**a**, **b**) Only one of the leaflet occluders (yellow arrows) is opening (note flow on CFD). The other leaflet occluder (red arrows) is stuck in a closed position. (**c**) After a second pump run and restoration of normal bileaflet occluder motion (white arrows). Yellow arrows point to fully open prosthesis orifices. Used with permission of Mayo Foundation for Medical Education and Research. All rights reserved. A, anterior; AV, aortic valve; CFD, color flow Doppler; L, lateral; LA, left atrium; M, medial; P, posterior

References

1. Lancelloti P, et al. Recommendations for the imaging assessment of prosthetic heart valves: a report from the European Association of Cardiovascular Imaging endorsed by the Chinese Society of Echocardiography, the Inter-American Society of Echocardiography, and the Brazilian Department of Cardiovascular Imaging. Eur Heart J Cardiovasc Imaging. 2016;17:2–47.
2. Spoon DB, Malouf JF, et al. Mitral paravalvular leak: description and assessment of in normal anatomical method of localization. JACC Cardiovasc Imaging. 2013;6(11):1212–4.
3. Tanis W, Habets J, Vanden Brink RBA, Symersky P, Budde RPJ, Chamuleau SAJ. Differentiation of thrombus from pannus as the cause of acquired mechanical prosthetic heart valve obstruction by non-invasive imaging: a review of the literature. Eur Heart J Cardiovasc Imaging. 2014;15:119–29.
4. Bonnichsen CR, Pellikka PA. Prosthetic valve thrombus versus pannus: progress with imaging. Circ Cardiovasc Imaging. 2015;18(12).
5. Maciejewski M, Piestrzeniewicz K, Dabrowa AB, Walczak A. Biological artificial valve dysfunction-single center, observational echocardiographic study in patient's operated on before age 65 year. Arch Med Sci. 2011;6:993–9.

16 3DE Assessment of Pathological Spectrum of Aortic Prosthesis Dysfunction: Incremental Value over 2DE

Joseph F. Maalouf

3D echocardiographic assessment of aortic valve prostheses (AVP) is more challenging than mitral prostheses [1, 2]. The resolution of 3D TTE remains suboptimal and anterior components of aortic valve prostheses are in the far field during transesophageal echocardiography (TEE). Moreover, there is degradation in echocardiographic image quality because of reverberation artifacts and acoustic shadowing by prosthetic material. None-the-less, despite these limitations, all aortic prosthesis components including sewing ring (SR) , bioprostheses cusps, and mechanical prostheses leaflets, can be readily seen enface on 3DTEE from both the aortic and left ventricular outflow perspectives, and from a single acoustic window without probe manipulation. Moreover, mechanical aortic prostheses leaflet occluder motion, frequently difficult to see on 2D echocardiography (2DE), can be readily appreciated on 3D TEE. Thus, 3DTEE not only complements the role of 2DE in the assessment of aortic valve prosthesis dysfunction, but may have an incremental value over 2DE. Gain and other image optimization tools including smoothing and avoidance of too low compression are helpful when imaging AVP with 3DE.

Aortic Periprosthetic Regurgitation

Aortic periprosthetic leak (PPL) or regurgitation is a potentially serious complication following surgical or transcatheter aortic valve replacement (TAVR) [3–7]. Patients can be very symptomatic either because of congestive heart failure or because of hemolytic anemia [4]. For surgical aortic PPL, the mechanism is incomplete seal between the sewing ring and surrounding annulus due to poor tissue quality related to friability from infection or calcification around the prosthetic valve [3]. Mechanisms of PPL associated with transcatheter heart valves (THV) include under sizing of the implanted THV, extensive calcifications in the device landing zone that preclude complete THV stent expansion, and incomplete sealing of the annulus by the THV skirt due to too high or too low positioning of the THV [2, 3].

Transcatheter PPL closure has emerged as the preferred and less invasive approach to closing such defects [3, 4]. Accurate determination of the number and locations of aortic PPL, and assessment of PPL shape and dimensions, analogous to mitral PPL, are therefore, critical for successful planning and execution of the procedure. With 2D echocardiography, this entails the use of multiple acoustic windows, x-Plane, and often off-axis probe manipulation [1, 2]. THV PPL may not be detected if the imaging plane is higher than the THV skirt, and because of the frequent "garden hose" effect of a PPL aortic regurgitation (AR) jet [2], imaging below the level of origin of a PPL may erroneously view AR jet spray rather than the AR vena contracta [1, 2]. Aortic prostheses PPL are also frequently multiple and eccentric, and PPL defects usually have irregular funnel shaped anatomy that is widest at origin of the PPL and narrowest where it exits into the left ventricular outflow tract (Fig. 16.1). These aortic prosthesis PPL characteristics also complicate imaging with 2DE.

3D TEE is ideally suited for imaging the entire aortic prosthesis from a single acoustic window and is very useful to exclude endocarditis. However, anteriorly located aortic PPL are in the far field for TEE and may be difficult to image because of acoustic shadowing and reverberation artifacts from the posterior surface of surgical aortic prostheses sewing ring cuff or TAVR stent [1, 2]. None-the-less, 3D TEE may be very useful in characterizing the geometry of posteriorly located aortic PPL (Fig. 16.2) and in localizing the site(s) of periprosthetic regurgitation (Fig. 16.3). Moreover,

Supplementary Information The online version of this chapter (https://doi.org/10.1007/978-3-030-72941-7_16) contains supplementary material, which is available to authorized users.

J. F. Maalouf (✉)
Professor of Medicine, Mayo Clinic College of Medicine; Director, Interventional Echocardiography; Consultant, Department of Cardiovascular Medicine, Mayo Clinic, Rochester, MN, USA
e-mail: maalouf.joseph@mayo.edu

J. F. Maalouf et al. (eds.), *Practical 3D Echocardiography*, https://doi.org/10.1007/978-3-030-72941-7_16

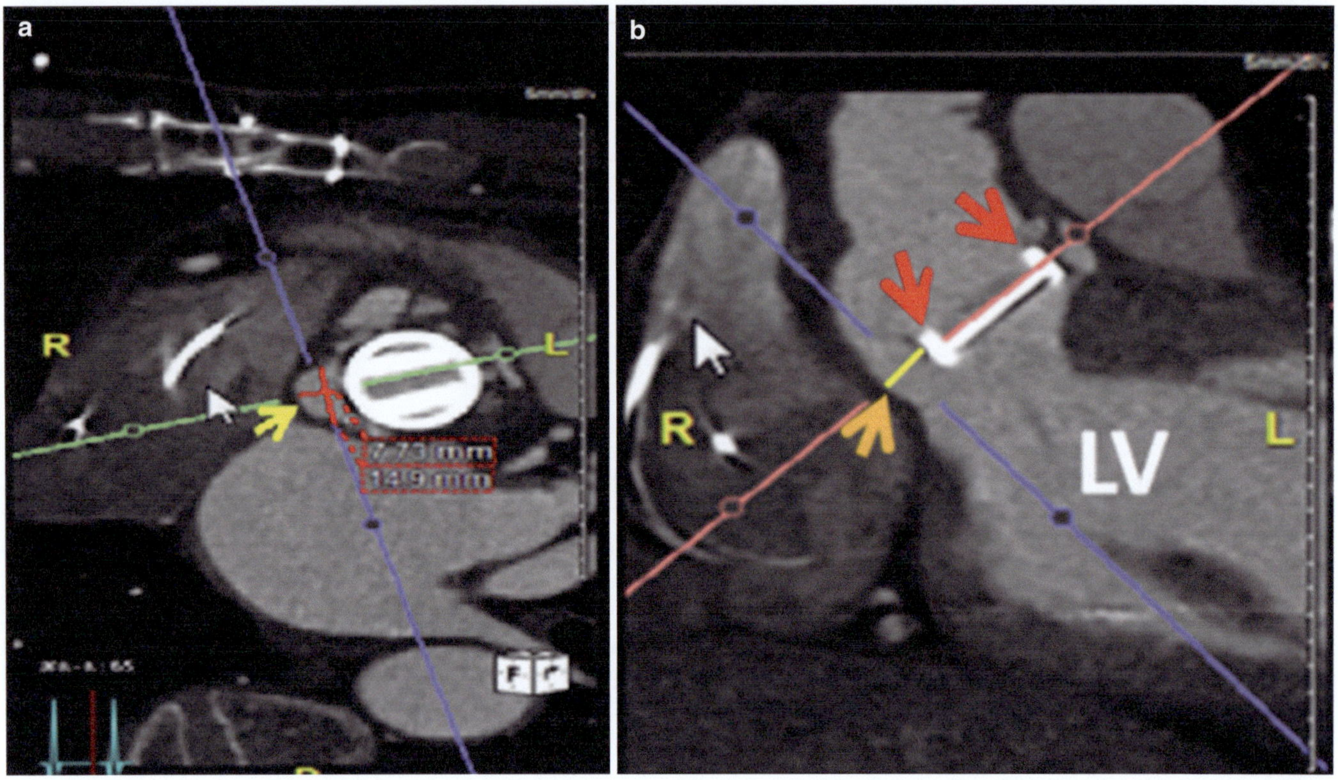

Fig. 16.1 CT scan of aortic PPL: Note the funnel shaped appearance of the periprosthetic defect with a wide crescent shaped inlet (**a**, yellow arrow) and narrower tubular component (**b**, orange arrow) that exits in the LV. The prosthesis sewing ring can be seen (red arrows). Used with permission of Mayo Foundation for Medical Education and Research. LV, left ventricle; PPL, periprosthetic leak

with multiplanar reconstruction (MPR) [8] of the 3D PPL color Doppler volume data set, severity of the PPL can be quantified by precisely identifying and measuring the vena contracta area a surrogate for the effective regurgitant orifice area (Fig. 16.4). A pitfall of MPR is color "bleed" blooming artifacts that can be exaggerated by inappropriately high color gain.

Other Causes of Aortic Prosthetic Valve Dysfunction

As with mitral prostheses, prosthesis thrombosis (Fig. 16.9) and pannus ingrowth account for the vast majority of non-infectious causes of aortic prosthetic valve dysfunction. However, pannus related prosthesis dysfunction is more common with aortic than mitral prostheses [9]. Pannus ingrowth is typically detected on the left ventricular side of surgical aortic prostheses where the sewing ring (SR) is implanted, but in rare cases, pannus ingrowth appears to grow from the aortic side of the prosthesis [9]. Pannus ingrowth arising from the SR may extend to the orifice and hinges of the prosthetic valve causing restriction of leaflet mobility and severe narrowing of the inflow orifice [9]. However, severe stenosis may also occur due to obstruction and narrowing of the left ventricular outflow tract by a circumscribed pannus without restricting leaflet motion [9]. In rare cases, the formation of pannus can lead to intermittent regurgitation caused by impairment of diastolic motion of one of the prosthetic leaflets [9]. Pannus arising from the aortic aspect of the prosthetic valve usually causes complete obstruction with immobility of leaflets [9].

Aortic bioprosthetic valve cusp degeneration can be in the form of prosthesis regurgitation due to cusp prolapse or perforation or prosthesis stenosis due to cusp calcification, pannus ingrowth or thrombosis, or a combination thereof (Figs. 16.5, 16.6, 16.7, 16.8, and 16.9). Aortic valve homograft failure usually presents with aortic regurgitation (Fig. 16.10) and dehiscence of aortic valved conduit can occur (Fig. 16.11).

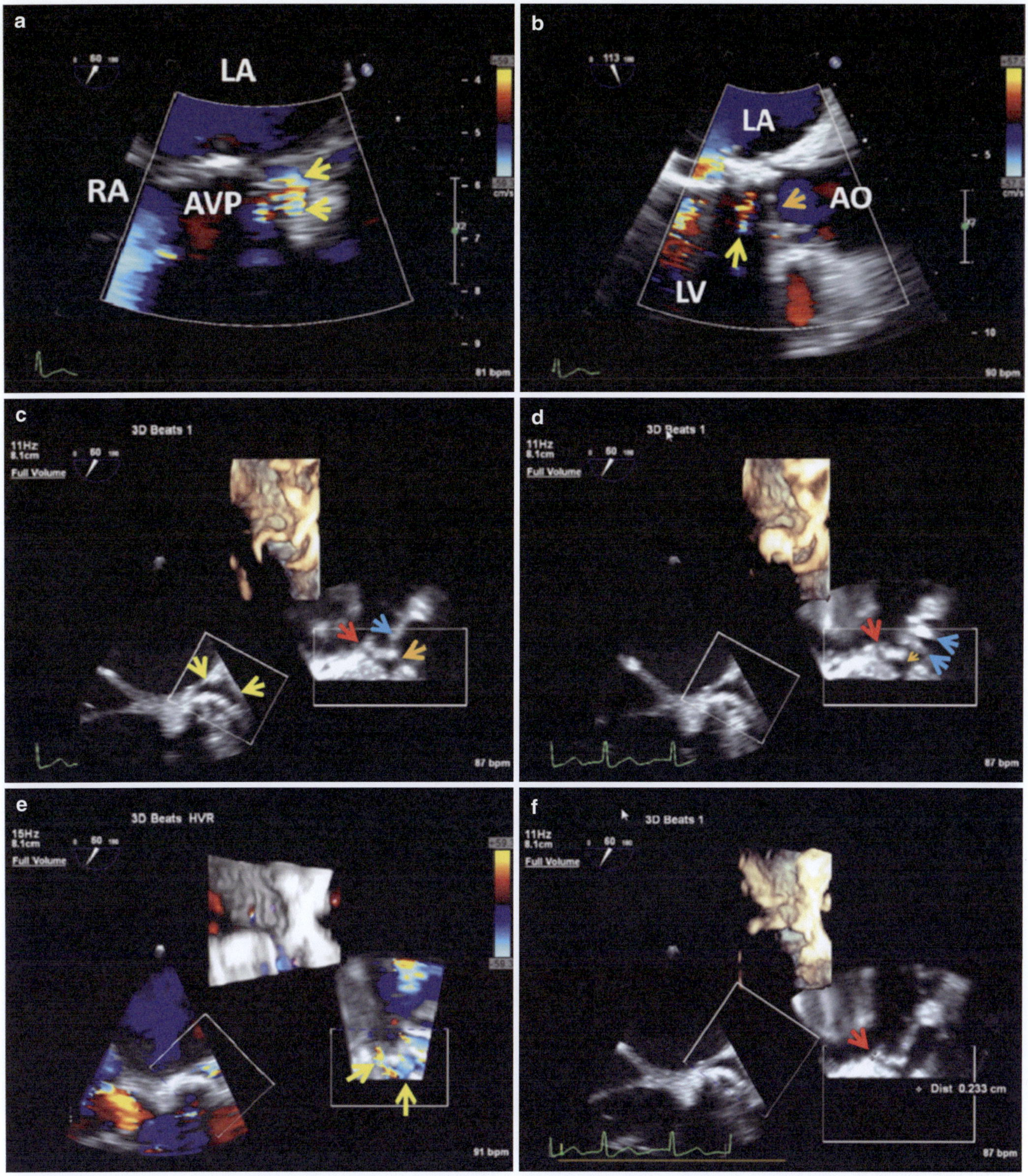

Fig. 16.2 PPL in another patient with a mechanical bileaflet aortic prostesis. **Top panel**: 2D TEE CFD views of the aortic prosthesis PPL. The origin of the periprosthetic AR jet (**a**, yellow arrows) and its exit in the the LVOT (**b**, yellow arrow) can be seen, but the anatomy of the PPL defect can not be discerned, and there is shadowing by prosthetic material. Orange arrow points to AVP. **Second panel**: MPR of the same aortic PPL as seen on 3D TEE both in diastole (**c**) and systole (**d**). The aortic periprosthetic defect has an irregular funnel shaped anatomy that is crescent shaped at the top (yellow arrows). It is also widest at its origin (orange arrows) and narrowest where it exits into the LVOT (red arrows). Blue arrows point to the bileaflet occluders. **Third panel**: As with any 3D defect, flow through the PPL channel on color Doppler (**e**, arrows) provides confirmation of pathology. The exit of the PPL into the LVOT measures 0.23 cm (**f**) . **Bottom panel**: (**g**) CT scan of same aortic PPL showing the entry (orange arrow) and exit (red arrow) sites for the PPL. (**h**) Mid PPL channel diameter measurement on CT. Blue arrows point to the bileaflet occluders and yellow arrows point to prosthesis SR. Used with permission of Mayo Foundation for Medical Education and Research. All rights reserved. AO, ascending aorta; AR, aortic regurgitation; AVP, aortic valve prosthesis; CFD, color flow Doppler; LA, left atrium; LV, left ventricle; LVOT, left ventricular outflow tract; MPR, multiplanar reconstruction; PPL, periprosthetic leak; RA, right atrium; SR, sewing ring

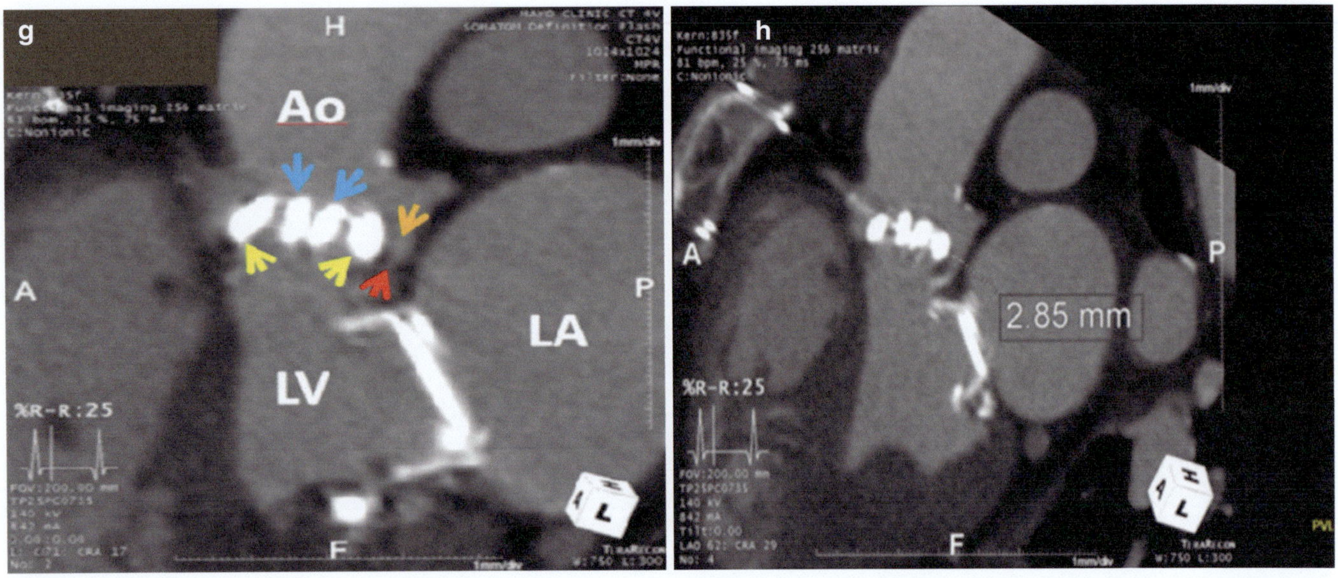

Fig. 16.2 (continued)

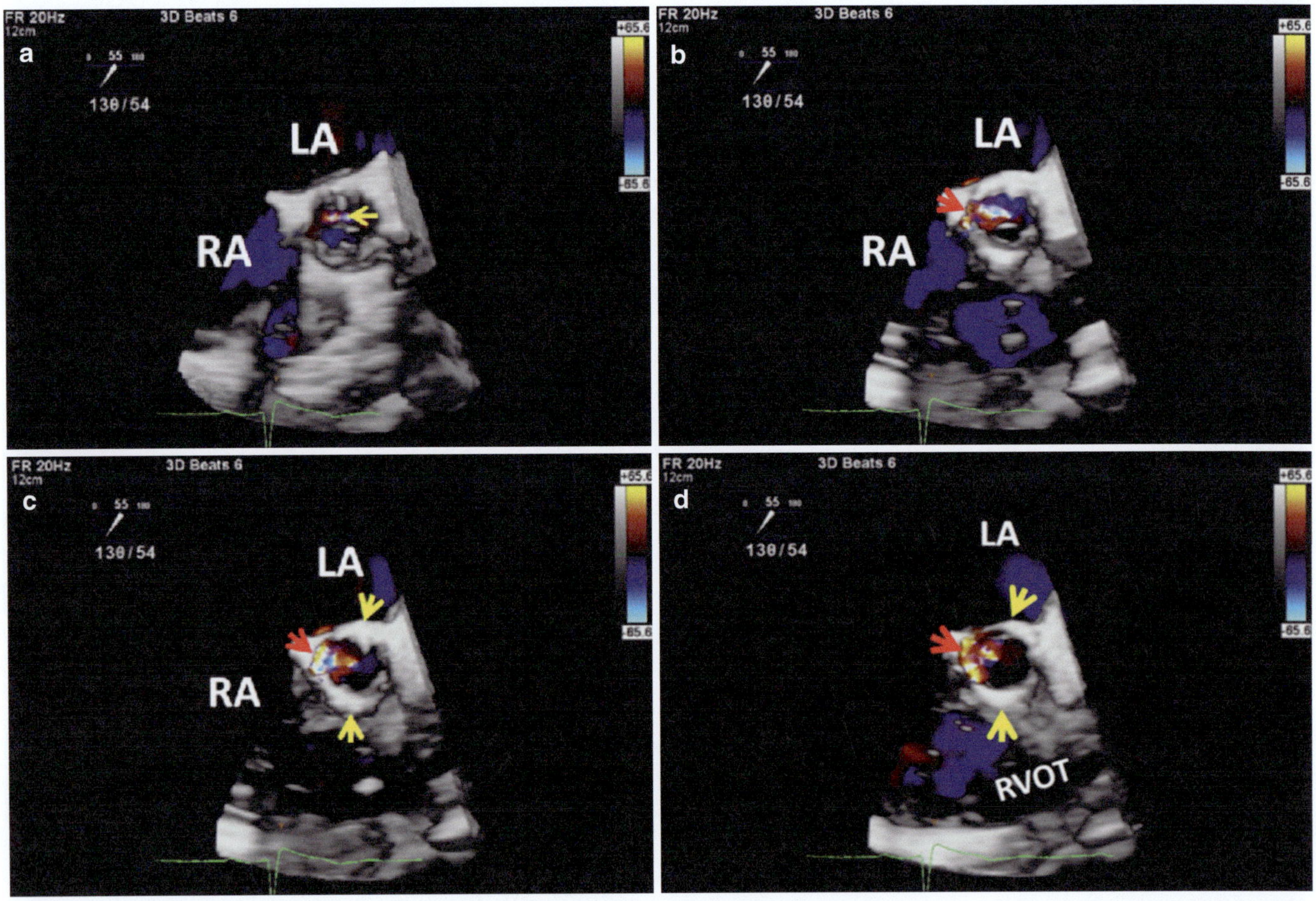

Fig. 16.3 3D TEE CFD enface aortic views of a THV PPL: **Top panel**: (**a**) the PPL is not seen. Arrow points to mild prosthesis regurgitation. (**b**) By cropping down towards the ventricular end of the THV stent the PPL (red arrow) begins to be seen and is single and posterior in location, adjacent to the atrial septum. **Bottom panel**: (**c**) The PPL and its circumferential extent (red arrow) are now clearly seen. (**d**) On further downward cropping , the PPL AR jet begins to splay (red arrow). Yellow arrows point to the ventricular end of the THV stent. Used with permission of Mayo Foundation for Medical Education and Research. All rights reserved. CFD, color flow Doppler; LA, left atrium; PPL, periprosthetic leak; RA, right atrium; RVOT, right ventricular outflow tract; THV, transcatheter heart valve

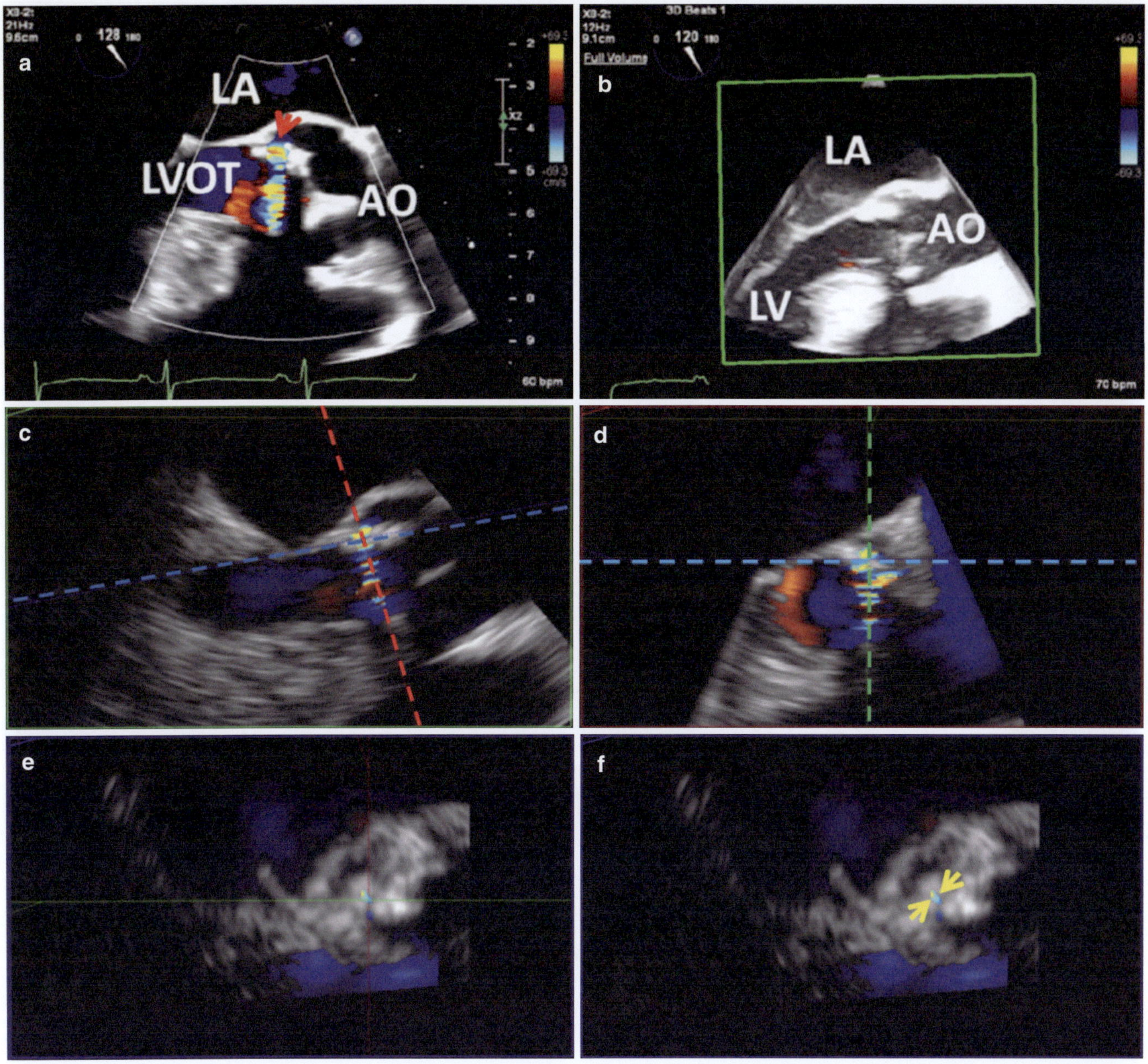

Fig. 16.4 Measurement of AVP PPLVC using MPR: **Top panel**: (**a**) 2D long axis view of the AVP showing the PPL (red arrow). (**b**) 3D FV CFD of the AVP. **Second panel**: MPR of 3D data set. (**c**) Coronal plane(green rectangle) showing alignment of the sagittal plane (dashed red line) and an orthogonal transverse plane (dashed blue line) at VC of the PPL AR jet. (**d**) Corresponding sagittal plane view (red rectangle) of the PPL with alignment of the coronal plane (dashed green line) with the transverse plane (dashed blue line). **Bottom panel**: PPL AR vena contracta (arrows) in the transverse plane with (**e**) and without (**f**) the reference sagittal and coronal plane lines. The VC area measured 0.04 cm.sq consistent with mild PPL. Note that compared with mitral PPL, aortic PPL are smaller. Used with permission of Mayo Foundation for Medical Education and Research. All rights reserved. AO, ascending aorta; AR, aortic regurgitation; AVP, aortic valve prosthesis; CFD, color flow Doppler; FV, full volume; LA, left atrium; LV, left ventricle; LVOT, left ventricular outflow tract; MPR, multiplanar reconstruction; PPL, periprosthetic leak; VC, vena contracta

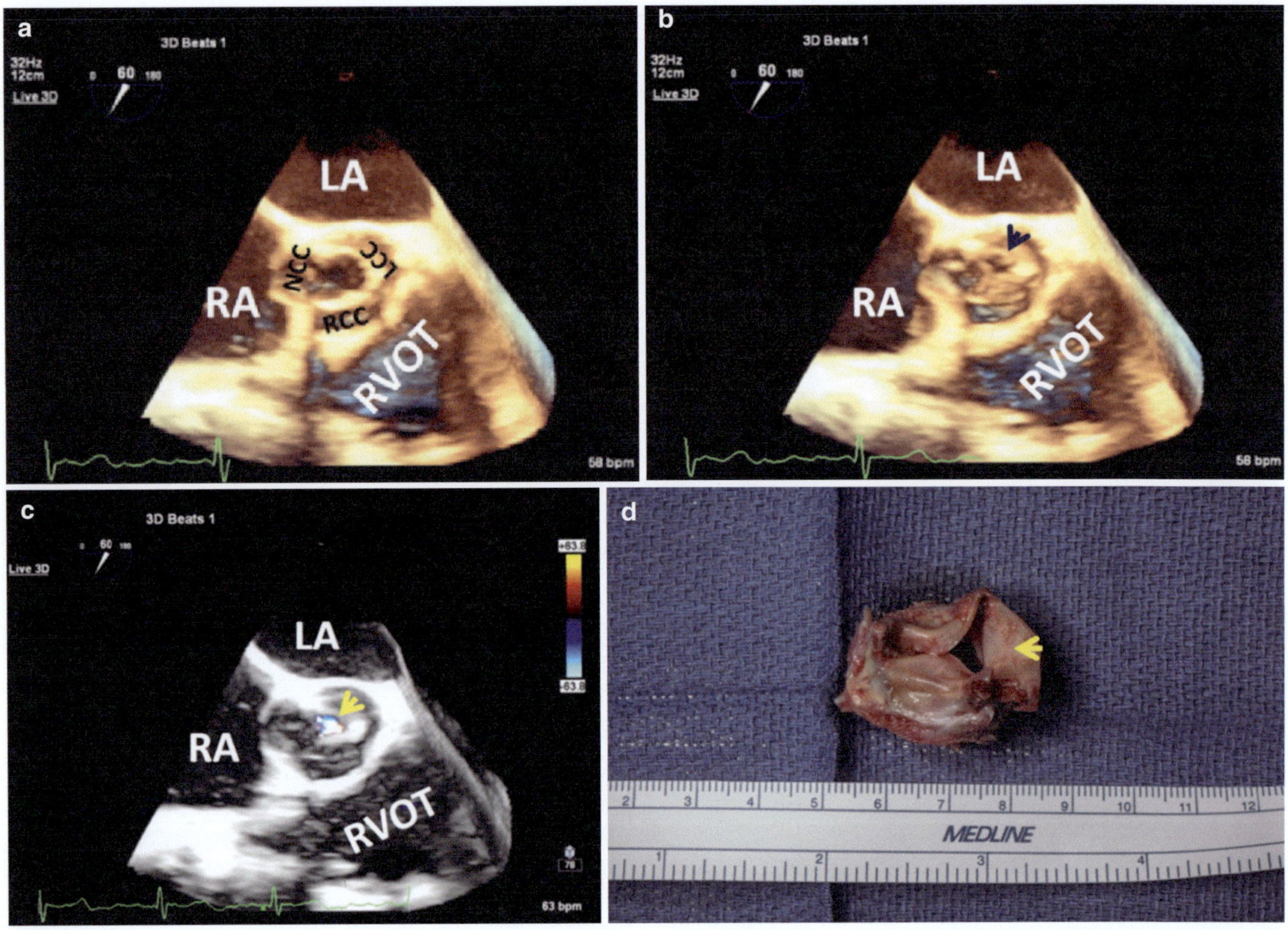

Fig. 16.5 3D TEE of a retracted aortic bioprosthesis cusp. **Top panel**: enface aortic views of the AVP showing the three cusps in systole (**a**) and diastole (**b**). Note that the prosthesis cusp that corresponds to the LCC does not close well in diastole resulting in a coaptation gap (arrow). **Bottom panel**: (**c**) 3D CFD showing aortic regurgitation through the coaptation gap (arrow). (**d**) Intraoperative image of explanted prosthesis showing retracted cusp (arrow). Used with permission of Mayo Foundation for Medical Education and Research. All rights reserved. AVP, aortic valve prosthesis; CFD, color flow Doppler; LA, left atrium; LCC, left coronary cusp; NCC, non-coronary cusp; RA, right atrium; RCC, right coronary cusp; RVOT, right ventricular outflow tract

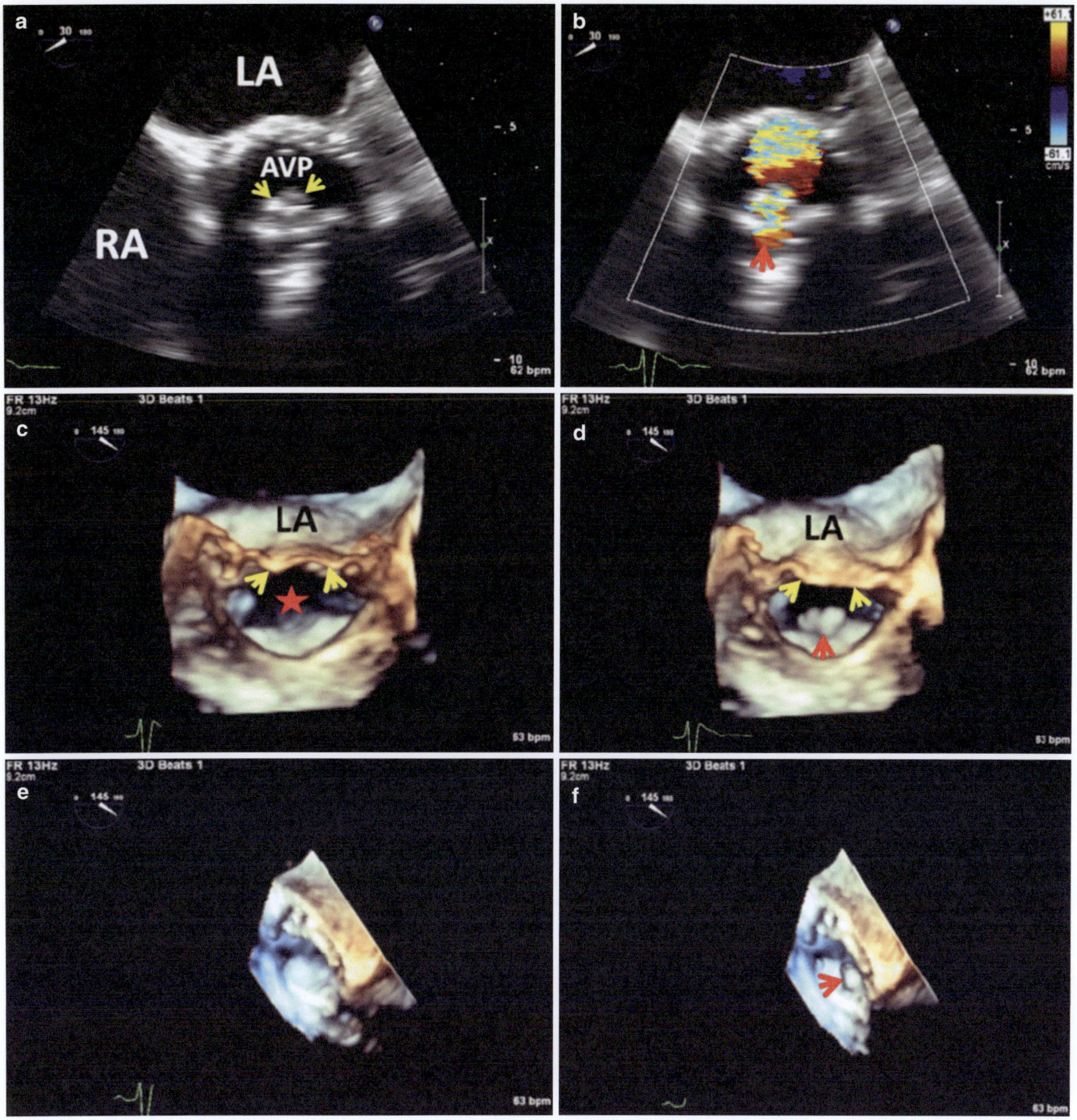

Fig. 16.6 Avulsion of AV bioprosthesis RCC: **Top panel**: 2D TEE short-axis diastolic views of the AVP showing an anterior echodensity (**a**; arrows) and an eccentric posteriorly directed jet of AR (**b**, arrow). **Middle panel**: 3D TEE enface LV views in systole (**c**) and diastole (**d**) showing prolapse of a segment of the RCC (red arrow) into the LVOT (star) in diastole. Yellow arrows point to tips of AML. **Bottom panel**: LVOT viewed sideways in systole (**e**) and end diastole (**f**) showing the avulsed cusp segment (red arrow). Used with permission of Mayo Foundation for Medical Education and Research. All rights reserved. AML, anterior mitral leaflet; AR, aortic regurgitation; AV, aortic valve; AVP, aortic valve prosthesis; CFD, color flow Doppler; LA, left atrium; LV, left ventricle; LVOT, left ventricular outflow tract; RA, right atrium; RCC, right coronary cusp

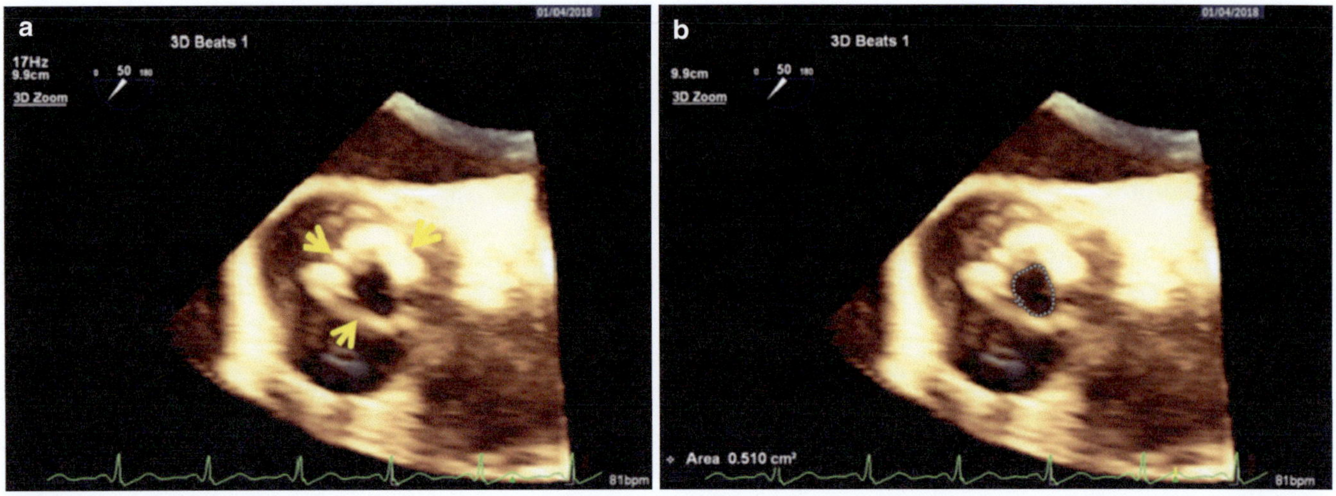

Fig. 16.7 (**a**, **b**) Degenerated AV bioprosthesis with severe stenosis (arrows). Valve area measured 0.51 cm.sq. on direct planimetry (**b**). Used with permission of Mayo Foundation for Medical Education and Research. All rights reserved

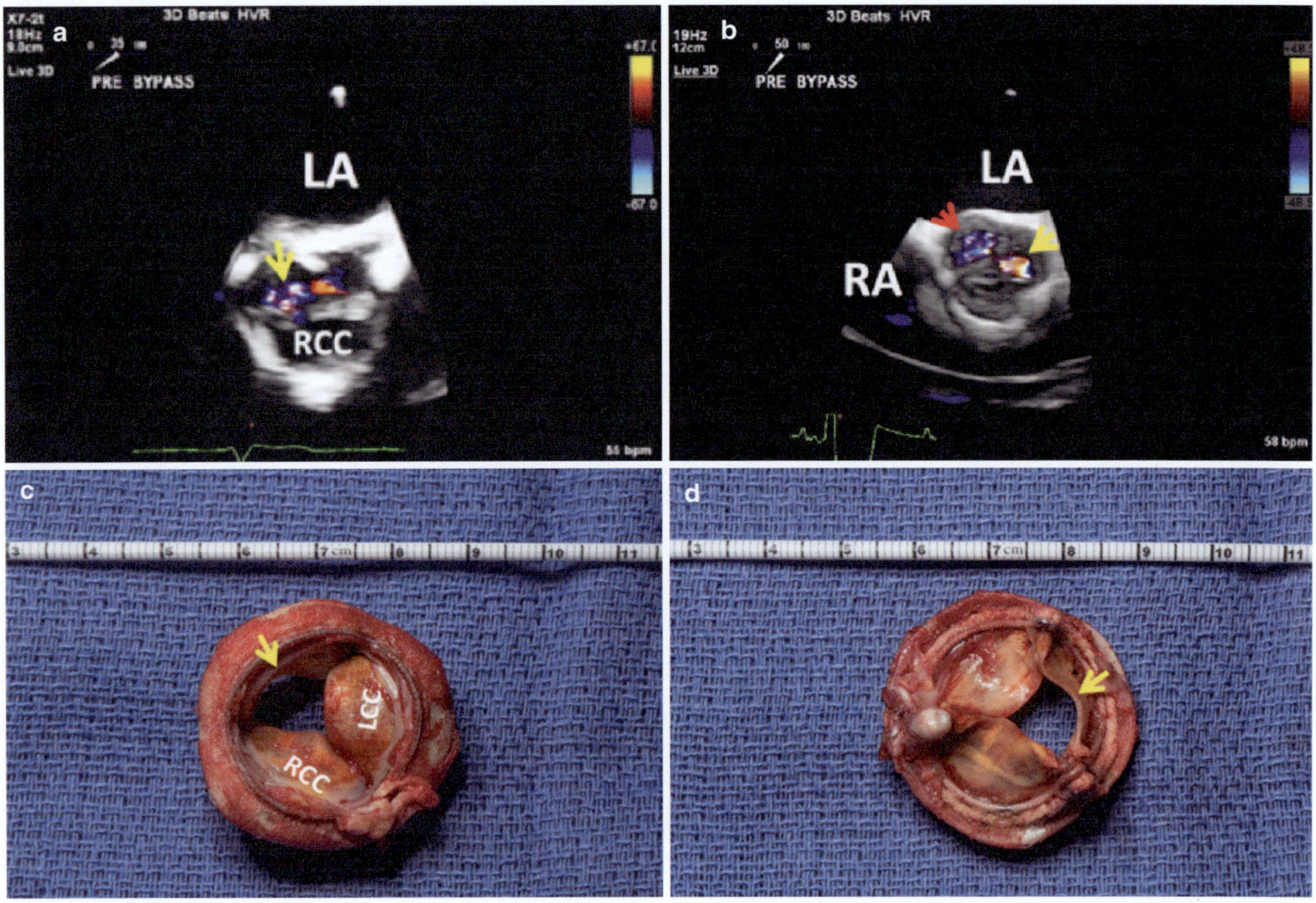

Fig. 16.8 **Top**: (**a**) 3D TEE of an AV bioprosthesis with prolapsed NCC and secondary AR (yellow arrow). (**b**) 3D TEE from a patient with native aortic valve perforations of the LCC (yellow arrow) and NCC (red arrow). Note the similarity in appearances of the NCC in the two images because both lesions cause regurgitation to go through the affected cusp. **Bottom panel**: IO photographs of the explanted AVP. (**c**) Aortic view showing a gap where the NCC should be (yellow arrow). (**d**) Ventricular view of the prosthesis showing the prolapsed cusp (yellow arrow). Used with permission of Mayo Foundation for Medical Education and Research. All rights reserved. AV, aortic valve; AVP, aortic valve prosthesis; AR, aortic regurgitation; IO, intraoperative; LA, left atrium; LCC, left coronary cusp; NCC, non coronary cusp; RA, right atrium; RCC, right coronary cusp

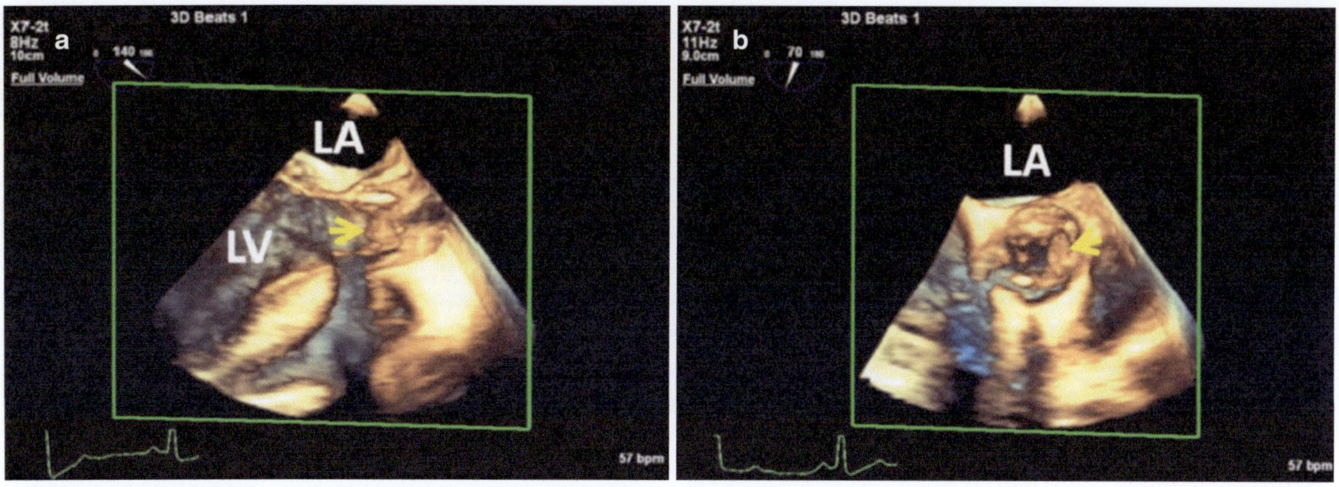

Fig. 16.9 Live FV 3D long axis (**a**) and short axis (**b**) views of AVP thrombus (yellow arrows). Used with permission of Mayo Foundation for Medical Education and Research. All rights reserved. AVP, aortic valve prosthesis; FV, Full Volume

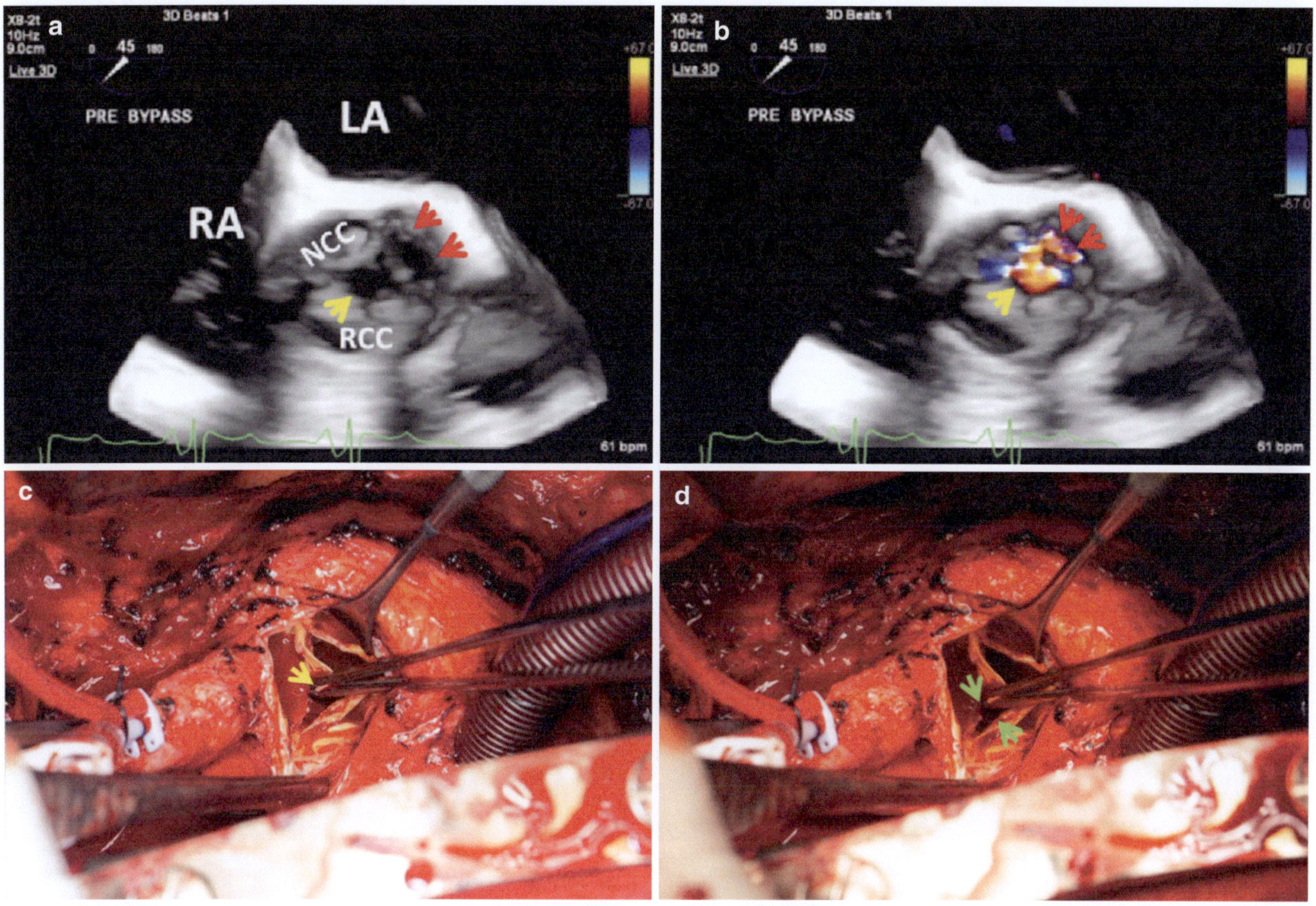

Fig. 16.10 **Top panel**: Live 3D in a patient with severe aortic homograft regurgitation. (**a**) Torn LCC (red arrows) and leaflet malcoaptation (yellow arrow). (**b**) Secondary severe aortic regurgitation (arrows). **Bottom panel**: (**c**, **d**) Intraoperative photographs showing torn edge of LCC that is held by the forceps (yellow arrow) and LCC leaflet gap (green arrows). Used with permission of Mayo Foundation for Medical Education and Research. All rights reserved. LA, left atrium; LCC, left coronary cusp; NCC, non coronary cusp; RA, right atrium; RCC, right coronary cusp

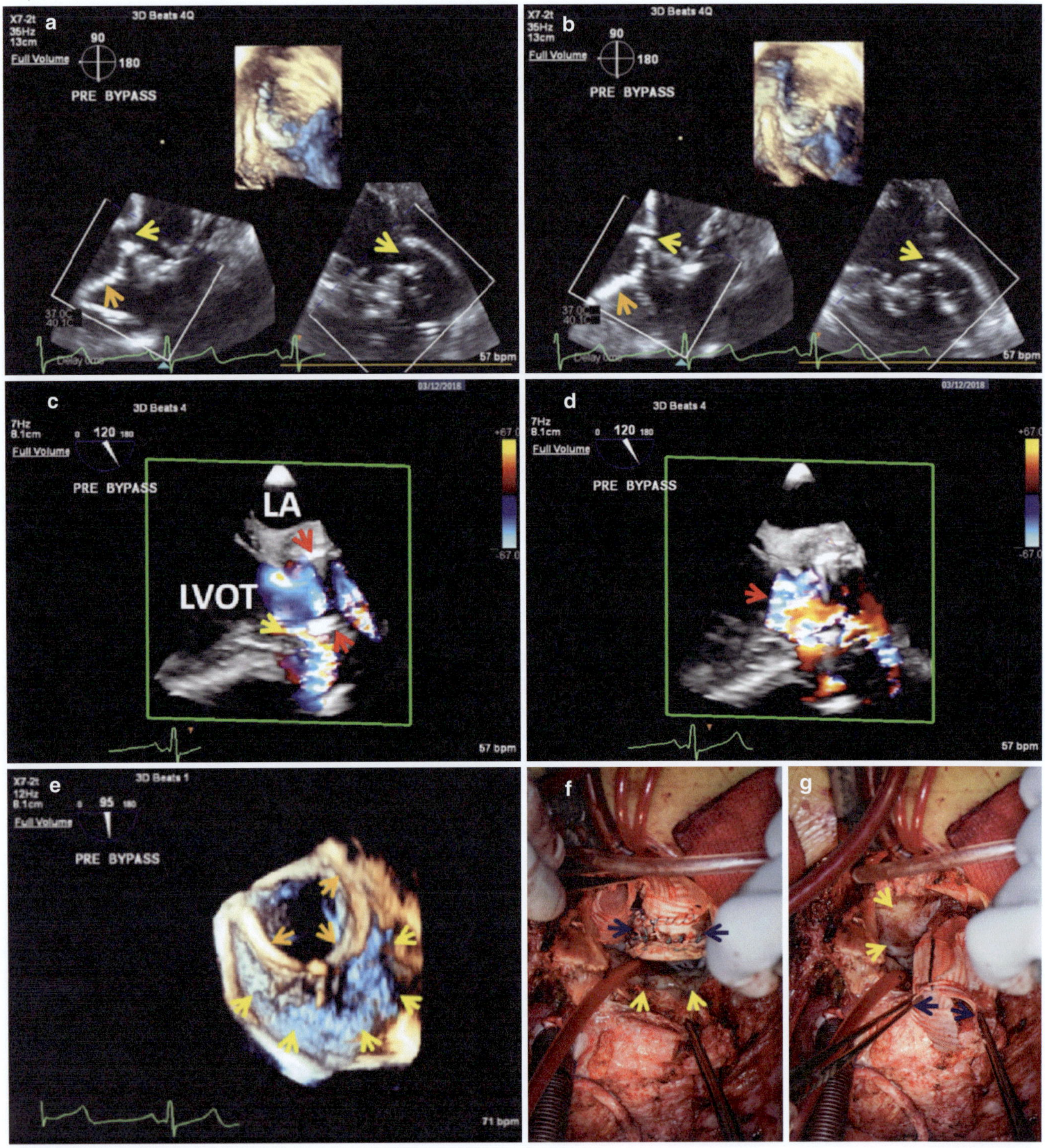

Fig. 16.11 Patient with dehiscence of a Bentall valved conduit and large aortic root pseudoaneurysm. **Top panel**: 3D TEE of dehised valved conduit (orange arrow) in systole (**a**) and diastole (**b**). Yellow arrows point to site of communication of dehised segment with LVOT. **Middle panel**: Autocropped multibeat 3D FV CFD showing blood flow in systole from LVOT into the pseudoaneurysm caused by dehiscence of the valved conduit (**c**; yellow arrow. Red arrows point to valved conduit) and flow regurgitation into the LV in diastole (**d**; red arrow). **Bottom panel**: (**e**) Live 3D FV short-axis view of the valved conduit (orange arrows) and pseudoaneurysm (yellow arrows). (**f**, **g**) IO photos of dehised conduit (dark blue arrows) and adjacent pseudoaneurysm (yellow arrows). Used with permission of Mayo Foundation for Medical Education and Research. All rights reserved. CFD, color flow Doppler; FV, Full Volume; LA, left atrium; LV, left ventricle; LVOT, left ventricular outflow tract

References

1. Zoghbi WA, et al. Guidelines for the evaluation of valvular regurgitation after percutaneous valve repair or replacement: a report from the American Society of Echocardiography developed in collaboration with the Society for Cardiovascular Angiography and Interventions, Japanese Society of Echocardiography, and Society for Cardiovascular Magnetic Resonance. JASE. 2019;32:431–75.
2. Lancelloti P, et al. Recommendations for the imaging assessment of prosthetic heart valves: a report from the European Association of Cardiovascular Imaging endorsed by the Chinese Society of Echocardiography, the Inter-American Society of Echocardiography, and the Brazilian Department of Cardiovascular Imaging. Eur Heart J Cardiovasc Imaging. 2016;17:1–47.
3. Kliger C, et al. Review of surgical prosthetic paravalvular leaks: diagnosis and catheter-based closure. Eur Heart J. 2013;34:638–48.
4. Rihal CS, Sorajja P, Booker JD, Hagler DJ, Cabalka AK. Principles of percutaneous paravalvular leak closure. JACC Cardiovasc Interv. 2012;5:121–30.
5. Wilczek K, Bujak K, Regula R, Chodor P, Osadnik T. Risk factors for paravalvular leak after transcatheter aortic valve implantation. Pol Junel Thorac Cardiovasc Surg. 2015;12:89–94.
6. Tarantini G, Gasparetto V, Napodano M, Fraccaro C, Gerosa G, Isabella G. Valvular leak after transcatheter aortic valve implantation: a clinician update on epidemiology, pathophysiology and the clinical implications. Am Gen Cardiovasc Dis. 2011;1:312–20.
7. Lerakis S, Hayek SS, Douglas PS. Paravalvular aortic leak after transcatheter aortic valve replacement: current knowledge. Circulation. 2013;127:397–407.
8. Franco E, Almería C, de Agustín JA, et al. Three-dimensional color Doppler transesophageal echocardiography for mitral paravalvular leak quantification and evaluation of percutaneous closure success. J Am Soc Echocardiogr. 2014;27:1153–63.
9. Darwazah A. Recurrence pannus formation causing prosthetic aortic valve dysfunction: is excision without valve re-replacement applicable. J Cardiothorac Surg. 2012;7:62–4.

Native and Prosthetic Valve Endocarditis: Incremental Value of 3DE over 2DE

17

Joseph F. Maalouf and Francesco F. Faletra

Two dimensional echocardiography (2DE) and in particular transesophageal echocardiography (TEE) plays a pivotal role in the diagnosis of infective endocarditis (IE), recognition of its associated complications, and guiding management [1–4]. 2DE is limited by its tomographic nature, however, and imaging can be challenging when there is valve calcification or prosthetic material [1–4]. These limitations can be overcome by three dimensional echocardiography (3DE) and in particular 3D TEE, that provides enface assessment of cardiac anatomy and pathology from a single imaging window. In patients with native and prosthetic valve endocarditis, 3D TEE not only complements 2D TEE by providing additional information and enhancing diagnostic accuracy, but may be superior to 2D TEE for identifying complications of IE [5–8]. Moreover, multiplanar reconstruction of the 3D volumetric data set, allows visualization of cardiac involvement by endocarditis from virtually any desired perspective.

Vegetations are the hall mark of endocarditis (Fig. 17.1). Berdejo et al. [9] showed that 2D TEE might underestimate the true size of a vegetation and its morphology, which was overcome with the use of 3D TEE. Hansalia et al. [10] compared 3D TEE to 2D TEE in 13 patients with valvular vegetations and concluded that 3D TEE was superior in determining the presence and site of valvular vegetations that were found during cardiac surgery. Moreover, the dimensions and volume of vegetations, and their spatial characterization, important determinants of embolic potential, can also be accurately determined by 3DE [10].

3D TEE is also the preferred imaging tool for diagnosis of a spectrum of endocarditis related complications (Figs. 17.2, 17.3, 17.4, 17.5, and 17.6). These include valve perforations and destruction (Figs. 17.2 and 17.4) [8, 11], and abscess formation (Figs. 17.5 and 17.6). Imaging of native aortic or mitral valve perforations can be very challenging with 2D TEE and may require imaging from unconventional acoustic windows and multiple probe manipulation. In contrast, enface views of the entire mitral or aortic valve from a single imaging window with 3D TEE allow for rapid diagnosis of leaflet perforation (Fig. 17.4) or valve destruction (Fig. 17.2) including extent of damage. In a large, retrospective case series of valve perforations reported by Thompson et al. [12], the use of 3D TEE was able to identify four cases of valve perforation not otherwise detected by standard 2D.

Abscess formation is usually associated with valve prostheses in particular in the aortic position. Because abscesses typically are not limited to specific tissue planes, they can extend in directions beyond the tomographic planes that are routinely acquired on 2D TEE [6, 7]. 3D TEE may be superior to standard 2D TEE for characterizing complex cardiac abscesses such as Intramural or intramyocardial abscesses (Figs. 17.5 and 17.6) [6].

Prosthetic valve sewing ring dehiscence (see Chap. 15) and mycotic aneurysms (Figs. 17.3 and 17.6) are other complications of IE that are readily detected on imaging with 3D TEE, particularly when the mitral valve is involved because it lends itself best to imaging with TEE [7]. Diagnosis and assessment of the extent of mitral prostheses sewing ring dehiscence using 2D imaging often requires extensive probe manipulation. With 3D TEE enface views of the mitral valve prosthesis and its bed from both the left atrium (surgeon's view) and left ventricular perspective can be readily obtained from a single acoustic window (see Chap. 15). This improves

Supplementary Information The online version of this chapter (https://doi.org/10.1007/978-3-030-72941-7_17) contains supplementary material, which is available to authorized users.

J. F. Maalouf (✉)
Professor of Medicine, Mayo Clinic College of Medicine; Director, Interventional Echocardiography; Consultant, Department of Cardiovascular Medicine, Mayo Clinic, Rochester, MN, USA
e-mail: maalouf.joseph@mayo.edu

F. F. Faletra
Director of Cardiac Imaging Lab, Cardiocentro Ticino Institute, Lugano, Switzerland
e-mail: Francesco.Faletra@cardiocentro.org

J. F. Maalouf et al. (eds.), *Practical 3D Echocardiography*, https://doi.org/10.1007/978-3-030-72941-7_17

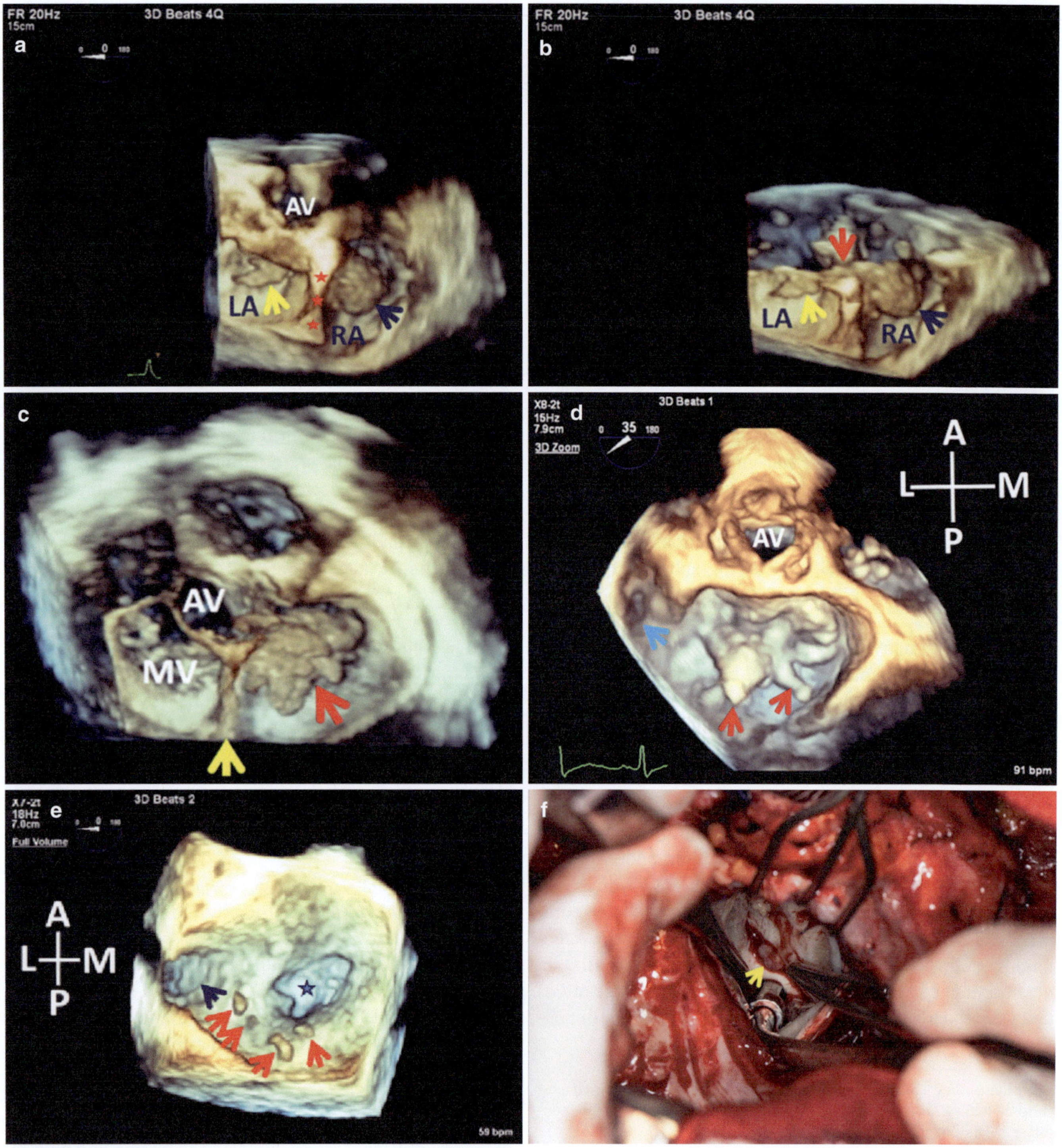

Fig. 17.1 **Top panel**: 3D TEE enface "surgeon's view" of the base of the heart. (**a**) Large right atrial vegetation (dark blue arrow) and smaller left atrial vegetation (yellow arrow). The atrial septum is marked by stars. (**b**) Cropped down image shows that the aforementioned vegetations are not distinct, but rather form a continuum through the internal cardiac crux (red arrow). **Middle panel**: (**c**) enface RA view showing a large TV vegetation (red arrow) .Yellow arrow points to atrial septum. (**d**) Flail AML with ruptured chordae (red arrows) secondary to streptococcus mitis endocarditis. Note that the appearance of ruptured chords can mimic vegetations particularly on 3DE because of blurring or amplification artifacts (see Chap. 3), and integration of clinical and other imaging data may be necessary. Light blue arrow points to ostium of LAA. **Bottom panel**: (**e**) Multiple small vegetations (red arrows), secondary to the commensal organism *Propionibacterium acnes*, on annuloplasty ring in a patient who had undergone surgical MV repair with insertion of a Carpentier-Edwards Physio ring 7 years earlier . The dark blue arrow points to orifice of LAA. Orifice of the MV is marked by a star. (**f**) One of the vegetations as seen intraoperatively (yellow arrow). Note the soft and fleshy appearance. Used with permission of Mayo Foundation for Medical Education and Research. All rights reserved. A, anterior; AML, anterior mitral leaflet; AV, aortic valve; L, lateral; LA, left atrium; LAA, left atrial appendage; M, medial; MV, mitral valve; P, posterior; RA, right atrium; TV, tricuspid valve

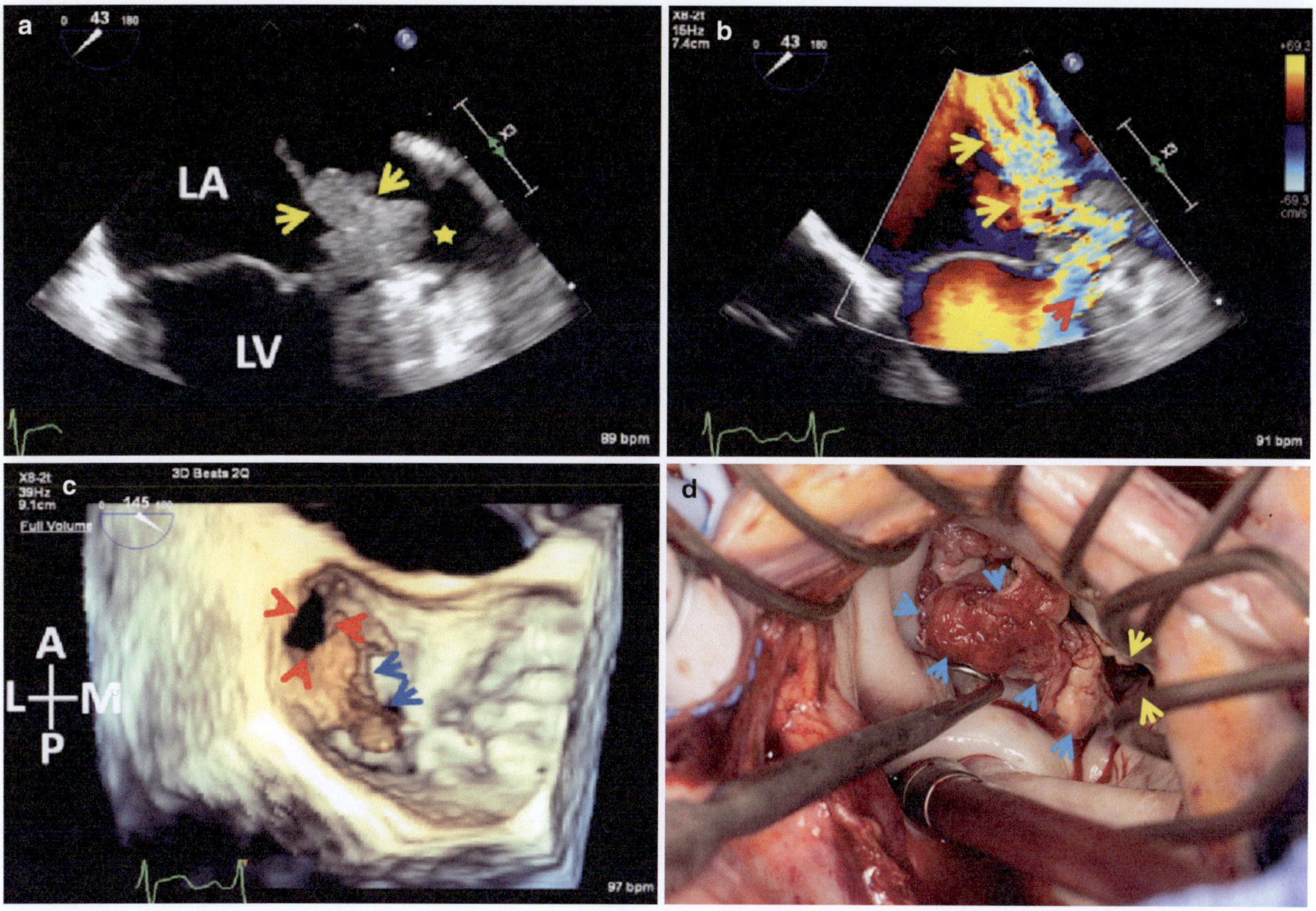

Fig. 17.2 36 year old male with MSSA endocarditis complicated by stroke. **Top panel**: (**a**) 2D TEE images showing a very large mitral valve vegetation (yellow arrows). (**b**) Severe MR (yellow arrows). Note that the origin of the jet (red arrow) is adjacent to the LAA (star). **Bottom panel**: (**c**) 3D TEE enface LA view of the MV showing a large anterolateral defect (red arrows) extending to the annulus. The blue arrows point to the vegetation. (**d**) Intraoperative photograph showing the large defect secondary to destructive endocarditis (yellow arrows) and the vegetation (blue arrows). Used with permission of Mayo Foundation for Medical Education and Research. All rights reserved. A, anterior; L, lateral; LA, left atrium; LAA, left atrial appendage; LV, left ventricle; M, medial; MR, mitral regurgitation; MSSA, methicillin sensitive *Staphylococcus aureus*; MV, mitral valve; P, posterior

communication with the treating team as the 3D image alleviates the need for "mental reconstruction" of the 2D images [7]. Accurate delineation of the extent of cardiac involvement by endocarditis also enables better risk stratification of patients with IE that can translate to better surgical decision making including timing of surgical intervention [7]. The information provided by 3D TEE also has important implications for preoperative surgical planning because it permits surgeons to further anticipate operative findings and plan the appropriate repair strategy [7]. Pseudoaneurysm is a rare yet well-known complication of endocarditis secondary to highly invasive organisms. When present, pseudoaneurysms are commonly secondary to abscesses in the region of the mitral-aortic intervalvular fibrosa (Figs. 17.5 and 17.6), also referred to as the aorto-mitral curtain, an avascular, fibrous area that separates the aortic valve from the anterior mitral leaflet [7, 13, 14]. Accurate characterization of the location, extent or fistulization of these aneurysms is key to guiding surgical management [7, 13, 14]. Newer 3D platforms now allow for higher temporal and spatial resolution, main limitations of earlier 3D technologies.

In patients with right sided IE (Fig. 17.1), 3D TEE provides additional delineation of IE involving right sided valves. In a study performed by Naqvi and colleagues [15], the use of real time 3D TEE in the setting of a tricuspid prosthetic valve or tricuspid annuloplasty was able to locate challenging right-sided vegetations despite artefact on traditional TTE and TEE. Another study by Utsunomiya et al.

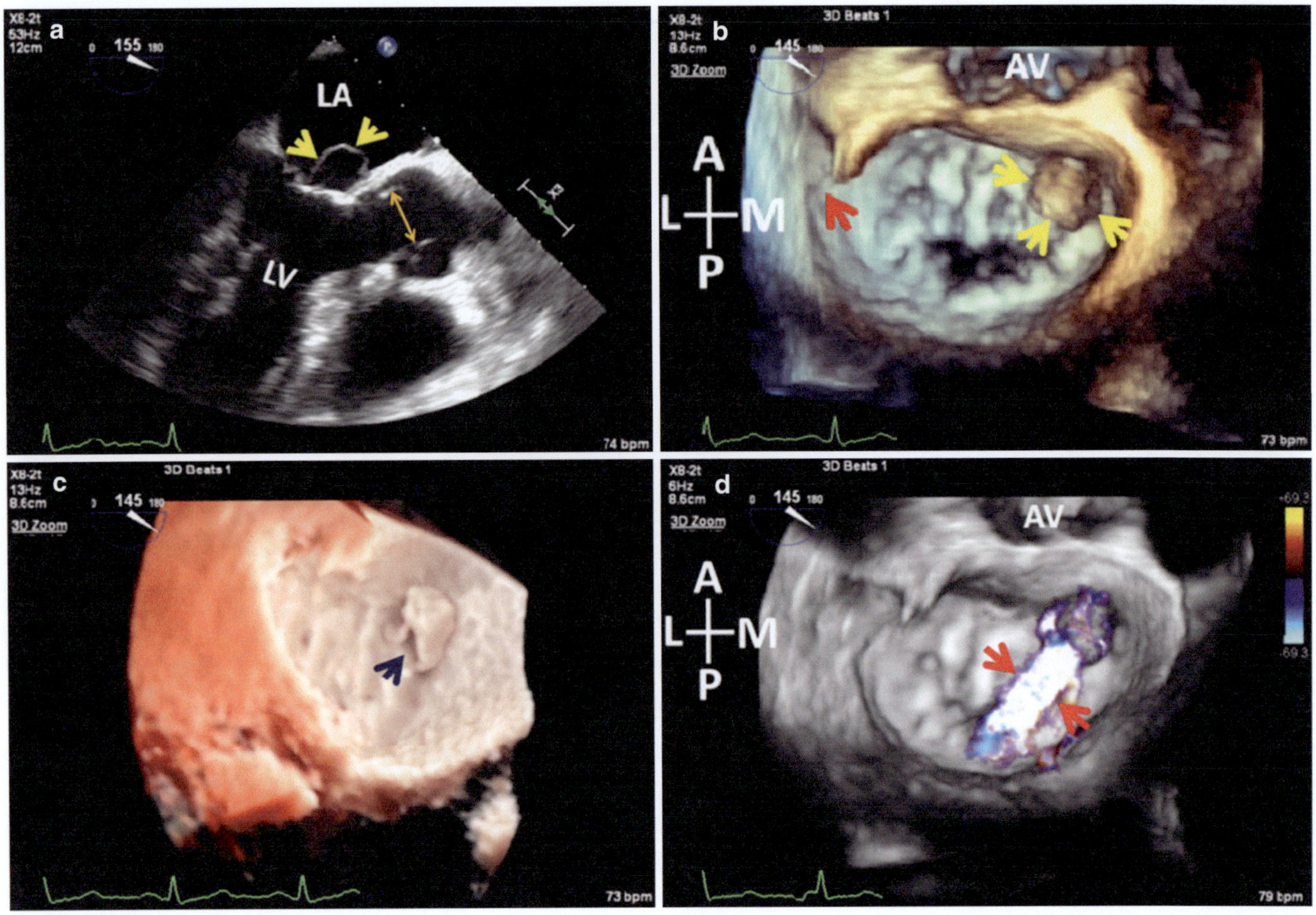

Fig. 17.3 **Top panel**: (**a**) 2D TEE in a 58 year old male with MRSA MV endocarditis. A large mycotic aneurysm is seen (yellow arrows). (**b**) 3D TEE enface LA view showing the mycotic aneurysm (yellow arrows) at base of A3 segment of the AML. Red arrow points to ostium of LAA. **Bottom panel**: (**c**) Site of rupture of the mycotic aneurysm into the LA (arrow) using TrueVue function (Philips Ultrasound) and adjusting depth of the light source on the 3D image. (**d**) 3D CFD showing MR (red arrows) through the ruptured mycotic aneurysm. Used with permission of Mayo Foundation for Medical Education and Research. All rights reserved. A, anterior; AML, anterior mitral leaflet; AV, aortic valve; CFD, color flow Doppler; L, lateral; LA, left atrium; LAA, left atrial appendage; LV, left ventricle; M, medial; MR, mitral regurgitation; MRSA, methicillin resistant *Staphylococcus aureus*; MV, mitral valve; P, posterior

[16] found that the maximum length of a vegetation in tricuspid valve endocarditis was a significant predictor of the occurrence of pulmonary embolism, and the additional use of 3D TEE with 2D TEE was believed to help identify those at high risk of recurrent pulmonary embolism. Similarly, the use of 3D TEE in patients who underwent surgery for native tricuspid valve endocarditis proved to be superior compared to standard 2D TEE allowing enhanced visualization of the tricuspid valve apparatus, vegetations and surrounding anatomy [16]. There is no clear advantage of 3DE over 2DE in the diagnosis of device lead endocarditis, but 3D TEE may improve the safety and outcome of complex transvenous lead extractions [17] in patients with endocarditis.

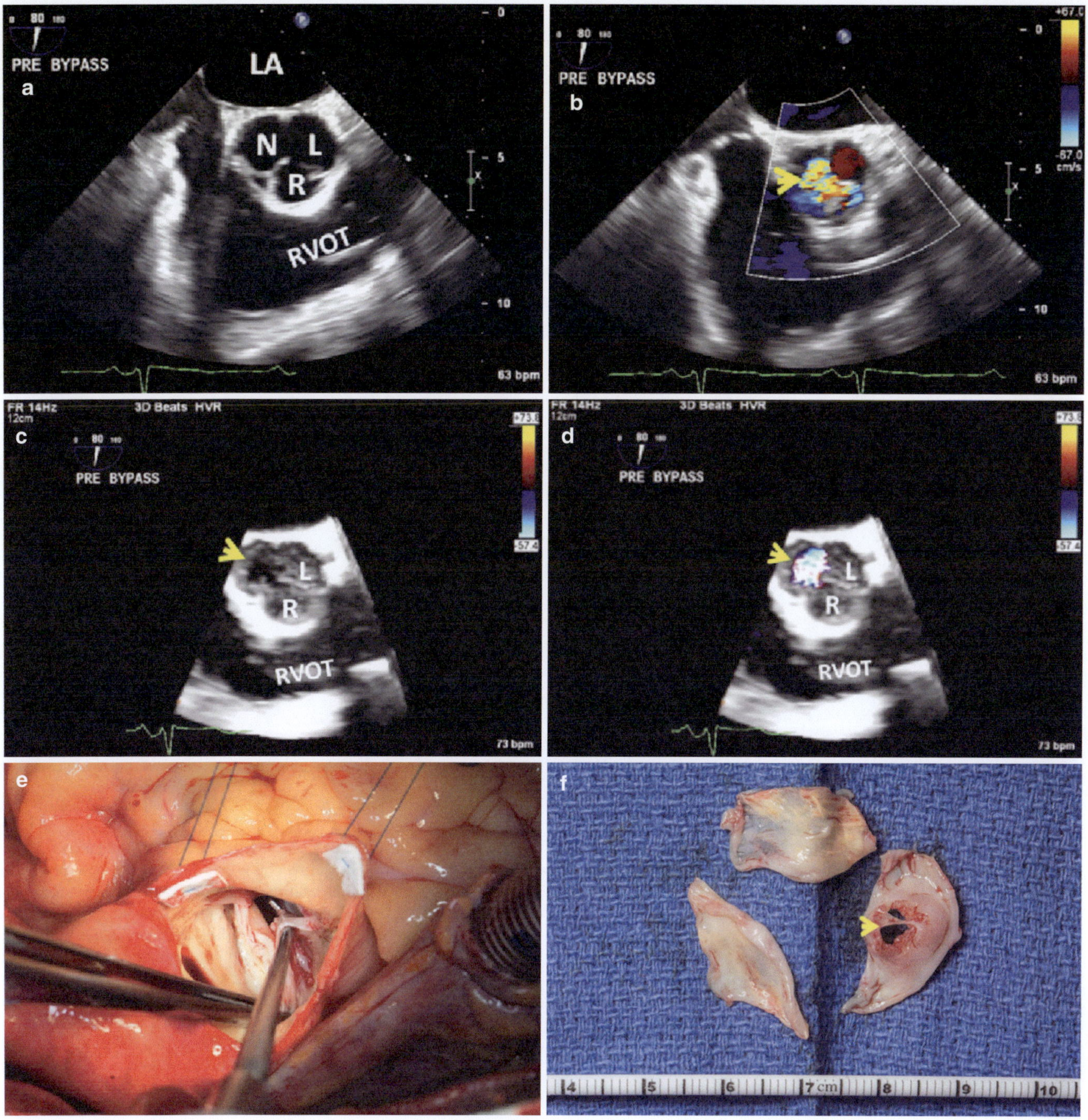

Fig. 17.4 Pre-bypass TEE in a 67 year old man with history of MSSA endocarditis and severe AR. **Top panel**: (**a**) 2D TEE mid-esophageal short-axis view of the AV; (**b**) CFD showing AR that appears to originate from the non-coronary cusp (arrow). **Middle panel**: (**c**) Live 3D CFD of AV with color suppress on showing a large perforation in the non-coronary cusp (arrow); (**d**) CFD shows regurgitant flow through the perforation (arrow). **Bottom panel**: (**e**) Intraoperative photo showing tip of forceps going through the perforation; (**f**) Excised AV cusps showing perforation (arrow) in non-coronary cusp. Used with permission of Mayo Foundation for Medical Education and Research. All rights reserved. AR, aortic regurgitation; AV, aortic valve; CFD, color flow Doppler; L, left coronary cusp; MSSA, methicillin sensitive *Staphylococcus aureus*; N, non-coronary cusp; R, right coronary cusp; RVOT, right ventricular outflow tract

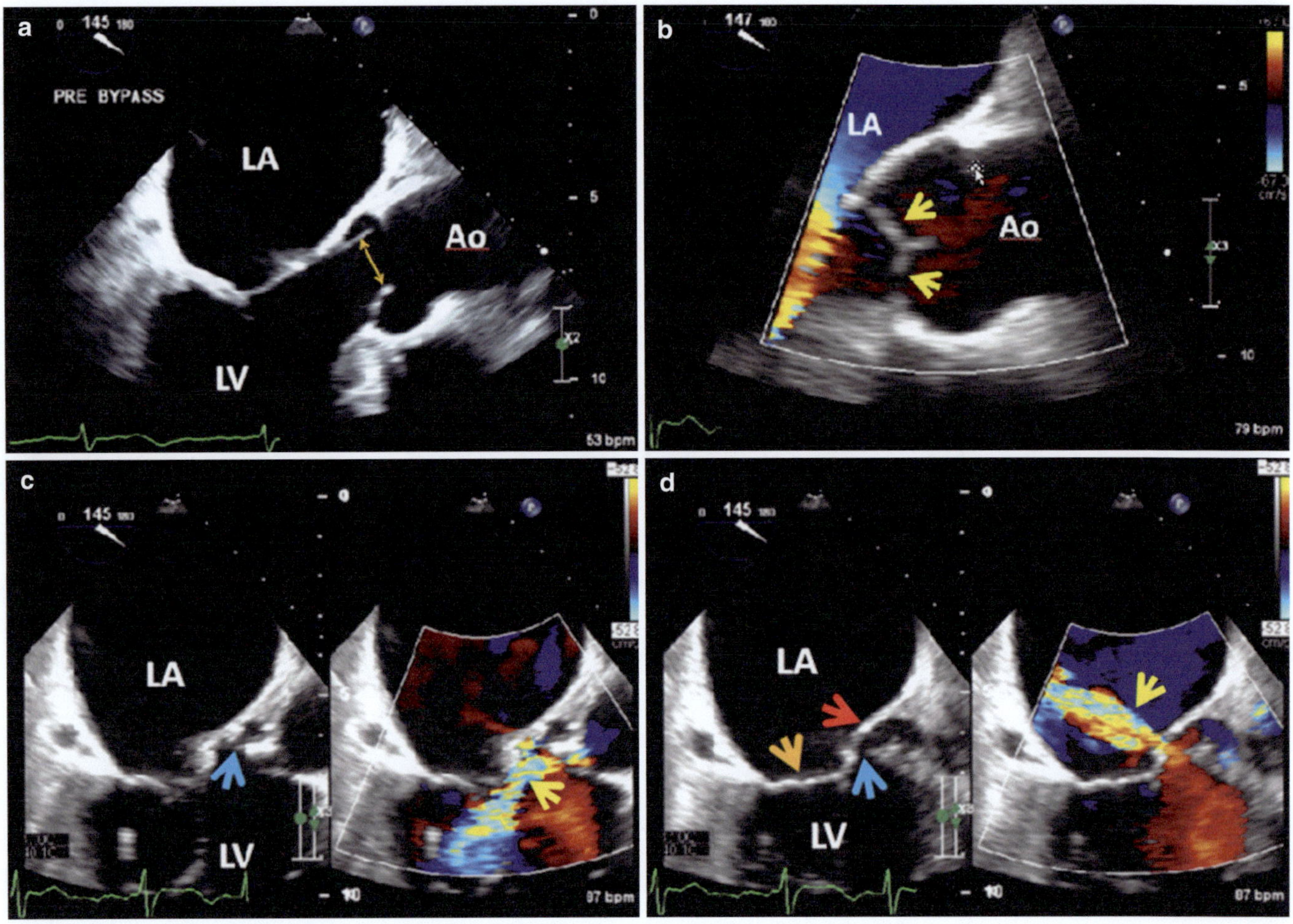

Fig. 17.5 Intraoperative pre-bypass TEE in a 71 year old man with complex MRSA endocarditis complicated by aortic root abscess and AML mycotic aneurysm that ruptured into the LA. **Top panel**: 2D TEE long-axis view of AV in systole (**a**, double headed arrow) and with CFD in diastole (**b**, arrows). The AV appears normal and there is no evidence of AR. **Second panel**: 2D TEE color-compare images from same angle of view (145°) but with off-axis imaging. (**c**) There is disruption of the aorto-mitral curtain (the intervening tissue between the mitral and aortic valves also known as MAIVF; light blue arrow); with diastolic flow from the MAIVF into the LV on CFD (yellow arrow). (**d**) Systolic flow (yellow arrow) from LV through the AML(red arrow) into the LA is appreciated on slight counterclockwise rotation of the ultrasound probe, orange arrow points to PML, and light blue arrow points to the discontinuity in the MAIVF. **Third panel**: Live 3D of same 2D image. (**e**) AML mycotic aneurysm (yellow arrow). Red double headed arrow points to AV leaflets; (**f**) The shape and size of the discontinuity in the MAIVF (dark blue arrow) can be appreciated on slight rotation of the image. Red arrow points to AML and orange arrow points to PML. **Bottom panel.** multibeat FV 3D. (**g**) "Surgeon's view" of cropped base of left heart showing an abscess cavity in the MAIVF (red arrows) posterior to the left coronary cusp (LC). The dark blue arrow points to ostium of LAA. (**h**) Spatial relationship of the AML mycotic aneurysm (yellow arrow) to the abscess cavity (red arrows) can be appreciated on 3D. The orthogonal 2D sector images at the bottom are derived from the FV 3D data set. Red arrow points to the abscess cavity adjacent to LAA (white arrow). The double headed red arrow points to the AV. Used with permission of Mayo Foundation for Medical Education and Research. All rights reserved. A, anterior; Ao, ascending aorta; AML, anterior mitral leaflet; AR, aortic regurgitation; AV, aortic valve; CFD, color flow Doppler; FV, full volume; L, lateral; LC, left coronary cusp; LA, left atrium; LAA, left atrial appendage; LV, left ventricle; M, medial; MAIVF, mitral aortic intervalvular fibrosa; MRSA, methicillin resistant *Staphylococcus aureus*; NC, non-coronary cusp; P, posterior; RC, right coronary cusp

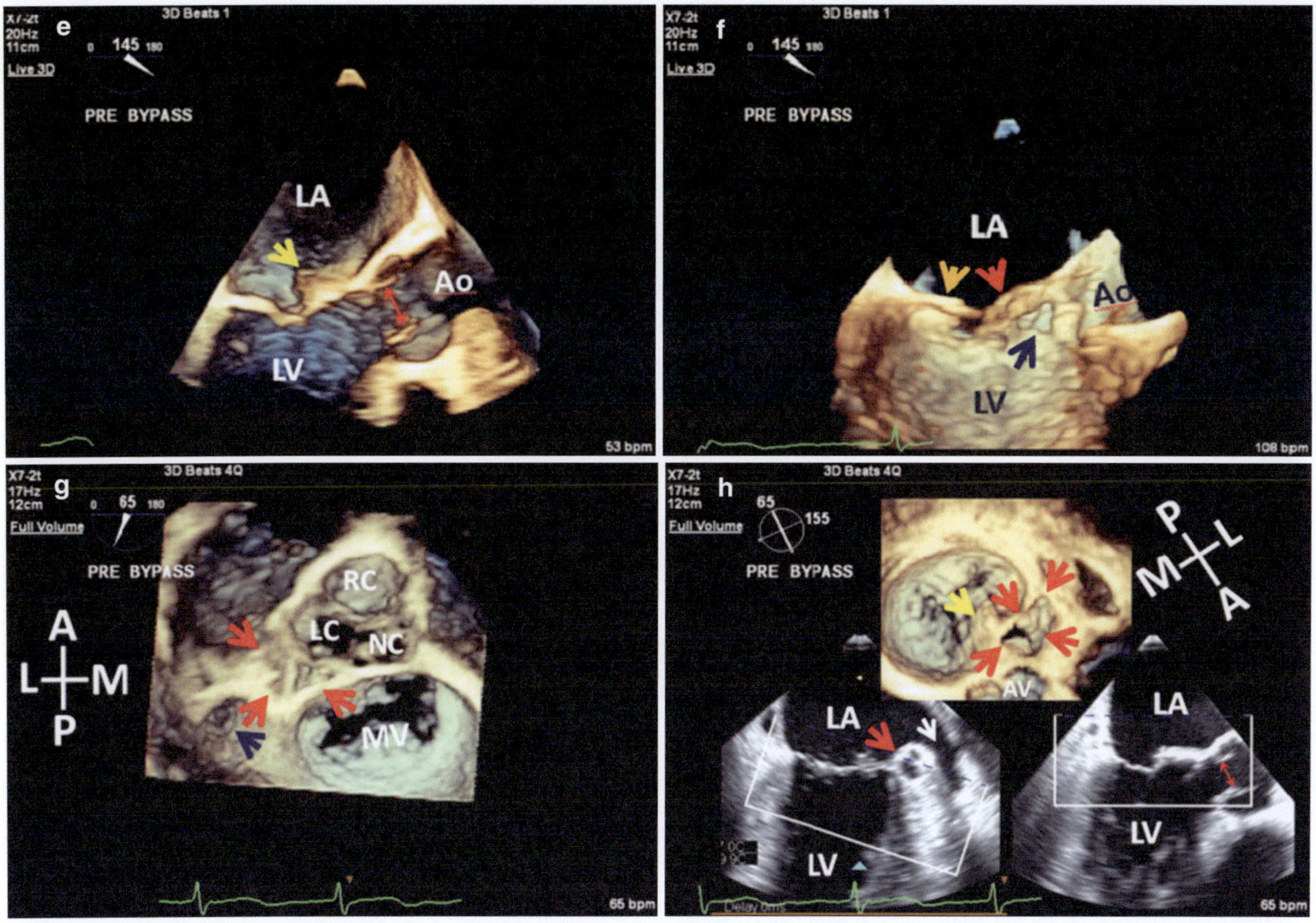

Fig. 17.5 (continued)

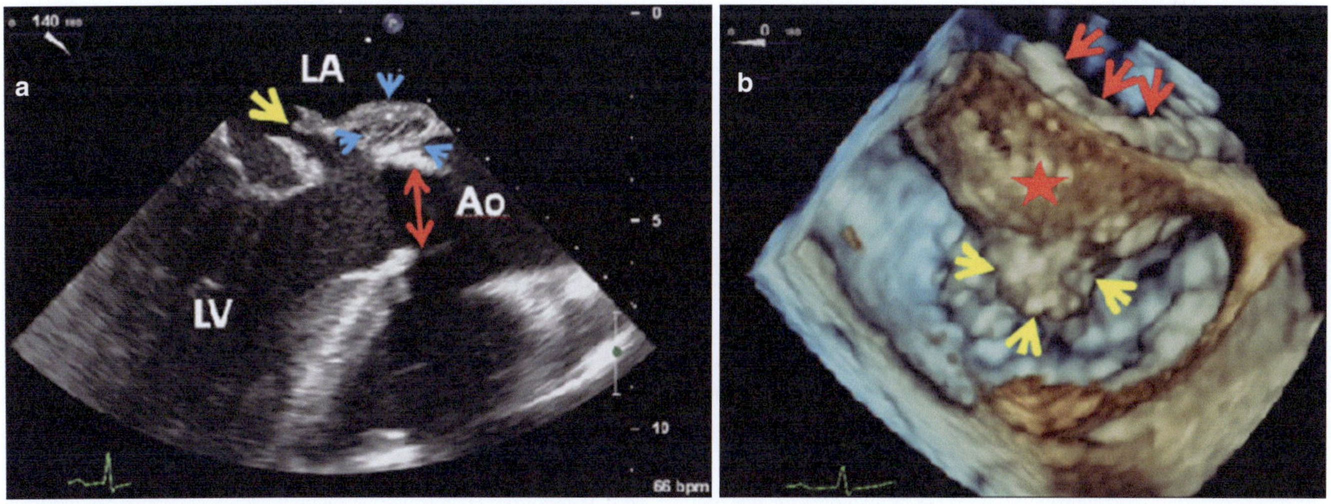

Fig. 17.6 Preoperative TEE in a patient with AVP *Haemophilus parainfluenzae* endocarditis with native MV involvement . **Top panel**: (**a**) 2D TEE long axis view of ascending aorta showing a posterior aortic root MAIVF abscess (blue arrows) and a ruptured mycotic aneurysm (yellow arrow). The double headed red arrow points to the AVP struts. (**b**) Enface "surgeon's view" of the mycotic aneurysm (yellow arrows) above the plane of the MV and the MAIVF abscess (star) that bulges into the LA. The red arrows are pointing to the AVP sewing ring. **Bottom panel**: (**c**) 3D enface view of the opening of the mycotic aneurysm (red arrows) into the LA and (**d**) intraoperative appearance of the ruptured mycotic aneurysm as seen in **c** (yellow arrows). Used with permission of Mayo Foundation for Medical Education and Research. All rights reserved. Ao, ascending aorta; AVP, aortic valve prosthesis; LA, left atrium; LV, left ventricle; MAIVF, mitral aortic intervalvular fibrosa; MV, mitral valve

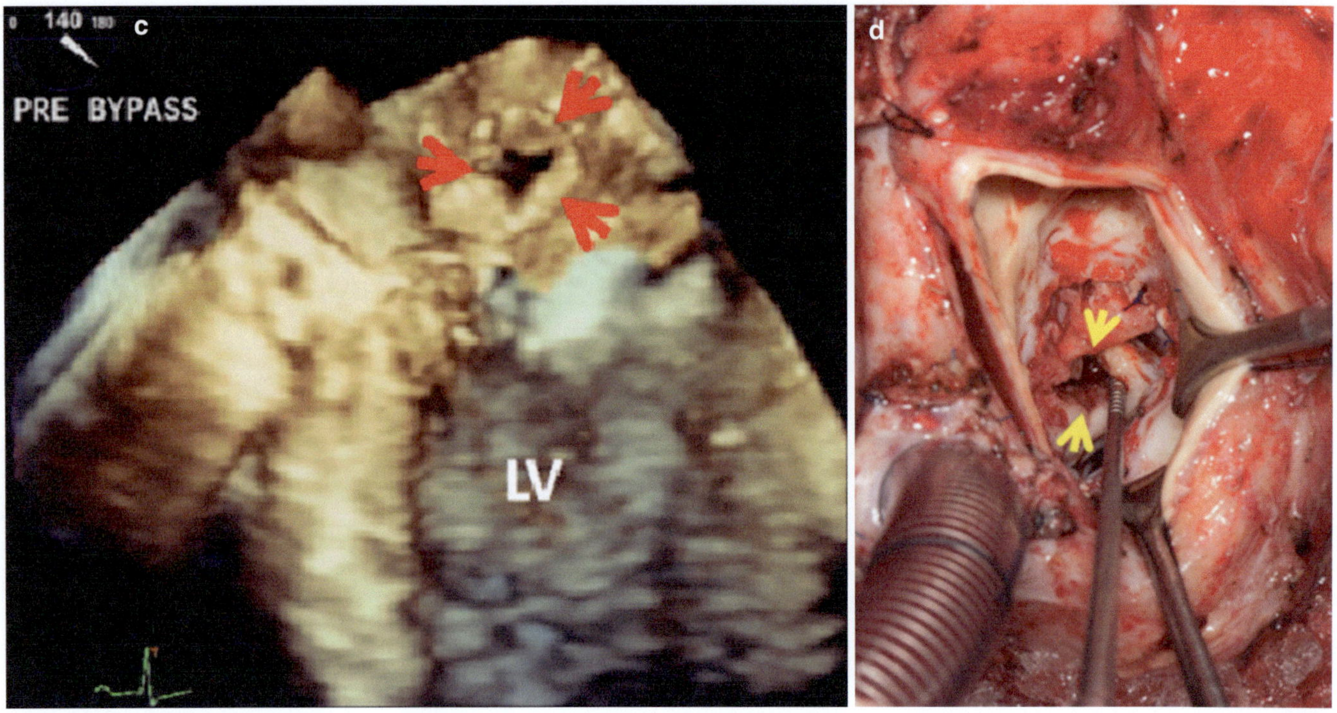

Fig. 17.6 (continued)

References

1. Erba PA, Pizzi MN, Roque A, Salaun E, Lancelloti P, Tornos P. Habib: multimodality imaging in infective endocarditis. Circulation. 2019;140:1753–65.
2. Habib G, Lancellotti P, Antunes MJ, Bongiorni MG, Casalta JP, Del Zotti F, Dulgheru R, El Khoury G, Erba PA, Iung B, Miro JM, Mulder BJ, Plonska-Gosciniak E, Price S, Roos-Hesselink J, Snygg-Martin U, Thuny F, Tornos Mas P, Vilacosta I, Zamorano JL, ESC Scientific Document Group. 2015 ESC Guidelines for the management of infective endocarditis: The Task Force for the Management of Infective Endocarditis of the European Society of Cardiology (ESC). Endorsed by: European Association for Cardio-Thoracic Surgery (EACTS), the European Association of Nuclear Medicine (EANM). Eur Heart J. 2015;36(44):3075–128.
3. Kini V, Logani S, Ky B, Chirinos JA, Ferrari VA, St John Sutton MG, Wiegers SE, Kirkpatrick JN. Transthoracic and transesophageal echocardiography for the indication of suspected infective endocarditis: vegetations, blood cultures and imaging. J Am Soc Echocardiogr. 2010;23(4):396–402.
4. Afonso L, Kottam A, Reddy V, Penumetcha A. Echocardiography in infective endocarditis: state of the art. Curr Cardiol Rep. 2017;19:127.
5. Brunn NE, Habib G, Thuny F, Sogaard P. Cardiac imaging in infective endocarditis. Eur Heart J. 2014;35:624–32.
6. Cacciapuoti F. Advantages of 3D echocardiography in the diagnosis of mitral valve endocarditis and its cardiac complications. J Cardiac Disord Ther. 2018;1:104.
7. Yong MS, Saxena P, Killu AM, Coffey S, Burkhart HM, Wan S-H, Malouf JF. The preoperative evaluation of infective endocarditis via 3-dimensional transesophageal echocardiography. Texas Heart Inst J. 2015;42(4):372–6.
8. Nemes A, Lagrand WK, McGhie JS, ten Cate FJ. Three-dimensional transesophageal echocardiography in the evaluation of aortic valve destruction by endocarditis. J Am Soc Echocardiogr. 2006;19:355.
9. Berdejo J, et al. Evaluation of vegetations size and its relationship with embolism infective endocarditis: A real-time 3-dimensional transesophageal echocardiography study. Circ Cardiovasc Imaging. 2014;7:149–54.
10. Hansalia S, et al. The value of live/real time three-dimensional transesophageal echocardiography in the assessment of valvular vegetations. Echocardiography. 2009;26:1264–73.
11. Alfonso L, Kottam A, Reddy V, Penumetcha A. Echocardiography an infective endocarditis: State of the art. Curr Cardiol Rep. 2017;19:127.
12. Thompson KA, Shiota T, Tolstrup K, Gurudevan SV, Siegel RJ. Utility of three-dimensional transesophageal echocardiography in the diagnosis of valvular perforations. Am J Cardiol. 2011;107(1):100–2.
13. Apostolidou E, Beale C, Poppas A, Stockwell P. Pseudoaneurysm of the mitral-aortic intervalvular fibrosa: a case series with literature review. CASE (Phila). 2017;1(6):221–6.
14. Çimen T, Doğan M, Kızıltepe U, Akyel A, Sunman H, Yeter E. Mitral-aortic intervalvular fibrosa pseudoaneurysm with rupture into the left atrium: a three-dimensional transesophageal echocardiographic approach. Anatol J Cardiol. 2016;15(12):1030–1.
15. Naqvi TZ, Rafie R, Ghalichi M. Real-time 3D TEE for the diagnosis of right-sided endocarditis in patients with prosthetic devices. JACC Cardiovasc Imaging. 2010;3(3):325–7.
16. Utsunomiya H, Berdejo J, Kobayashi S, Mihara H, Itabashi Y, Shiota T. Evaluation of vegetation size and its relationship with septic pulmonary embolism in tricuspid valve infective endocarditis: a real time 3DTEE study. Echocardiography. 2017;34:537–48.
17. Strachinaru M, et al. Multiplane/3D transesophageal echocardiography monitoring to improve the safety and outcome of complex transvenous lead extractions. Echocardiography. 2019;36(5):980–6.

CT and MRI Correlations with 3DE in Assessment of Prosthetic Valves Including New Trends

18

Kathleen A. Young, Korosh Sharain, Nandan S. Anavekar, and Thomas A. Foley

Valvular heart disease is a significant cause of morbidity and mortality in the cardiovascular patient [1–3]. As the population is aging, the number of valve interventions is also increasing [4, 5]. Surgical or catheter-based interventions for native valvular heart disease is commonly viewed as an exchange of one valve disease for another, as prosthetic heart valves require ongoing monitoring due to a number of potential complications which can result in prosthetic valve dysfunction [6].

Typically, echocardiography is the first-line modality to evaluate prosthetic valve function [7, 8]. However, in the setting of a prosthetic valve, echocardiography may have limitations due to shadowing and artifact. Cardiac computed tomography (CT) and magnetic resonance imaging (MRI) are increasingly utilized to aide in diagnosis and management of common causes of prosthetic valve dysfunction [4, 9].

For prosthetic heart valves, assessment for both prosthetic and periprosthetic regurgitation is an imperative component of the postoperative echocardiographic exam. Frequently, transesophageal echocardiography (TEE) is needed to localize and fully assess degree of regurgitation when present [8, 10]. Independently, cardiac CT and MRI are inadequate for detection of prosthetic regurgitation [4]. However, cardiac CT is a helpful adjunct in the procedural planning for perivalvular leak closure. The perivalvular leak is often detected by visualization of contrast agent extravasation (Fig. 18.1, [4]).

When prosthetic valve obstruction is suspected, prosthetic valve leaflet motion is an important assessment which may be difficult to assess on echocardiography. Cardiac CT has been shown to be very accurate in assessment of leaflet motion [4]. In addition, cardiac CT can add further information on the presence or absence of prosthetic valve thrombus or pannus (Fig. 18.2). Tissue differentiation based on CT attenuation is not well established; however, higher attenuation has been found with pannus formation versus thrombus [4, 11].

Prosthetic valve infective endocarditis is a dreaded complication, of which the diagnosis can be challenging. There are often limits to the assessment of the valve prosthesis and surrounding structures by echocardiography and multimodality imaging approaches are increasing utilized. Cardiac CT in particular is integral in the assessment for periprosthetic extension of infection (Fig. 18.3, [12]).

In summary, there is an increasing role for multimodality imaging in the assessment of prosthetic valves. Cardiac MRI is beneficial and complementary for evaluation of cardiac dimensions, volumetric assessment of heart chambers, assessment of leaflet motion, and detection of regurgitation [4, 9]. In comparison, the role of cardiac CT is perhaps more vast and has been included in recent valve guidelines for various applications including: assessment of leaflet motion, evaluation for thrombus or pannus, imaging of valve cusps in the setting of bioprosthesis degeneration, and structural evaluation in suspected periprosthetic infection [4, 7, 8].

K. A. Young
Instructor in Medicine, Mayo Clinic College of Medicine; Resident, Department of Cardiovascular Medicine, Mayo Clinic, Rochester, MN, USA
e-mail: Young.Kathleen1@mayo.edu

K. Sharain
Assistant Professor in Medicine, Mayo Clinic College of Medicine; Resident, Department of Cardiovascular Medicine, Mayo Clinic, Rochester, MN, USA
e-mail: Sharain.Korosh@mayo.edu

N. S. Anavekar
Professor of Medicine, Mayo Clinic College of Medicine; Consultant, Department of Cardiovascular Medicine, Mayo Clinic, Rochester, MN, USA
e-mail: Anavekar.Nandan@mayo.edu

T. A. Foley (✉)
Assistant Professor of Radiology, Mayo Clinic College of Medicine; Consultant, Division of Cardiovascular Radiology, Department of Radiology, Mayo Clinic, Rochester, MN, USA
e-mail: Foley.Thomas@mayo.edu

J. F. Maalouf et al. (eds.), *Practical 3D Echocardiography*, https://doi.org/10.1007/978-3-030-72941-7_18

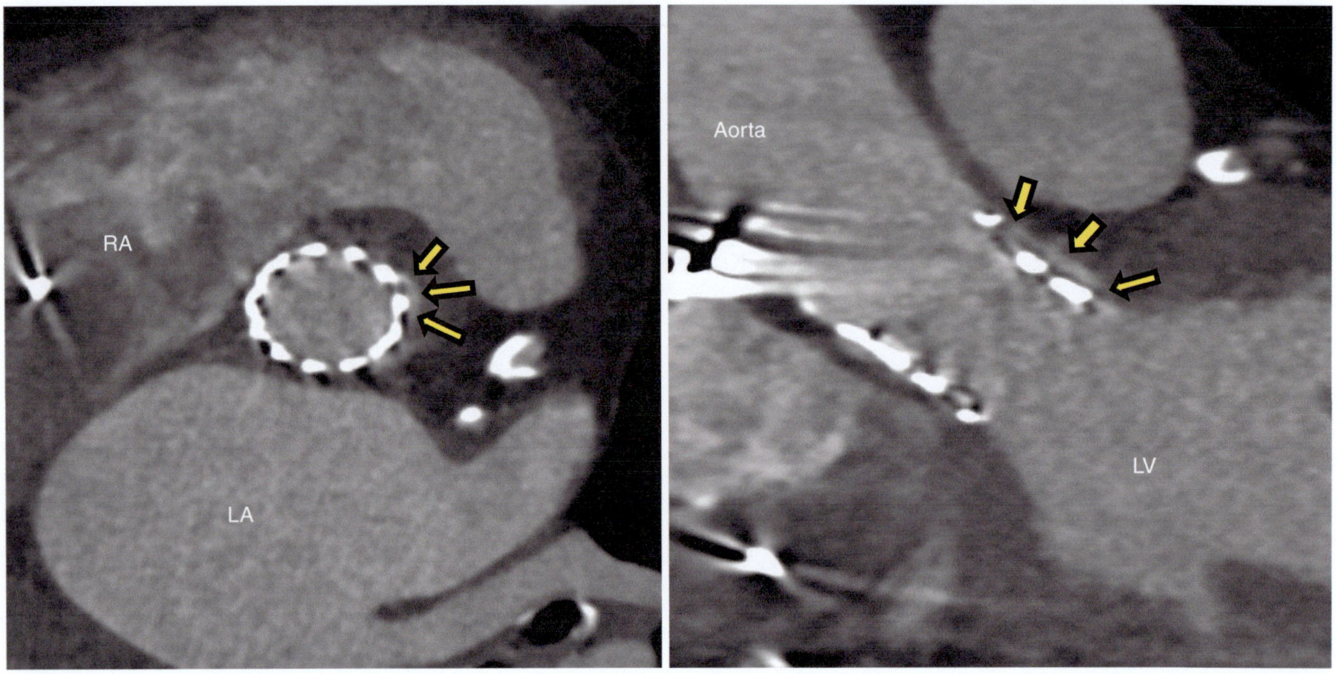

Fig. 18.1 Periprosthetic Leak: Patient was found to have severe periprosthetic leak on transthoracic echocardiography after transcatheter heart valve placement. Retrospective gated cardiac computed tomography was performed for preprocedural planning of perileak closure. Left panel (axial reconstruction view of the prosthetic aortic valve)—the metal frame of the prosthetic valve is well visualized as the centrally located bright signal circular structure. There is a contrast filled channel external to the transcatheter heart valve in the 2–3 O'clock position (arrows). Right panel (coronal reconstruction view)—there is a contrast filled channel which extends from the superior portion of the prosthetic aortic valve caudally into the left ventricular outflow tract (arrows). These findings were consistent with the known periprosthetic leak. The channel measured 3 mm in caliber in diastole and the location was clearly visualized as described above. Used with permission of Mayo Foundation for Medical Education and Research. All rights reserved. LA, left atrium; LV, left ventricle; RA right atrium

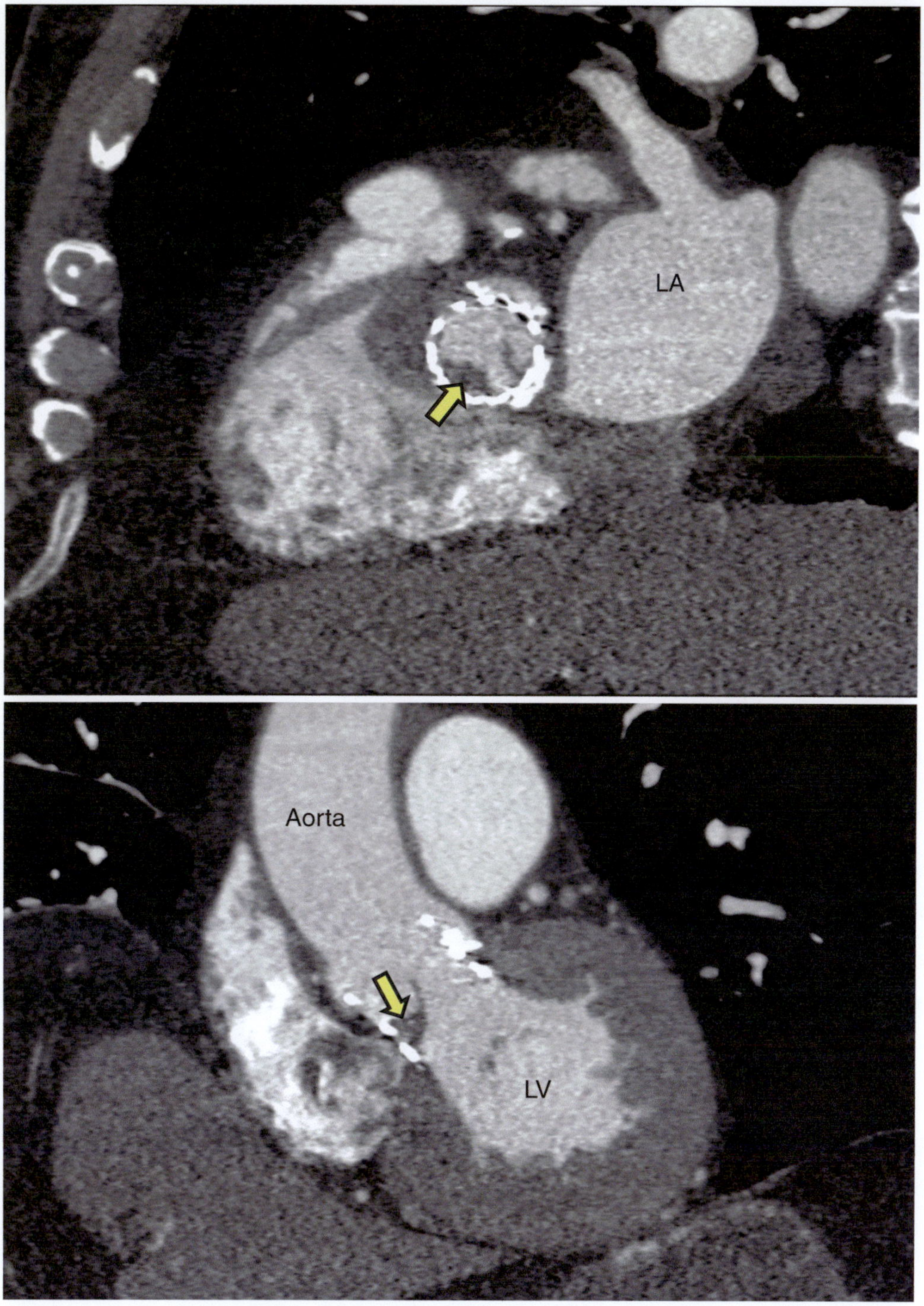

Fig. 18.2 Prosthetic Valve Thrombus/Pannus. This patient presented with dyspnea on exertion 12 months after his transcatheter heart valve procedure, and was found to have an increased gradient across the prosthetic aortic valve by transthoracic echocardiography (post-procedure gradient of 13 mmHg increased to 32 mmHg). Retrospective gated cardiac computed tomography was performed to evaluate aortic valve cusp anatomy and motion. **Top panel** (axial reconstruction view)—the metal frame of the prosthetic valve is well visualized as the centrally located bright signal circular structure. In systole, the right coronary cusp remained in a semi-fixed closed position and there was a hypoattenuating density present on the cusp (arrow). **Bottom panel** (coronal reconstruction view)—again seen is the right coronary cusp remaining in a semi-closed position in systole with the hypoattenuating density on the cusp (arrow). On cine imaging, the right coronary cusp was relatively immobile. These findings were consistent with valve thrombosis of the right coronary cusp. The patient's aortic valve gradient improved to 15 mmHg after 3 months of anticoagulation. Used with permission of Mayo Foundation for Medical Education and Research. LA, left atrium; LV, left ventricle

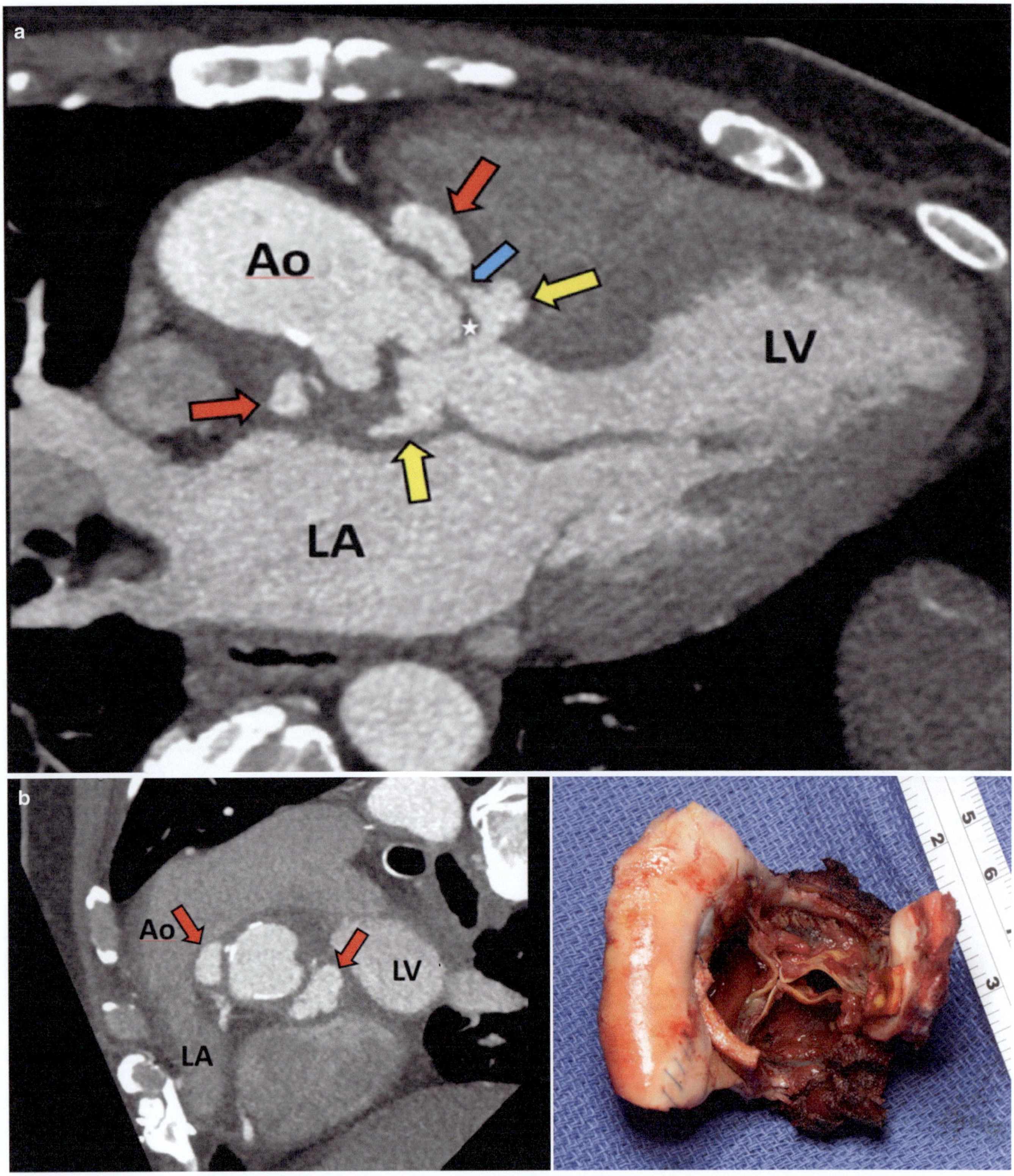

Fig. 18.3 Prosthetic Valve Endocarditis and Aortic Root Abscess: Patient with a history of bioprosthetic aortic valve replacement presented with weight loss, fevers, and a rash concerning for endocarditis. Transesophageal echocardiogram demonstrated aortic root abscess with likely prosthetic valve dehiscence. Retrospective gated cardiac computed tomography was performed to evaluate the extent of the abscess and for surgical planning. Top panel (three chamber view)—there was a near circumferential aortic root abscess (red arrows). There were also anterior and posterior pseudoaneurysms of the left ventricular outflow tract (yellow arrows). Additionally, the right coronary cusp can be seen prolapsing into the left ventricular outflow tract (white star) with just a small attachment point to the aortic root (blue arrow) which is consistent with prosthetic valve dehiscence. Middle panel. Left: (axial reconstruction view)—the near circumferential root abscess is again visualized (red arrows). Right: Surgical specimen demonstrating significant destruction of the bioprosthetic valve. Used with permission of Mayo Foundation for Medical Education and Research. Ao, aorta; LA, left atrium; LV, left ventricle

References

1. Benjamin EJ, et al. Heart disease and stroke Statistics-2018 update: a report from the American Heart Association. Circulation. 2018;137(12):e67–e492.
2. Iung B, Vahanian A. Epidemiology of valvular heart disease in the adult. Nat Rev Cardiol. 2011;8(3):162–72.
3. Nkomo VT, et al. Burden of valvular heart diseases: a population-based study. Lancet. 2006;368(9540):1005–11.
4. Sucha D, et al. Multimodality imaging assessment of prosthetic heart valves. Circ Cardiovasc Imaging. 2015;8(9):e003703.
5. Yacoub MH, Takkenberg JJ. Will heart valve tissue engineering change the world? Nat Clin Pract Cardiovasc Med. 2005;2(2):60–1.
6. Singh M, et al. ACC/AHA versus ESC guidelines on prosthetic heart valve management: JACC guideline comparison. J Am Coll Cardiol. 2019;73(13):1707–18.
7. Nishimura RA, et al. 2014 AHA/ACC guideline for the Management of Patients with Valvular Heart Disease: a report of the American College of Cardiology/American Heart Association task force on practice guidelines. Circulation. 2014;129(23):e521–643.
8. Zoghbi WA, et al. Recommendations for evaluation of prosthetic valves with echocardiography and doppler ultrasound: a report from the American Society of Echocardiography's Guidelines and Standards Committee and the Task Force on Prosthetic Valves, developed in conjunction with the American College of Cardiology Cardiovascular Imaging Committee, Cardiac Imaging Committee of the American Heart Association, the European Association of Echocardiography, a registered branch of the European Society of Cardiology, the Japanese Society of Echocardiography and the Canadian Society of Echocardiography, endorsed by the American College of Cardiology Foundation, American Heart Association, European Association of Echocardiography, a registered branch of the European Society of Cardiology, the Japanese Society of Echocardiography, and Canadian Society of Echocardiography. J Am Soc Echocardiogr. 2009;22(9):975–1014. quiz 1082-4
9. Lancellotti P, et al. Recommendations for the imaging assessment of prosthetic heart valves: a report from the European Association of Cardiovascular Imaging endorsed by the Chinese Society of Echocardiography, the inter-American Society of Echocardiography, and the Brazilian Department of Cardiovascular Imaging. Eur Heart J Cardiovasc Imaging. 2016;17(6):589–90.
10. Blauwet LA, Miller FA Jr. Echocardiographic assessment of prosthetic heart valves. Prog Cardiovasc Dis. 2014;57(1):100–10.
11. Gunduz S, et al. Sixty-four-section cardiac computed tomography in mechanical prosthetic heart valve dysfunction: thrombus or pannus. Circ Cardiovasc Imaging. 2015;8(12):e003246.
12. Erba PA, et al. Multimodality imaging in infective endocarditis: an imaging team within the endocarditis team. Circulation. 2019;140(21):1753–65.

Part III

Atria and Atrial Septum

Normal 3DE Anatomy of Atrial Septum: Image Display and Anatomical Specimen Correlations

19

Francesco F. Faletra, Laura A. Leo, Susanne A. Schlossbauer, Vera L. Paiocchi, Elisa Gherbesi, and Marco Valgimigli

Interatrial Septum

Atrial Septation

Atrial septation begins with the appearance of a thin crescent ridge of connective tissue that grows from the atrial roof and is called *septum primum (SP)*. The free edge of the SP is covered by mesenchymal cells (mesenchymal cup). The SP descends towards the endocardial cushions and the gap between the leading edge of the SP and the endocardial cushions is called *ostium primum (OP)*. Before the fusion between SP and endocardial cushions takes place, in the upper part of the SP, cell apoptosis results in multiple small holes which eventually coalesce creating a new communication between the right and left sides of the primitive atrium: the *ostium secundum (OS)*. The OS allows blood flow passage from the right to the left heart through the primitive septation once the OP is obliterated. At the same time, a "folding" of the atrial wall, appears to the right side of the SP progressively extending in anterior, superior, posterior and inferior directions overlapping and encircling the SP: this folding takes the name of *septum secundum (SS)*. Thus, seen from a right atrial perspective, the SP becomes the floor of the fossa ovalis (FO), while the SS is the muscular part of the IAS, on all sides of the SP [1]. In fetal life, the SP works as a flap valve guiding blood flow from right atrium to left atrium through the OS. After birth, pressure increase in the left atrium pushes the flap valve against the muscular rim, leading to functional closure of the OS (see Chap. 27).

The Adult IAS

With the body in anterior-posterior position, the right atrium lies anterior and to the right, whilst the left atrium is posterior and slightly to the left. The position of atrial cavities determines the orientation of the IAS with respect to the body planes. With the body in anterior-posterior orientation, the plane of the IAS is oriented obliquely extending from right-superior to left-anterior position with an angle approximately of 60°. Of note, this angle may change with pathological left and right atrial enlargement.

Cadaveric hearts remain the state-of-the-art for describing anatomy of the IAS [2]. However, two/three-dimensional transesophageal echocardiography (2D/3D TEE) and cardiac magnetic resonance (CMR) today allow visualization of all anatomical details of the IAS either in cross section or in "en face" view. Particularly, 3D TEE has the unique ability of showing the surfaces of the IAS from both the left and right-atrial perspectives (Fig. 19.1). As viewed from the left atrium, the IAS is almost featureless (Fig. 19.1a). In contrast, the IAS from the right atrium appears as an extensive muscular area interposed between the two atrial cavities and surrounding the fossa ovalis (FO). Boundaries of this area are the orifice of the inferior vena cava, (IVC), the right atrial appendage, the superior vena cava (SVC), and insertion of the septal leaflet of the tricuspid valve (TV). Several anatomic structures can be recognized: the FO with its crater-shaped feature, the Eustachian valve (EV), and the orifice of the coronary sinus (CS) (Fig. 19.1b). Particularly relevant is the fact that the so-called triangle of Koch can be imaged on the right side of the IAS. Named by German pathologist and cardiologist Walter Karl Koch in 1909 [3], this triangle is an anatomic area limited by the superior margin of the coronary sinus orifice, septal leaflet of the tricuspid valve and by the tendon of Todaro. This

F. F. Faletra (✉)
Director of Cardiac Imaging Lab, Cardiocentro Ticino Institute, Lugano, Switzerland
e-mail: Francesco.Faletra@cardiocentro.org

L. A. Leo · S. A. Schlossbauer · V. L. Paiocchi · E. Gherbesi
Cardiac Imaging Lab, Cardiocentro Ticino Institute, Lugano, Switzerland
e-mail: lauraanna.leo@cardiocentro.org; Susanne.schlossbauer@cardiocentro.org; vera.paiocchi@cardiocentro.org; elisa.gherbesi@cardiocentro.org

M. Valgimigli
Professor, Division of Cardiology, Cardiocentro Ticino Institute, Lugano, Switzerland
e-mail: marco.valgimigli@cardiocentro.org

J. F. Maalouf et al. (eds.), *Practical 3D Echocardiography*, https://doi.org/10.1007/978-3-030-72941-7_19

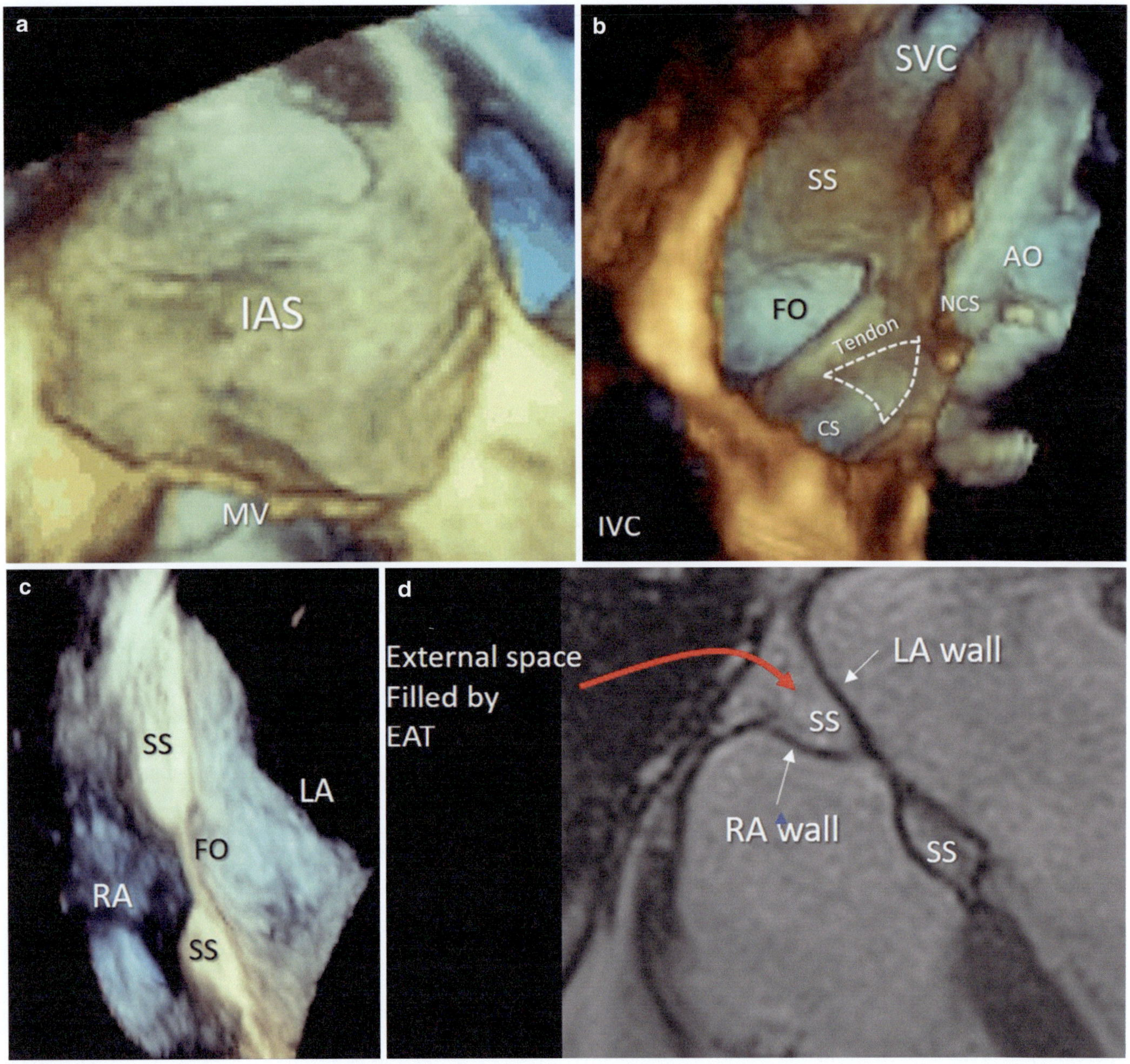

Fig. 19.1 (**a**) 3D TEE image of the left side of the IAS appearing as an extensive interposed structure in between the two atrial cavities (**b**) 3D TEE image of the right side of the IAS showing several landmarks (see text). The dotted triangle represents the triangle of Koch (**c**) 3D TEE cross section of the IAS in anatomical position. This image shows the septum secondum (SS) as a muscular protuberance dividing the right atrium (RA) from the left atrium (LA); (**d**) CMR cine sequence, showing that the SS is an enfolding of the atrial wall with a three-layered configuration (i.e. the two atrial walls and the epicardial adipose tissue (EAT) in between). AO, Aorta; CS, coronary sinus; FO, fossa ovalis; IAS, interatrial septum; IVC, inferior vena cava; NCS, non-coronary sinus; LA, left atrium; MV, mitral valve; NCS, noncoronary sinus; RA, right atrium; SP, septum primum; SS, septum secodum; SVC, superior vena cava

latter is a collagen band, which runs antero-superiorly within the sub-endocardium of the right atrium, travelling between the FO and the orifice of the CS and ending nearby the membranous septum. However, while the coronary sinus orifice and the hinge line of septal leaflet of the tricuspid valve are easily recognizable, the tendon of Todaro is not visible on the gross anatomic specimen or during surgical inspection. Although only seen microscopically, the tendon of Todaro in the operating room can be virtually traced as the continuation of the Eustachian ridge. Though an "imaginary" geometrical figure, the triangle of Koch is an important landmark for cardiac surgeons to localize the compact AV node (located near the apex of the triangle) and the His bundle (located below the inferior margin of the membranous septum, where the tendon ends).

Anatomists describe the IAS as a partition between the two atria. Consequently, removal or puncturing this area is supposed to create a communication between the two atrial cavities without producing an exit from the heart. Following this anatomical criterion, only the floor of the FO, i.e. the SP, should be labelled IAS. Indeed, as briefly mentioned in the paragraph "atrial septation", the muscular area, surrounding the posterior, superior and inferior margins of the FO, called SS, is a folding of the atrial wall. Removal or puncturing this region causes an exit from the cavities of the heart into epicardial fat or into the extra-cardiac space. This folding, was first described in the nineteenth century by Waterston and today it is known as the Waterston groove or interatrial groove. It is filled with epicardial adipose tissue (EAT) and contains the sinus node artery [4].

In conclusion, the SS is a three-layered structure formed by the muscular tissue of the two atrial walls with the epicardial adipose tissue (EAT) located in between. 2D and3D TEE usually fail to identify the adipose tissue inside the folding (Fig. 19.1c). Without any doubt, the best imaging modality to illustrate the SS architecture is CMR. This technique allows a clear distinction between muscular and adipose tissue when a specific pulse sequence, called Steady State Free Precession (SSFP) is used. SSFP provides a strong signal from the blood and fat, and a weak signal from the muscular tissue and is therefore capable of distinguishing the adipose tissue located within the fold of the atrial walls from the atrial walls themselves (Fig. 19.1c, d).

The FO may have different sizes depending on the variable extension of the folding, and on the dimension of the atrial cavities. Defining the size of FO is important because the only site for safest transseptal crossing is through the FO. Though formed by a folding of the atrial wall, the SS undeniably contributes to a septation between the atrial cavities and can properly be labelled as "septum".

Drop Out Artifacts

Although 3D TEE is very consistent in visualizing the IAS according to an "en face" perspective, "false" defects especially at the level of the FO may appear on 3D images. These defects are technically named "drop out artifacts" [5] (see Chap. 3). There are two main reasons for this phenomenon. The first is that the FO is much thinner than the surrounding SS. Although the ultrasound beams in TEE echocardiography have a very high frequency (5 MHz), the wavelength may be not short enough to intersect this very thin structure. Thus, reflection of return echoes may be substantially absent in some areas of the FO. The second reason is that not infrequently the FO is rather oblique or even parallel to the ultrasound beam. As a result, the FO reflects weak and scattered rather than strong specular echoes. Scattered echoes are not strong enough to allow perfect reconstruction of the FO surface and, consequently, the thin FO connective tissue is represented on the echocardiographic image with anatomical discontinuities which may be erroneously interpreted as defects (Fig. 19.2).

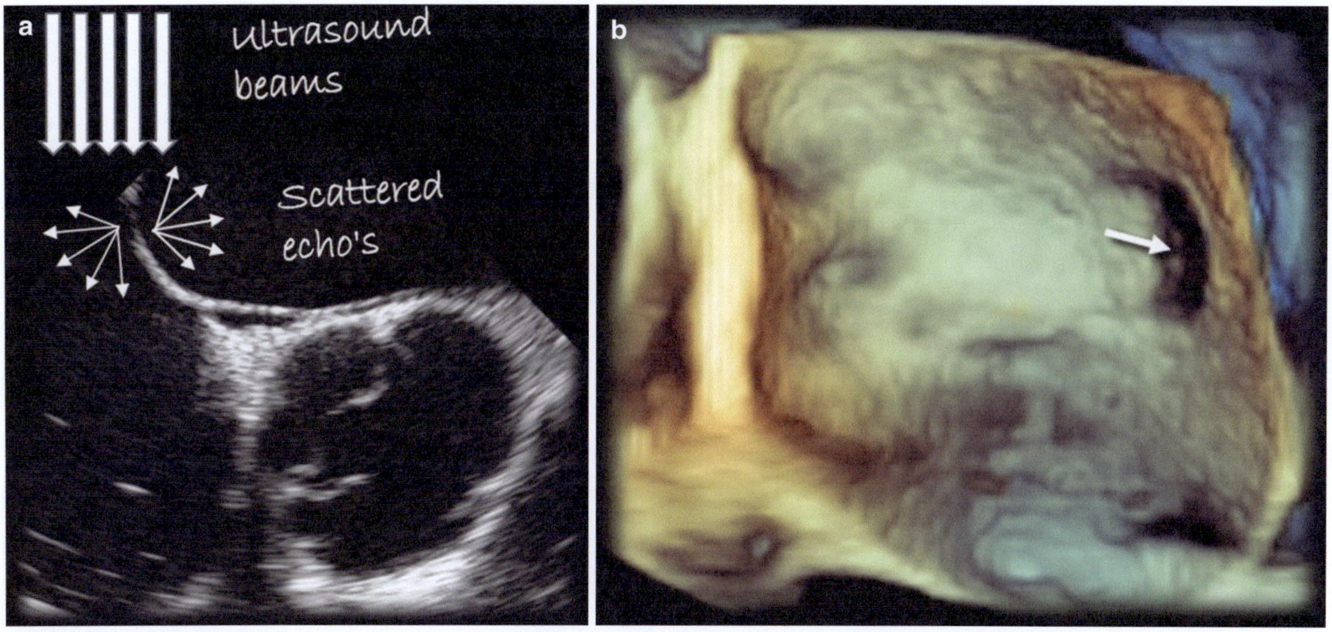

Fig. 19.2 (**a**) 2D TEE showing that the IAS is partially parallel to the ultrasound beam (thick arrows). As a result, the FO reflects weak and scattered echos (thin arrows) rather than specular echoes, which may create apparent defects inside the FO. (**b**) 3D TEE images of the IAS from the left atrial perspective. The arrow points to the defect created by dropout artifacts. FO, fossa ovalis; IAS, interatrial septum

Misnomers

Some misnomers, which derive from incomplete understanding of the peculiar anatomy of the SS, are outlined below:

1. The term "lipomatous hypertrophy" of the IAS, coined by Prior in 1964 [6], is incorrect for several reasons: (a) the term "lipomatous" is itself misleading because, unlike a true lipoma, this lipomatous tissue is not encapsulated; (b) Also the term "hypertrophy" is misleading since the accumulation of fat is due to an increased number of adipocytes (hyperplasia) and not to an increased size of individual adipocyte (hypertrophy). (c) the accumulation of adipocytes is not an adipose "infiltration" of the IAS, as often described, but just the presence of an abnormal amount of extracardiac fat that occupies the folding of the SS in continuity with the epicardial adipose tissue (Fig. 19.4a). Thus, rather than labeling this entity as a disease, tumor, or disorder, as often described in the literature, it should be simply considered an "anatomical variant". It is however believed that large amount of fat accumulation may sporadically cause geometrical distortion of the atrial walls and atrial arrhythmias or, very rarely, presents as a protruding atrial mass which may partially obstruct the IVC inflow. Echocardiographers, surgeons, interventional cardiologists and electrophysiologists should therefore know that the so-called "lipomatous hypertrophy" of the IAS is nothing other than an excess accumulation of extracardiac fat within the folds of the SS [7].
2. Among the subtypes of atrial septal defects only the septum secundum type, should be labelled as an interatrial "septal" communication. The other subtypes (i.e. sinus venousus, ostium primum, unroofed coronary sinus) should be considered more correctly as interatrial "extra-septal" communications, since the shunt between the atrial chambers occurs outside the border of the true atrial septum.
3. The old classification of septal aneurysm as "limited" to the fossa ovalis or "involving the entire septum" is highly misleading. Indeed, septal aneurysms are always limited to the FO, and may be small or large according the size of the FO, considering that a three-layered structure of fat-filled muscular sandwich cannot be part of an aneurysmal formation (Fig. 19.4b).

The Septal Pouch

The septal pouch was described by Krushnan and Salazar [8] as a new anatomic entity. These investigators examined 94 autopsied hearts focusing on the pattern of fusion between SP and SS. They found that 27% had a PFO. Among the remaining 68 hearts without PFO, only 27 had complete fusion, whereas in 41 the fusion was incomplete with a Kangaroo-like pocket opening into the left atrium in 37 anatomic specimens, and in 4 into the right atrium. They named this blind ended pocket septal pouch. These authors hypothesized that fusion between SP and SS starts at the caudal margin of the zone of overlap and continues in a cranial direction. The more frequent location of a left sided pouch due to incomplete fusion can be explained by the fact the SP is a left sided structure. Whether the stagnant blood in the pouch may be a site of blood stasis and thrombus formation, analogous to the left atrial appendage, remains unclear. Indeed, case reports have shown the presence of thrombus within the pouch in patients with cryptogenic stroke. However, epidemiological studies remain contradictory. While a meta-analysis performed in 2017 detected no difference in left septal pouch prevalence between controls and patients with ischemic stroke, more recent studies showed that the presence of a left septal pouch (Figs. 19.3 and 19.4c) was associated with an increased risk for cryptogenic stroke [9–13]. Certainly, a better understanding and awareness of the role played by the septal pouch, espe-

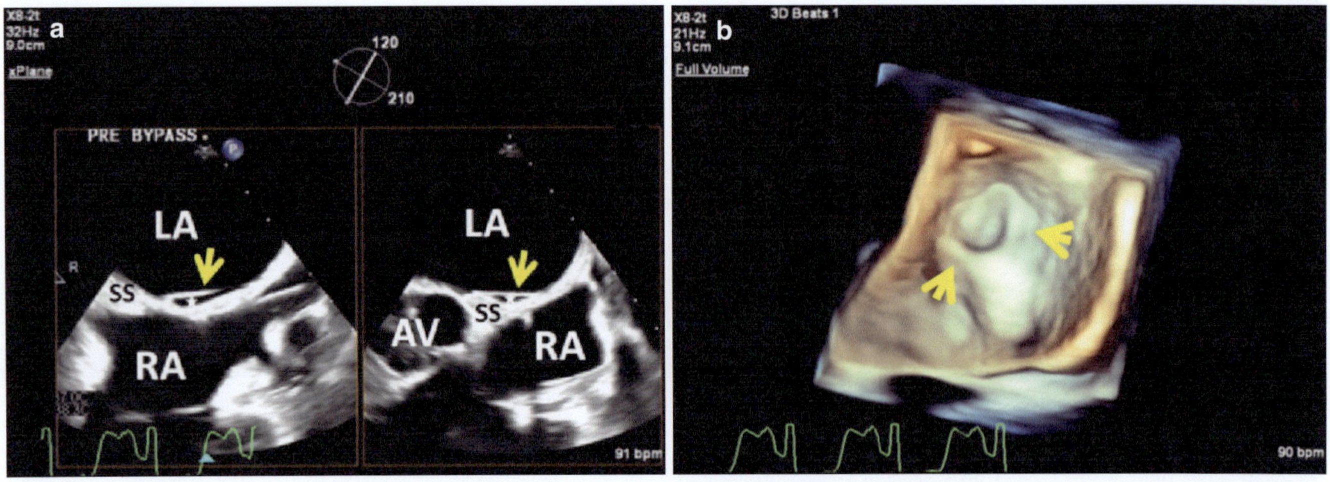

Fig. 19.3 Left side atrial septal pouch (Used with permission of Mayo Foundation for Medical Education and Research. All rights reserved): (**a**) xPlane of atrial septum showing an apical pouch (astersiks) between the septum primum (arrows) and septum secondum (SS). (**b**) 3D view of the left sided Kangaroo-like septal pouch (arrows). AV, aortic valve; LA, left atrium; RA, right atrium

cially if left-sided, may potentially expand our knowledge of cardio-embolic stroke, considering that the septal pouch may be a novel contributor to thrombus formation within the left atrium.

Ridges

The left side of the IAS, with the exception of the septal pouch, is almost featureless. Rarely, a prominent ridge-like formation runs laterally to the oval fossa and extends to the atrial free wall [13]. Whether this ridge, which potentially may interfere with the septal puncture or catheter navigation into the left atrium, is acquired or due to a kind of "irregular" fusion between septum primum and septum secundum remains speculative (Fig. 19.4d).

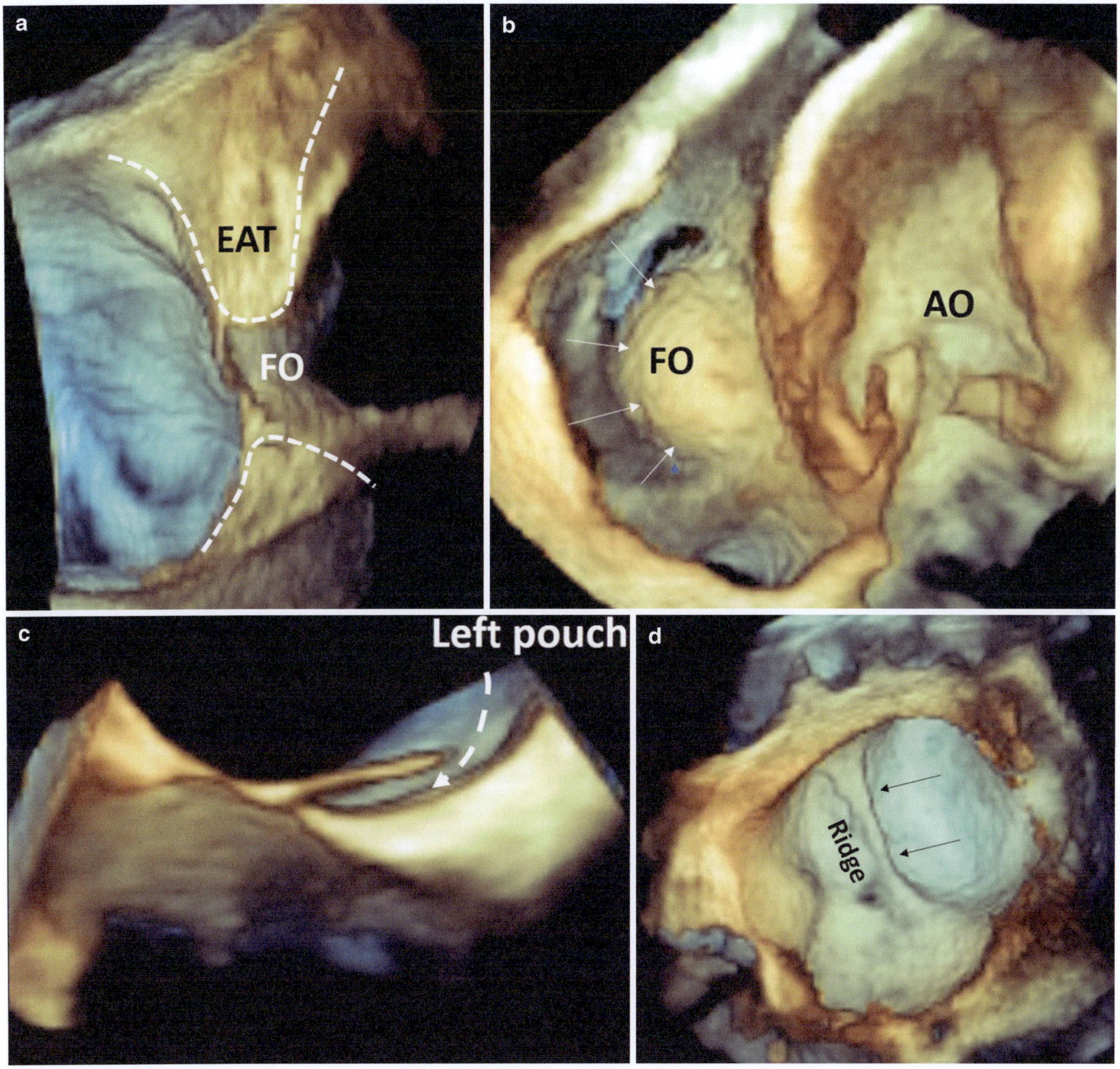

Fig. 19.4 (**a**) 3D TEE image obtained cropping longitudinally the so-called lipomatous septum. The image clearly shows how the epicardial adipose tissue (EAT) penetrates the folding of the SS (dotted line). (**b**) 3D TEE image showing a FO aneurysm (arrows). (**c**) 3D TEE image showing a septal pouch (dotted arrow). (**d**) 3D TEE image showing a ridge on the left atrial surface of the IAS (arrows). AO, ascending aorta; FO, fossa ovalis; IAS, interatrial septum

The Atrio-Ventricular Junction

The name *atrio-ventricular junction*, refers the junction between septa and the hinge line of atrioventricular valves. This region is also named "crux cordis". Silverman and Shiller in a paper entitled "apex echocardiography" described this region using 2D transthoracic echocardiography [14]. With the transducer placed on the apex of the heart, they obtained a cross-section where the four chambers of the heart were visualized simultaneously. This section, now well-known as apical four-chamber view, is today one of the most informative echocardiographic cross-sections and is available in almost every case. The most peculiar anatomical feature of this area is the hinge line of the tricuspid septal leaflet, which is positioned more apically than the corresponding hinge of the mitral leaflet. In the normal adult, the distance between the two hinge lines should not exceed 8–9 mm/m^2. The tricuspid valve is always associated with the morphologic right ventricle. Thus, the low insertion of the tricuspid septal leaflet is a useful marker to recognize the morphological right ventricle in complex congenital heart disease. Given this arrangement, the portion of septum between the two hinge lines is termed atrio-ventricular septum (AVS) because it is placed between the right atrium and the left ventricle. The AVS, was described in the past as a muscular partition between right atrium and left ventricle. More recent anatomical observations have shown that the AVS is formed by the atrial wall on the right side and the crest of the interventricular septum on the left side. Between these two muscular partitions, there is a small amount of adipose tissue originating from the inferior pyramidal space [15]. The inferior pyramidal space is a three-dimensional pyramidal-shaped extracardiac area containing epicardial adipose tissue (EAT) situated in between the atrial walls and the ventricular walls in the posterior-inferior epicardial surface of the heart (the so-called cardiac crux). Recently this area was re-named "atrio-ventricular muscular sandwich" with the adipose tissue in between the two muscular tissue representing the "meat" in the sandwich. Current non-invasive imaging techniques can clearly illustrate the atrio-ventricular region, but they fail to distinguish this fine anatomical arrangement since it is beyond their spatial resolution power. However, in some cases, where the adipose tissue is abundant enough to separate the atrial wall from the ventricular crest this sandwich arrangement can be appreciated by using the SSFP sequences of CMR (Fig. 19.5).

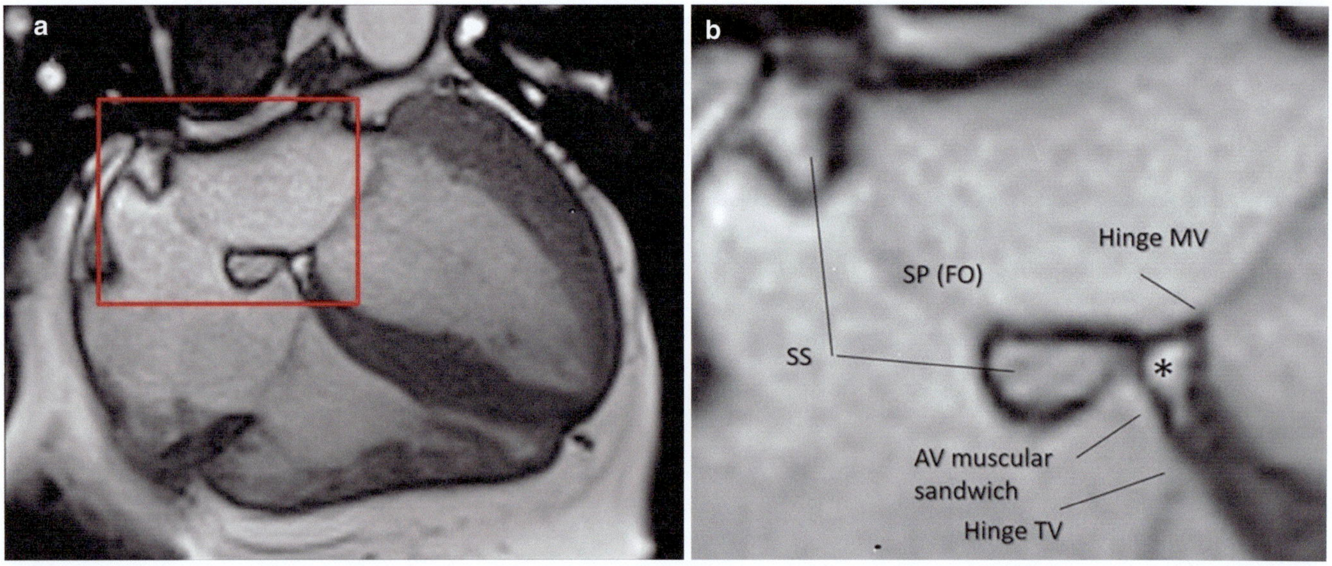

Fig. 19.5 Modified with permission from Faletra et al: in "Atlas of non-invasive imaging in cardiac anatomy" page 59 from Springer Nature Switzerland 2020. The (**a**) and (**b**) panels show in four-chamber view the anatomical architecture of the septum primum (SP) corresponding to the fossa ovalis (FO), the septum secundum (SS) and the atrioventricular (AV) muscular sandwich, the anatomic and histological specimens shown in panels (**c**) and (**d**) show the same structures. The asterisks in panel (**b**), (**c**), (**d**) mark small amount of adipose tissue originating from the inferior pyramidal space (see text)

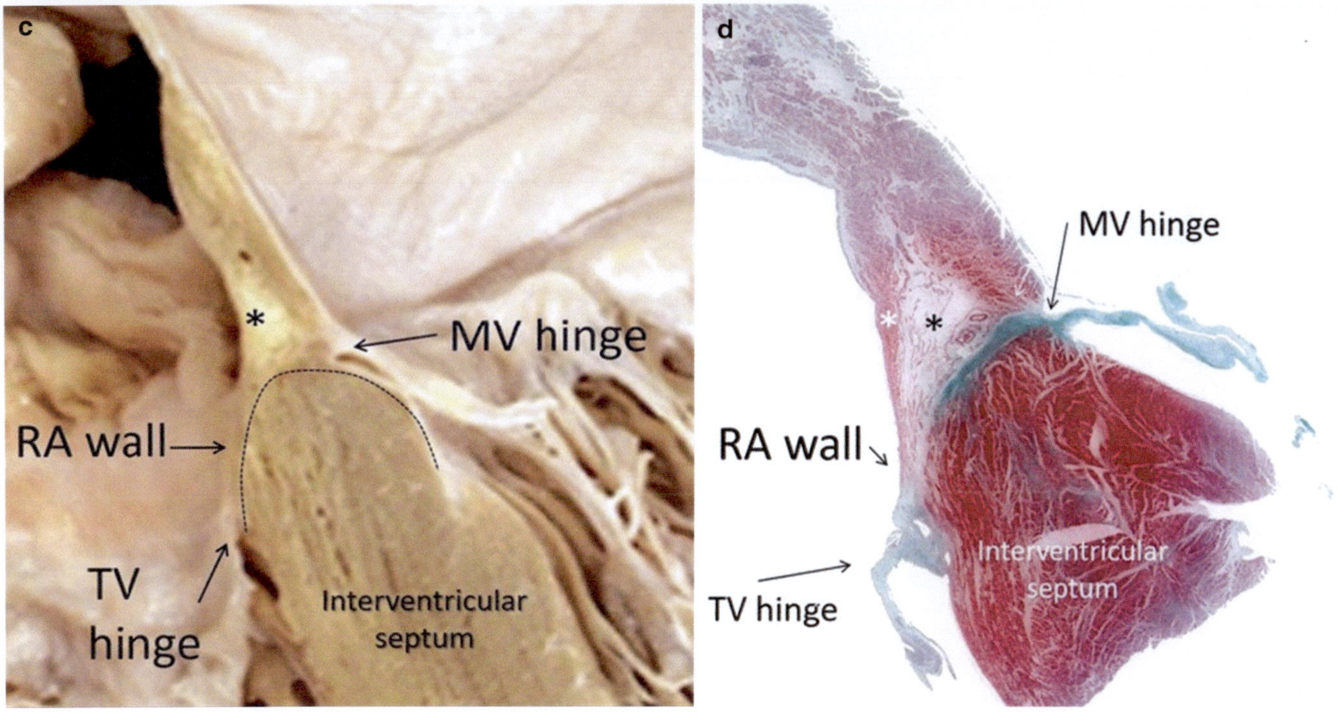

Fig. 19.5 (continued)

References

1. Anderson RH, Brown NA, Webb S. Development and structure of the atrial septum. Heart. 2002;88:104–10.
2. Breithardt OA, Papavassiliu T, Borggref M. Clinical anatomy of the atrial septum with reference to its developmental components. Clin Anat. 1999;12:362–74.
3. Koch W. Weiter Mitteilungen über den Sinusknoten des Herzens. Verh Dt Ges Pathol. 1909;13:85–92.
4. Klimek-Piotrowska W, Hołda MK, Koziej M, Piątek K, Hołda J. Anatomy of the true interatrial septum for transseptal access to the left atrium. Ann Anat. 2016;205:60–4.
5. Faletra FF, Ramamurthi A, Dequarti MC, Leo LA, Moccetti T, Pandian N. Artifacts in three-dimensional transesophageal echocardiography. J Am Soc Echocardiogr. 2014;27(5):453–62.
6. PRIOR JT. Lipomatous hypertrophy of interatrial septum. A lesion resembling hibernoma, lipoblastomatosis and infiltrating lipoma. Arch Pathol. 1964;78:11–5.
7. Ribeiro RNF, Ribeiro BNF, Martins WA, Antunes LO, Marchiori E. Lipomatous hypertrophy of the interatrial septum. Radiol Bras. 2018;51(2):130–1.
8. Krishnan SC, Salazar M. Septal pouch in the left atrium: a new anatomical entity with potential for embolic complications. JACC Cardiovasc Interv. 2010;3:98–104.
9. Tugcu A, Okajima K, Jin Z, Rundek T, Homma S, Sacco RL, et al. Septal pouch in the left atrium and risk of ischemic stroke: a case-control study. JACC Cardiovasc Imaging. 2010;3(12):1276–83.
10. Shimamoto K, Kawagoe T, Dai K, et al. Thrombus in the left atrial septal pouch mimicking myxoma. J Clin Ultrasound. 2014;42:185–8.
11. Wong JM, Lombardo D, Handwerker J, et al. Cryptogenic stroke and the left atrial septal pouch: a case report. J Stroke Cerebrovasc Dis. 2014;23:564–5.
12. Chandrashekhar Y, Narula J. LA septal pouch as a source of thromboembolism: innocent until proven guilty? JACC Cardiovasc Imaging. 2010;3:1296–8.
13. Zisa D, Faletra FF, Wessler BS, et al. Ridges and pouches: a case series of anomalous atrial septal fusion. CASE (Phila). 2019;4(1):7–17.
14. Silverman NH, Schiller NB. Apex echocardiography. A two-dimensional technique for evaluating congenital heart disease. Circulation. 1978;57:503–11.
15. Becker AE, Anderson RH. Atrioventricular septal defect. What's in a name? J Thorac Cardiovasc Surg. 1982;83:461–9.

Atrial Septal Defects: 2DE vs 3DE and Anatomic Specimen

20

Francesco F. Faletra, Vera L. Paiocchi, Laura A. Leo, Susanne A. Schlossbauer, and S. Yen Ho

Atrial septal defects (ASDs) embrace a group of congenital cardiac anomalies that allow communication between the left and right atrial cavities. These defects are among the most common congenital heart anomaly with an approximate birth prevalence of 1.6 in 1000 individuals [1]. There are four types of ASDs: secundum ASD (S-ASD), sinus venosus ASD (SV-ASD), unroofed coronary sinus ASD (UCS-ASD) and primum ASD (P-ASD). Figure 20.1 is a 3D TEE image of the interatrial septum visualized from a right atrial perspective with superimposed locations of the aforementioned defects.

Most patients with ASD, even when large, remain asymptomatic throughout most of childhood. In the majority of cases, the diagnosis is made incidentally by an echocardiogram required because of a heart murmur or because of abnormal findings on the electrocardiogram or chest X-ray. Until the third decade of life, shortness of breath with exercise or palpitations are uncommon. Conversely, in the fourth/fifth decades, patients with large ASD may complain of fatigue, exercise intolerance and/or arrhythmias [2, 3].

The decision to repair an ASD is based on clinical and echocardiographic information which include (a) size and location of ASD; (b) hemodynamic impact of the left-to-right shunt and associated right ventricular volume overload (this typically occurs when the Qp:Qs ratio is greater than 1.5 to 1) and (c) the presence and degree of pulmonary hypertension.

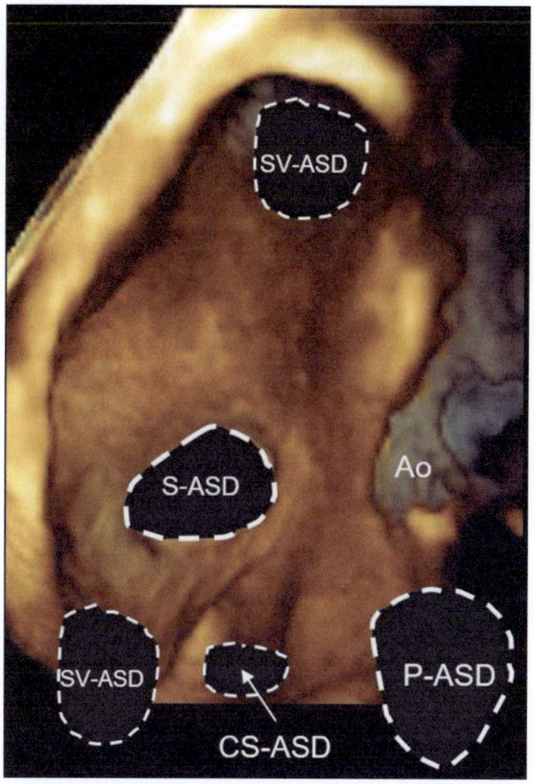

Fig. 20.1 3D TEE images of the right side of the interatrial septum. Superimposed are the locations of subtypes of atrial septal defect (ASD). SV-ASD, sinus venous ASD; S-ASD, secundum ASD; CS-ASD, coronary sinus ASD; P-ASD, primum ASD; Ao, ascending aorta

Pulmonary hypertension (PH), defined as a mean pulmonary artery pressure ≥25 mm Hg, pulmonary capillary wedge pressure ≤15 mm Hg, and pulmonary vascular resistance ≥3 Wood units) is a significant complication in adults with large ASD and has been noted in 6–30%, while severe PH (systolic pressure >60 mmHg) is seen in 9–22% of cases [2]. These patients have more severe symptoms such as, syncope, thromboembolism and cyanosis. Of note preoperative PH remains predictive of mortality, heart failure, and arrhythmias even after closure of the ASD. According to the guide-

F. F. Faletra (✉)
Director of Cardiac Imaging Lab, Cardiocentro Ticino Institute, Lugano, Switzerland
e-mail: Francesco.Faletra@cardiocentro.org

V. L. Paiocchi · L. A. Leo · S. A. Schlossbauer
Cardiac Imaging Lab, Cardiocentro Ticino Institute, Lugano, Switzerland
e-mail: vera.paiocchi@cardiocentro.org; lauraanna.leo@cardiocentro.org; susanne.schlossbauer@cardiocentro.org

S. Yen Ho
Professor, Cardiac Morphology Unit, Royal Brompton Hospital and Imperial College, London, UK
e-mail: yen.ho@imperial.ac.uk

J. F. Maalouf et al. (eds.), *Practical 3D Echocardiography*, https://doi.org/10.1007/978-3-030-72941-7_20

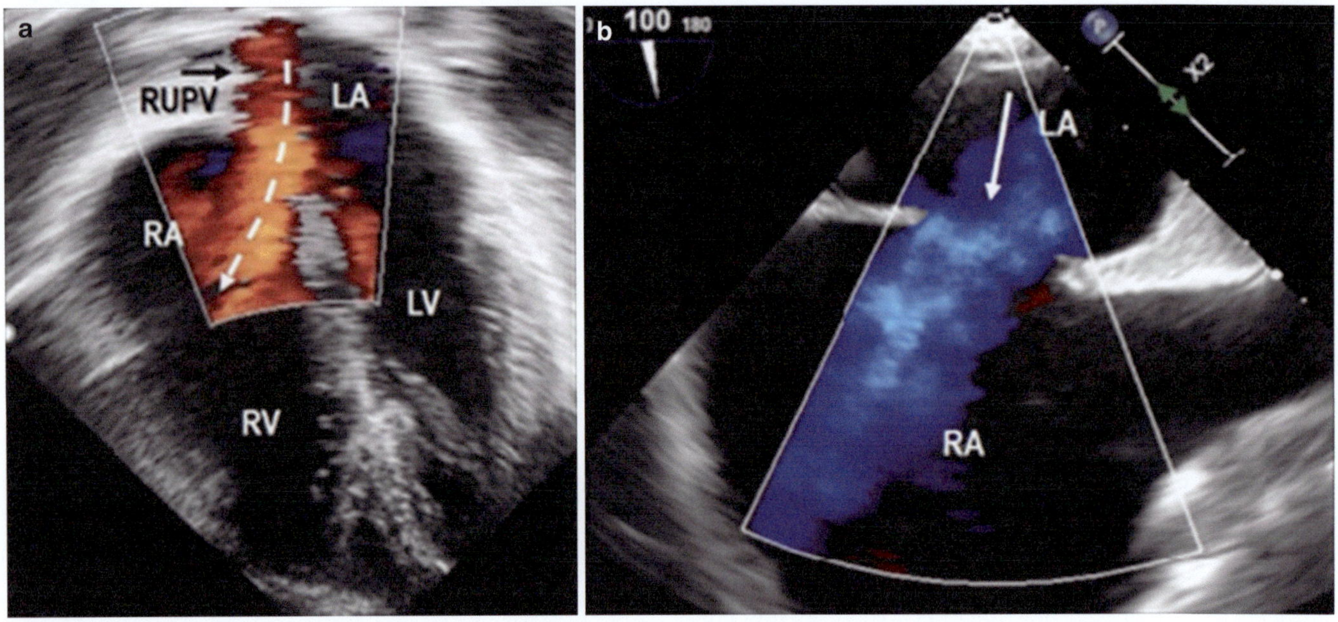

Fig. 20.2 (**a**) 2D TTE four chamber view color Doppler in correct anatomical orientation. The image shows flow crossing the S-ASD (dotted arrow) from left atrium (LA) to right atrium (RA). Please note that flow from the right superior pulmonary vein (RSPV) runs directly through the defect. (**b**) 2D TEE cross section bi-caval view showing the flow (arrow) crossing the S-ASD from the LA into the RA. RV, right ventricle, LV, left ventricle

lines, large defects with prevalent systemic to pulmonary shunting and without cyanosis at rest are correctable when the indexed pulmonary vascular resistance (PVRi) is <4 WU m^2, and ASDs with PVRi >8 WU/m^2 should not be repaired. Repair of ASDs with PVRi between 4–8 WU m^2 may be considered individually, after carefully weighing the risks and benefits of the procedure, particular patient characteristics, institutional expertise, and local postoperative care resources [4].

Specific ASD

Secundum ASD

S-ASD is the most common type accounting for about 75% of all ASDs and is more common in females than males [1]. As described in Chap. 19, the floor of the fossa ovalis (FO) is formed by the septum primum which developmentally, grows down from the roof of the common atrium to cover the enfolded muscular rim formed by the septum secundum. As it descends, the upper part of the septum primum breaks down to form the ostium secundum [5]. S-ASD is an interatrial communication at this site, caused by an excessive resorption (through apoptosis) of the septum primum and therefore it is located within the borders of the FO. Its size varies from a few millimeters in diameter to more than 3 cm and its shape may be variable. With the largest S-ASD, the septum primum may be virtually absent. The diagnosis of a S-ASD and its hemodynamic consequences can be established by 2D transthoracic echocardiography (TTE) and color Doppler in the majority of cases. Figure 20.2 shows two of the classic transthoracic and transesophageal approaches for the diagnosis of S-ASD.

Cardiac catheterization, CT and CMR may provide additional hemodynamic data and visualization of associated anomalies. However, 3D TEE is today necessary for detailing the ASD anatomy and sizing. 3D TEE allows for accurate visualization of the size and shape of the defect and its rims (see Chap. 27) on unique en face views either from right or from left side. Figure 20.3 shows four 3D TEE still frames of a S-ASD with different angulation from left side to right side.

Interestingly, its margins being surrounded by atrial muscular tissue confers on the S-ASD its own unique "dynamicity". Indeed, while the other types of ASD maintain almost the same dimensions during the cardiac cycle, the size of S-ASD varies depending on the contraction and relaxation of the atrial musculature. Thus, at ventricular end-diastole following atrial contraction, the size of S-ASD reaches its minimal dimensions. In contrast, at ventricular end-systole, the S-ASD reaches its maximal dimensions due to atrial filling and the increase in atrial volume (Fig. 20.4).

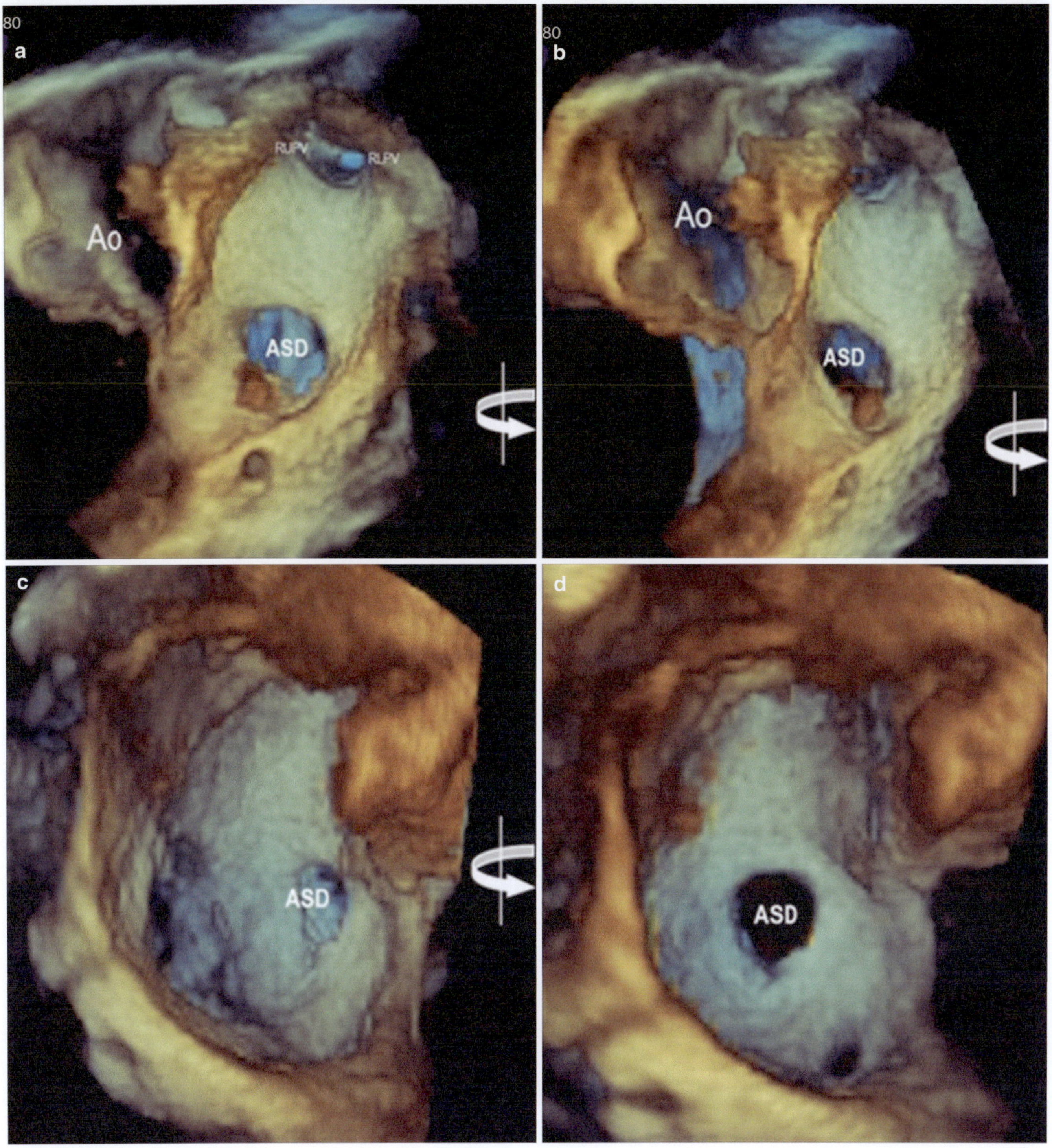

Fig. 20.3 3D TEE still images of a S-ASD shown in different angulations from LA (panel **a**), to RA (panel **d**). Panels **b** and **c** show intermediate images obtained by rotating the volumetric data set from right to left around the y-axis (curved arrows). LA, left atrium; RA, right atrium; Ao, ascending aorta; RLPV, right lower pulmonary vein; RUPV, right upper pulmonary vein

3D TEE color Doppler provides beautiful images of flow crossing the ASD, precisely delineating the margins of the defect (Fig. 20.5a, b). Moreover, color Doppler is invaluable for distinguishing between true defects and drop out artifacts (Figs. 20.5c, d and 20.6). In some cases, residual strands of the septum primum tissue may cross the S-ASD creating two or multiple defects (Figs. 20.5c, d and 20.6).

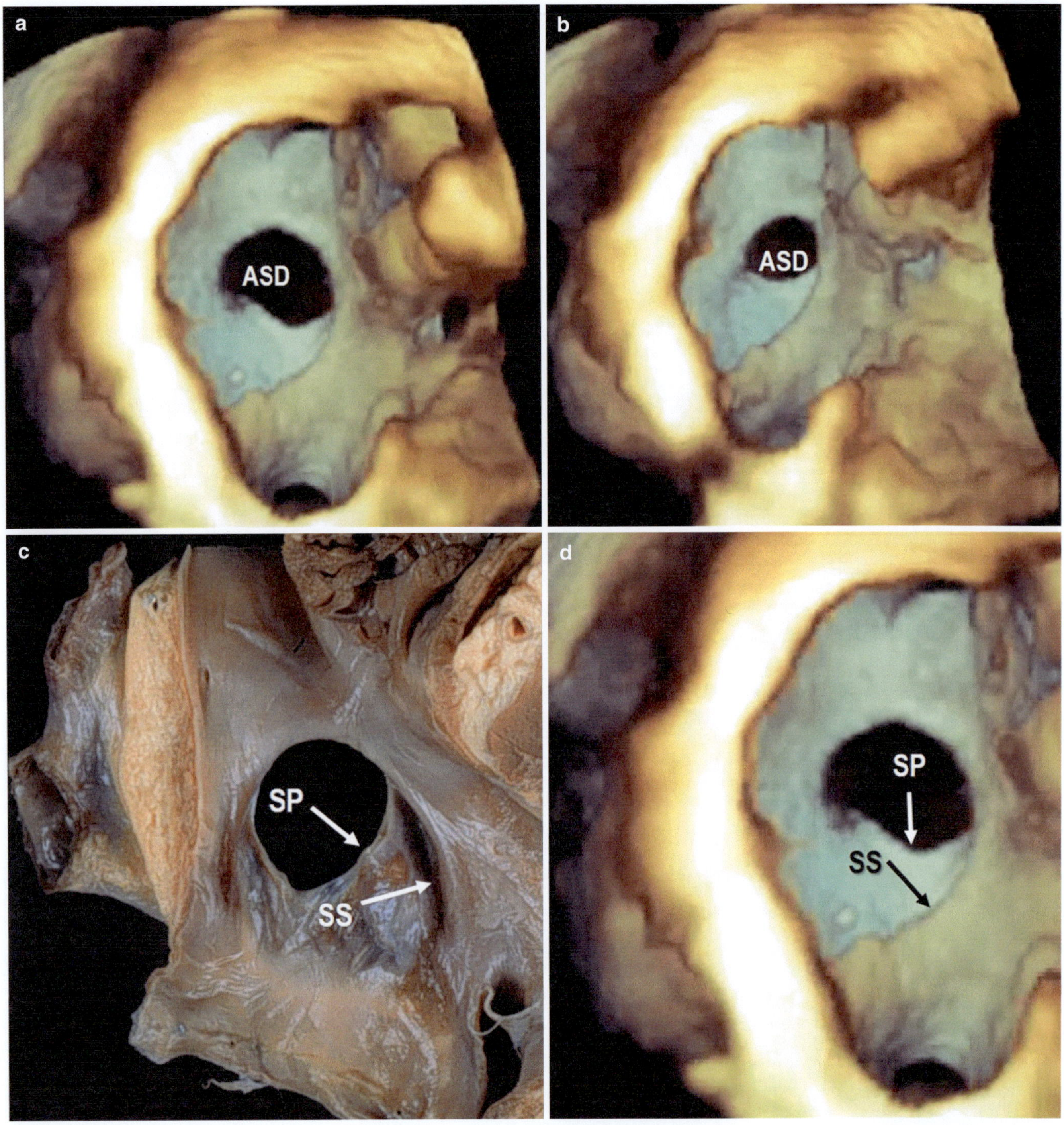

Fig. 20.4 3D images showing a secundum ASD from the right atrial perspective. The size of the defect varies significantly from atrial filling (panel **a**) to atrial contraction (Panel **b**). (**c**) Anatomic specimen (Courtesy of Dr. William D. Edwards –Mayo Clinic) and (**d**) similar 3D TEE image showing an ASD and malalignment of the septum primum (SP) and septum secundum (SS)

A new surface 3D rendering algorithm using a movable source of light creates shadowing that allows for delineating more clearly the margins of the defect. Figure 20.7a, b shows a S-ASD "illuminated" with this new rendering algorithm from the left and right atrial perspectives, while panels c and

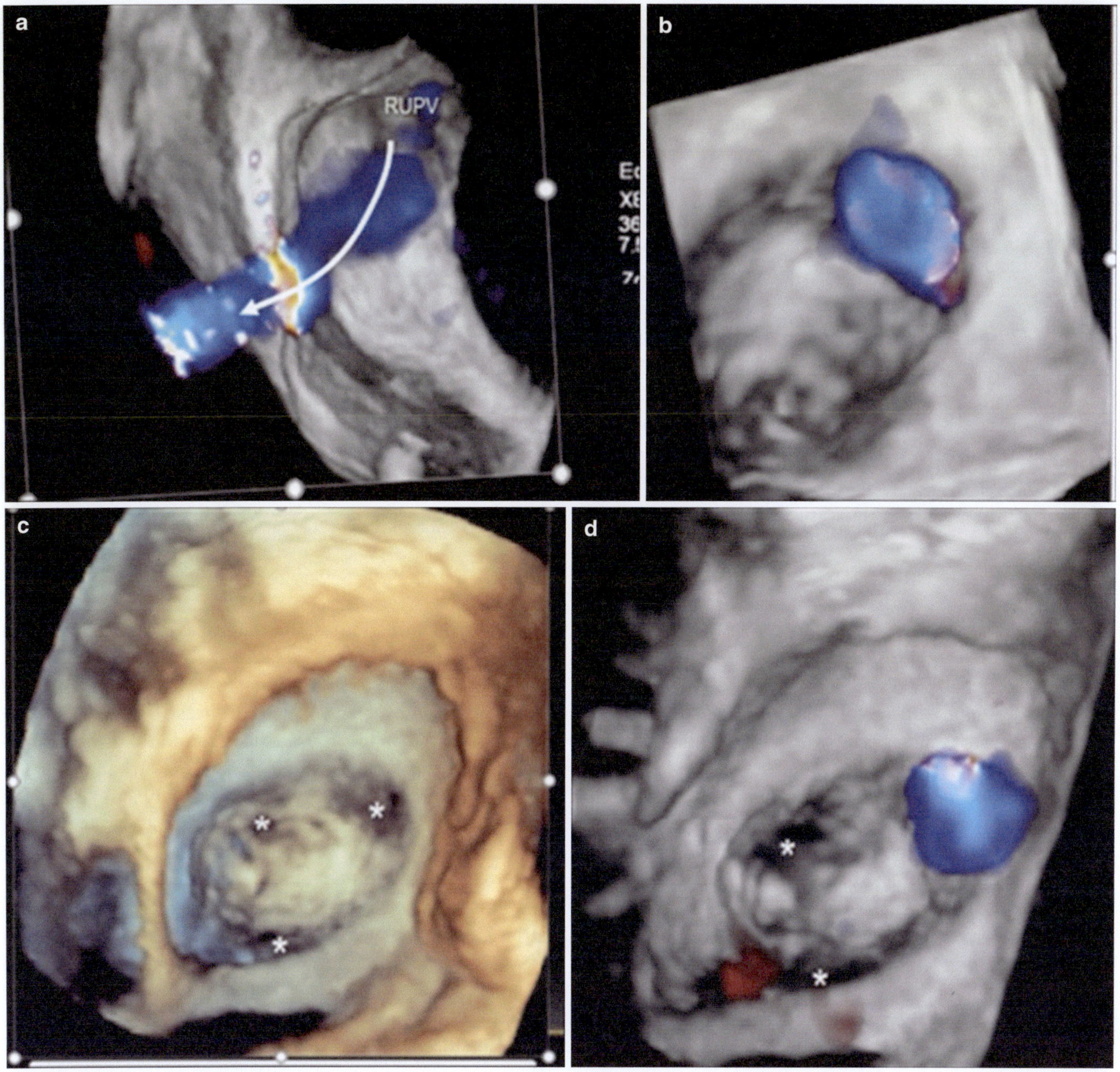

Fig. 20.5 3D TEE color Doppler showing (**a**) flow from the right upper pulmonary vein (RUPV) running through the S-ASD (curved arrow) from the left atrium (LA) to the right atrium (RA). (**b**) Flow crossing the ASD seen in "en face" view. The margins of the defect are well defined. (**c**) 3D TEE of the interatrial septum seen from a right atrial perspective. The image show three defects (asterisks). From this image it is difficult to establish the true ASD from drop-out artifacts (see text). (**d**) With color Doppler, the distinction is clear

d show the same S-ASD after percutaneous closure with an Amplatzer device.

Medium-sized S-ASDs (i.e. <30 mm of maximum diameter) with sufficient rims (2–5 mm) are amenable to percutaneous closure, while S-ASDs which exceed the above-mentioned dimensions should undergo surgical repair. Technical Details for percutaneous closure of S-ASD are described in Chap. 27.

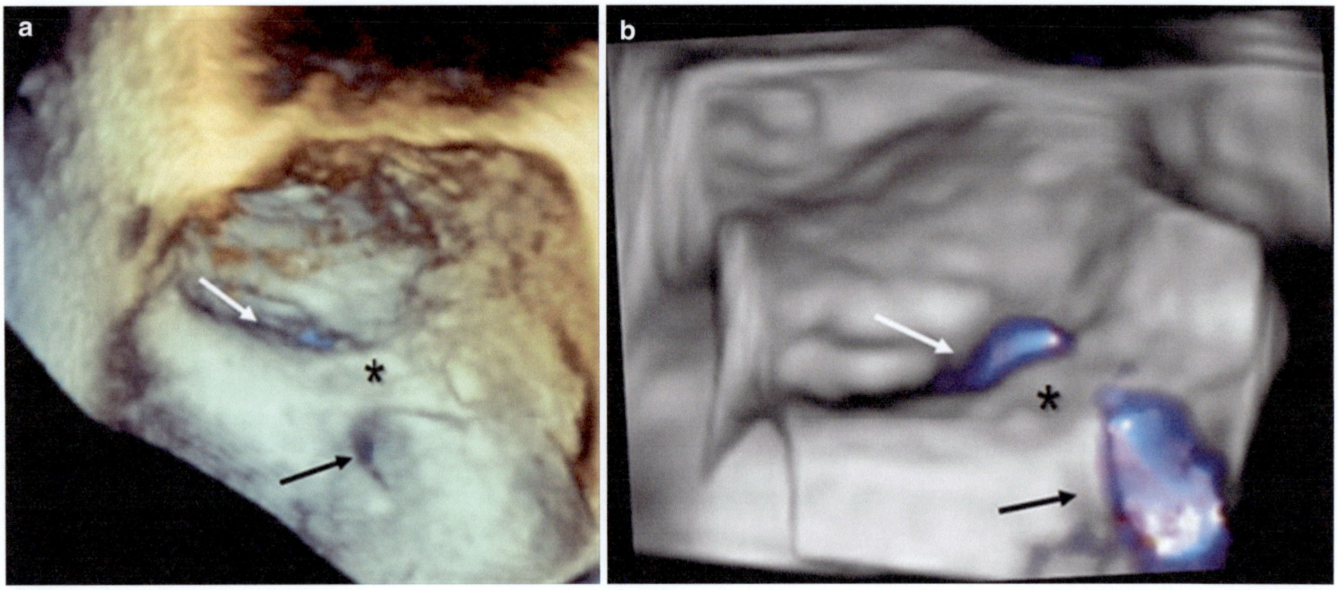

Fig. 20.6 3D TEE images without (**a**) and with (**b**) color Doppler showing a S-ASD divided by a string of septal tissue (asterisk) into two defects (arrows)

Sinus Venous Atrial Septal Defect

SV-ASD, originally described in 1858 by Peacock [6], encompasses approximately 4–11% of atrial septal defects and is situated at the interface between the right atrium (RA) and the embryological sinus venosus. About 80–90% of these defects are located immediately below the orifice of the superior vena cava (SVC; Fig. 20.8), while the remaining 10–20% are next to the orifice of the inferior vena cava (IVC). Both are very often associated with anomalous return of one or more pulmonary veins.

As described earlier, only the floor of the fossa ovalis (FO) is the true septum. Recognition of this particular anatomical architecture is important for making the distinction between septal and extra-septal communication. The anatomical configuration of SV-ASD is that of an interatrial-extra-septal-communication due to a deficiency outside the true septum. The orifice of the SVC (or IVC) overrides to various extents the enfolded muscular border of the FO. Typically, the right pulmonary veins open into the SVC near its junction with the right atrium producing an additional left-to-right shunt. However, this associated anomaly is not a "*conditio-sine-qua-non*" for the diagnosis of SV-ASD because abnormal connections of pulmonary veins are present in most but not in all SV-ASDs. SV-ASD close to the IVC is rare and often is difficult to distinguish from a large S-ASD extending posterior-inferior near the orifice of inferior vena cava. SV-ASD is typically associated with a large shunt that usually requires surgical or percutaneous closure [7].

Surgical correction is the standard of care and, until recently, was the only treatment option. The classic approaches are by median sternotomy or right anterolateral thoracotomy; however, other mini-invasive approaches are used as well in an effort to reduce morbidity. If the anomalous pulmonary venous drainage is to the atrium and adjacent to the ASD then the repair is relatively simple and the same as for secundum ASDs. In the presence of anomalous venous drainage into the superior vena cava, the so-call "two-patch technique" is required with one patch to close the ASD and one patch to close the right atriotomy at the caval-atrial junction in such a fashion as to avoid SVC-right atrial stenosis [8]. The overall survival is similar to that of matched population, with a low rate of perioperative morbidity and mortality and need for redo surgery. Post-operative symptomatic improvement occurs in the majority of patients. However, older age and class NYHA III or IV symptoms, are independent predictors of new-onset postoperative atrial fibrillation and late mortality.

More recently, a transcatheter repair technique consisting of a covered stent which replaces the deficient posterior wall of the SVC, closing the SV-ASD and redirecting the anomalous pulmonary veins into the LA, has been proposed. Suitability for transcatheter SV-ASD closure must be assessed by a multimodality stepwise approach, including evaluation with 2-dimensional and 3D cross-sectional imaging. Ex-vivo simulation of stent implantation with printed or virtual 3D models helps to avoid potential areas of residual shunt or obstruction to the pulmonary venous pathway

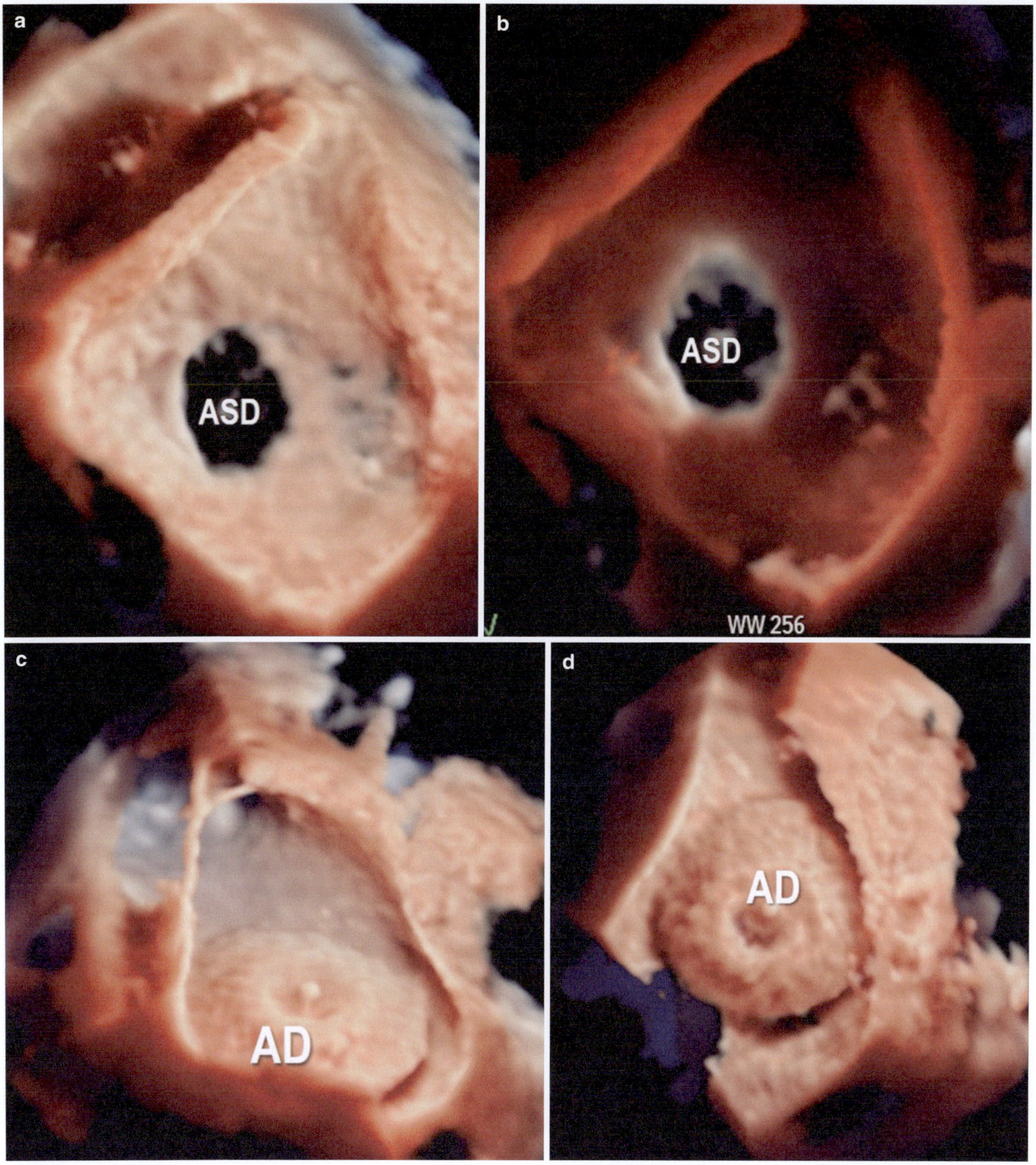

Fig. 20.7 3D TEE with a new rendering algorithm which uses a movable source of light showing an ASD from left (**a**) and right (**b**) atrial perspectives. This novel rendering modality allows highlighting of the ASD's well-defined margins. (**c** and **d**) Same patient after percutaneous closure with Amplatzer device (AD) shown from a slightly different perspective

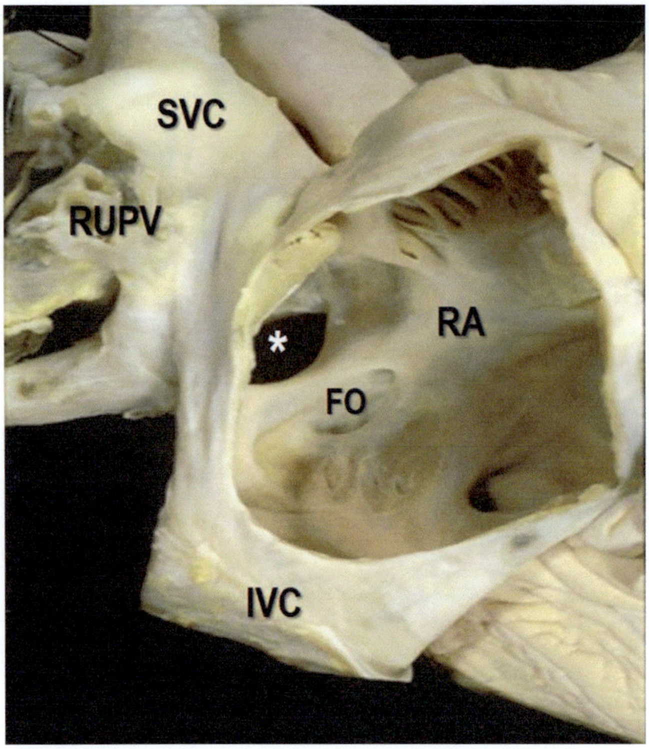

Fig. 20.8 Right-lateral view of right atrium in heart specimen showing separation of the superior SV-ASD (asterisk) from the fossa ovale (FO) by a muscular rim. IVC, inferior vena cava; FO, fossa ovalis; RA, right atrium; RUPV, right upper pulmonary vein; SVC, superior vena cava

behind the stent. Although in its infancy, percutaneous repair of SV-ASD may become, in suitable patients, an alternative to surgery [9, 10].

Coronary Sinus ASD

CS-ASD is the rarest form of interatrial communication accounting for <1% overall. The communication occurs between the left atrium (LA) and the coronary sinus (CS) as a result of a single or multiple focal fenestrations or complete absence of the left atrial wall and the adjoining wall of the CS channel [11]. The presence of a persistent left superior vena cava (LSVC) is almost constant in this form of atrial defect. The left-to-right shunt occurs because the oxygenated LA blood enters into the right atrium, through the incomplete roof of the CS. Associated anomalous pulmonary venous return has also been described. The clinical diagnosis is often difficult because of non-specific clinical features, and before the "echocardiographic era" the diagnosis was only possible during surgery or at autopsy. Angiographic study of the anomalous systemic venous connection was the procedure of choice for demonstration of the morphology as well as associated defects. Today the diagnosis relies on echocardiography or other imaging techniques. The presence of a dilated CS is an important clue for establishing the diagnosis. The communication between the LA and CS can be demonstrated by color Doppler, and injection of saline solution into a left arm peripheral vein will show microbubbles reaching the unroofed coronary sinus from the LSVC. More sophisticated imaging techniques such as 3D TEE or CMR, have facilitated the noninvasive diagnosis of UCS-ASD. Surgically patch closure can be accomplished through a left atriotomy. Very rarely the LSVC drains into the LA in absence of CS. Surgical closure is the only treatment option.

Primum ASD

Primum ASD (P-ASD) is part of a group of malformations called atrioventricular septal defects (AVSD), previously known as atrio-ventricular canal defect or endocardial cushion defect [12, 13]. The anatomic hallmark of AVSD is a common atrio- ventricular junction, upon which is inserted a single atrioventricular valve. The common junction being more or less oval in shape results in anterior displacement of the aortic outflow tract and 'unwedged' location of the aortic valve compared to the normal heart. The common atrioventricular valve consists of five leaflets (Fig. 20.9). Two of them (superior and inferior bridging leaflets) override the crest of the interventricular septum. Of the remaining three, one is inserted in the left segment (left mural leaflet) and the other two on the right segment (right inferior and right superior leaflets) of the common junction. In the case of primum ASD (also called partial AVSD), the superior and inferior bridging leaflets are fused with the crest of the interventricular septum, separating the common valve into two half valves and creating "de facto" two orifices (Fig. 20.9). Of note, the tissue continuity between the left and right segments of the bridging leaflets is maintained. As a consequence, the left half-valve comprises three leaflets: the half superior and inferior bridging leaflets and the mural left leaflet, thus it is misleading to label the left half valve as mitral valve. It is equally misleading to call the line of apposition between the left half of the two bridging leaflets a mitral valve "cleft". This line of apposition may close in systole effectively preventing any regurgitation or may leave a gap with consequent regurgitation. Similarly, the right half of the common valve has four leaflets: the two right segments of the bridging leaflets and the superior-anterior and posterior right leaflets. Thus, it is inappropriate to label this half valve as tricuspid.

As mentioned above, in P-ASD the bridging leaflets are fused directly on the crest of the interventricular septum, leaving only an interatrial communication. In some cases, the bridging leaflets adhere to the crest of the interventricular septum through short chordae. In such cases there may be a hemodynamically insignificant interventricular communication through the small spaces between chordae. By contrast, the bridging leaflets in the complete type of AVSD, as will be described in more details below, are not fused together and not adherent to the ventricular septum, thereby allowing for both interatrial and interventricular communications. A variant of this situation is the intermediate type in which the bridging leaflets are fused together, still permitting interatrial and interventricular communications. A further type of AVSD is when the bridging leaflets are fused to the free edge of the atrial septum, leaving an interventricular communication, which is similar to an inlet VSD. Finally, in rare cases, there is a fibrous membrane at the site of the defect without any detectable communication. These cases are erroneously labelled as isolated mitral valve cleft although they have all the other features of AVSD.

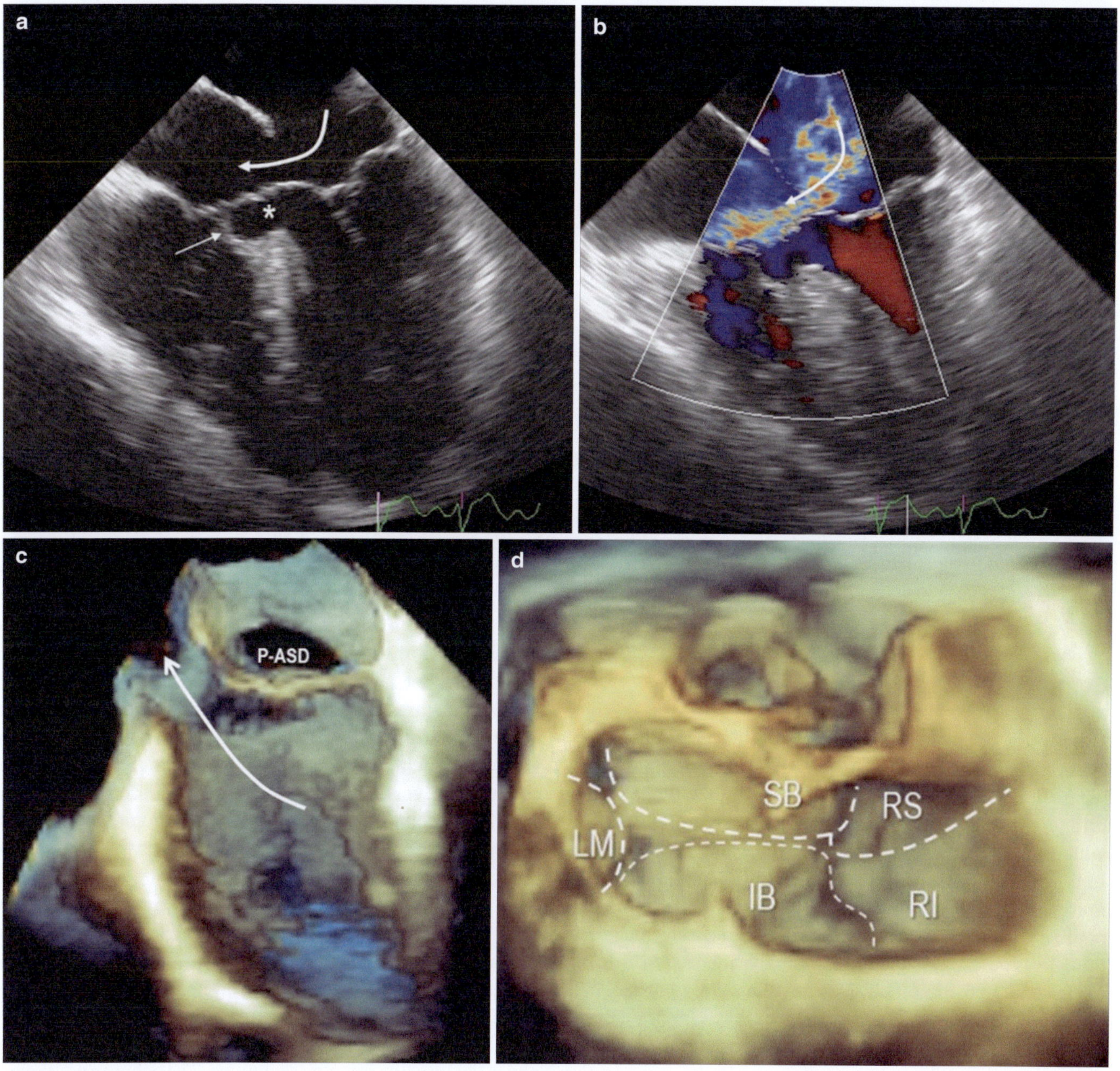

Fig. 20.9 (**a**) 2D TEE image four chamber cross-section view showing a P-ASD (curved arrow). The asterisk points at a previous small ventricular septal defect closed by valve tissue forming a small aneurysm (arrow). (**b**) Same image with color Doppler. (**c**) Primum ASD (P-ASD) seen "en face" from a left atrial perspective. The curved arrow outlines the elongated left ventricular outflow tract. (**d**) 3D Images from an atrial perspective showing the five leaflets: superior bridging (SB), inferior bridging (IB), left mural (LM) Right superior (RS) and right inferior (RI). In systole the coaptation line between leaflets is marked by a dotted line. (**e**) and (**f**) are anatomical specimens displayed in similar perspectives as (**c**) and (**d**). Note the elongated outflow tract in (**e**) and the 'unwedged' location of the aortic valve in (**f**)

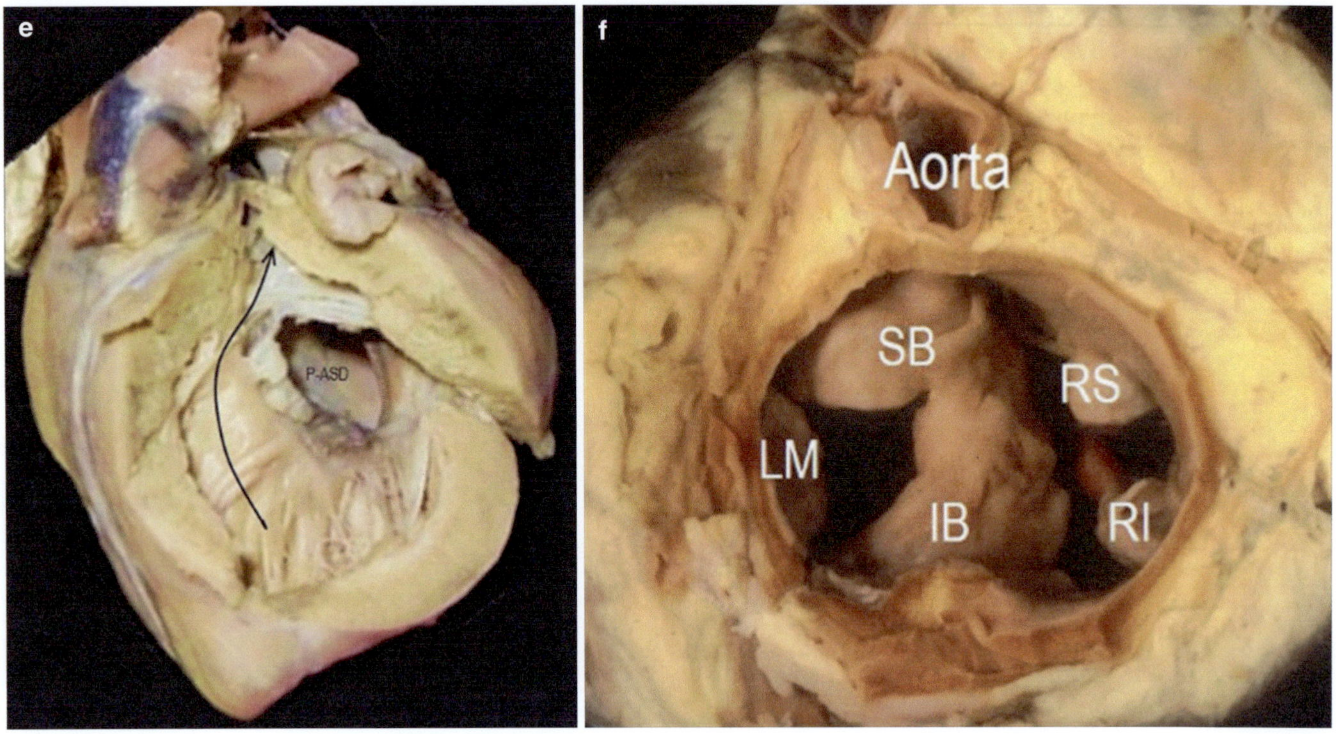

Fig. 20.9 (continued)

While in a normal heart the aorta is 'wedged' between the tricuspid and mitral orifices, in AVSD the aortic valve is displaced anteriorly in an unwedged position. This arrangement produces an elongated and intrinsically narrow aortic outflow tract giving the characteristic "goose-neck" appearance of the left ventricle seen on angiography.

Complete AVSD

Description of the patho-morphology of the complete AVSD, is beyond the scope of this chapter. Herein, for completeness, we include consideration of the extent that the superior bridging leaflet reaches into the right ventricular cavity which forms the basis for the revised Rastelli classification. In type A the superior (and anterior) bridging leaflet, shows minimal extension into the right ventricle and the medial papillary muscle (PM) is located in an almost normal position. In type B the superior bridging leaflet extends to an intermediate position (half guarding the right ventricle, half the left ventricle) and its right component is supported by an anomalous papillary muscle arising from the trabecula septomarginalis. Finally, in type C, the superior bridging leaflet extends more into the right than in the left cavity and its right component is supported by an anterior right PM arising from the right ventricular wall. In these cases, the bridging leaflet is often free floating. The variable morphology of the inferior bridging leaflet is not described based on the extent of leaflet tissue impingement upon the right ventricle. Indeed, from a surgical point of view, it is essential whether or not an interventricular communication is present underneath the leaflet. In all three modified Rastelli types, the posterior bridging leaflets is almost always attached to the crest of the interventricular septum either directly or by a short membrane or by chordae. Thus, usually the amount of shunt across the two ventricles mainly depends on the arrangement of the superior bridging leaflet.

Other features of AVSD should be addressed. For instance, the atrioventricular leaflets may appear dysplastic leading to valve regurgitation or stenosis. When more than 75% of the common valve is committed to one ventricle, the atrioventricular connection becomes by definition a double-inlet ventricle with a common valve. There may be a marked disproportion between the ventricles depending on whether or not the common AV valve may be dominantly committed to one or to another ventricle. In extreme cases one ventricle is too small to support the circulation and the anomaly shifts into the spectrum of hypoplastic left heart syndrome.

Although other non-invasive techniques may be useful to establish the diagnosis, it is indisputable that echocardiography is the first line imaging technique. The echocardiographic examination should establish: (a) the diagnosis of AVSD and the level of shunting (interatrial, interventricular or both); (b) the adequacy of ventricular sizes; (c) the regurgitation (or stenosis) of the common valve; (d) the function of both ventricles; (e) the presence of sub-aortic obstruction.

While 2D TTE and TEE are able to illustrate almost all the anomalies of AVSD, 3D TTE/TEE has the unique ability to show "en face" the defects that depict almost all the pathomorphological aspects of AVSD.

References

1. Hoffman JIE, Kaplan S. The incidence of congenital heart disease. J Am Coll Cardiol. 2002;39:1890–900.
2. Green CE, Gottdiener JS, Goldstein HA. Atrial septal defect. Semin Roentgenol. 1985;20(3):214–25.
3. Thompson E. Atrial septal defect. JAAPA. 2013;26(6):53–4.
4. Supomo S, Arjana AZ, Darmawan H. Predictive model for secundum atrial septal defect closure with pulmonary artery hypertension in adult: When to close. Heart Surg Forum. 2018;21(2):E108–11.
5. Naqvi N, McCarthy KP, Ho SY. Anatomy of the atrial septum and interatrial communications. J Thorac Dis. 2018;10(Suppl 24):S2837–47.
6. Peacock TB. Malformations of the heart. In: Peacock TB, editor. On Malformations, &c., of the human heart: With original cases. London: John Churchill; 1858. p. 11–102.
7. Attenhofer Jost CH, Connolly HM, Danielson GK, et al. Sinus venosus atrial septal defect: long-term postoperative outcome for 115 patients. Circulation. 2005;112(13):1953–8.
8. Elzein C, Abdulkarim M, Abbas U, Vricella L, Ilbawi M. Repair of superior sinus venosus atrial septal defect using a modified two-patch technique. Ann Thorac Surg. 2020;109(2):583–7.
9. Abdullah HAM, Alsalkhi HA, Khalid KA. Transcatheter closure of sinus venosus atrial septal defect with anomalous pulmonary venous drainage: Innovative technique with long-term follow-up. Catheter Cardiovasc Interv. 2020;95(4):743–7.
10. Riahi M, Velasco Forte MN, Byrne N, et al. Early experience of transcatheter correction of superior sinus venosus atrial septal defect with partial anomalous pulmonary venous drainage. EuroIntervention. 2018;14(8):868–76.
11. Zieliński P, Konka M, Hoffman P, Różański J, Michałowska I. Unroofed coronary sinus atrial septal defect. J Card Surg. 2019;34(1):41–2.
12. Sadeghi AM, Laks H, Pearl JM. Primum atrial septal defect. Semin Thorac Cardiovasc Surg. 1997;9(1):2–7.
13. Anderson RH, Mohun TJ, Brown NA. Clarifying the morphology of the ostium primum defect. J Anat. 2015;226(3):244–57.

CT and MRI Correlations of Atria and Atrial Septum

21

Prajwal Reddy, Korosh Sharain, Thomas A. Foley, and Nandan S. Anavekar

Patent foramen ovale (PFO) is the most commonly encountered atrial septal abnormality which is present in approximately 25% of adults [1, 2]. This finding is typically asymptomatic, but increases the risk of a paradoxical embolism in patients with large defects and those with atrial septal aneurysm. 2D transthoracic (TTE) and transesophageal echocardiography (TEE) are normally sufficient to detect these abnormalities. Given their asymptomatic nature, they are often incidentally noted and can be suspected on ECG-gated CT completed for other diagnoses such as coronary artery disease. A jet of contrast from the left to right atrium can suggest this abnormality (Figs. 21.1 and 21.2) [3].

Secundum and primum atrial septal defects (ASD) are typically well assessed with TTE and TEE. Sinus venosus ASD along with the associated partial anomalous venous connections (PAPVR) can be more challenging to identify. CT and MRI offer the added advantage of a comprehensive assessment of abnormal pulmonary venous drainage (Fig. 21.3). In addition, right ventricular size can be more accurately determined as this is often the indication for closure. Moreover, recent MRI studies have gone further to assess shunt fraction (Qp/Qs) with 4D flow MRI techniques [4, 5]. In recent years, as more percutaneous devices for closure of these defects became available computed tomography was found to be particularly useful in identifying post procedural complications such as access site issues or damage to surrounding structures following these interventions.

It is difficult to establish a tissue diagnosis for masses seen on TTE or TEE even with ultrasound enhancing agents. Pathologic diagnosis remains the gold standard; however MRI with tissue characterization can narrow the differential diagnosis. Versatility of imaging planes, assessment of cardiac and extra cardiac structures, analysis of tissue characteristics with T1 and T2 weighted images, and contrast enhancement improve the diagnostic power in assessment of atrial masses (Figs. 21.4 and 21.5) [6, 7].

P. Reddy
Cardiovascular Disease, Mayo Clinic, Rochester, MN, USA
e-mail: reddy.prajwal@mayo.edu

K. Sharain
Assistant Professor in Medicine, Mayo Clinic College of Medicine; Resident, Department of Cardiovascular Medicine, Mayo Clinic, Rochester, MN, USA
e-mail: sharain.korosh@mayo.edu

T. A. Foley
Assistant Professor of Radiology, Mayo Clinic College of Medicine; Consultant, Division of Cardiovascular Radiology, Department of Radiology, Mayo Clinic, Rochester, MN, USA
e-mail: foley.thomas@mayo.edu

N. S. Anavekar (✉)
Professor of Medicine, Mayo Clinic College of Medicine; Consultant, Department of Cardiovascular Medicine, Mayo Clinic, Rochester, MN, USA
e-mail: anavekar.nandan@mayo.edu

J. F. Maalouf et al. (eds.), *Practical 3D Echocardiography*, https://doi.org/10.1007/978-3-030-72941-7_21

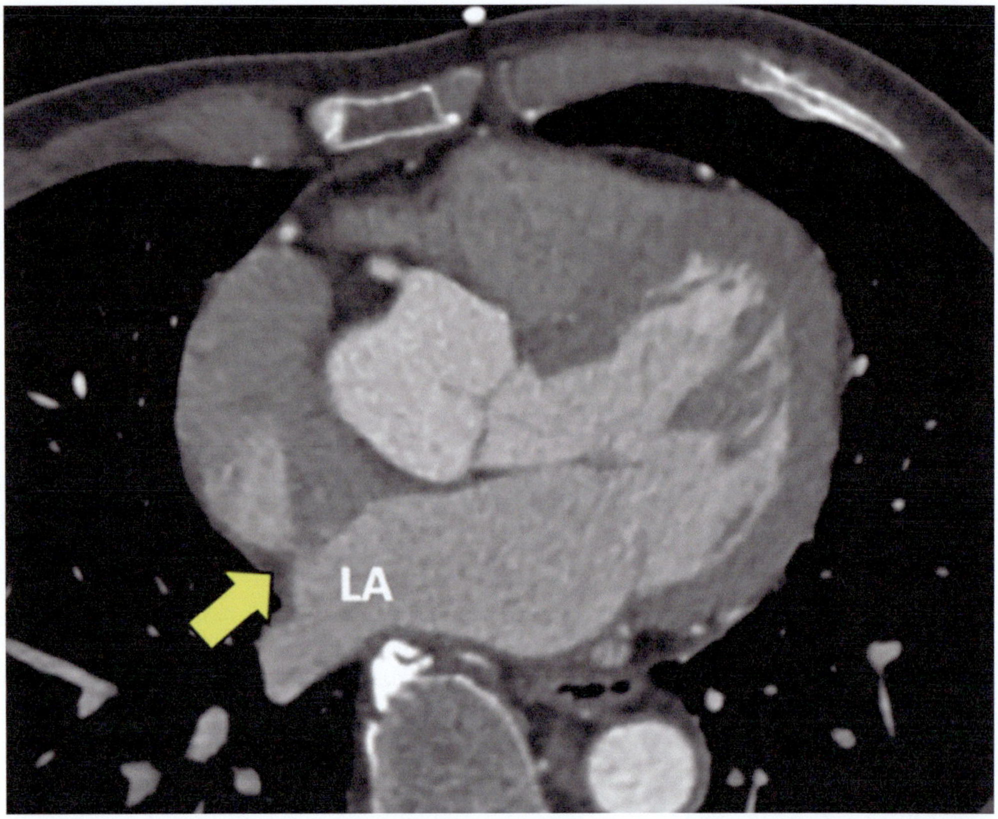

Fig. 21.1 An intermediate risk female with atypical chest pain underwent cardiac CTA to evaluate her coronary arteries. On cine imaging contrast is seen squirting from the left atrium to the right atrium consistent with a patent foramen ovale (yellow arrow). She did not have any coronary artery disease. The cause for her chest pain was not forthcoming on the examination. Used with permission of Mayo Foundation for Medical Education and Research. All rights reserved. LA, left atrium

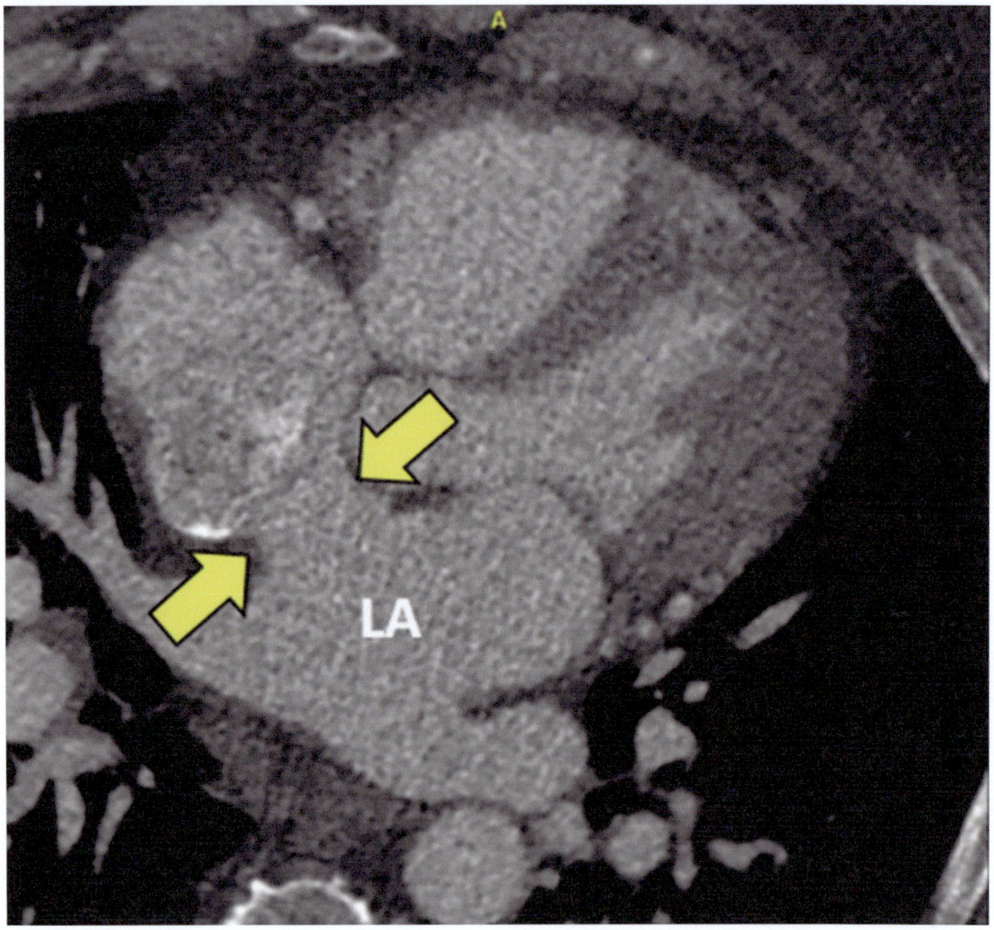

Fig. 21.2 A middle-aged male was found to have a secundum ASD on transthoracic echocardiography. He underwent cardiac CT for further evaluation of the defect along with preoperative coronary evaluation. The patient had a 3 cm secundum ASD (arrows). He had no coronary artery disease. He underwent surgical patch closure. Used with permission of Mayo Foundation for Medical Education and Research. All rights reserved. LA, left atrium

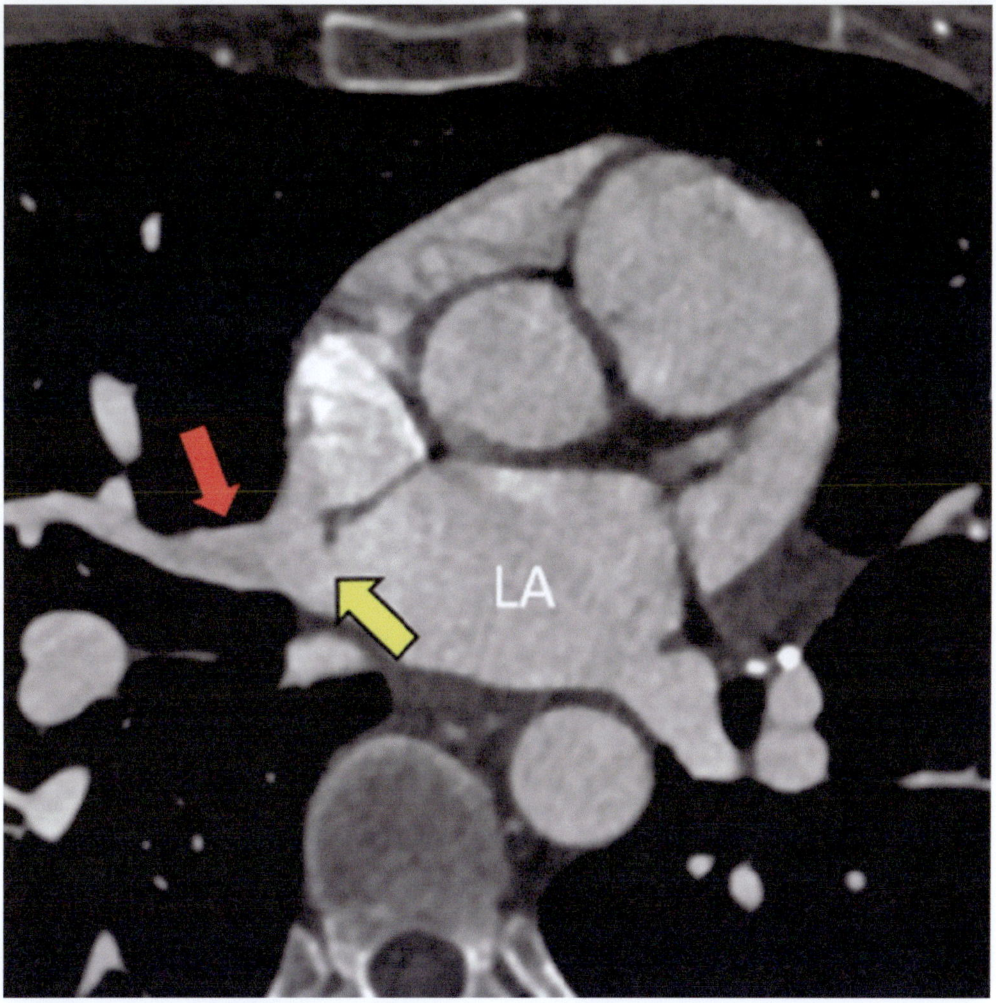

Fig. 21.3 A middle-aged female underwent transthoracic echocardiography after accessory pathway ablation. Her right ventricle appeared larger in size compared to an echocardiogram from 2 years prior. Saline bubble study was positive for right to left shunt with near-simultaneous opacification of both atria suggestive of sinus venosus atrial septal defect. Computed tomography was performed to evaluate the level of the shunt and evaluate for partial anomalous pulmonary venous return (PAPVR). The CT identified a sinus venosus ASD (yellow arrow) with PAPVR of the right upper pulmonary vein (red arrow). Given the enlarging right ventricle, the patient underwent ASD patch closure and baffling of the PAPVR into the left atrium. Used with permission of Mayo Foundation for Medical Education and Research.

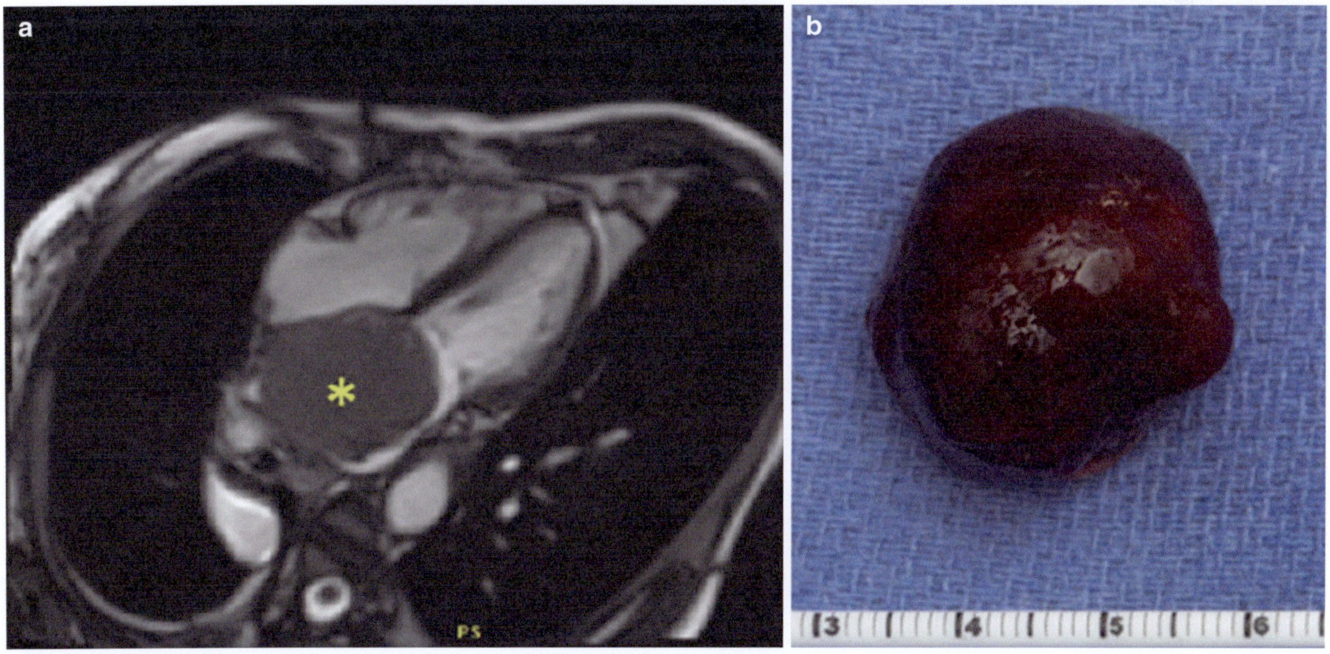

Fig. 21.4 An elderly female with night sweats and weight loss was found to have a large left atrial mass on transthoracic echocardiography. Cardiac MRI was obtained for further tissue characterization. Steady state free precession imaging identified the large left atrial mass (**a**; yellow asterisk). The mass arose from the interatrial septum, and was hypointense on T1-weighted images, hyperintense on T2-weighted imaging, and had heterogeneous gadolinium enhancement. These findings were consistent with myxoma which was confirmed on pathology (**b**; gross surgical specimen). Used with permission of Mayo Foundation for Medical Education and Research. LA, left atrium; ASD, atrial septal defect

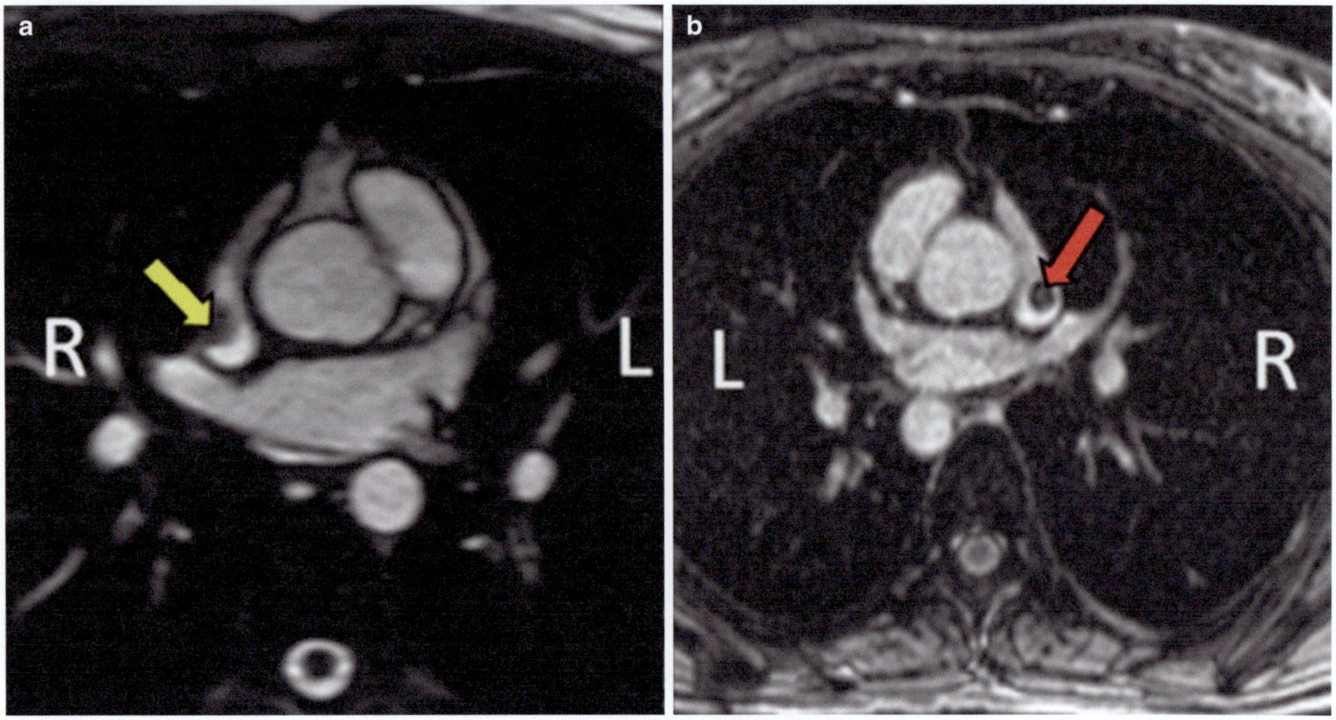

Fig. 21.5 A middle-aged female with metastatic malignant melanoma underwent cardiac MRI after PET scan demonstrated indeterminate FDG uptake in the right atrium. MRI demonstrated a 10 mm T2 hyper-intense mass at the junction of superior right atrium just distal to the superior vena cava (**a**; yellow arrow) with mild central gadolinium enhancement within the mass (**b**; red arrow) suggestive of malignant etiology and most suspicious for metastatic melanoma given the patient's history. Used with permission of Mayo Foundation for Medical Education and Research. All rights reserved. L, left; R, right

References

1. Nicolay S, et al. CT imaging features of atrioventricular shunts: what the radiologist must know. Insights Imaging. 2016;7(1):119–29.
2. Jujo T, et al. Importance of carefully interpreting computed tomography images to detect partial anomalous pulmonary venous return. Respir Investig. 2016;54(1):69–74.
3. Kim YJ, et al. Patent foramen ovale: diagnosis with multidetector CT--comparison with transesophageal echocardiography. Radiology. 2009;250(1):61–7.
4. Chelu RG, et al. Evaluation of atrial septal defects with 4D flow MRI-multilevel and inter-reader reproducibility for quantification of shunt severity. MAGMA. 2019;32(2):269–79.
5. Yamasaki Y, et al. One-stop shop assessment for atrial septal defect closure using 256-slice coronary CT angiography. Eur Radiol. 2017;27(2):697–704.
6. Lapinskas T, et al. Cardiac MRI quantitative tissue characterization of right atrial mass using mDixon and parametric mapping. Clin Res Cardiol. 2017;106(10):840–5.
7. Motwani M, et al. MR imaging of cardiac tumors and masses: a review of methods and clinical applications. Radiology. 2013;268(1):26–43.

Part IV

Ventricles and Ventricular Septum

How to Acquire and Calculate 3D LV and RV Volumes and Ejection Fraction (Three Vendors)

22

Hyun Suk Yang and Krishnaswamy Chandrasekaran

Introduction

Left and right ventricular chamber quantification is essential in clinical practice. The current techniques have limitations in meeting this need and 3-dimensional echocardiography (3DE) is increasingly utilized for this purpose [1, 2]. For assessment of left ventricular (LV) and right ventricular (RV) morphology and function, three acquisition modes can be chosen: (1) simultaneous multiple two-dimensional (2D) planes, (2) live or single-beat 3D full-volume (large volume), and (3) multi-beat ECG-gated 3D acquisition.

Although Live or real time 3D (that is, single-beat) imaging grants freedom from stitch artifacts and expands the applications beyond regular rhythm, chamber quantification involves acquisition of a large 3D volumetric data set which often leads to insufficient volumes per second (VPS) when acquired Live. Hence the usual need for multi-beat (typically 6) ECG-gated 3D Full Volume (Philips Healthcare) or Large (GE Healthcare) acquisition. Subsequent 3D analysis offers better visualization and quantification of chamber volumes and function without speculative geometric assumptions. Furthermore, the advances in 3D myocardial deformation analysis allow more accurate and reproducible results than conventional 2D strain analysis [3]. The EAE/ASE recommendations [4] are helpful for beginners in 3D echocardiography; this section will discuss a few more recent developments and practical tips for 3D echo to assess LV and RV volume and function.

Supplementary Information The online version of this chapter (https://doi.org/10.1007/978-3-030-72941-7_22) contains supplementary material, which is available to authorized users.

H. S. Yang
Professor, Research institute of Medical Science, Konkuk University School of Medicine, Department of Cardiovascular Medicine, Konkuk University Medical Center, Neungdong-ro, Gwangjin-gu, Seoul, Korea
e-mail: yang.hyun@kuh.ac.kr

K. Chandrasekaran (✉)
Professor of Medicine, Mayo Clinic College of Medicine; Consultant, Department of Cardiovascular Medicine, Mayo Clinic, Rochester, MN, USA
e-mail: kchandra@mayo.edu

Left Ventricle

Three commercially available echocardiographic platforms (EPIQ CVx, Vivid E95, and Acuson SC2000) are summarized in Table 22.1. Traditionally one must change probes from 2D to 3D, but many newer systems with newer probes (e.g., the GE 4Vc and Philips X5–1 TTE probes, and all TEE probes) dispose of this requirement. Although both transthoracic and transesophageal approaches are feasible for LV imaging, clinically one of the major functions of TTE is LV function assessment, and so this chapter will focus on 3D TTE for LV volumetric or functional analysis. After proper image acquisition, 3D volume data can be stored digitally for on-cart or offline analysis using vendor-specific software (QLAB; EchoPAC; SC2000 workplace) or TomTec workstation (TomTec 4D-LV function, Munich, Germany). The vendor-specific analysis features are summarized in Table 22.2.

Image Acquisition

For 3D LV imaging, three different modes can be applied using a vendor-specific transducer (Table 22.1). Switching the probe from 2D to 3D is necessary for GE or Siemens 3D TTE; continuous 3D imaging following 2D without changing transducers works with all 3D transesophageal probes and the Philips 3D TTE probe. Optimization of 2D images, focusing on the desired target anatomy (adjusting depth, sector angle; gain, compression, and time-gain compensation) with an ECG signal is crucial for optimal 3D image acquisition.

J. F. Maalouf et al. (eds.), *Practical 3D Echocardiography*, https://doi.org/10.1007/978-3-030-72941-7_22

Table 22.1 3D LV volume acquisition

	PHILIPS	GE	SIEMENS
Model	EPIQ CVx (Philips healthcare, Andover, MA)	Vivid E95 (GE Healthcare, Wauwatosa, WI)	ACUSON SC2000 (Siemens Healthcare Mountain view, CA)
3D TTE probe	X5-1 (combined 2D/3D)	4Vc (combined 2D/3D)	4Z1c
3D TEE probe	X8-2T	6VT-D	Z6Ms
Acquisition			
Bi- or tri-plane	xPlane (biplane), iRotate	Multi-D (bi-,triplane)	Bi-plane+ (TEE)
Single-beat 3D full volume	[HM ACQ] single-beat on A4C (includes LA)	[4D default] single-beat	[4D default] single-beat; 3–5 cardiac cycles
Sector, L × E	Up to 100° × 100°	Medium: 35° × 35°large: 60° × 60°; up to 90° × 90°	Up to 90° × 90°
VPS	22 (80° × 80°, 15 cm) 25 (70° × 70°, 15 cm)	12–24 (80° × 80°, 12 cm) 15–30 (70° × 70°, 12 cm)	T2: 51 (90° × 90°, 12 cm) T1: 35 (80° × 80°, 12 cm) T1: 51 (70° × 70°, 12 cm)
ECG gated 3D full volume	4 or 6 beats	2, 3, 4, or 6 beats	No
Sector, L × E	Up to 100° × 95°	Up to 90° × 90°	
VPS (4 beats)	46 (80° × 80°, 12 cm) 68 (70° × 70°, 12 cm)	23 (80° × 80°, 12 cm) 31 (70° × 70°, 12 cm)	
VPS (6 beats)	56 (80° × 80°, 12 cm) 100 (70° × 70°, 12 cm)	34 (80° × 80°, 12 cm) 52 (70° × 70°, 12 cm)	

The VPS expressed as number (sector L × E, depth). T1 and T2, grades of temporal resolution (T1 < T2). Used with permission of Mayo Foundation for Medical Education and Research.

Abbreviations: *3D* three-dimensional, *TTE* transthoracic echocardiography, *TEE* transesophageal echocardiography, *L × E* Lateral plane sector angle × Elevation plane sector angle, *VPS* volume per second, *ECG* electrocardiography, *2D* two-dimensional, *LA* left atrium

Bi- or Triplane Mode

The key to biplane or triplane imaging using a 3D probe is making optimal cut-off planes in the same cardiac cycle, thereby shortening imaging time [5] and overcoming rhythm disturbances. Biplane with various angles of approach are feasible on the EPIQ CVx (x-Plane or iRotate); triplane images are available with the Vivid E95 (Fig. 22.1).

Table 22.2 3D LV volume analysis

Analysis	PHILIPS	GE	SIEMENS
Workstation	QLAB	EchoPAC	SC2000 workplace
3D cropping	iCrop, quick Vue	2 click-crop, 4D views	D' art
Extract 2D slices	iSlice, MultiSlice	FlexiSlice, MultiSlice	3 × 3 screen
LV volume software	HeartModel[A.I.]	4D auto LVQ	eSie LVA
LV EDV, ESV, EF	**HMQ**: Single-beat 3D (A4C); fully automated; global or regional editing (ED, ES); LA volume (ES); analysis of up to 5 cardiac cycles **3DQ**: Template mitral annulus and LV apex (ED, ES) from biplane MOD volume; manual editing	3D full-volume (VPS >12); align views; auto initial or two-click points of apex and mid-base (ED, ES) to define endocardial border; regional editing; volume waveform; followed by LV mass and strain	Single-beat 3D (VPS >20); one-click fully automated; consecutive beat-to-beat LV volume, and EF (3 cardiac cycles)
LV EDV, ESV, EF, timing, dyssynchrony index	**3DQ-adv**: Single-beat or gated 3D; manual MPR axis align; five reference points of the mitral septal, lateral, anterior, inferior annulus, apex (ED, ES) from the biplane volume; manual editing; sequence analysis		
LV mass	**HMQ:** Check "compute LV mass"; ED mass **3DQ**: Go to preference to check display LV mass; endocardial and epicardial border ROI from the biplane volume	LV mass: Editing epicardial border at ED	No
3D/4D strain	No	4D strain ROI: Editing epicardial border at ES (VPS >25)	No
Characteristics	– TrueVue, light source – HMQ: Fully automatic LV as well as LA volume	– True confocal imaging – HDlive imaging – Laser lines	– Sequential 3 beats EF – 3D color analysis – eSie flow

Used with permission of Mayo Foundation for Medical Education and Research.

Abbreviations: *3D* three-dimensional, *2D* two-dimensional, *LV* left ventricular, *EDV* end-diastolic volume, *ESV* end-systolic volume, *EF* ejection fraction, *4D* four-dimensional, *A4C* apical 4-chamber view, *LA* left atrium, *ED* end-diastole, *ES* end-systole, *MOD* the Simpson rule method of discs, *MPR* multi-planar reconstruction, *VPS* volume per second, *ROI* region of interest

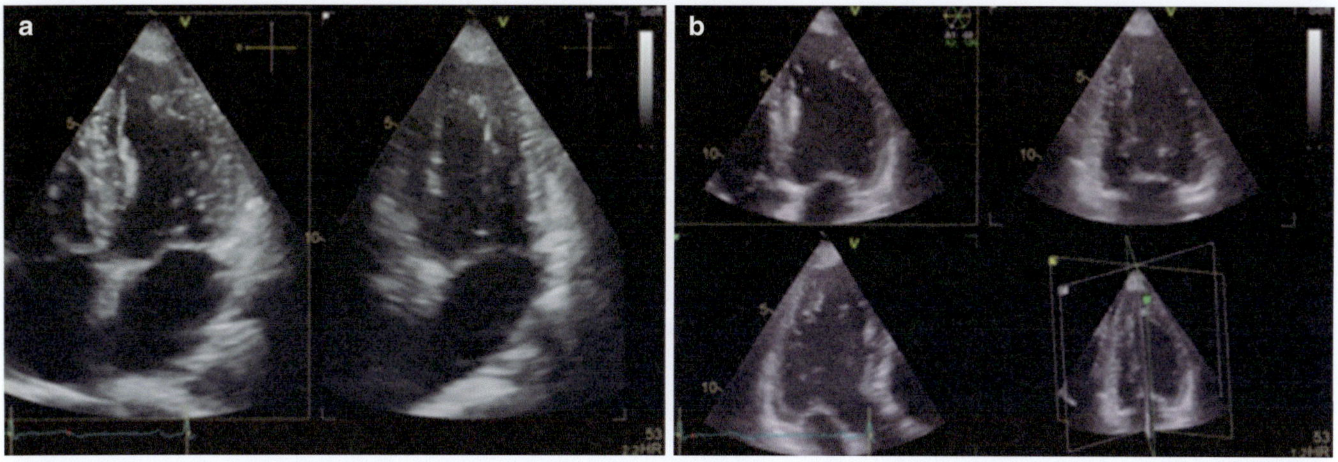

Fig. 22.1 Simultaneous biplane (**a**) and triplane (**b**) imaging using 3D transthoracic echo probe. Used with permission of Mayo Foundation for Medical Education and Research.

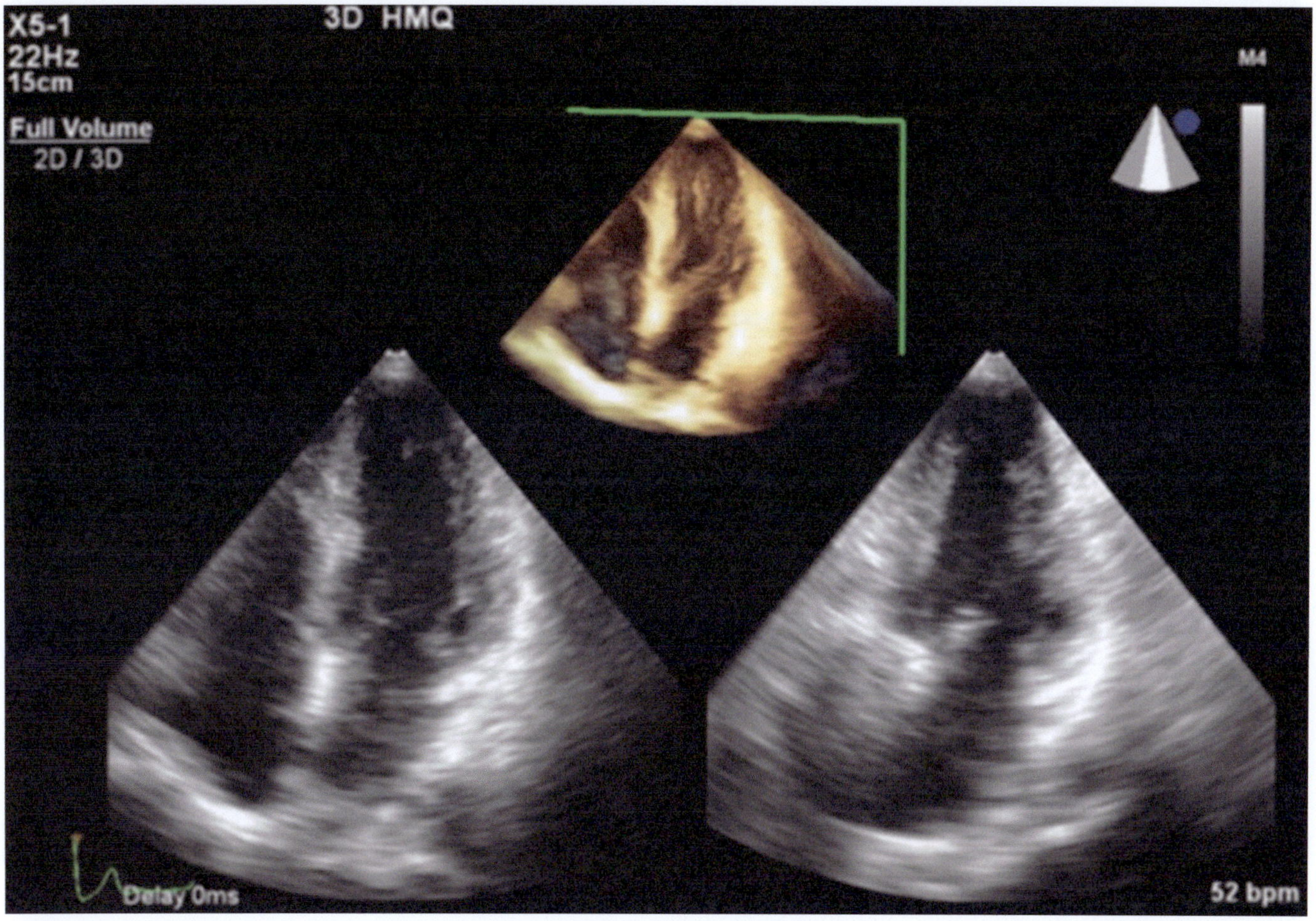

Fig. 22.2 Biplane-guided 3D Full-Volume acquisition (Left bottom, lateral plane; Right bottom, elevation plane). Used with permission of Mayo Foundation for Medical Education and Research.

Live 3D or Single-Beat 3D Full-Volume Mode

First, from the LV focused apical four chamber orientation, imaging depth and sector angle should be optimized. Fundamentally, the minimum depth and sector angle necessary to encompass the LV cavity will achieve the highest possible volumes per second (VPS). It is important to make sure the sector angle is sufficient to enclose the whole LV chamber, along with the biplane (Philips, GE) or triplane (Siemens) guided previsioned 3D before the volume acquisition (Fig. 22.2). Care must be taken to avoid common drop-

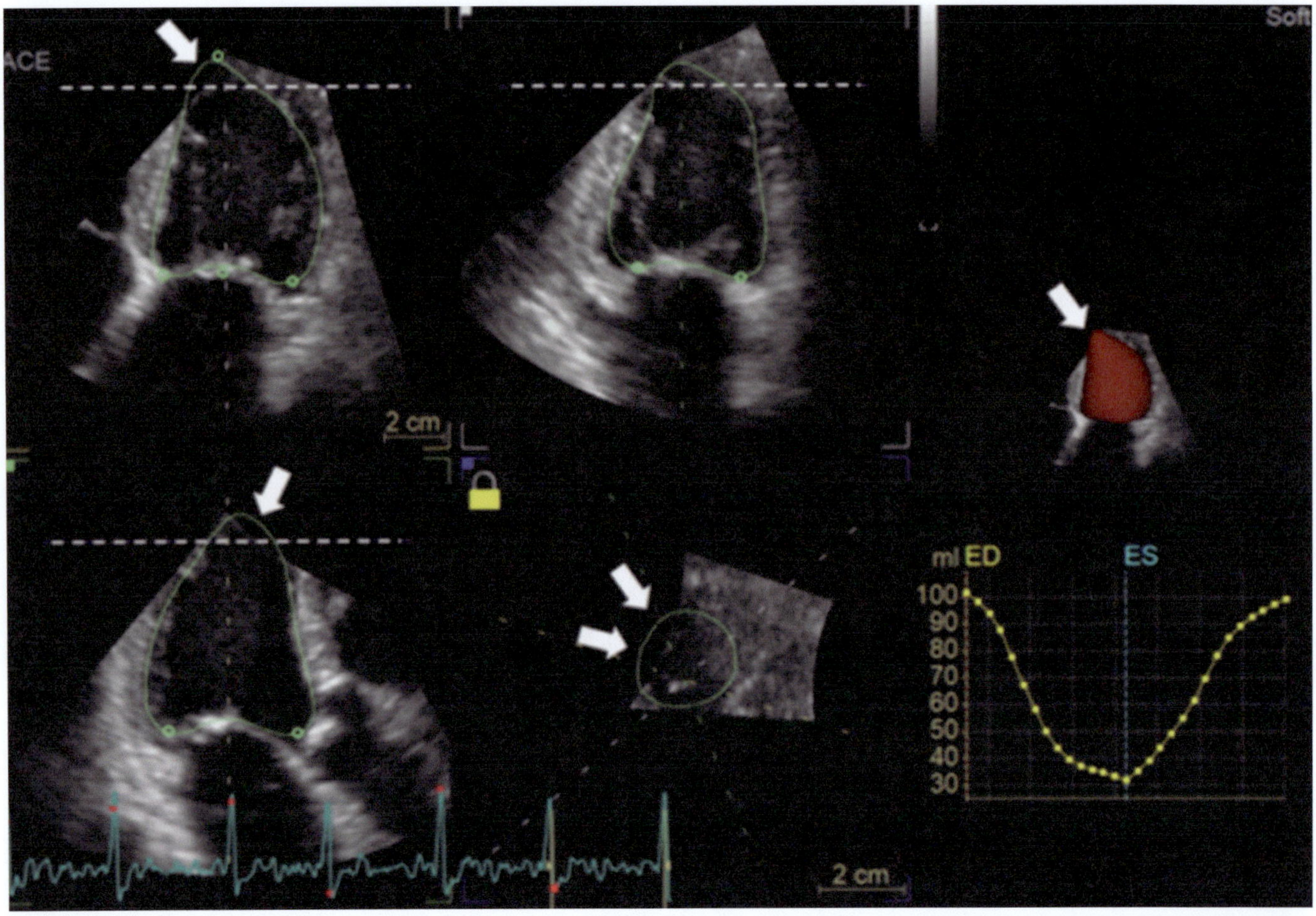

Fig. 22.3 Dropout artifacts in some part of the left ventricular apex (arrows). Used with permission of Mayo Foundation for Medical Education and Research.

out artifacts in the LV apex or lateral wall (Fig. 22.3). A breath-hold is not required for live 3D acquisition. **Second,** vendor-specific features should be considered. With the EPIQ CVx (Philips Healthcare), the depth should be adjusted also to include the left atrium from the standard apical four-chamber window, and acquiring five consecutive cardiac cycles with a breath-hold is required for beat-to-beat analysis; using the Vivid E95 (GE Healthcare), LV strain measurement feature requires at least 25 VPS, sometimes requiring a frame-rate-knob adjustment. The depth adjustment is not necessary with Vivid 95 (GE Healthcare). With the Acuson SC2000 (Siemens), obtain live 3D full-volume images for at least three consecutive cardiac cycles from the apical four chamber orientation for subsequent beat-to-beat ejection fraction (EF) analysis. With Vivid 95, it is important to check in multislice whether the LV fits into the chosen 4D sector size. **Third**, in patients with atrial fibrillation, due to the greater cardiac motion complexity, acquiring at least five consecutive cardiac beats with a breath-hold is recommended, either for trimming a proper single cardiac cycle (Philips, or GE) or averaging three cardiac cycles (Siemens).

Multi-Beat ECG-Gated 3D Large(GE) or Full-Volume(Philips) Mode

The acquisition should be performed during a breath-hold and requires a relatively stable R–R interval to minimize translation artifacts (Fig. 22.4) between the acquired sub-volumes. This multi-beat (2–6 beats) acquisition is required especially in patients with dilated cardiomyopathy if a wide-angle, single-beat, Large or Full-Volume scan cannot achieve sufficient VPS, or even in regional scans to get higher temporal resolution. Among the vendors, the Acuson SC2000 has the highest VPS to accommodate the LV in a single-beat, up to 51 (90° × 90°, at 12 cm depth), not necessarily requiring ECG-gated multi-beat acquisition.

Data Analysis

Visualization of Segmental LV Wall Motion

From the LV volume, nine parallel, simultaneous, uniformly spaced 2D slices can be extracted horizontally (iSlice and MultiSlice, Philips) or arbitrarily orientated (MultiSlice, GE)

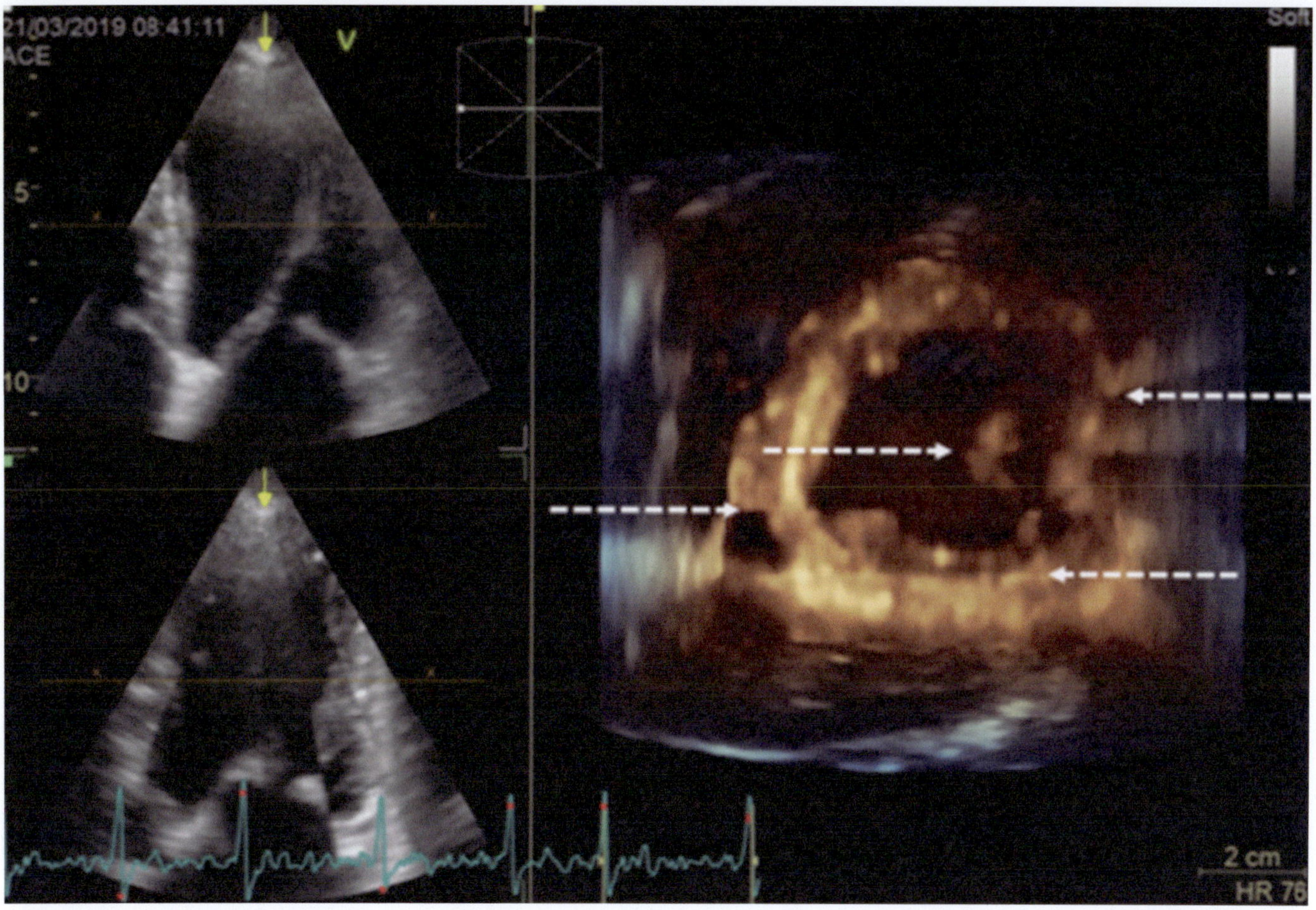

Fig. 22.4 Stich artifacts (arrows) on a multibeat ECG-gated 3D acquisition (GE Healthcare). Used with permission of Mayo Foundation for Medical Education and Research.

(Fig. 22.5). This facilitates detailed visual evaluation of LV regional wall motion abnormalities.

LV Volume, Ejection Fraction (EF), and Dyssynchrony

LV volume and function quantification is the main purpose of 3D transthoracic echocardiography [1, 2]. Freeing medical analysis from visual foreshortening or sometimes-inaccurate geometric assumptions, 3D is more accurate and reliable than 2D and well-validated with cardiac magnetic resonance (CMR). Despite its superiority over 2D in visual presentation, its time-consuming quantification workflow has hampered its use in clinical practice. Fortunately, recent developments of fully automatic quantification algorithms and "artificial intelligence" for ultrasound make 3D quantification easy, fast, and reproducible. The vendor-specific software features are summarized in Table 22.2.

Philips' new artificial intelligence model-based algorithm output (HeartModel, Philips Ultrasound) is shown in Fig. 22.6. From a single-beat 3D Full-Volume scan, just click one-button (HM ACQ) to produce preliminary output of LV volumes {both end-diastole (ED) and end-systole (ES), stroke volume (SV), EF, and left atrial volume [6, 7]}. If the initial contours are not satisfactory, global or regional editing is available for the 12 LV planes (apical or short axis; ED or ES). Beat-to-beat volume and EF quantification are also available, incorporating a maximum of five beats. For regional timing or synchronicity, 3DQ Adv (Philips Healthcare) software is helpful with a higher frame rate Full-Volume scan (such as multi-beat ECG-gated 3D Full-Volume image), as follows: (1) Find the ED frame and manually align the multi-planar reconstruction (MPR) axis, (2) Enter five ED reference points (septal, lateral, anterior, inferior and apex) and edit borders if necessary, (3) Find the ES frame, (4) Enter five ES reference points, and finally (5) Click Sequence Analysis (Fig. 22.7).

GE Healthcare's automatic LV analysis software (4D Auto LVQ) produces results presented in Fig. 22.8. Using a 3D Large volume scan (VPS > 12), the software sequentially offers output ranging from 3D LV volume and mass computation to the 3D strain [3, 8]. It begins with volumetric analysis: (1) Manually align views, (2) Select the endocardial

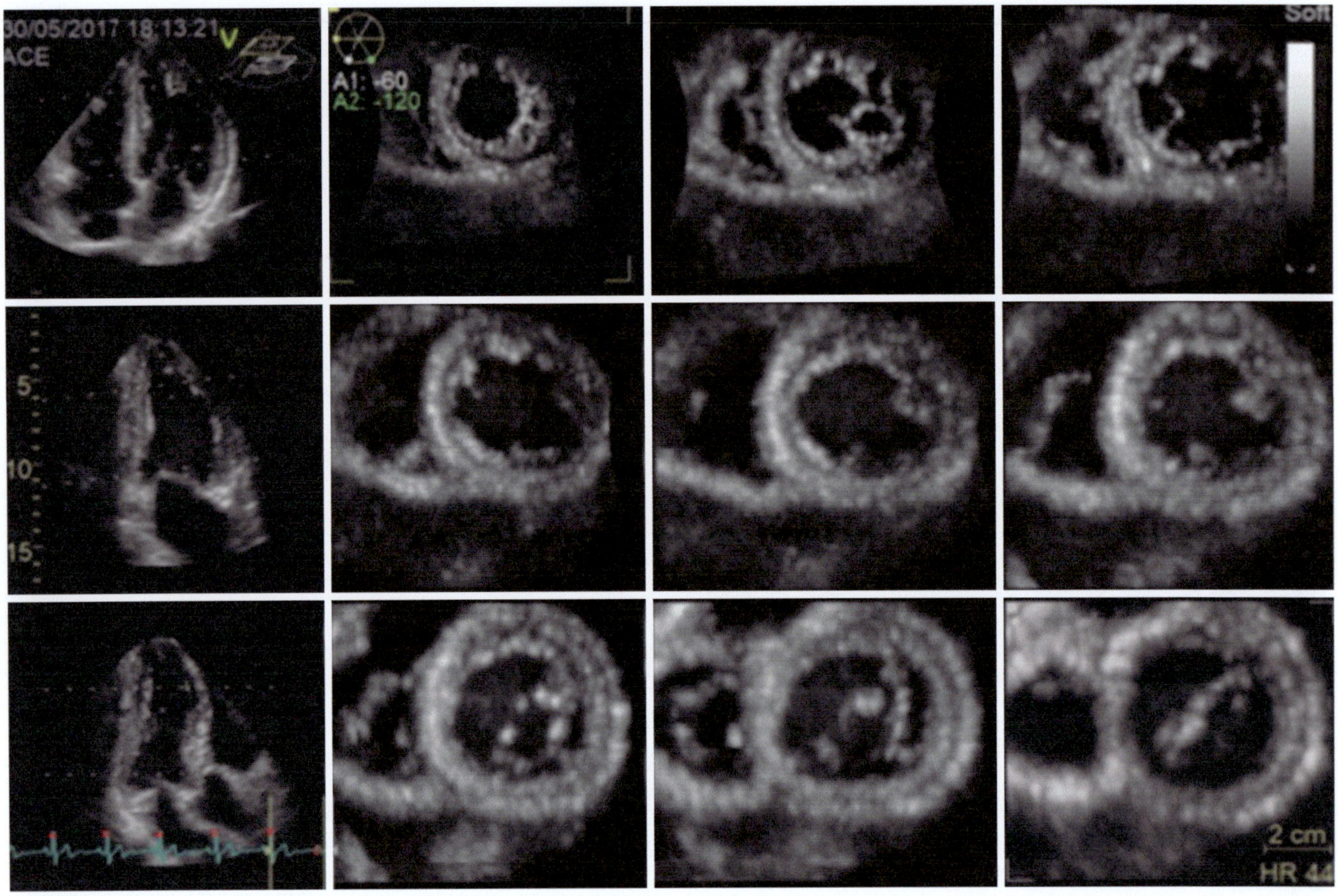

Fig. 22.5 Simultaneous multi-slice (3 × 3 planes) visualization of LV from a Large 3D (GE Healthcare) volume dataset. Used with permission of Mayo Foundation for Medical Education and Research. All rights reserved

border at ED, either auto-initialize or click two reference points (apex and mid-base) and follow with regional editing if necessary, (3) In the same way, select the endocardial border at ES, and (4) Click volume waveform.

Siemens Healthcare's fully automatic LV volumetric analysis of eSie LVA is presented in Fig. 22.9. Select the sequential single-beat 3D large volume option and one-click automatically computes beat-to-beat EF, SV, and LV volumes, either as three individual cycles or a single average of the three cycles [9]. A reliable systolic dyssynchrony index of 16 or 17 segments is generally available because of the Acuson SC2000's high VPS. Especially the sequential beat-to-beat EF or average 3D volume quantification has advantages in patients with an irregular rhythm.

Fundamentally, the superiority of various inter- or even intra-vendor differences, such as fully automatic algorithms versus semiautomatic border tracking and manual editing, is debatable. A head-to-head comparison of the different 3D platforms (3DQ ADV on QLAB 9.0 for iE33 data; 4D Auto LVQ on EchoPAC; BT12 for Vivid E9 data; eSie LVA on SC2000 workplace for Acuson SC2000 data sets) in measuring LV volume [10], concluded that the three systems' results are comparable, but the fully automatic features provide smaller and less accurate LV volumes than do the manually edited measurements, so that manual editing is the preferred option for patients with dilated or distorted geometry.

LV Mass

In principle, LV mass calculation is feasible in any 3D-volume-capable software based on subtracting the LV endocardial volume from the LV epicardial volume multiplied by the specific density of myocardial tissue (1.05 g/cm^3) [11]. A convenient LV mass measuring option is available via tracing the endocardial and epicardial borders during the 3D volumetric analysis. For example, in HeartModel (Philips Healthcare), clicking a check box to compute the LV mass leads to automatic endocardial and also epicardial border tracing, and in 3DQ (Philips Healthcare), check the box 'display LV mass' in preferences before sequential volumetric analysis (which gives endo/epicardial border region of interest), and the semi-automatic border tracing outputs the mass as well as the volume of the LV (Fig. 22.10). In 4D Auto LVQ (GE Healthcare), after LV endocardial volume quantification, just click LV mass to draw automatically the

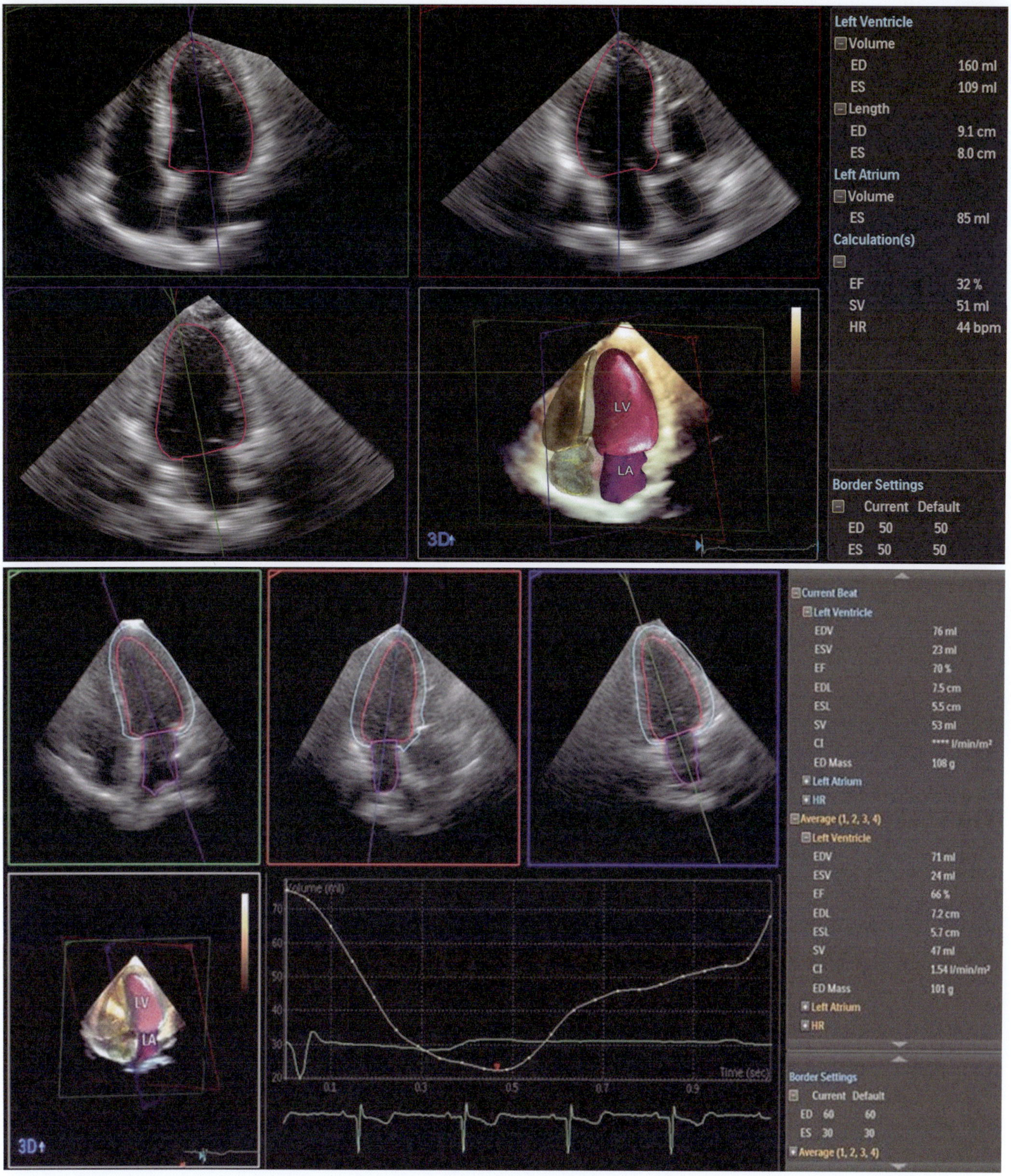

Fig. 22.6 Examples of 3D Heart Model quantification (Philips Healthcare). **Top panel**: A fully automatic LV endocardial contour tracing on the 2D cuts derived from the 3D data sets are shown. Final outcome displays the left ventricular as well as the left atrial volume. **Bottom panel**: Same as in top panel from another patient, but also showing LV mass quantification. Used with permission of Mayo Foundation for Medical Education and Research.

epicardial contours in ED, manually edit if necessary, and then the LV mass is computed as in Fig. 22.10.

LV Strain

LV mechanics are by nature complex 3D phenomena. Conventional 2D strain measurement is limited to tracking the out-of-plane motion of speckles, and the final 2D global longitudinal strain will not reliably represent simultaneous segmental peaks. Recent developments of ultrasound technology have allowed the simultaneous 3D longitudinal, circumferential, radial, and area strain measurements, which were well-validated by sonomicrometry [12, 13]. The Vivid E95 (GE Healthcare) is so far, the only commercially available 3D myocardial deformation measurement platform. Simply follow the extension to the 4D LV Mass tool to calculate both global and regional strain values based upon a spatial speckle-tracking algorithm in the 4D Auto LVQ software. The information is presented in a strain bullseye plot accompanied by time-strain curves (Fig. 22.11). The Acuson SC2000 is also reported to have an upcoming version of its eSie Mechanics software to analyze 3D strain [14].

Normal References

Normal reference ranges of 3D echocardiographic LV parameters are presented in Table 22.3 [15–21]. The 3D volumes or mass are normalized for body surface area. Ideally, the echocardiographic parameters obtained from different echo techniques (e.g. EF in 2D and 3D) should be the same, but so far echo reports tend to show the individual results separately (e.g. 2D EF or 3D EF), making comparison inconvenient. One must be careful not to simply adopt a 3D normal range from a 2D analysis, or vice versa, though theoretically the 3D EF should be preferable to other EF measures. Further studies are warranted to find cut-off points and their clinical strength, especially for 3D-specific parameters such as global area strain or for newly developed quantification software [22].

Right Ventricle

The complex geometry of the RV presents a major challenge for 2D interpretation and a larger benefit from 3D echocardiography. The guidelines for the echocardiographic assessment of the adult RV from the American Society of Echocardiography [23] describe the echocardiographic parameters for assessing RV size and function. 2D-derived estimates of the RV EF are not recommended because of the heterogeneity of methods and the numerous geometric assumptions. 3D echocardiographic measurements using the disc method may be used to report the RV EF in selected patients with RV dilatation, using a lower reference limit of 44% [23]. The 3D RV volume measurements have been validated in animal models [24]. Compared with CMR, RV volumes by 3D echo are lower, but the RV EF difference is insignificant [25]. Next we describe how to assess the 3D RV volume and EF using commercially available software.

Triplane Imaging and Analysis

Simultaneous RV cavity imaging using triplane acquisition (Fig. 22.12a) is helpful to assess the RV volume and EF. For manual tracing of the triplane RV end-diastolic and end-systolic volumes on the Vivid E95, select Measure, then Volume, and then Tri Plane.

RV 3D Imaging

For RV volume imaging, we recommend the RV focused apical 4-chamber view or RV modified apical 4-chamber orientation [17, 26]. The image acquisition proceeds as with 3D LV imaging by either the single-beat live 3D Large (GE) or Full Volume (Philips) or the ECG gated multi-beat 3D mode. Make sure to include the entire RV cavity with a frame rate over 12 VPS.

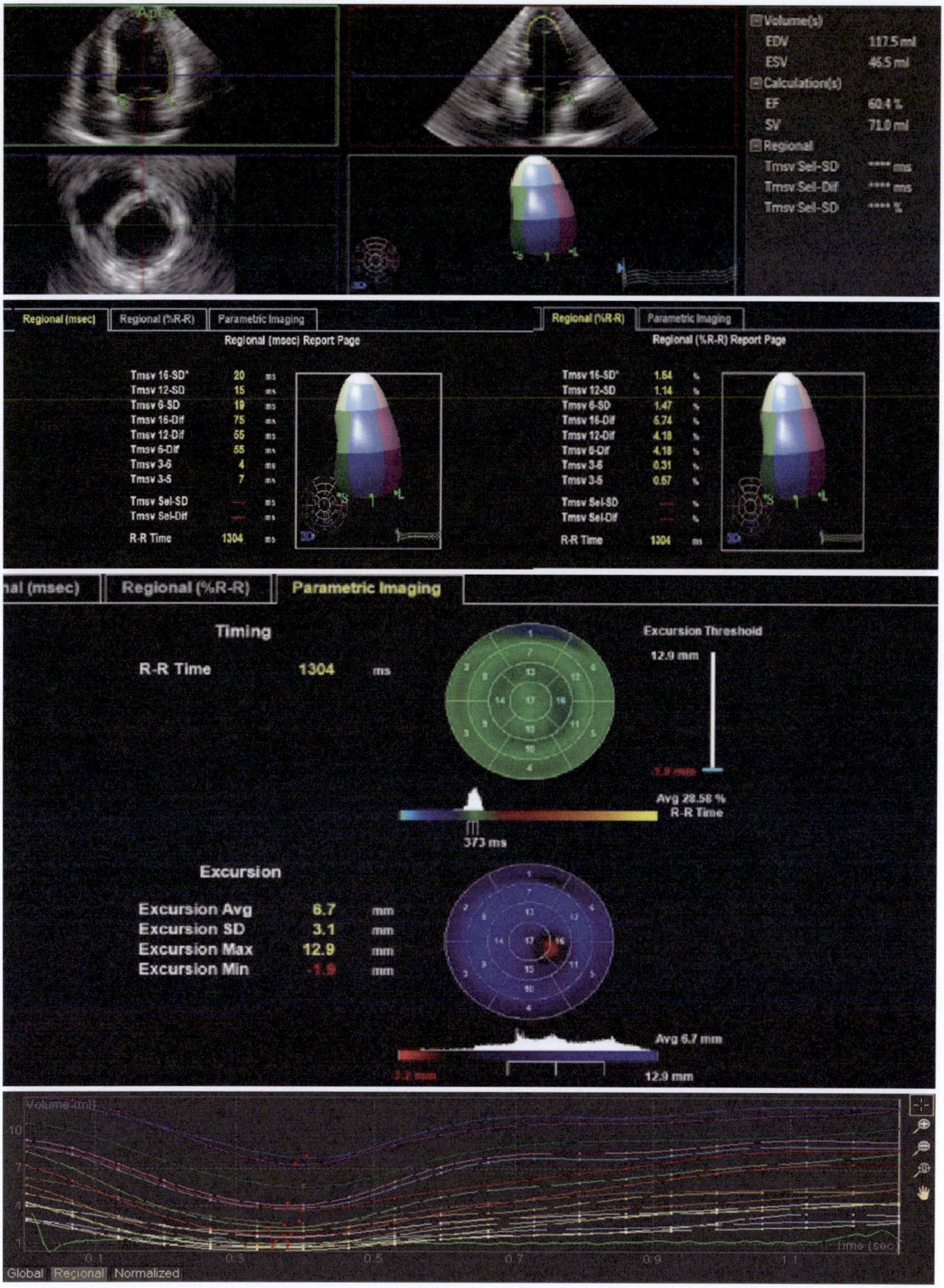

Fig. 22.7 An example of a regional volume and dyssynchrony analysis by QLAB 3DQadv (Philips Healthcare).**Top panel:** End-diastolic and end-systolic LV volumes and ejection fraction. **Second panel:** Regional volume-time data denotes the time to reach minimum systolic volume (MSV). "Tmsv 16SD" means standard deviation of time difference to reach MSV of the 16 segments, either %RR or millisecond calculation. **Third panel:** Parametric imaging showing two bullseye plots of regional timing and excursion. **Bottom panel:** Regional volume-time curves of 16 LV segments. Used with permission of Mayo Foundation for Medical Education and Research.

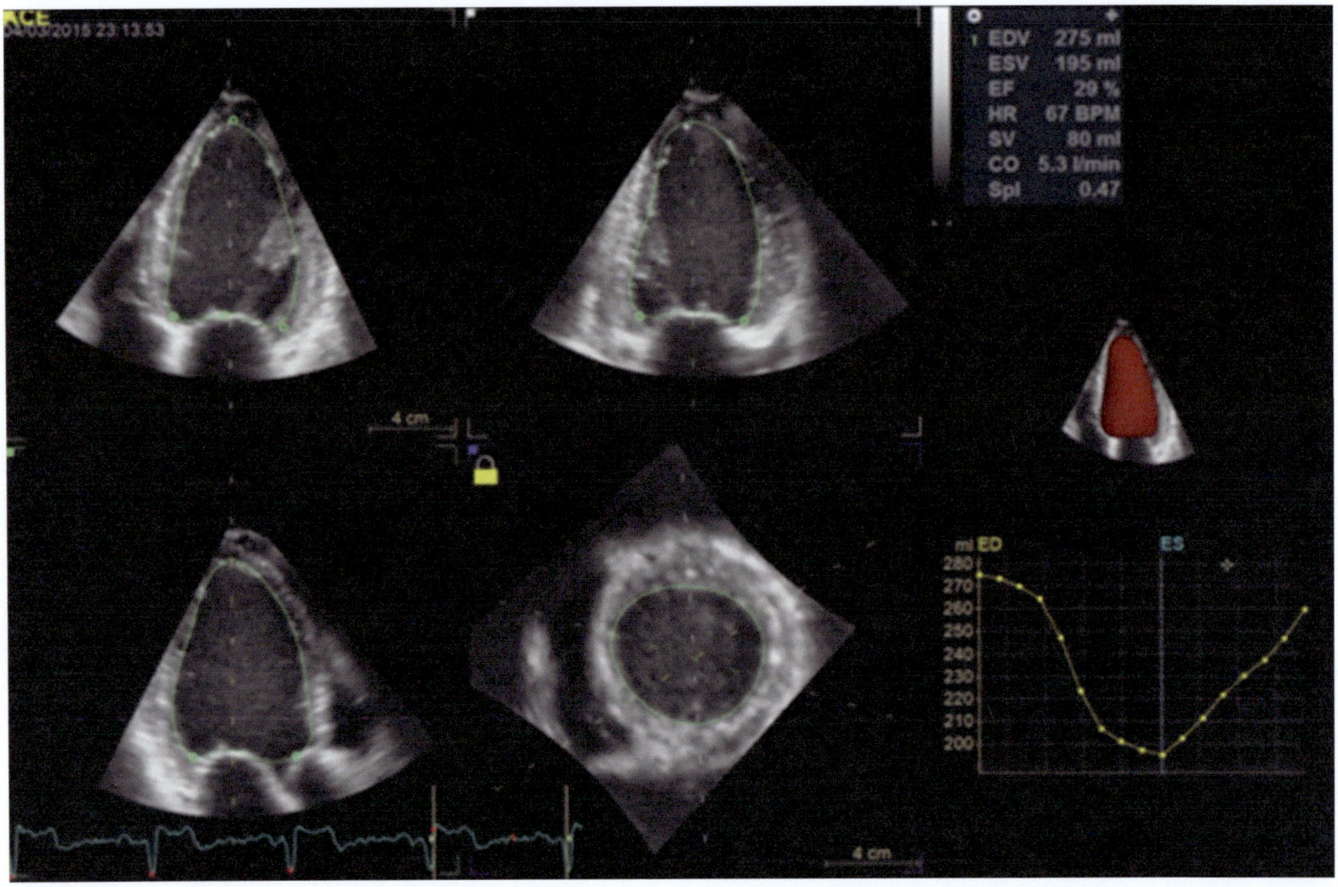

Fig. 22.8 An example of the 4D Auto LVQ software outcome (GE Healthcare). A semi-automatic LV endocardial contouring results in end-diastolic volume (EDV), end-systolic volume (ESV), ejection fraction (EF), stroke volume (SV), cardiac output (CO), and spherical index (SpI). Used with permission of Mayo Foundation for Medical Education and Research.

RV 3D Analysis

From a RV 3D acquisition, post-processing simultaneous visualization of 2D RV walls using the multi-slice option is helpful to analyze RV regional wall motion (Fig. 22.12b). For RV volumetric analysis on the Vivid E95 (GE Healthcare), the RV-specific software of '4D Auto RVQ' can be used. In sequence, select (1) Measure, (2) Volume, (3) 4D auto RVQ, (4) Align the views and set landmarks (tricuspid annulus free wall, septal, RV apex; LV/RV posterior, LV/RV anterior, RV free wall) with a reference image, (5) Manually adjust the initial results if necessary, (6) Select results. This semi-automatic surface-detecting algorithm displays the RV volume, EF, tricuspid annular plane systolic excursion, and fractional area change (Fig. 22.13). With the ACUSON SC2000 (Siemens), eSie RVA has a one-click fully automated algorithm resulting in the RV volume and EF (Fig. 22.14). Normal values of 3D RV volume and function are in Table 22.4 [17, 23, 27, 28]. With Philips EPIQ CVx platform Dynamic Heart Model, the 3D Auto RV application identifies the borders of and aligns the views of the right ventricle, enabling quantification.

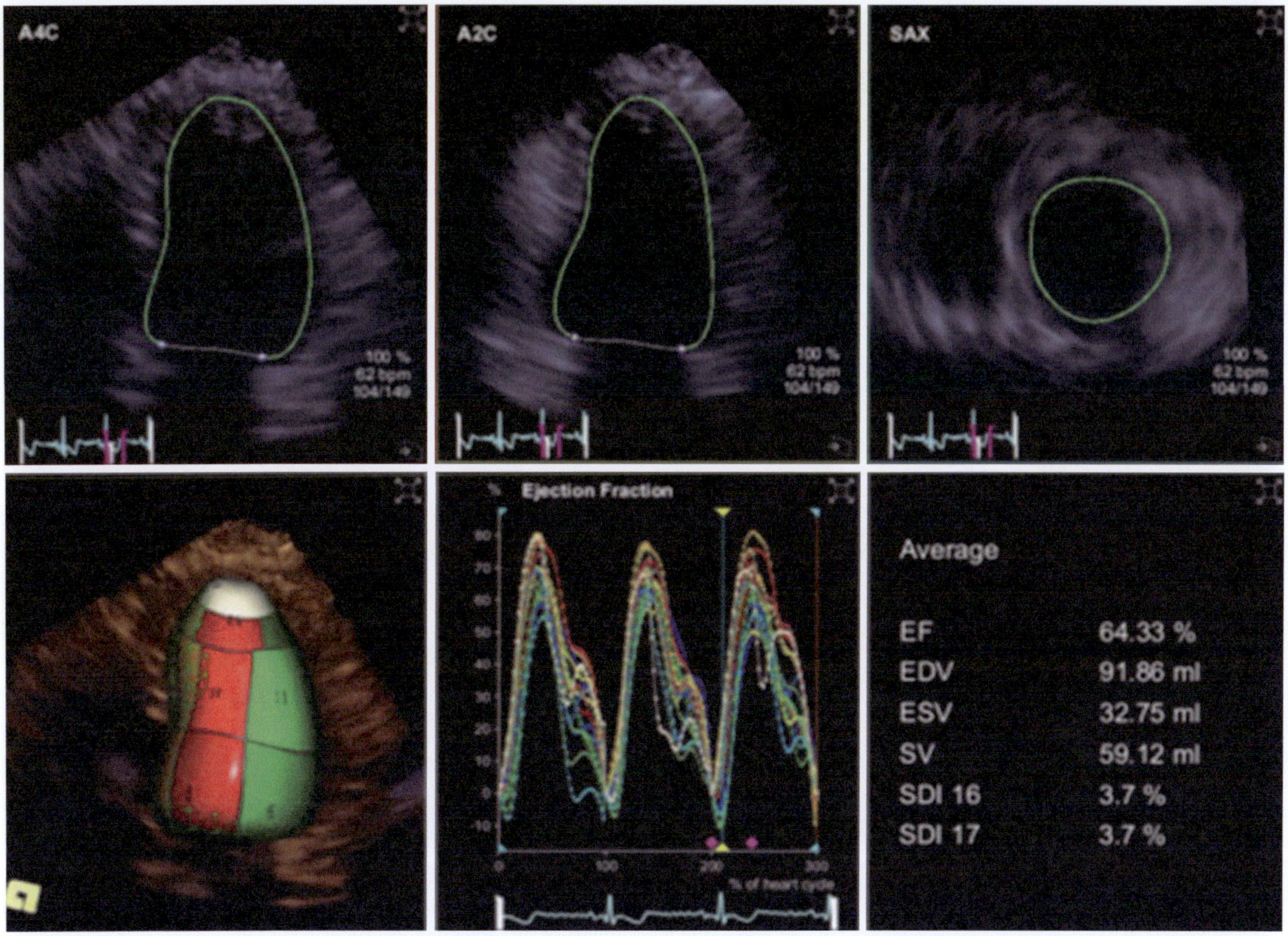

Fig. 22.9 An example of 3D eSie LVA quantification (Siemens). A fully automatic LV endocardial contouring analysis of sequential three cardiac cycles shows beat-to-beat ejection fractions and a single average of the three cycles. Used with permission of Mayo Foundation for Medical Education and Research. All rights reserved. EF, ejection fraction; EDV, end-diastolic volume; ESV, end-systolic volume; SV, stroke volume; SDI, systolic dyssynchrony index

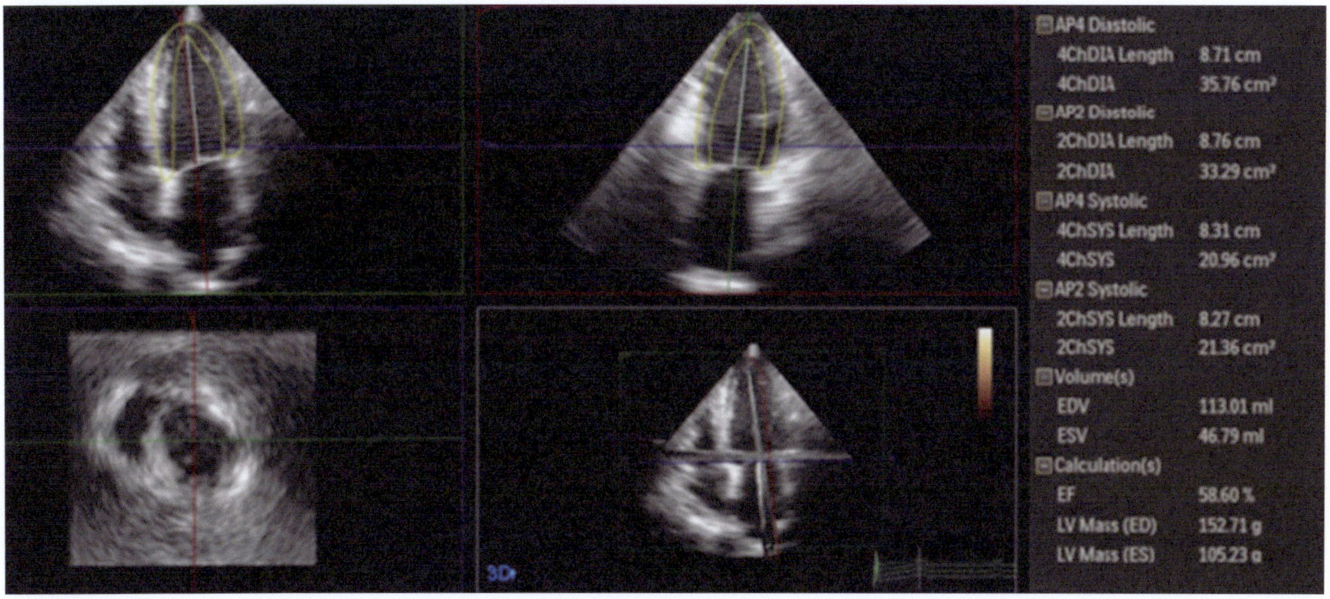

Fig. 22.10 Measurement of the left ventricular mass on the basis of semi-automated identification of endocardial and epicardial contour from a 3D dataset. Used with permission of Mayo Foundation for Medical Education and Research. All rights reserved

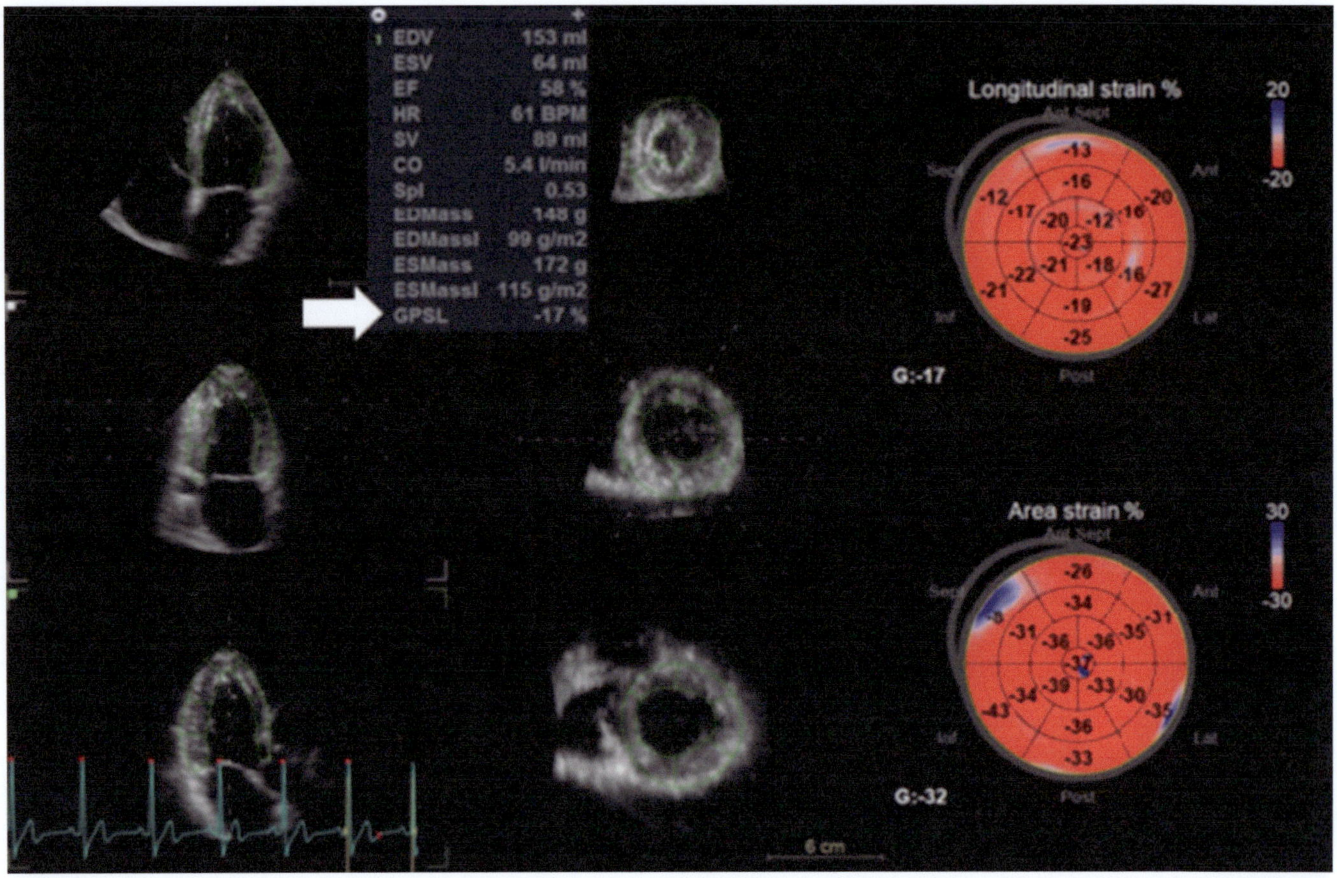

Fig. 22.11 An example of 3D speckle-tracking strain analysis in a healthy subject (GE Healthcare). Both endocardial and epicardial meshes from a 3D Large volume are displayed (left and middle) with 17-segment bullseye maps of longitudinal (right top) and area strain (right bottom). An arrow indicates the global peak longitudinal strain (GPSL). Used with permission of Mayo Foundation for Medical Education and Research.

Table 22.3 Normal values of 3D echocardiographic LV volumes, mass, and function

		NORRE study [15]	Mizukoshi et al. [16]		ASE, EACVI [17]	Muraru et al. [18]	Chahal et al. [19]		Fukuda et al. [20]	Aune et al. [21]
Publication year		2016	2016		2015	2014	2012		2012	2010
Number		440	230	160	.	265	499	479	410	166
Nationality		European	Japanese	American	.	European	European	Indian	Japanese	Scandinavian
LV EDVi (mL/m²)	M	69 (41, 97)	64 (45, 83)	66 (41, 90)	<80	63 (41, 85)	49 (31, 67)	41 (23, 59)	50 (26, 74)	66 (46, 86)
	W	60 (39, 82)	58 (40, 76)	57 (38, 75)	<72	57 (39, 75)	42 (26, 58)	39 (23, 55)	46 (28, 64)	58 (42, 74)
LV ESVi (mL/m²)	M	28 (15, 42)	24 (15, 34)	26 (15, 36)	<33	24 (14, 34)	19 (9, 29)	16 (6, 26)	19 (9, 29)	29 (17, 41)
	W	24 (13, 35)	20 (12, 29)	21 (12, 30)	<29	20 (12, 28)	16 (8, 24)	15 (7, 23)	17 (9, 25)	23 (13, 33)
LV EF (%)	M	58 (50, 67)	62 (56, 69)	61 (53, 69)	52–72*	62 (54, 70)	61 (49, 73)	62 (52, 72)	61 (53, 69)	57 (49, 65)
	W	60 (51, 69)	65 (57, 73)	64 (56, 71)	54–74*	65 (57, 73)	62 (52, 72)	62 (52, 72)	63 (55, 71)	61 (49, 73)
LV mass (g/m²)	M	.	.	.	50–102*	77 (57, 97)	.	.	64 (40, 88)	.
	W	.	.	.	44–88*	73 (57, 89)	.	.	56 (34, 78)	.
LV GLS (%)	M	−20 (−26, −15)	.	.	≤−20*	<−15	.	.	.	.
	W	−21 (−26, −17)	.	.		<−15	.	.	.	.

Values are presented as mean (LLN, ULN). LLN, Lower limit of normality, ULN, Upper limit of normality, LLN and ULN are defined as mean ± 2SD. *based on 2D echocardiography. Used with permission of Mayo Foundation for Medical Education and Research.
Abbreviations: *LV* left ventricular, *EDVi* end-diastolic volume index, *ESVi* end-systolic volume index, *EF* ejection fraction, *GLS* Global longitudinal strain, *M* men, *W* women, *NORRE* Normal Reference Ranges for Echocardiography, *ASE* American Society of Echocardiography, *EACVI* European Association of Cardiovascular Imaging

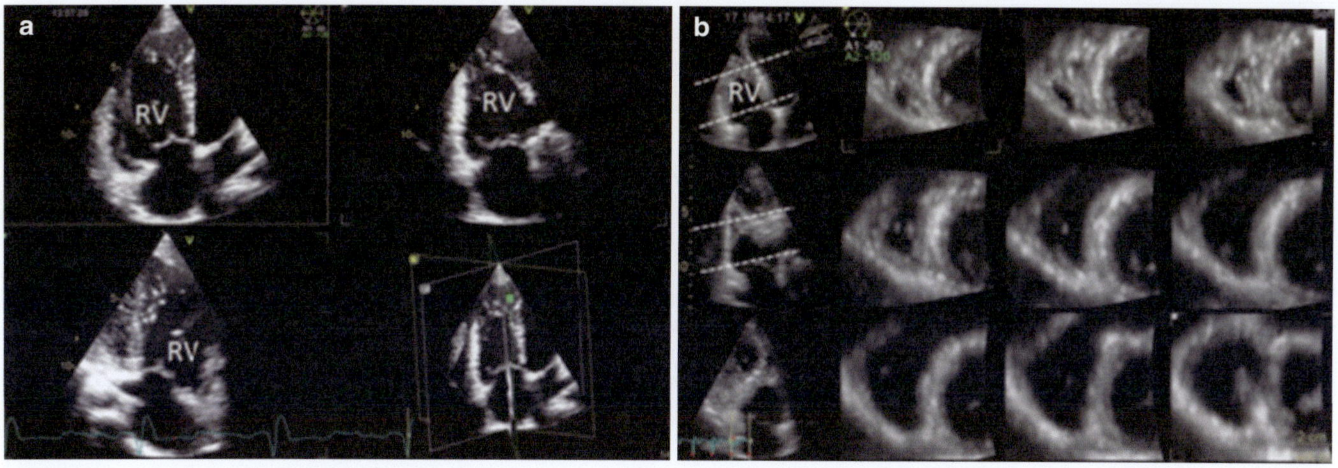

Fig. 22.12 (**a**) Simultaneous triplane imaging by a 3D transthoracic echo probe, (**b**) Post-processing multi-slice 2D planes visualization from a single 3D right ventricular (RV) Large volume acquisition Used with permission of Mayo Foundation for Medical Education and Research.

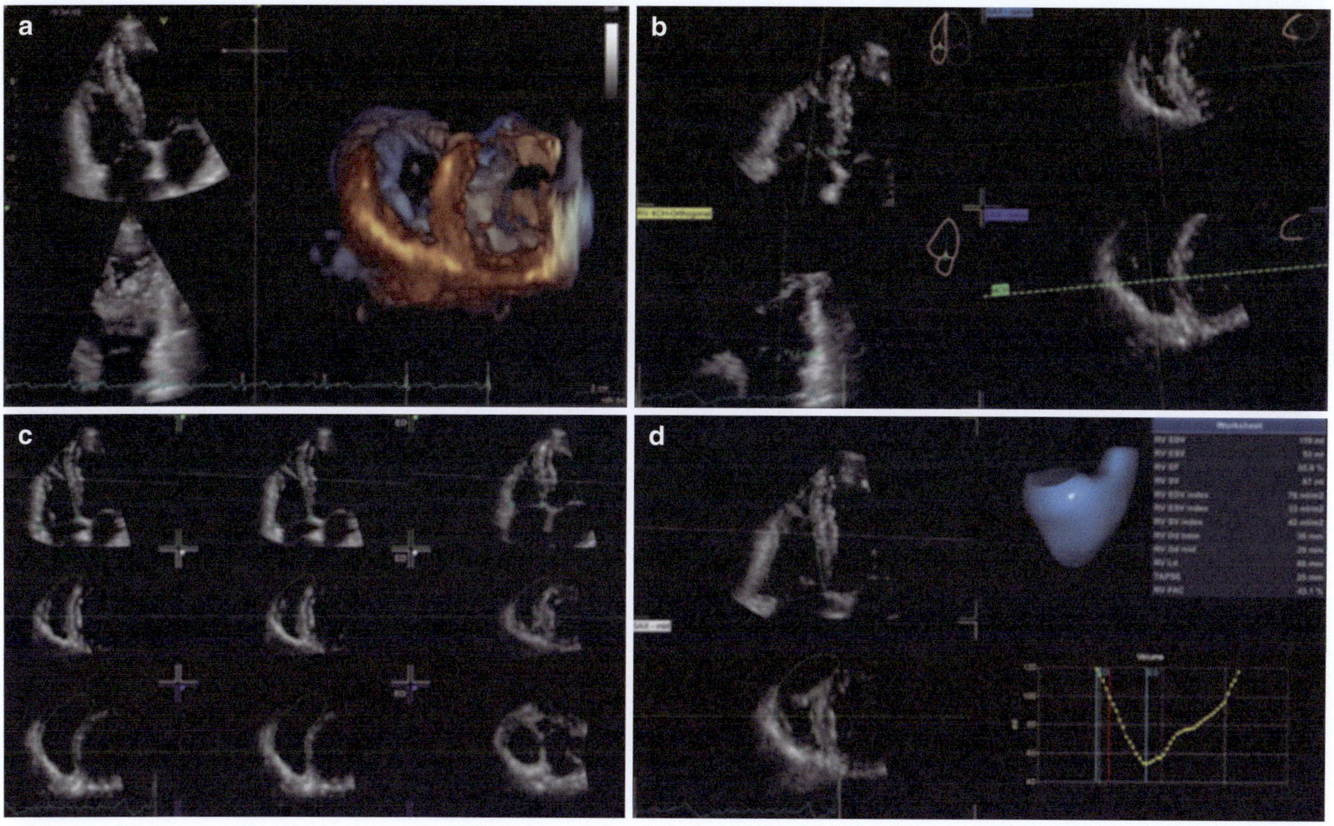

Fig. 22.13 Right ventricular (RV) 3D imaging and analysis using the 4D Auto RVQ software (GE Healthcare). (**a**) RV focused apical 4-chamber view oriented, biplane-guided 3D RV dataset acquisition. (**b**) Align views following the reference images in the right upper corner of each 2D cut. (**c**) Setting the six landmarks and manually editing from the automatic initial endocardial tracing. (**d**) Final results show a global volume-time curve and RV parameters: EDV, end-diastolic volume; ESV, end-systolic volume; EF, ejection fraction; SV, stroke volume; TAPSE, tricuspid annular plane systolic excursion; FAC, fractional area change. Used with permission of Mayo Foundation for Medical Education and Research.

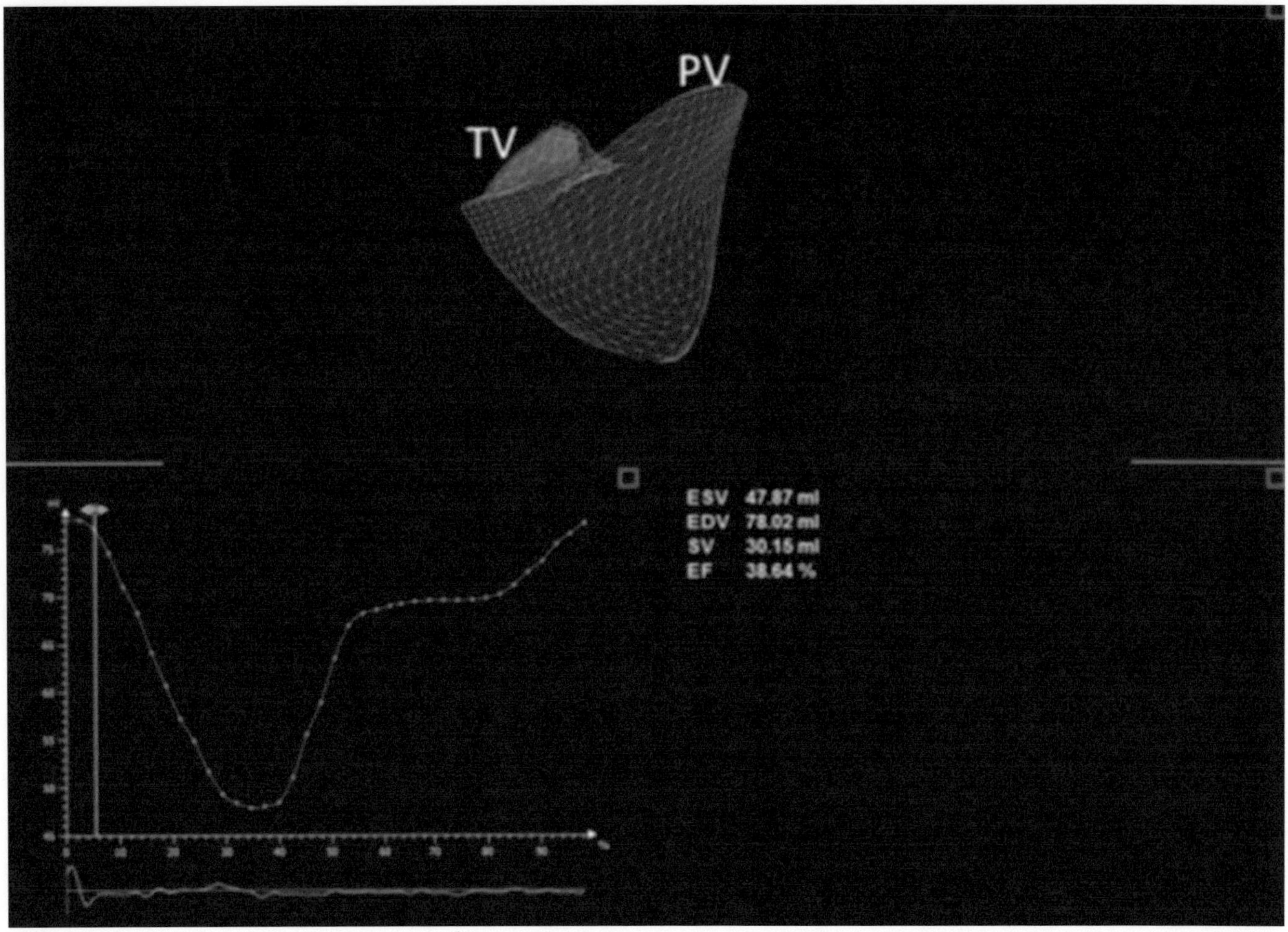

Fig. 22.14 Right ventricular 3D volumetric analysis using the eSie RVA software (Siemens). ESV, end-systolic volume; EDV, end-diastolic volume; SV, stroke volume; EF, ejection fraction; TV, tricuspid valve; PV, pulmonary valve. Used with permission of Mayo Foundation for Medical Education and Research. All rights reserved

Table 22.4 Normal values of 3D echocardiographic RV volumes and function

		ASE, EACVI [17]	ASE [23]	Gopal et al. [27]	Maffessanti et al. [28]
Publication year		2015	2010	2007	2013
Number of subject		.	.	71	540
RV EDVi (mL/m²)	M	61 (35, 87)	65 (40, 89)	75 (49, 100)	EDV, mL: 107 (74, 163)
	W	53 (32, 74)		65 (39, 92)	EDV, mL: 81 (58, 120)
RV ESVi (mL/m²)	M	27 (10, 44)	28 (12, 45)	38 (23, 53)	ESV, mL: 44 (22, 80)
	W	22 (8, 36)		29 (8, 51)	ESV, mL: 30 (15, 52)
RV EF (%)	M	58 (45, 71)	57 (44, 69)	49 (30, 58)	60 (45, 75)
	W			56 (38, 65)	63 (49, 79)

Values are presented as mean (LLN, ULN). LLN, Lower limit of normality, ULN, Upper limit of normality, LLN and ULN are defined as mean ± 2SD. Used with permission of Mayo Foundation for Medical Education and Research. All rights reserved

Abbreviations: *RV* right ventricular; *EDVi* end-diastolic volume index, *ESVi* end-systolic volume index, *EF* ejection fraction, *M* men, *W* women, *ASE* American Society of Echocardiography, *EACVI* European Association of Cardiovascular Imaging

References

1. Yang HS, Bansal RC, Mookadam F, Khandheria BK, Tajik AJ, Chandrasekaran K. Practical guide for three-dimensional transthoracic echocardiography using a fully sampled matrix array transducer. J Am Soc Echocardiogr. 2008;21:979–89. quiz 1081-2
2. Lang RM, Addetia K, Narang A, Mor-Avi V. 3-dimensional echocardiography: latest developments and future directions. JACC Cardiovasc Imaging. 2018;11:1854–78.
3. Xu TY, Sun JP, Lee AP, Yang XS, Qiao Z, Luo X, et al. Three-dimensional speckle strain echocardiography is more accurate and efficient than 2D strain in the evaluation of left ventricular function. Int J Cardiol. 2014;176:360–6.
4. Lang RM, Badano LP, Tsang W, Adams DH, Agricola E, Buck T, et al. EAE/ASE recommendations for image acquisition and display using three-dimensional echocardiography. J Am Soc Echocardiogr. 2012;25:3–46.
5. Yang HS, Pellikka PA, McCully RB, Oh JK, Kukuzke JA, Khandheria BK, et al. Role of biplane and biplane echocardiographically guided 3-dimensional echocardiography during dobutamine stress echocardiography. J Am Soc Echocardiogr. 2006;19:1136–43.
6. Tsang W, Salgo IS, Medvedofsky D, Takeuchi M, Prater D, Weinert L, et al. Transthoracic 3D echocardiographic left heart chamber quantification using an automated adaptive analytics algorithm. JACC Cardiovasc Imaging. 2016;9:769–82.
7. Otani K, Nakazono A, Salgo IS, Lang RM, Takeuchi M. Three-dimensional echocardiographic assessment of left heart chamber size and function with fully automated quantification software in patients with atrial fibrillation. J Am Soc Echocardiogr. 2016;29:955–65.
8. Muraru D, Badano LP, Peluso D, Dal Bianco L, Casablanca S, Kocabay G, et al. Comprehensive analysis of left ventricular geometry and function by three-dimensional echocardiography in healthy adults. J Am Soc Echocardiogr. 2013;26:618–28.
9. Thavendiranathan P, Liu S, Verhaert D, Calleja A, Nitinunu A, Van Houten T, et al. Feasibility, accuracy, and reproducibility of real-time full-volume 3D transthoracic echocardiography to measure LV volumes and systolic function: a fully automated endocardial contouring algorithm in sinus rhythm and atrial fibrillation. JACC Cardiovasc Imaging. 2012;5:239–51.
10. Muraru D, Cecchetto A, Cucchini U, Zhou X, Lang RM, Romeo G, et al. Intervendor consistency and accuracy of left ventricular volume measurements using three-dimensional echocardiography. J Am Soc Echocardiogr. 2018;31:158–168.e1.
11. Volpato V, Mor-Avi V, Narang A, Prater D, Goncalves A, Tamborini G, et al. Automated, machine learning-based, 3D echocardiographic quantification of left ventricular mass. Echocardiography. 2019;36:312–9.
12. Hjertaas JJ, Fossa H, Dybdahl GL, Gruner R, Lunde P, Matre K. Accuracy of real-time single- and multi-beat 3-d speckle tracking echocardiography in vitro. Ultrasound Med Biol. 2013;39:1006–14.
13. Bouchez S, Heyde B, Barbosa D, Vandenheuvel M, Houle H, Wang Y, et al. In-vivo validation of a new clinical tool to quantify three-dimensional myocardial strain using ultrasound. Int J Cardiovasc Imaging. 2016;32:1707–14.
14. Zhou X, Thavendiranathan P, Chen Y, Cheng L, Qian Z, Liu S, et al. Feasibility of automated three-dimensional rotational mechanics by real-time volume transthoracic echocardiography: preliminary accuracy and reproducibility data compared with cardiovascular magnetic resonance. J Am Soc Echocardiogr. 2016;29:62–73.
15. Bernard A, Addetia K, Dulgheru R, Caballero L, Sugimoto T, Akhaladze N, et al. 3D echocardiographic reference ranges for normal left ventricular volumes and strain: results from the EACVI NORRE study. Eur Heart J Cardiovasc Imaging. 2017;18:475–83.
16. Mizukoshi K, Takeuchi M, Nagata Y, Addetia K, Lang RM, Akashi YJ, et al. Normal values of left ventricular mass index assessed by transthoracic three-dimensional echocardiography. J Am Soc Echocardiogr. 2016;29:51–61.
17. Lang RM, Badano LP, Mor-Avi V, Afilalo J, Armstrong A, Ernande L, et al. Recommendations for cardiac chamber quantification by echocardiography in adults: an update from the American Society of Echocardiography and the European Association of Cardiovascular Imaging. J Am Soc Echocardiogr. 2015;28:1–39.e14.
18. Muraru D, Cucchini U, Mihaila S, Miglioranza MH, Aruta P, Cavalli G, et al. Left ventricular myocardial strain by three-dimensional speckle-tracking echocardiography in healthy subjects: reference values and analysis of their physiologic and technical determinants. J Am Soc Echocardiogr. 2014;27:858–871.e1.
19. Chahal NS, Lim TK, Jain P, Chambers JC, Kooner JS, Senior R. Population-based reference values for 3D echocardiographic LV volumes and ejection fraction. JACC Cardiovasc Imaging. 2012;5:1191–7.
20. Fukuda S, Watanabe H, Daimon M, Abe Y, Hirashiki A, Hirata K, et al. Normal values of real-time 3-dimensional echocardiographic parameters in a healthy Japanese population: the JAMP-3D study. Circ J. 2012;76:1177–81.
21. Aune E, Baekkevar M, Rodevand O, Otterstad JE. Reference values for left ventricular volumes with real-time 3-dimensional echocardiography. Scand Cardiovasc J. 2010;44:24–30.
22. Yuda S, Sato Y, Abe K, Kawamukai M, Kouzu H, Muranaka A, et al. Inter-vendor variability of left ventricular volumes and strains determined by three-dimensional speckle tracking echocardiography. Echocardiography. 2014;31:597–604.
23. Rudski LG, Lai WW, Afilalo J, Hua L, Handschumacher MD, Chandrasekaran K, et al. Guidelines for the echocardiographic assessment of the right heart in adults: a report from the American Society of Echocardiography endorsed by the European Association of Echocardiography, a registered branch of the European Society of Cardiology, and the Canadian Society of Echocardiography. J Am Soc Echocardiogr. 2010;23:685–713. quiz 786-8
24. Linker DT, Moritz WE, Pearlman AS. A new three-dimensional echocardiographic method of right ventricular volume measurement: in vitro validation. J Am Coll Cardiol. 1986;8:101–6.
25. Greiner S, Andre F, Heimisch M, Aurich M, Steen H, Katus HA, et al. A closer look at right ventricular 3D volume quantification by transthoracic echocardiography and cardiac MRI. Clin Radiol. 2019;74(6):490.e7–490.e14.
26. Medvedofsky D, Addetia K, Patel AR, Sedlmeier A, Baumann R, Mor-Avi V, et al. Novel approach to three-dimensional echocardiographic quantification of right ventricular volumes and function from focused views. J Am Soc Echocardiogr. 2015;28:1222–31.
27. Gopal AS, Chukwu EO, Iwuchukwu CJ, Katz AS, Toole RS, Schapiro W, et al. Normal values of right ventricular size and function by real-time 3-dimensional echocardiography: comparison with cardiac magnetic resonance imaging. J Am Soc Echocardiogr. 2007;20:445–55.
28. Maffessanti F, Muraru D, Esposito R, Gripari P, Ermacora D, Santoro C, et al. Age-, body size-, and sex-specific reference values for right ventricular volumes and ejection fraction by three-dimensional echocardiography: a multicenter echocardiographic study in 507 healthy volunteers. Circ Cardiovasc Imaging. 2013;6:700–10.

Is 3D Better than 2D During Stress Echo?

23

Hyun Suk Yang and Krishnaswamy Chandrasekaran

Introduction

Conventional two-dimensional (2D) stress echocardiography (SE) has been well established as a noninvasive imaging method for the diagnosis and prognosis of ischemic heart disease. However, obtaining the exact plane matching the various stages, is a limitation at times [1–3]. Compared to 2D, three-dimensional (3D) SE has the theoretical advantages of encompassing the entire left ventricle (LV) within a single dataset and obtaining precise, anatomically correct tomographic sections, matching them at different stages of stress with less operator-dependence [4, 5] (Table 23.1). Mainly, 3D multiplane imaging markedly shortens image acquisition time compared with conventional 2D imaging [5] (Fig. 23.1). During exercise SE, time efficiency in acquisition of 3D datasets is more beneficial because increasing the time between exercise termination and image acquisition reduces diagnostic sensitivity [6]. Historically, there have been more published reports on 3D pharmacological stress because previous multi-beat full-volume imaging resulted in more stitching artifacts from hyperventilation with exercise stress [5, 7].

Recent advances in 3D ultrasound technology offer superior image quality, higher frame rate, single beat acquisition of whole 3D datasets without stich artifacts, and user-friendly post-processing software which makes 3D attractive for routine SE.

H. S. Yang
Professor, Research institute of Medical Science, Konkuk University School of Medicine, Department of Cardiovascular Medicine, Konkuk University Medical Center, Neungdong-ro, Gwangjin-gu, Seoul, Korea
e-mail: yang.hyun@kuh.ac.kr

K. Chandrasekaran (✉)
Professor of Medicine, Mayo Clinic College of Medicine; Consultant, Department of Cardiovascular Medicine, Mayo Clinic, Rochester, MN, USA
e-mail: kchandra@mayo.edu

Table 23.1 Advantages and disadvantages of 3D stress echocardiography

	Advantages	Disadvantages
Image acquisition	• Reduced image acquisition time	• Lower image resolution
	• Single-beat acquisition of a whole dataset, especially good for arrhythmias	• Lower frame rate (volumes per second)
	• Avoids apical foreshortening	• Stich artifacts from multi-beat full-volume acquisition
	• Encompasses the entire left ventricle	
	• Improves reproducibility	
	• Reduces operator dependency	
Data analysis	• Volumetric data allows many different planes and slices simultaneously available	• Time requirement for further postprocessing
	• Optimal visualization of the LV apex with true tomographic imaging of all segments • Choice between similar-plane rest and stress for comparison	
	• Accurate assessment of volume or ejection fraction	
	• Parametric imaging	
	• 3D strain	

3D SE Image Acquisition

Generally, 3D SE image acquisition based on a routine SE protocol [1] can be accomplished using either exercise or pharmacologic stress. The core echo images to be obtained at baseline and at peak stress include whole LV walls, and care should be given to ensure a high-quality electrocardiogram (ECG). Along with ECG, heart rate (HR), and blood pressure monitoring, continuous echo imaging allows detection of the ischemic threshold using dobutamine SE (DSE). The standard DSE protocol involves infusion of dobutamine at 10,

J. F. Maalouf et al. (eds.), *Practical 3D Echocardiography*, https://doi.org/10.1007/978-3-030-72941-7_23

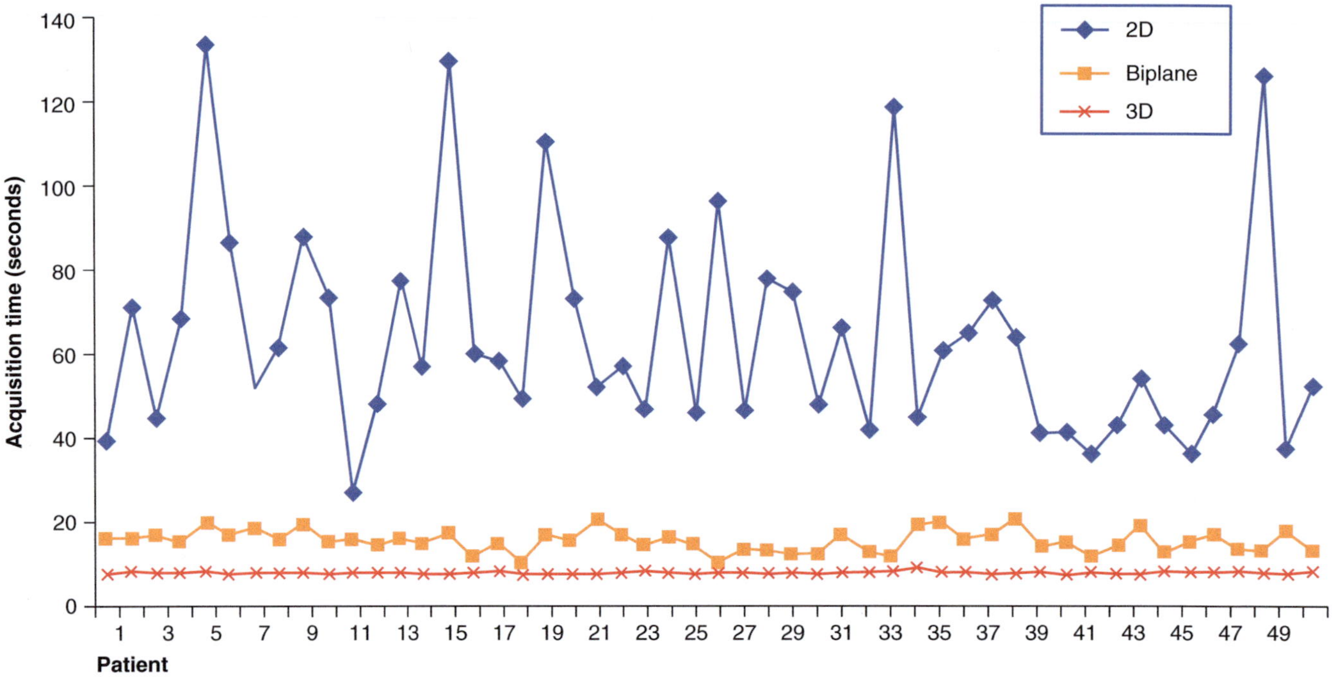

Fig. 23.1 Imaging acquisition time at peak stress: the imaging acquisition time is significantly shorter in 3D or biplane than 2D (3D vs 2D: 1.9 ± 0.2 vs. 60 ± 27 seconds; Biplane vs. 2D: 9.3 ± 2.8 vs. 60 ± 27 seconds, all, $P < 0.001$) [5]. Used with permission of Mayo Foundation for Medical Education and Research.

20, 30, and 40 mg/kg/min at every 3-minute stage, and additional atropine (0.5–2.0 mg) is used to achieve a target HR of 85% of the age-predicted maximal HR. Endpoints for termination include achievement of the target HR, hypotension, new or worsening wall motion abnormalities, significant arrhythmias, severe hypertension, and intolerable symptoms [1]. Contrast agent for left ventricular opacification is recommended when two or more contiguous segments of any coronary territory cannot be adequately visualized [1] which increases yield of 3D DSE [8, 9].

Specifically in 3D SE, first, make sure to choose the 3D-capable matrix-array transthoracic transducer from the vendor [Philips EPIQ CVx for X5–1 (combined 2D/3D); GE Vivid E95 for 4Vc (combined 2D/3D); Siemens Acuson SC2000 for 4Z1c]. Secondly, fix the probe in the optimal apical position, no longer needing to move to another parasternal echo window position.

Modes of 3D SE

Multi-Plane, or Multi-Slice Imaging

Biplane SE can be performed from the apical window (60- and 120-degree planes) imaging two apical views simultaneously (Fig. 23.2), leading to a significant reduction in acquisition time without compromising image quality or diagnostic yield compared with 2D SE [5]. Bi- or triplane imaging permits capture of multiple "2D" images from different planes in the same beat, providing superior frame rates as compared to 3D volumetric imaging [5, 10]. Multi-slice SE permits simultaneous presentation of standard long axis (apical 4-chamber, 2-chamber, and 3-chamber) and short axis views (apex, mid, and base levels), sorted by stage (Fig. 23.3).

Real-Time 3D Full Volume (Multi-Beats, or Single Beat)

Using the matrix array transducer, real-time 3D full volume datasets are obtained from the apical window with the volume-size adjusted to encompass the entire LV. The multi-beat 3D full-volume acquisition requires several consecutive ECG-gated conical sub-volumes to develop one full volume. One has to make sure the breath is held at end-expiration to avoid stich artifacts between the sub volumes (Fig. 23.4). Recently available single beat live 3D full volume acquisition can accommodate the entire LV within a sizable single sector (up to 100° × 100° degrees) with an acceptable frame rate range (up to 51 volumes per seconds). This actual live 3D full volume image avoids stich artifacts, overcomes rhythm disturbances, and reduces acquisition time.

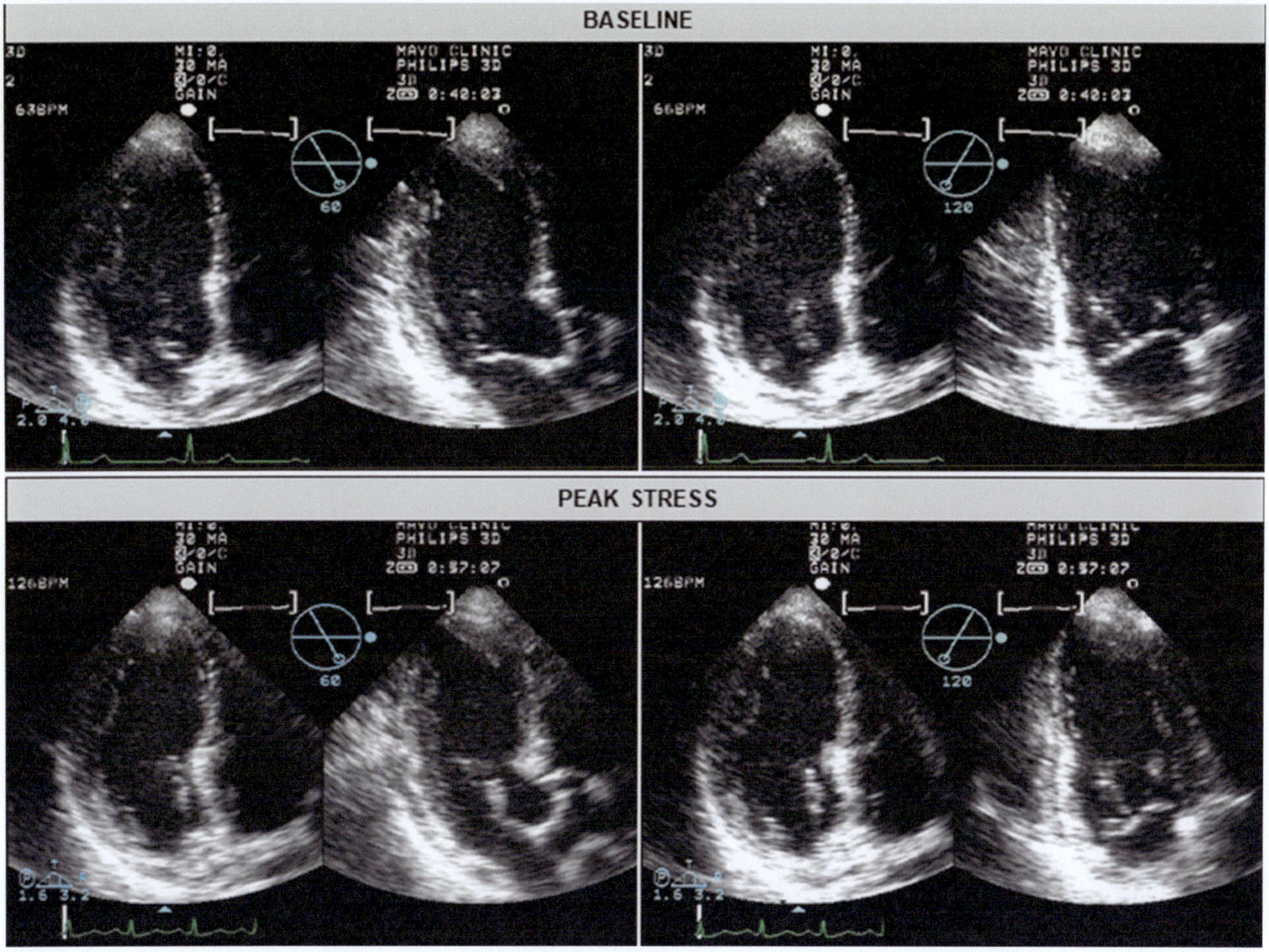

Fig. 23.2 Biplane images of the LV obtained from apical window at 60 and 120 degrees, at baseline and peak stress. Used with permission of Mayo Foundation for Medical Education and Research.

Integrated 2D/3D Mode

Integrated 2D- and 3D-mode approaches to SE may improve the diagnostic yield while maximizing image quality and choosing the optimal imaging plane [11]. Biplane-guided volumetric 3D SE helps avoid losing any LV walls [5]. Single transducers can acquire both 2D and 3D studies, eliminating an early limitation of 3D SE that required switching transducers in an integrated 2D and 3D protocol (X5-1 of EPIQ CVx, 4Vc of Vivid E95).

3D SE Data Analysis: LV Wall Motion Abnormality

The 3D SE analysis for myocardial ischemia depends on standard 2D slices using a 16- or 17- segment wall motion analysis model following American Society of Echocardiography guidelines [1]. The 3D volume datasets can be auto-extracted and visualized on-cart during the SE (Fig. 23.3). Sorting and comparison options are generally available either by stage or by view. Volumetric data can be exported to vendor-specific workstations for rendering and further analysis (QLAB for Philips, Echo PAC for GE, SC200 workplace for Siemens). The 3D full volume can be cropped as apical 4-chamber, apical long-axis, and apical 2-chamber views and then as short-axis views at various levels from the LV apex to base, and can be rendered as a 9-slice simultaneous display [5, 12] (Fig. 23.4). Most clinically performed 3D SE for diagnosis and prognosis of myocardial ischemia is based on detection of new or worsening regional wall motion abnormalities (RWMA) by qualitative analysis. Good feasibility and accuracy for angiographic ischemic heart disease has been reported in both exercise and dobutamine 3D SE [5, 6, 13]. Further quantitative 3D SE analysis may be followed as an adjuvant to LV wall motion analysis [14, 15].

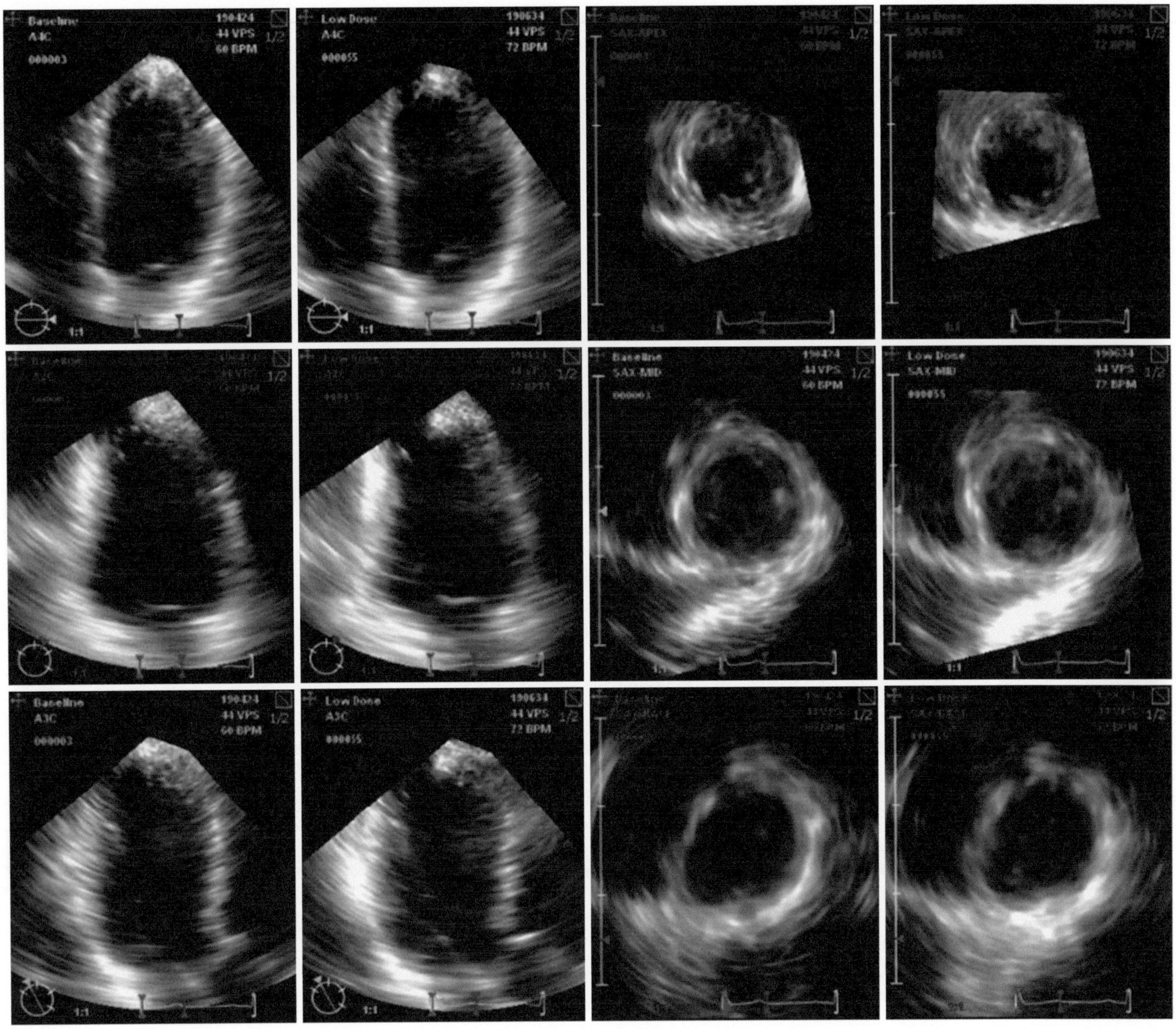

Fig. 23.3 Auto extracted long- and short-axis standard images of the LV, compared by stage (baseline, low dose). Used with permission of Mayo Foundation for Medical Education and Research. All rights reserved

Beyond LV Wall Motion

In addition to visualizing new or worsening RWMA, 3D SE can provide more accurate quantitative data regarding LV volumes and ejection fraction, both at baseline and peak stress (Fig. 23.5). A low resting-LV ejection fraction or an absence of LV contractile reserve (<5% increase in ejection fraction) are negative prognostic markers in SE [16].

Limitations

Disadvantages of 3D SE are summarized in Table 23.1. Low temporal resolution is more problematic in contrast 3D SE [9]. Stich artifacts from respiration (it's hard to ask patients to stop breathing at end-expiration during peak exercise), cardiac motion, and irregular cardiac rhythms often limit image quality in multibeat ECG-gated full volumes which a single-beat acquisition can overcome.

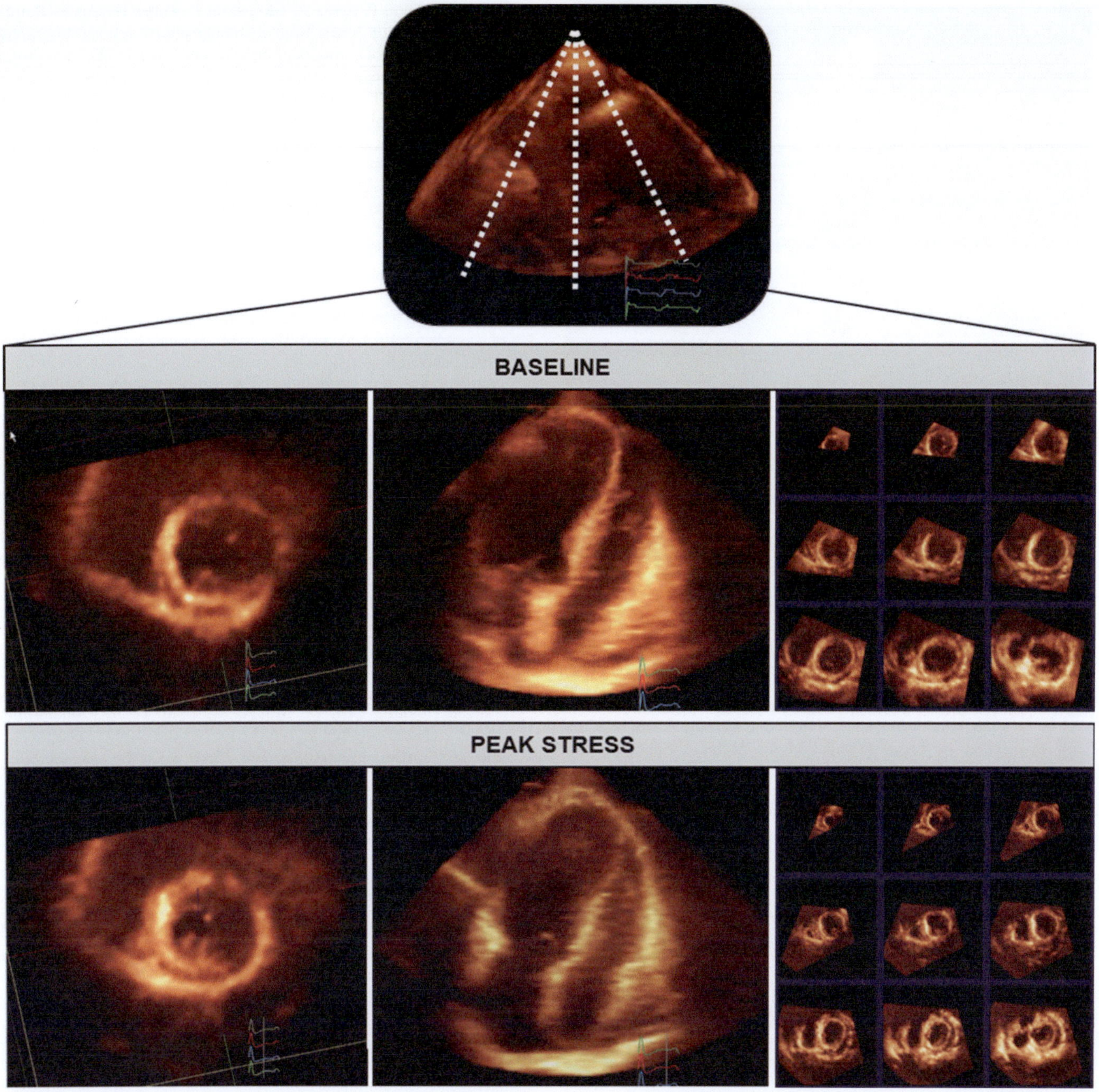

Fig. 23.4 Real-time 3D full volume image from four conical subvolume summation. Post-processing of the volumetric dataset allows visualizing the orthogonal short and true LV apex using optimal side-by-side display of rest and stress images, and 9-slice displays as well. Used with permission of Mayo Foundation for Medical Education and Research. All rights reserved

Future Direction

Until now, 3D SE has not been widely performed worldwide. Smaller-footprint matrix transducers (combined 2D and 3D) and single beat 3D full volume modes with wider sector angles and higher frame rates will improve image quality, and the ease of obtaining 3D datasets may increase the utility of 3D during stress. 3D SE software providing automated side-by-side- analysis of multiple sections at each stage will save post-processing analysis time. In addition, analysis of segmental volumetric changes, or parametric imaging with myocardial deformation (strain or strain rate) will allow objective assessment of the segmental myocardial ischemia [15, 17]. Furthermore, 3D fusion with CT or MRI or true 3D visualization with virtual reality or holography [18] may extend 3D communication to a more general, less technical audience.

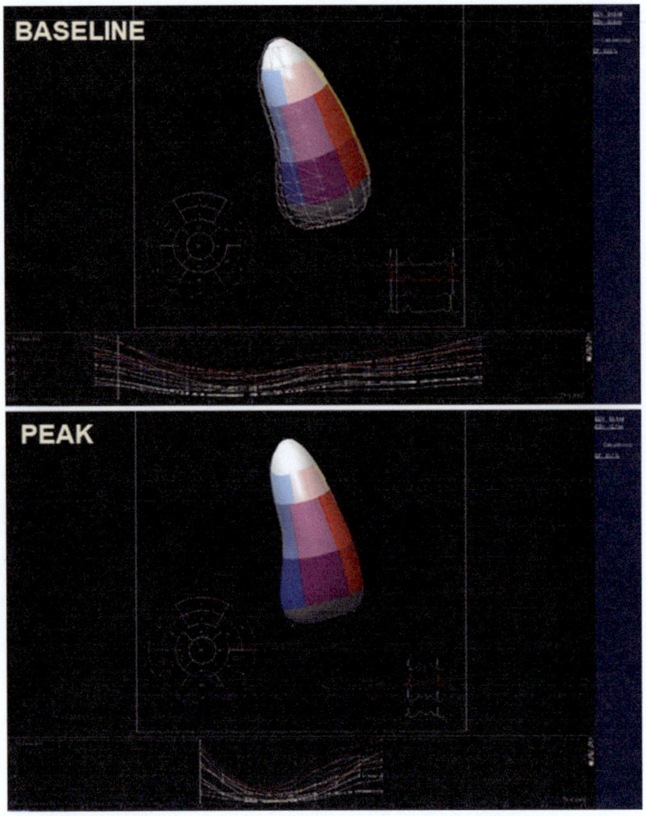

Fig. 23.5 3D volumetric images at rest and peak stress permit evaluation of LV global and segmental volumes and ejection fractions. Used with permission of Mayo Foundation for Medical Education and Research.

References

1. Pellikka PA, Arruda-Olson A, Chaudhry FA, Chen MH, Marshall JE, Porter TR, et al. Guidelines for performance, interpretation, and application of stress echocardiography in ischemic heart disease: from the American society of echocardiography. J Am Soc Echocardiogr. 2020;33(1):1–41.e8.
2. Steeds RP, Wheeler R, Bhattacharyya S, Reiken J, Nihoyannopoulos P, Senior R, et al. Stress echocardiography in coronary artery disease: a practical guideline from the British Society of Echocardiography. Echo Res Pract. 2019;6(2):G17–g33.
3. Gurunathan S, Senior R. Stress echocardiography in stable coronary artery disease. Curr Cardiol Rep. 2017;19(12):121.
4. Berbarie RF, Dib E, Ahmad M. Stress echocardiography using real-time three-dimensional imaging. Echocardiography. 2018;35(8):1196–203.
5. Yang HS, Pellikka PA, McCully RB, Oh JK, Kukuzke JA, Khandheria BK, et al. Role of biplane and biplane echocardiographically guided 3-dimensional echocardiography during dobutamine stress echocardiography. J Am Soc Echocardiogr. 2006;19(9):1136–43.
6. Peteiro J, Piñon P, Perez R, Monserrat L, Perez D, Castro-Beiras A. Comparison of 2- and 3-dimensional exercise echocardiography for the detection of coronary artery disease. J Am Soc Echocardiogr. 2007;20(8):959–67.
7. Ahmad M, Xie T, McCulloch M, Abreo G, Runge M. Real-time three-dimensional dobutamine stress echocardiography in assessment stress echocardiography in assessment of ischemia: comparison with two-dimensional dobutamine stress echocardiography. J Am Coll Cardiol. 2001;37(5):1303–9.
8. Aggeli C, Felekos I, Roussakis G, Kazazaki C, Lagoudakou S, Pietri P, et al. Value of real-time three-dimensional adenosine stress contrast echocardiography in patients with known or suspected coronary artery disease. Eur J Echocardiogr. 2011;12(9):648–55.
9. Takeuchi M, Otani S, Weinert L, Spencer KT, Lang RM. Comparison of contrast-enhanced real-time live 3-dimensional dobutamine stress echocardiography with contrast 2-dimensional echocardiography for detecting stress-induced wall-motion abnormalities. J Am Soc Echocardiogr. 2006;19(3):294–9.
10. Eroglu E, D'Hooge J, Herbots L, Thijs D, Dubois C, Sinnaeve P, et al. Comparison of real-time tri-plane and conventional 2D dobutamine stress echocardiography for the assessment of coronary artery disease. Eur Heart J. 2006;27(14):1719–24.
11. Johri AM, Chitty DW, Hua L, Marincheva G, Picard MH. Assessment of image quality in real time three-dimensional dobutamine stress echocardiography: an integrated 2D/3D approach. Echocardiography. 2015;32(3):496–507.
12. Yang HS, Bansal RC, Mookadam F, Khandheria BK, Tajik AJ, Chandrasekaran K. Practical guide for three-dimensional transthoracic echocardiography using a fully sampled matrix array transducer. J Am Soc Echocardiogr. 2008;21(9):979–89. quiz 1081-2
13. Shivalkar B, De Keersmaeker A, Van Hoeck N, Belkova P, Van de Heyning CM, De Maeyer C, et al. Is 3D Dobutamine stress echocardiography ready for prime time? Diagnostic and prognostic implications. Eur Heart J Cardiovasc Imaging. 2020;21(4):428–36.
14. Hoogslag GE, Joyce E, Bax JJ, Ajmone Marsan N, Delgado V. Assessment of global left ventricular excursion using three-dimensional dobutamine stress echocardiography to identify significant coronary artery disease. Echocardiography. 2016;33(10):1532–8.
15. Parker KM, Clark AP, Goodman NC, Glover DK, Holmes JW. Comparison of quantitative wall-motion analysis and strain for detection of coronary stenosis with three-dimensional dobutamine stress echocardiography. Echocardiography. 2015;32(2):349–60.
16. Lancellotti P, Pellikka PA, Budts W, Chaudhry FA, Donal E, Dulgheru R, et al. The clinical use of stress echocardiography in non-ischaemic heart disease: recommendations from the European Association of Cardiovascular Imaging and the American Society of Echocardiography. Eur Heart J Cardiovasc Imaging. 2016;17(11):1191–229.
17. Tanaka H, Oishi Y, Mizuguchi Y, Emi S, Ishimoto T, Nagase N, et al. Three-dimensional evaluation of dobutamine-induced changes in regional myocardial deformation in ischemic myocardium using ultrasonic strain measurements: the role of circumferential myocardial shortening. J Am Soc Echocardiogr. 2007;20(11):1294–9.
18. Lang RM, Addetia K, Narang A, Mor-Avi V. 3-dimensional echocardiography: latest developments and future directions. JACC Cardiovasc Imaging. 2018;11(12):1854–78.

Congenital and Acquired Ventricular Septal Defects

24

Francesco F. Faletra, Krishnaswamy Chandrasekaran, and Joseph F. Maalouf

Introduction

A full understanding of congenital ventricular septal defects (VSDs), [location, structure relationships with adjacent muscular or fibrous septum and/or surrounding atrioventricular or semilunar valves], requires a certain familiarity with septation of the ventricles and *normal* post-natal appearance of the interventricular septum (IVS). Indeed, the IVS is a complex three-dimensional non-planar partition between the right ventricle (RV) and left ventricle (LV), running obliquely (with respect to coronal plane of the body) from the anterior to posterior interventricular groove. Due to this angulation, the RV lies anteriorly and the LV posteriorly. Most of the surface of the IVS is muscular. Only a small segment, located just below the aorta, is made up of fibrous tissue. This region is termed membranous septum (MS). The muscular and MS have different developmental origins. This chapter will start with a concise description of the septation of the ventricles and normal aspects of the IVS.

Interventricular Septum Development

A comprehensive depiction of the septation of the ventricles is beyond the scope of this chapter. Herein, readers will find a brief and necessarily simplified portrayal of IVS development. Before septation, two distinct chambers in the heart tube (Fig. 24.1) contribute to the adult ventricles [1]. They are called the bulbus cordis and primitive ventricle. The bulbus cordis is composed of three segments: a proximal 1/3 which becomes the truncus arteriosus that gives rise to the pulmonary artery and aorta, a middle 1/3 conus segment that forms the LV and RV outflow tracts, and a caudal 1/3 from which most of the right ventricle is derived. The common ventricular cavity is formed by fusion of the primitive ventricle with the caudal 1/3 of the bulbus cordis, and the circular constriction or sulcus separating the two is named the bulbo-ventricular fold or sulcus that develops into the interventricular sulcus or groove. A muscular sheet grows upwards from the floor of the common ventricle dividing it into right and left halves, and forms the muscular part of the IVS (muscular sep-

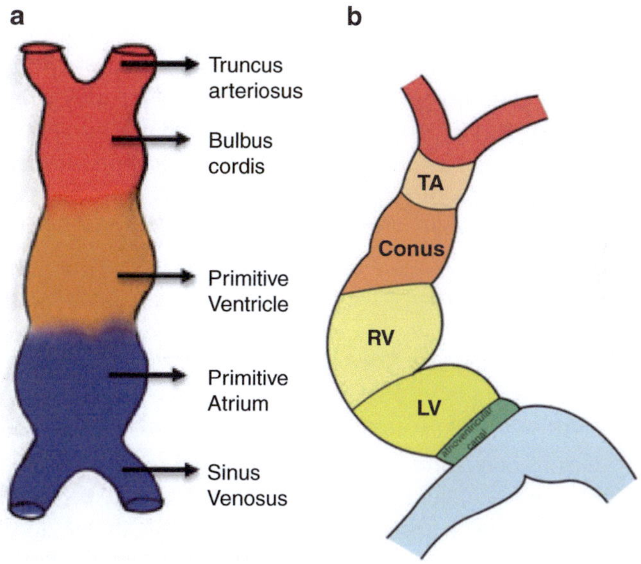

Fig. 24.1 (**a** and **b**) Illustrations of the heart tube used with permission from Core Concepts of Pediatrics, second Edition, Ashraf Aly, MD and Soham Dasgupta, MBBS, September 2020 (**a**), and adapted with permission from ThoracicKey.com General Considerations of Cardiac Embryology (**b**). The bulbus cordis gives rise to the proximal truncus arteriosus (TA), a middle conus segment, and a distal segment from which most of the right ventricle is derived (see text)

F. F. Faletra (✉)
Director of Cardiac Imaging Lab, Cardiocentro Ticino Institute, Lugano, Switzerland
e-mail: Francesco.Faletra@cardiocentro.org

K. Chandrasekaran
Professor of Medicine, Mayo Clinic College of Medicine; Consultant, Department of Cardiovascular Medicine, Mayo Clinic, Rochester, MN, USA
e-mail: kchandra@mayo.edu

J. F. Maalouf
Professor of Medicine, Mayo Clinic College of Medicine; Director, Interventional Echocardiography; Consultant, Department of Cardiovascular Medicine, Mayo Clinic, Rochester, MN, USA
e-mail: maalouf.joseph@mayo.edu

J. F. Maalouf et al. (eds.), *Practical 3D Echocardiography*, https://doi.org/10.1007/978-3-030-72941-7_24

tum). Meanwhile a partition named conal septum divides the upper 2/3 of the bulbus cordis and grows downwards. The muscular septum and the conal septum approximate each other leaving in between a small space named interventricular foramen. This foramen is filled up by a proliferation of the mesenchymal cells from endocardial cushion and conal septum. The MS takes origin from this fusion. Because the future tricuspid valve is more apical than the mitral valve, a small portion of the membraneous septum separates the future right atrium from the LV and is called the atrio-ventricular (AV) septum.

Thus, the post-fetal IVS has three origins, (1) upwards proliferation of muscular cells from the floor of the common ventricle (2) downwards proliferation of muscular cells from the conal septum and (3) proliferation of mesenchymal cells derived from the AV endocardial cushions or the conal septum. Muscular and membranous VSDs either isolated or part of more complex congenital malformations take origin from a deficient growth of one or more of these components.

Anatomy of IVS

The Membranous Septum

The MS is a thin, roughly quadrangular fibrous area about 10 mm in maximum length. When viewed from a left ventricular perspective, the MS is positioned in the space of a fibrous triangular area between the hinge line of the aortic right coronary and non-coronary leaflets [named interleaflet triangle (ILT)]. The superior margin of the MS merges with the fibrous tissue of the ILT while the inferior margin, inserts on the crest of the muscular IVS (Fig. 24.2).

The MS is in fibrous continuity with the right fibrous trigone. These two fibrous structures form the central fibrous body. The hinge line of the septal leaflet of the tricuspid valve divides the MS into two parts. The cranial component is the atrio-ventricular membranous septum (AVMS), separating the right atrium from the left ventricle, and is also referred to as the fibrous AV septum. The caudal part is the interventricular membranous septum (IVMS) which is a fibrous partition between the two ventricles. The size of the AVMS and IVMS is variable depending on the insertion of the septal leaflet: the higher the leaflet's insertion the smaller the AVMS (Fig. 24.3).

Muscular Septum

The muscular septum is an extensive non-planar muscular partition between the two ventricles. In cross-section, the muscular septum has a curved-shaped arrangement. The convex surface is towards the RV (which wraps around the LV extending from the anterior to the posterior interventricular groove), and concave surface towards the LV. consequently, the right surface is larger than the left surface (Fig. 24.4a and b). Although real anatomic boundaries do not exist, the muscular septum can be empirically divided into three components: an inlet, an apical trabeculated, and an outlet component. *The inlet part* is inferior-posterior to the membranous septum. It begins at the level of the atrioventricular valves and ends approximately at level of chordal attachment. The *trabecular part* is mainly limited to the apex, and *the infundibular part is* smooth-walled and separates the right ventricular outflow tract from the left ventricular outflow tract. The right side of the infundibular septum is more extensive than its left counterpart, and is bordered superiorly by the

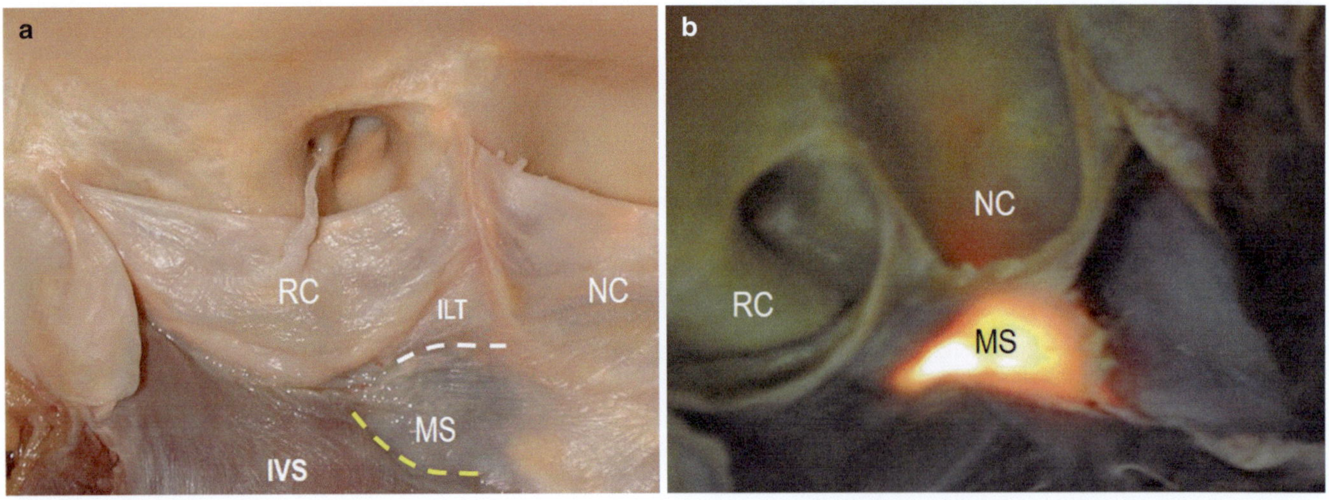

Fig. 24.2 With the permission of Edgardo Bonacina, Niguarda hospital Milan. (**a**) Anatomic specimen showing the membranous septum (MS) located in the caudal space of the interleaflet triangle (ILT) between the right coronary (RC) and noncoronary (NC) aortic leaflets hinge lines. The superior border of the MS inserts into the fibrous tissue of the ILT (white dotted line) while the inferior border inserts on the crest of the interventricular septum (IVS-yellow dotted line). (**b**) The margins of the MS are well-delineated through transillumination

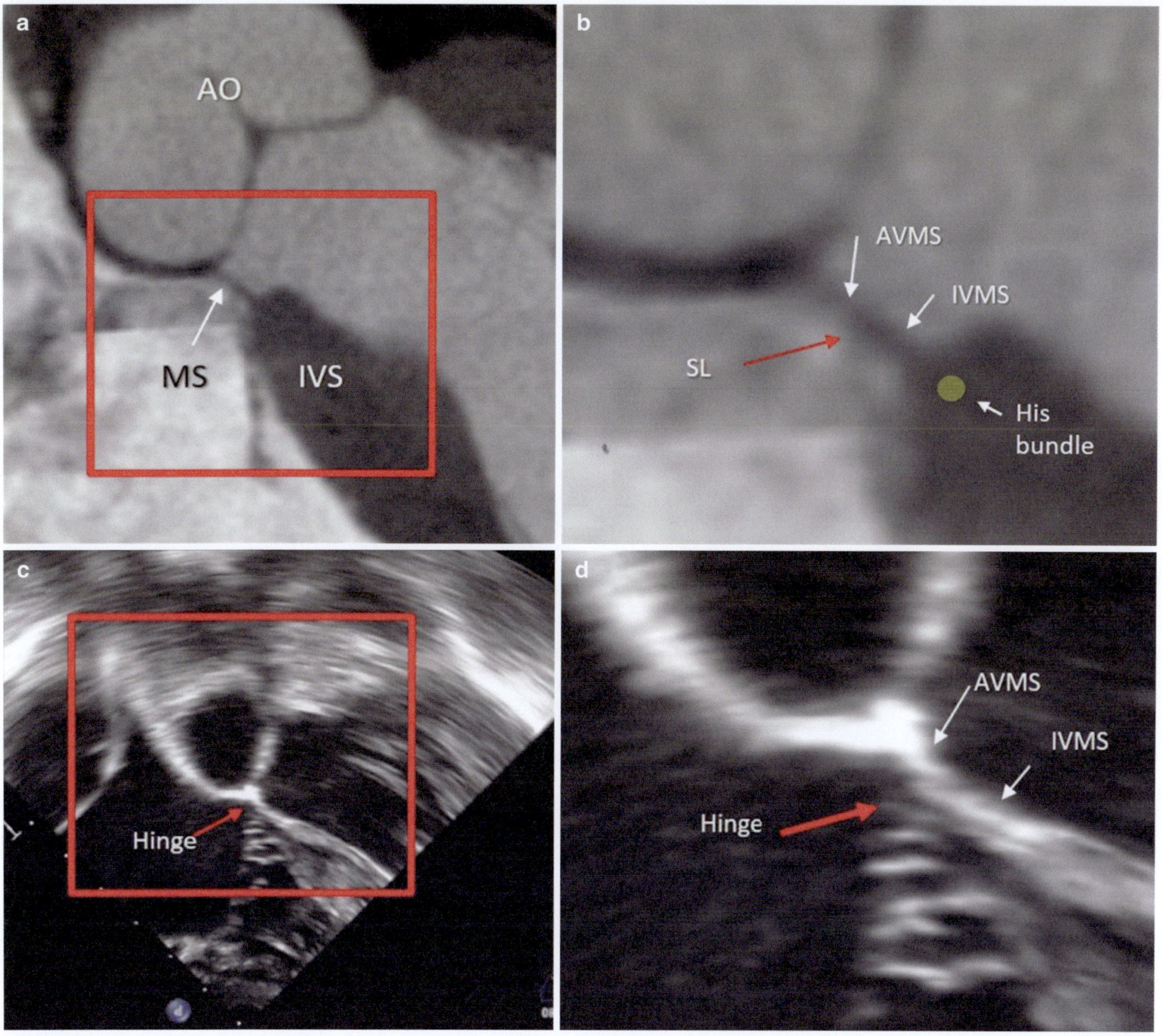

Fig. 24.3 With the permission of Faletra et al. in "Atlas of non-invasive imaging in cardiac anatomy" Springer Nature Switzerland 2020, Page 60–61. (**a**, **c**) CT scan and 2D TTE longitudinal cross-section of the aortic valve, membranous septum (MS), and interventricular septum (IVS) (**b**, **d**). Magnified images of the areas inside the red square, showing the MS divided by the insertion of the septal leaflet (SL) of the tricuspid valve (hinge), into two parts the atrio ventricular membranous septum (AVMS) and the interventricular membranous septum (IVMS). Of note the bundle of His (pale-green circle) runs between the inferior border of the MS and the crest of the IVS (panel B)

pulmonary semilunar valves, while the inferior border is delimited by the crista supraventricularis. This segmentation, though anatomically not existing, allows a more rational and easier classification of VSDs. CMR and CT cross-sectional images show the curved arrangement of the IVS (Fig. 24.4a and b). 3D TEE is able to visualize the muscular IVS from a unique "en face" view either from the LV or RV perspectives that is unavailable when using 2D cross-sectional imaging. (Fig. 24.4c and d).

Isolated Congenital VSDs

Congenital VSDs are the most common congenital defects both in children and adults apart from the bicuspid aortic valve [2]. They can exist in isolation, but are also found as integral components of other cardiac anomalies, such as tetralogy of Fallot, double outlet right ventricle, or common arterial trunk. In this chapter we focus on isolated VSDs. They may vary greatly in site, size and consequently in clini-

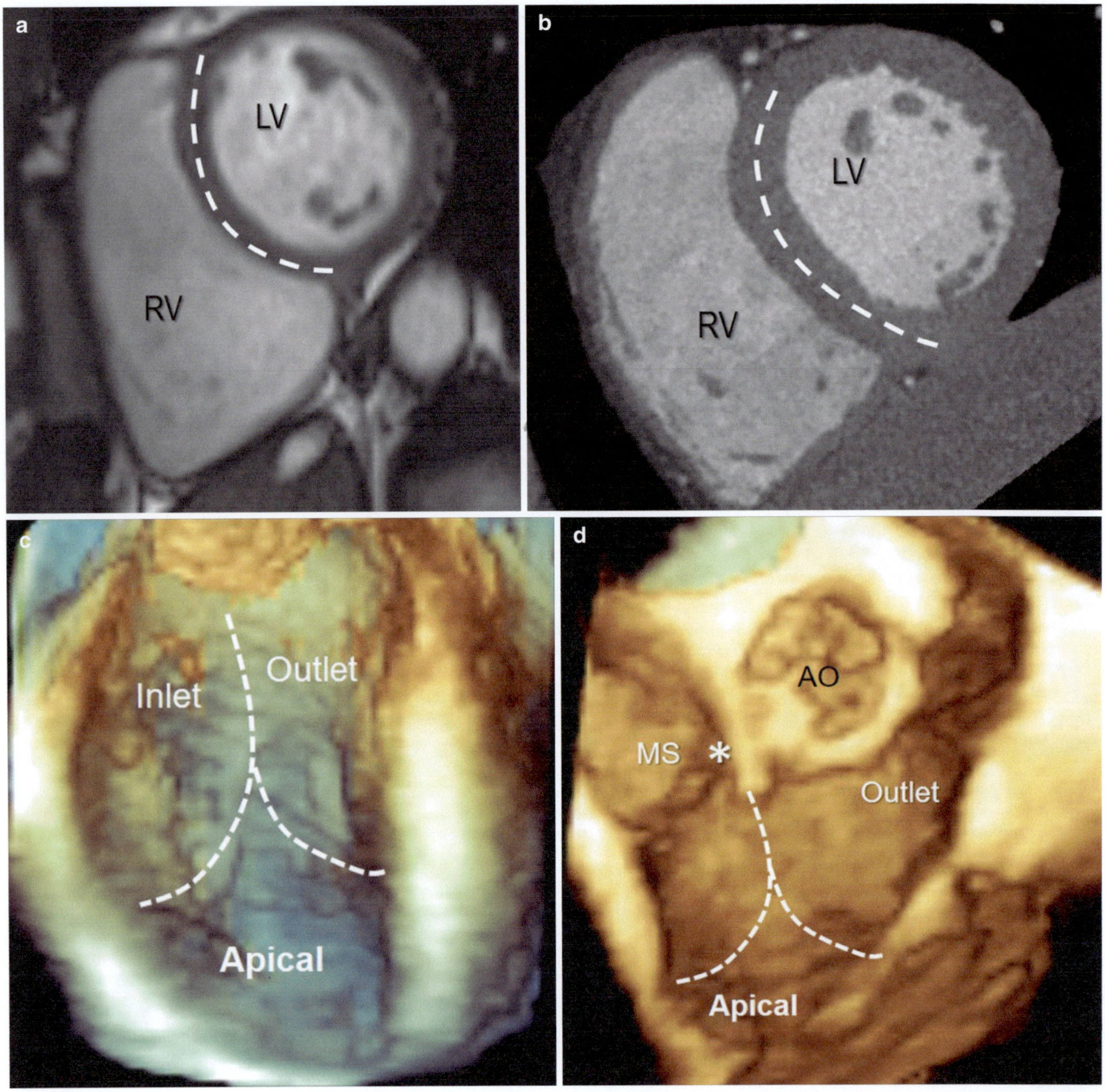

Fig. 24.4 (**a**, **b**) CMR (**a**) and CT (**b**) cross section images of the interventricular septum (IVS, dotted line) showing that the septum is convex towards the right ventricle (RV) and concave towards the left ventricle (LV). (**c**, **d**) Modified images with the permission of Faletra et al. in "Real time interventional echocardiography" Springer-Verlag London 2014, Page 139. Images show the left surface (**c**) and the right surface (**d**) of the IVS "en face". Conventional subdivision of the IVS into inlet, trabeculated apical and outlet. The dotted lines mark the arbitrary boundaries between them. Asterisk marks the position of the membranous septum (MS)

cal presentation and natural history. In the ensuing paragraphs we illustrate nomenclature, basic physiopathology and the anatomical arrangement of the most common isolated VSDs.

Nomenclature Unfortunately, there is no full agreement on how to classify isolated VSDs [3]. This lack of uniformity is due at least to two factors: first, there are different interpretations regarding the anatomy of the VSD, second when there is agreement on the patho-morphology, authors have used different names for indicating the same type of VSD. Classically, there are two ways for classifying VSDs, one is based on their location within the septum from right ventricular perspective (geographic approach), the other is based on the type of VSD borders and the relationships to adjacent septum and/or surrounding fibrous structures (border approach). Both approaches are useful. Classifying the VDSs based on the geographic approach allows determination of the site of surgical incision (for instance through the atrium, or through the RV or pulmonary artery). Whereas the border approach helps to define the structures adjacent to the defect, for instance pathway of conduction system, arterial or atrio-ventricular leaflets, in order to avoid injuries during surgery.

Pathophysiology Analogous to ASDs, the size of the VSD, the amount of shunt and the pulmonary and systemic vascular resistances are the key factors for determining the patho-physiological consequences and clinical scenarios in patients with VSD. There is a spectrum of patho-physiological states and the aforementioned geographic or border classifications can be coupled to a classification based on patho-physiology. At one end of the spectrum are ***restrictive VSDs***. This term refers to small VSDs (also called "maladie de Roger") in which the size of the defect is less than 1/3 of the size of the aortic annulus and a significant gradient between left and right ventricle (>60 mmHg) can be measured. Both pulmonary pressure and pulmonary vascular resistances are normal. These VSDs are usually benign, and, apart of the risk of infective endocarditis, children with restrictive VSDs remain asymptomatic and spontaneous closure and normal growth can be expected. On the other end of the spectrum are the ***non-restrictive VSDs.*** The term refers to large VSDs in which the pulmonary circulation is subjected to an increase in pulmonary flow early in the course of the disease. Over few years (but also over few months depending on how large the VSD is) the majority of patients develop irreversible pulmonary vascular changes (such us thickened adventitia, medial hypertrophy and vascular endothelial changes) leading to a progressive increase in pulmonary vascular resistance with a consequent reduction in the left-to-right shunt. With disease progression, equalization of pressures between the two ventricles with cessation of the shunt occurs. This may be followed by development of irreversible severe pulmonary hypertension (Eisenmenger syndrome) with right-to-left shunting across the VSD. In between these two extremes there are VSDs called ***moderately restrictive VSD*** in which the size of the VSD is about half of the aortic annulus and the pulmonary pressure and resistances are increased but not at systemic levels. Characteristically these VSDs result in left atrial and left ventricular dilation due to volume overload, and patients may present with shortness of breath due to excessive pulmonary blood flow. In the following paragraphs we describe the anatomic appearance of the most common types of VSD: perimebranous VSD, Gerbode defect, muscular and infundibular VSD.

Perimembranous VSDs are located in the area of the interventricular part of the MS and therefore, below the septal leaflet of the tricuspid valve at level of the antero-septal commissure (Fig. 24.5a and b). This defect is the most common VSD subtype occurring in 75–80% of all cases of isolated VSD and is due to deficiency of membranous septum along with variable portion of the surrounding muscular septum. Characteristically part of the border of this defect is lined by the border of residual MS itself or by fibrous tissue of the superior interleaflet triangle (Fig. 24.5c). The remaining borders are muscular with variable extension towards the inlet, trabeculated or outlet septum. It is very unlikely for the perimebranous defect to exist completely inside the interventricular membranous septum without a muscular border. Of note, the His bundle, courses along the posterior-inferior rim. When the defect extends underneath the commissure between the right and non-coronary aortic leaflets, one of the leaflets may prolapse thorough the defect, accidentally closing (or reducing) the size of the defect but, at the same time, distorting the valve with consequent aortic regurgitation (Fig. 24.5d). It has been recognized for years that this type of defect is associated with so-called aneurysm of the membranous septum. Angiographically this is a pouch like structure with well-defined margins protruding for some extent into the right ventricle. Imaging of this anatomic arrangement can be obtained using CT or TTE (Fig. 24.5e and f). A hemodynamically large perimebranous VSD in infancy may progress to a smaller defect later in childhood with the formation of such aneurysm. The presence of the aneurysm has therefore, been considered a marker for the defect that is likely to close or become smaller and hemodynamically and clinically irrelevant [4]. The substrate of this anatomical arrangement has been in the past subjected to numerous studies and is still controversial. The hypothesis that this pouch-like deformation may originate from the membranous septum itself appears rather questionable. Indeed, the membranous septum is made up from compact and robust fibrous tissue resistant to left ventricular pressure and it is unlikely (unless there is connective tissue deficiency of the MS itself, which is improbable) that it may progress to aneurysm formation. Most likely the aneurysm derives from the juxtaposition of tricuspid leaflet tissue around the defect. The septal leaflet may, in fact, be injured by the high-velocity jet crossing the defect. Jet lesions may, in turn, cause inflammation, de-endothelization and adherence of leaflet tissue around the border of the defect, partially (or entirely) closing the defect and creating the aneurysm [5].

Gerbode Defect While a perforation through the IVMS connects the two ventricles, a perforation of the AVMS connects the LV with the right atrium (RA). This rare congenital communication is called a Gerbode defect, after the name of

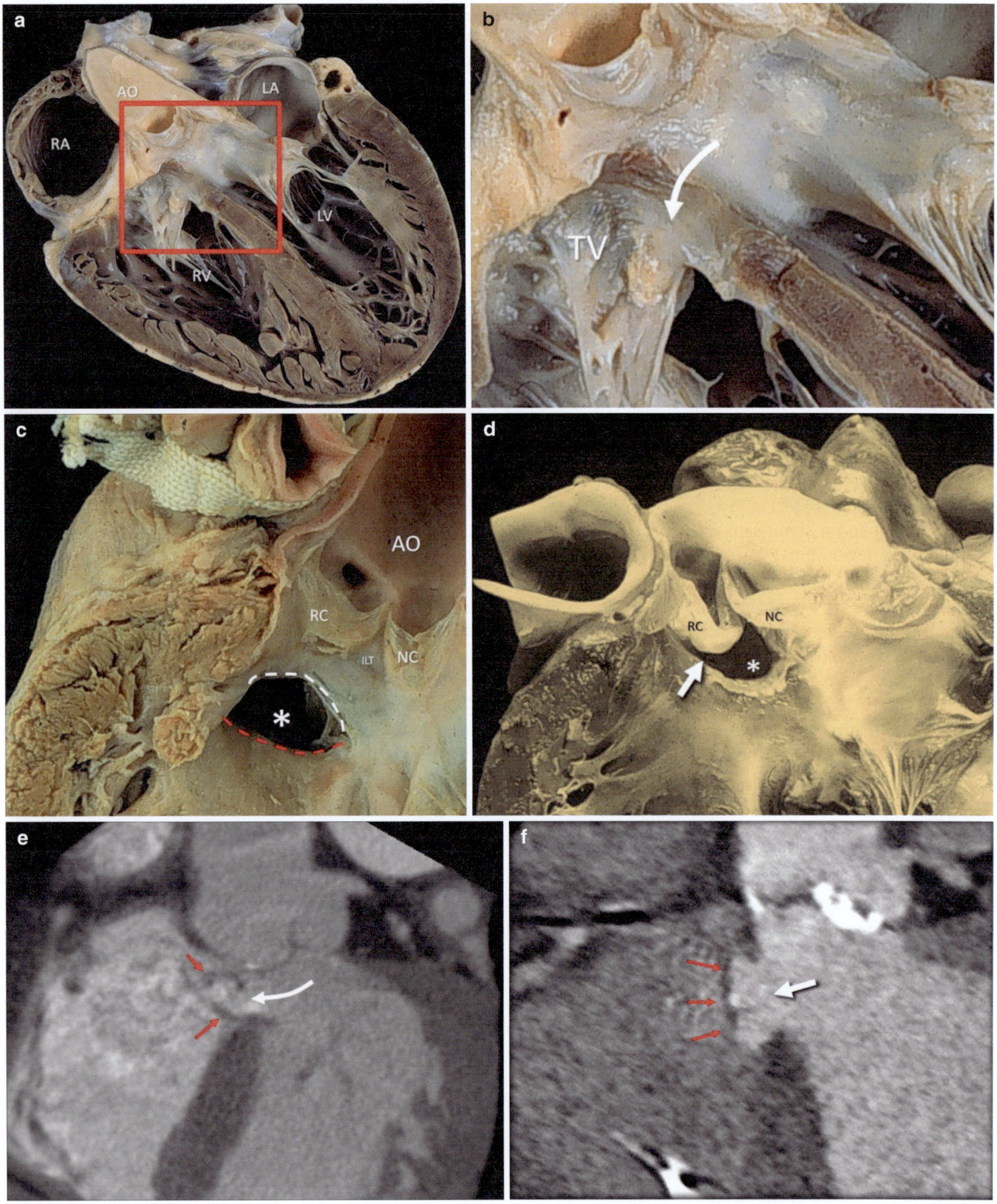
a
AO
LA
RA
LV
RV
b
TV
c
AO
RC
ILT
NC
*
d
RC
NC
*
e
f

Fig. 24.5 (**a–d**) Anatomic specimens courtesy Dr. William D. Edwards. Cross section cut "five chamber view" showing the aorta (AO), right atrium (RA), left atrium (LA) Right ventricle (RV) and left ventricle (LV). (**b**) Magnified image of the structures inside the red square in panel a. The image shows a perimebranous defect (arrow) immediately below the tricuspid valve leaflets (TV). (**c**) Anatomic images of a perimebranous defect (asterisk). The superior-anterior margin is made up from the residual membranous septum immediately below the interleaflet triangle (ILT) between the non-coronary (NC) and right coronary (RC) cusps (white dotted line), while the inferior margin is made up from muscular tissue (red dotted line). (**d**) Perimebranous defect (asterisk) extending to the commissure between the RC and NC cusps. The right coronary cusp prolapses (arrow) into the defect likely causing aortic regurgitation (see text). (Images **a–d** were used with permission of Mayo Foundation for Medical Education and Research. All rights reserved) (**e**). CT scan in long axis view showing a perimebranous defect (white curved arrow) partially closed by tricuspid tissue (red arrows). (**f**) CT scan in long axis view of a perimebranous defect (white arrow) totally closed by tricuspid tissue (red arrows)

the cardiac surgeon who first successfully performed the closure [6]. Three types of congenital patho-morphological arrangements may connect the LV to the RA. The classic one is perforation of the AVMS and is called supra-valvular or direct, the second type, called infra-valvular is likely due to a perimembranous defect accompanied by structural changes of septal leaflet as a result of the aneurysmal pouch. This defect connects the LV either with RA or with RV (see previous paragraph on perimembranous defect); the third type is a combination of supra and infra-valvular communications. Although known as congenital, LV to RA communications may be iatrogenic. Surgical aortic and mitral valve replacements, tricuspid annuloplasty ring insertion, and percutaneous cardiac interventions such as AV node ablation, and endomyocardial biopsies may accidentally result in damage to the MS with consequent perforation and LV-to-RA shunt. Finally, non-congenital, non-iatrogenic Gerbode defects are those caused by infective endocarditis or blunt cardiac trauma.

The Muscular Inlet VSDs maintain a muscular rim all around the defect and are located in the inlet portion of the muscular septum. The inlet VSDs that have no rim between the defect and the atrioventricular annulus and include abnormalities of the atrio-ventricular valves are referred to as atrio-ventricular septal defects (see Chap. 20).

The Trabecular VSDs are located in the trabecular part of the septum. Some of these defects have multiple holes visible on both side of the IVS. These defects can be further classified according their location in mid-septal, apical, posteroinferior and anterosuperior.

The Outlet VSDs are located in the muscular part of the infundibular septum and are rimmed completely by muscular tissue. In some outlet VSDs the superior part of the defect is adjacent to the aortic annulus, pulmonary annulus or both (Fig. 24.6). These defects are termed supracristal, conal subpulmonary or double-committed. Right coronary cusp prolapse into the VSD can occur analogous to perimembranous VSDs.

Ventricular Septal Rupture

Post acute myocardial infarction (AMI) ventricular septal rupture (VSR) is a potentially devastating complication that occurs 1–8 days after the AMI, and is caused by complete occlusion of a major coronary artery that supplies the IVS and results in transmural septal infarction. The incidence of VSR has decreased from 1 to 3% in the pre-reperfusion era to 0.17–0.31% following primary percutaneous coronary intervention [7]. In fact, reperfusion of the infarct-related artery within the first 6 h of AMI limits the necrotic area which helps prevent the occurrence of VSR. Several mechanisms may cause VSR (1) a large intramural hematoma may "dissect" the necrotic tissue leading to an abrupt laceration within the first 24 h. (2) Lytic enzymes produced by neutrophils in the infarcted area, may erode the wall with subsequent tear and (3) A perforation may occur in the central portion of a thin septal aneurysm. It is interesting to note that delayed reperfusion (after 6–10 h) may contribute to the genesis of VSR. Indeed, in this time frame, the myocardium undergoes coagulation necrosis and edema, and the capillary network begins to be disrupted. In this histopathological setting, torrential blood flow (due to the opening of the epicardial infarct-related artery into myocardial tissues) may itself cause an intramural hematoma with potential risk of VSR. Septal rupture in anterior AMI tends to be apical with a discrete simple defect. Conversely, in inferior-posterior AMI the VSR is usually located in the basal portion of the posterior septum and often has a more complex, serpiginous course (Fig. 24.7).

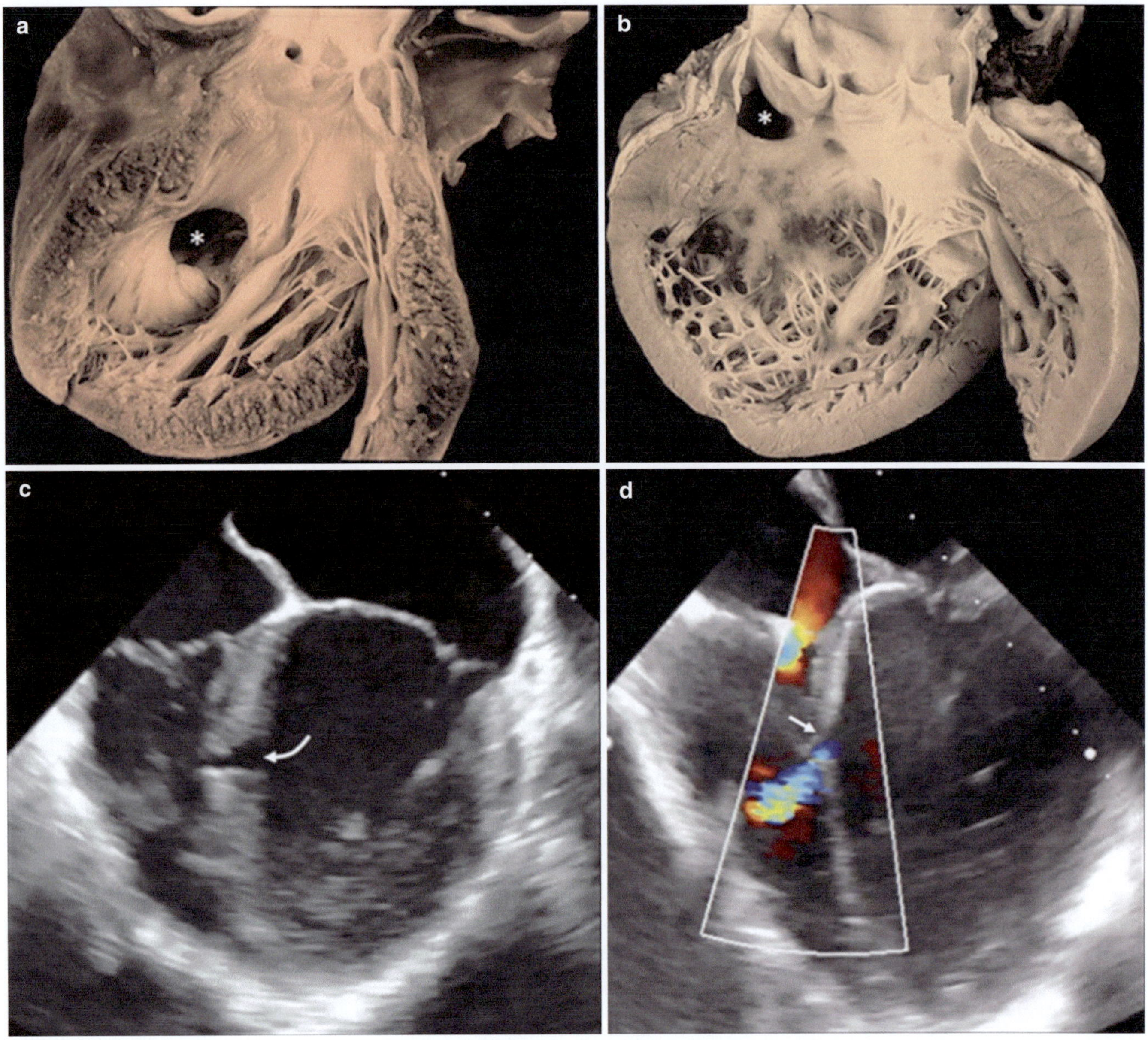

Fig. 24.6 (**a**, **b**) anatomic specimens showing a large trabecular muscular VSD (**a**) and a large infundibular VSD (**b**). Courtesy William D. Edwards (Mayo Clinic). (Images **a** and **b** were used with permission of Mayo Foundation for Medical Education and Research. All rights reserved). The defects are marked with asterisks. (**c**) 2D TEE showing a trabecular VSD (arrow). (**d**) Same VSD with color Doppler, the jet is seen crossing the defect (arrow)

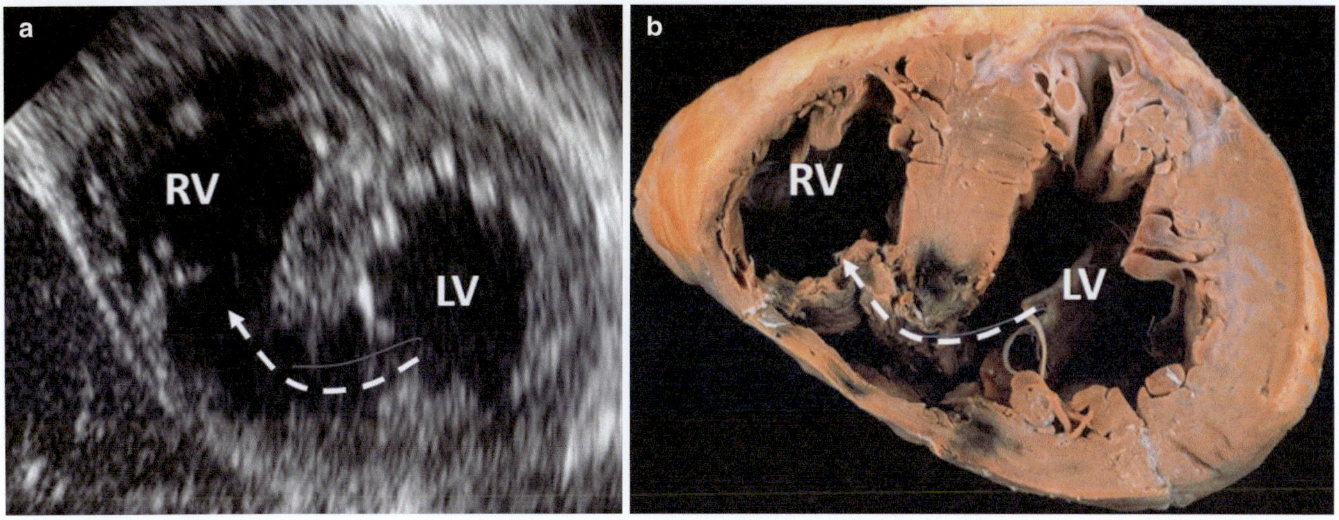

Fig. 24.7 (**a**) 2D TEE short axis transgastric view showing a huge VSR (dotted arrow) in the inferior septum. (**b**) Similar image anatomic specimen (Image **b** used with permission of Mayo Foundation for Medical Education and Research. All rights reserved). LV, left ventricle; RV, right ventricle

The size of the defect may vary from few millimeters to several centimeters and is the primary cause of the magnitude of the left-to-right shunt. Large defects lead to the development of right ventricular dysfunction, pulmonary hypertension, congestive heart failure, low cardiac output and fatal cardiogenic shock.

References

1. Wenink AC. Embryology of the ventricular septum. Separate origin of its components. Virchows Arch A Pathol Anat Histol. 1981;390(1):71–9.
2. Spicer DE, Hsu HH, Co-Vu J, Anderson RH, Fricker FJ. Ventricular septal defect. Orphanet J Rare Dis. 2014;9:144. Published 2014 Dec 19
3. Anderson RH, Spicer DE, Mohun TJ, Hikspoors JPJM, Lamers WH. Remodeling of the embryonic interventricular communication in regard to the description and classification of ventricular septal defects. Anat Rec (Hoboken). 2019;302(1):19–31.
4. Li X, Ren W, Song G, Zhang X. Prediction of spontaneous closure of ventricular septal defect and guidance for clinical follow-up. Clin Cardiol. 2019;42(5):536–41.
5. Ilmaz AT, Ozal E, Arslan M, Tatar H, Oztürk OY. Aneurysm of the membranous septum in adult patients with perimembranous ventricular septal defect. Eur J Cardiothorac Surg. 1997;11(2):307–11.
6. Saker E, Bahri GN, Montalbano MJ, et al. Gerbode defect: a comprehensive review of its history, anatomy, embryology, pathophysiology, diagnosis, and treatment. J Saudi Heart Assoc. 2017;29(4):283–92.
7. Menon V, Webb JG, Hillis LD, Sleeper LA, Abboud R, Dzavik V, Slater JN, Forman R, Monrad ES, Talley JD, Hochman JS. Outcome and profile of ventricular septal rupture with cardiogenic shock after myocardial infarction: a report from the SHOCK trial registry. SHould we emergently revascularize occluded coronaries in cardiogenic shocK? J Am Coll Cardiol. 2000;36:1110–6.

CT and MRI of Ventricles and Ventricular Septum

25

Kathleen A. Young, Korosh Sharain, Thomas A. Foley, and Nandan S. Anavekar

Both cardiac computed tomography (CT) and magnetic resonance imaging (MRI) are adjuncts to echocardiography in the assessment of cardiac structure and function. In this chapter, we demonstrate how cross-sectional imaging with CT or MRI vastly improves the understanding of both acquired and congenital structural defects of the ventricles and ventricular septum.

Left ventricular pseudoaneurysms are cardiac ruptures which are contained by the pericardium or scar tissue, without involvement of myocardium or endocardium [1, 2]. They can occur as a complication of myocardial infarction (Fig. 25.1), cardiac surgery, chest trauma (Fig. 25.2), or endocarditis [1, 2]. On imaging, they generally have a narrow neck compared to the body of the aneurysm [2]. On cardiac CT and MRI, they generally appear as contrast or fluid-filled saccular or fusiform outpouchings, and may also include thrombus [3]. Surgical or transcatheter closure is usually considered [1, 4]. Both cardiac CT and MRI can provide information regarding the anatomy and involvement of adjacent structures to aide procedural planning [3, 4].

Identification and characterization of congenital or acquired defects within the ventricular septum is greatly enhanced by the use of cross-sectional imaging. For example, in congenital ventricular septal defects, either MRI or CT can be helpful to define surrounding anatomy, identify associated lesions, and confirm anatomy of defects less well visualized by echocardiography (Fig. 25.3, [5, 6]). Similarly, in acquired ventricular septal defects, such as what can occur as a complication of an acute myocardial infarction, iatrogenic following aortic or mitral valve surgery (Fig. 25.4), or due to infection or trauma; a multimodality imaging approach with cardiac CT or MRI can provide crucial information for surgical or transcatheter procedural planning [7, 8].

K. A. Young
Instructor in Medicine, Mayo Clinic College of Medicine; Resident, Department of Cardiovascular Medicine, Mayo Clinic, Rochester, MN, USA
e-mail: young.kathleen1@mayo.edu

K. Sharain
Assistant Professor in Medicine, Mayo Clinic College of Medicine; Resident, Department of Cardiovascular Medicine, Mayo Clinic, Rochester, MN, USA
e-mail: sharain.korosh@mayo.edu

T. A. Foley
Assistant Professor of Radiology, Mayo Clinic College of Medicine; Consultant, Division of Cardiovascular Radiology, Department of Radiology, Mayo Clinic, Rochester, MN, USA
e-mail: foley.thomas@mayo.edu

N. S. Anavekar (✉)
Professor of Medicine, Mayo Clinic College of Medicine; Consultant, Department of Cardiovascular Medicine, Mayo Clinic, Rochester, MN, USA
e-mail: anavekar.nandan@mayo.edu

J. F. Maalouf et al. (eds.), *Practical 3D Echocardiography*, https://doi.org/10.1007/978-3-030-72941-7_25

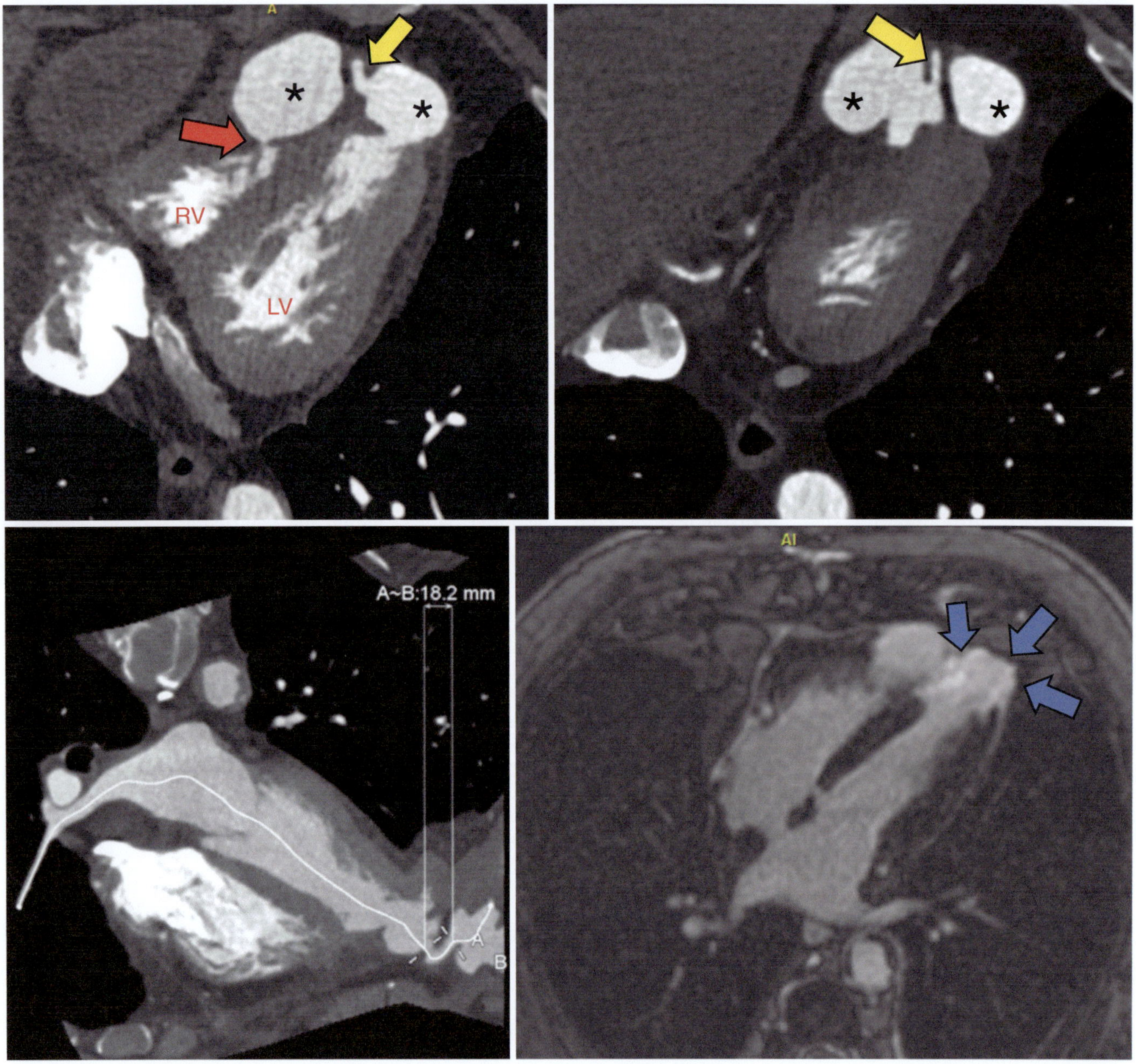

Fig. 25.1 Ventricular Pseudoaneurysm: patient had a history of NSTEMI and was found to have severe multivessel disease for which he underwent urgent revascularization with coronary artery bypass grafting. He presented 4 months later with dyspnea and an apical systolic murmur was heard. Transthoracic echocardiography identified a complex-appearing left ventricular pseudoaneurysm. Computed tomography was performed to evaluate the extent of the pseudoaneurysm. **Top two panels**—The patient had a bi-lobed LV pseudoaneurysm (asterisks) that communicated with each other by a thin tract (yellow arrows) which ultimately connected to the right ventricle (red arrow). **Bottom panel—Left:** curved planar reformatting provided better visualization of the tract into the right ventricle. The tract connecting the bilobed pseudoaneurysm (A–B) was measured for pre-procedural planning. No intracardiac thrombus was identified. Additionally, CT provided the ability to evaluate the coronary artery bypass grafts which were all patent. **Right:** Cardiac MRI demonstrating thinning and transmural delayed enhancement (blue arrows) of the apex. Used with permission of Mayo Foundation for Medical Education and Research. All rights reserved. *LV* left ventricle, *RV* right ventricle

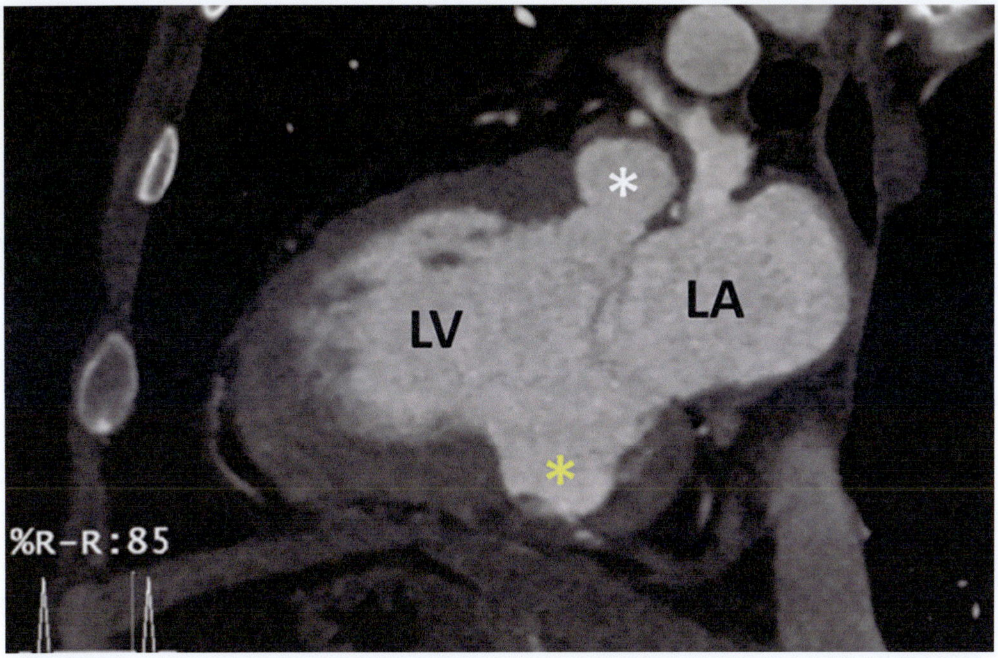

Fig. 25.2 Traumatic Ventricular Pseudoaneurysm: Patient presented after a high-speed head on motor vehicle accident. Cardiac CT demonstrated a pseudoaneurysm of the basal anterior wall (white asterisk) and an aneurysm of the basal inferior wall (yellow asterisk) suspected to be post-traumatic in nature. Of note, no intracardiac thrombus was identified on CT. The CT also evaluated his coronary arteries which were without disease. He also developed flail mitral and tricuspid valves requiring repair. Used with permission of Mayo Foundation for Medical Education and Research. All rights reserved. LA, left atrium; LV, left ventricle

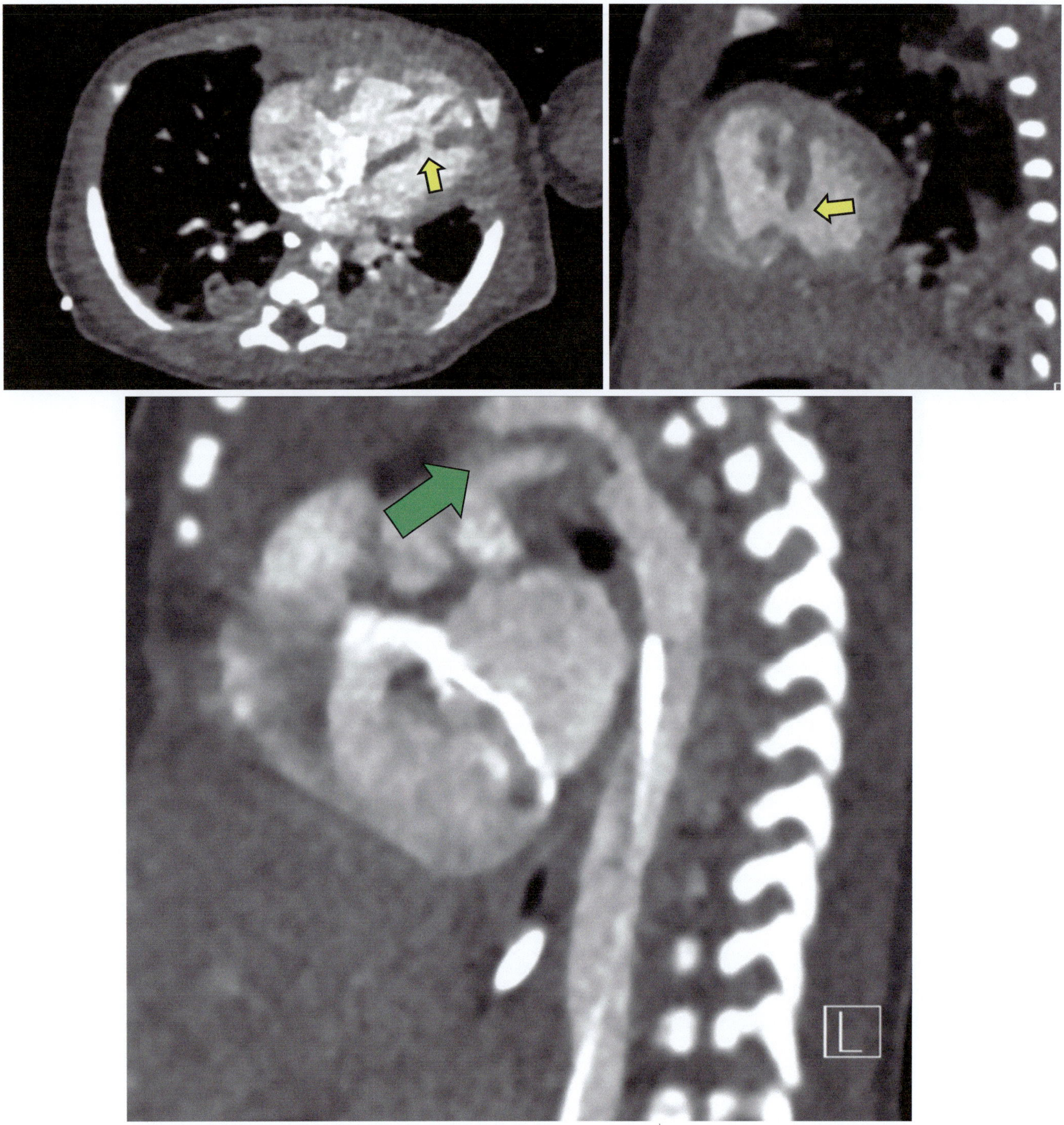

Fig. 25.3 Congenital Ventricular Septal Defect: A baby was born with desaturations and a loud systolic murmur. Echocardiography identified a VSD and possible patent ductus arteriosus (PDA). Computed tomography was obtained to evaluate for any other congenital heart disease. The muscular ventricular septal defect was better characterized and measured 3 mm in the axial view (top left panel—yellow arrow) and short axis view (top right panel—yellow arrow). Additionally, the baby was found to have coarctation of the aorta (bottom panel—green arrow). No patent ductus arteriosus or partial anomalous pulmonary venous return was identified. The baby underwent coarctation and VSD repair. *VSD*, ventricular septal defect

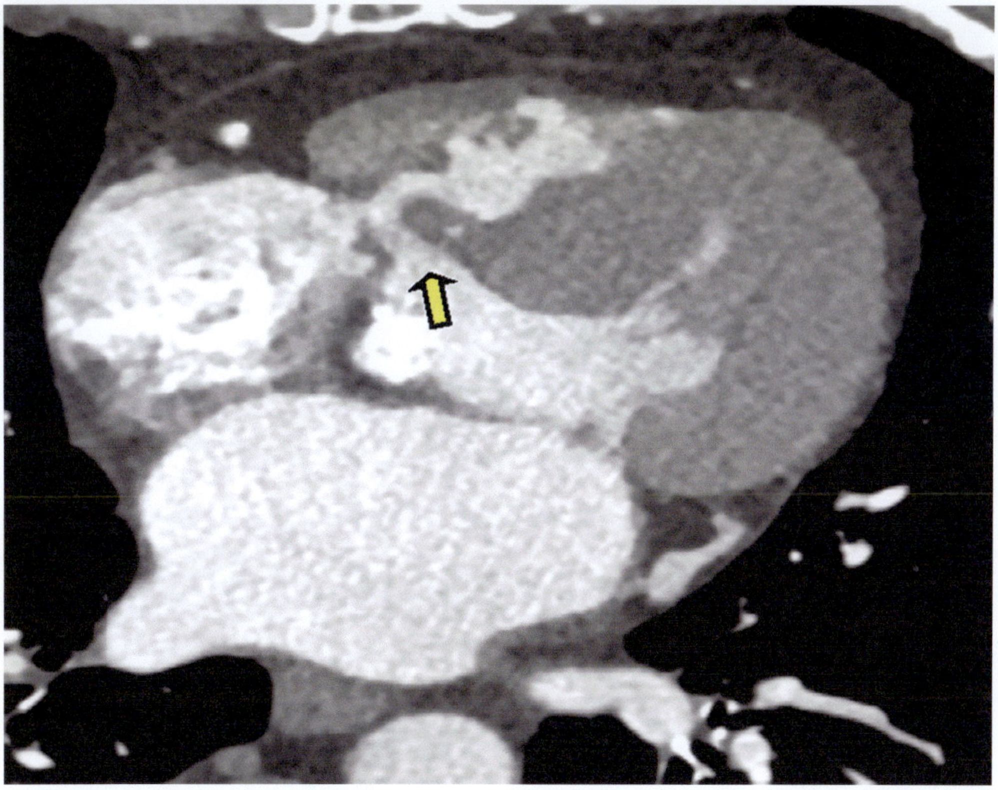

Fig. 25.4 Acquired Ventricular Septal Defect: Membranous VSD identified in a patient who underwent transcatheter aortic valve replacement (arrow). Used with permission of Mayo Foundation for Medical Education and Research. All rights reserved. VSD, ventricular septal defect

References

1. Frances C, Romero A, Grady D. Left ventricular pseudoaneurysm. J Am Coll Cardiol. 1998;32(3):557–61.
2. Yeo TC, et al. Clinical profile and outcome in 52 patients with cardiac pseudoaneurysm. Ann Intern Med. 1998;128(4):299–305.
3. Rajiah P, et al. Multimodality imaging of complications of cardiac valve surgeries. Radiographics. 2019;39(4):932–56.
4. Kumar PV, et al. Percutaneous therapeutic approaches to closure of cardiac pseudoaneurysms. Catheter Cardiovasc Interv. 2012;80(4):687–99.
5. Kim AM, et al. Imaging in congenital and hereditary abnormalities of the interventricular septum: clinical anatomy and diagnostic clues. J Thorac Imaging. 2018;33(3):147–55.
6. Warnes CA, et al. ACC/AHA 2008 guidelines for the management of adults with congenital heart disease: a report of the American College of Cardiology/American Heart Association task force on practice guidelines (Writing Committee to Develop Guidelines on the Management of Adults With Congenital Heart Disease). Developed in Collaboration With the American Society of Echocardiography, Heart Rhythm Society, International Society for Adult Congenital Heart Disease, Society for Cardiovascular Angiography and Interventions, and Society of Thoracic Surgeons. J Am Coll Cardiol. 2008;52(23):e143–263.
7. Giblett JP, Jenkins DP, Calvert PA. Transcatheter treatment of postinfarct ventricular septal defects. Heart. 2020;106(12):878–884.
8. DeClue C, Donatelli JM, Rojas CA. Noncongenital ventricular septal defects: a pictorial review. J Thorac Imaging. 2018;33(4):W22–9.

Part V

Cardiac Masses

26 Role of 3DE in Assessment of Cardiac Masses: Incremental Value over 2DE

Hyun Suk Yang, Tae-Yop Kim, Joseph F. Maalouf, and Krishnaswamy Chandrasekaran

Introduction

Three-dimensional (3D) echocardiography offers incremental value to two-dimensional (2D) echocardiography in the evaluation of intra-cardiac masses (thrombi, tumors, and vegetations), by providing real time and post-processing assessments of size, shape, inner composition, and relationships with surrounding structures [1] (Figs. 26.1 and 26.2). Transthoracic echocardiography (TTE) is the preferred method for initial assessment, but transesophageal echocardiography (TEE) is often the imaging modality of choice for better delineation due to its superior resolution. 3D TEE provides unprecedented anatomic detail of intra-cardiac masses with en-face views [2]. In serial size comparisons, 3D TTE reliably permits exactly the same 2D tomographic planes from volumetric data allowing accurate measurement of mass changes over times.

Supplementary Information The online version of this chapter (https://doi.org/10.1007/978-3-030-72941-7_26) contains supplementary material, which is available to authorized users.

H. S. Yang · T.-Y. Kim
Professor, Research institute of Medical Science, Konkuk University School of Medicine, Department of Cardiovascular Medicine, Konkuk University Medical Center, Neungdong-ro, Gwangjin-gu, Seoul, Korea
e-mail: yang.hyun@kuh.ac.kr

J. F. Maalouf
Professor of Medicine, Mayo Clinic College of Medicine; Director, Interventional Echocardiography; Consultant, Department of Cardiovascular Medicine, Mayo Clinic, Rochester, MN, USA
e-mail: maalouf.joseph@mayo.edu

K. Chandrasekaran (✉)
Professor of Medicine, Mayo Clinic College of Medicine; Consultant, Department of Cardiovascular Medicine, Mayo Clinic, Rochester, MN, USA
e-mail: kchandra@mayo.edu

Thrombi

Intra-cardiac thrombus typically occurs where there is blood stasis (e.g. left ventricular (LV) apical aneurysm with a myocardial infarction; left atrial appendage (LAA) in atrial fibrillation), a mechanical prosthesis with suboptimal anticoagulation, or hypercoagulable states. The LAA is the most common location for atrial thrombus formation, and its multi-lobular structure with pectinate muscles often mimic thrombi [2]. Conventional 2D TEE is the typical diagnostic choice for LAA thrombi. However, biplane TEE imaging of the LAA targeting the region of interest (ROI) allows multiple simultaneous measurements of the mass in a fast and convenient manner (Fig. 26.3). Live 3D echocardiography further enhances identification of intra-cardiac thrombi. The focused 3D zoom or live 3D Full-Volume acquisition, and subsequent post-processing cropping planes help to identify the accessary lobes or inner thrombi (Fig. 26.4). Live 3D echocardiography also enhances visualization of intraaortic atheromatous plaque related thrombus (Fig. 26.5).

Tumors

Primary cardiac tumors are rare with a reported incidence of 1.38 per 100,000 inhabitants per year [3]. The majority (75%) of primary cardiac tumors are benign, predominantly being myxoma (50–70%), followed by papillary fibroelastoma, lipoma, and fibroma [3, 4]. Routine 2D echocardiography can evaluate the location, appearance, size, and mobility of cardiac tumors. Color and spectral Doppler are useful in determining the hemodynamic consequences resulting from the tumor. Simultaneous biplane or focused live 3D imaging of the cardiac tumor allows better visualization of the extent, size, shape, and point of attachment.

J. F. Maalouf et al. (eds.), *Practical 3D Echocardiography*, https://doi.org/10.1007/978-3-030-72941-7_26

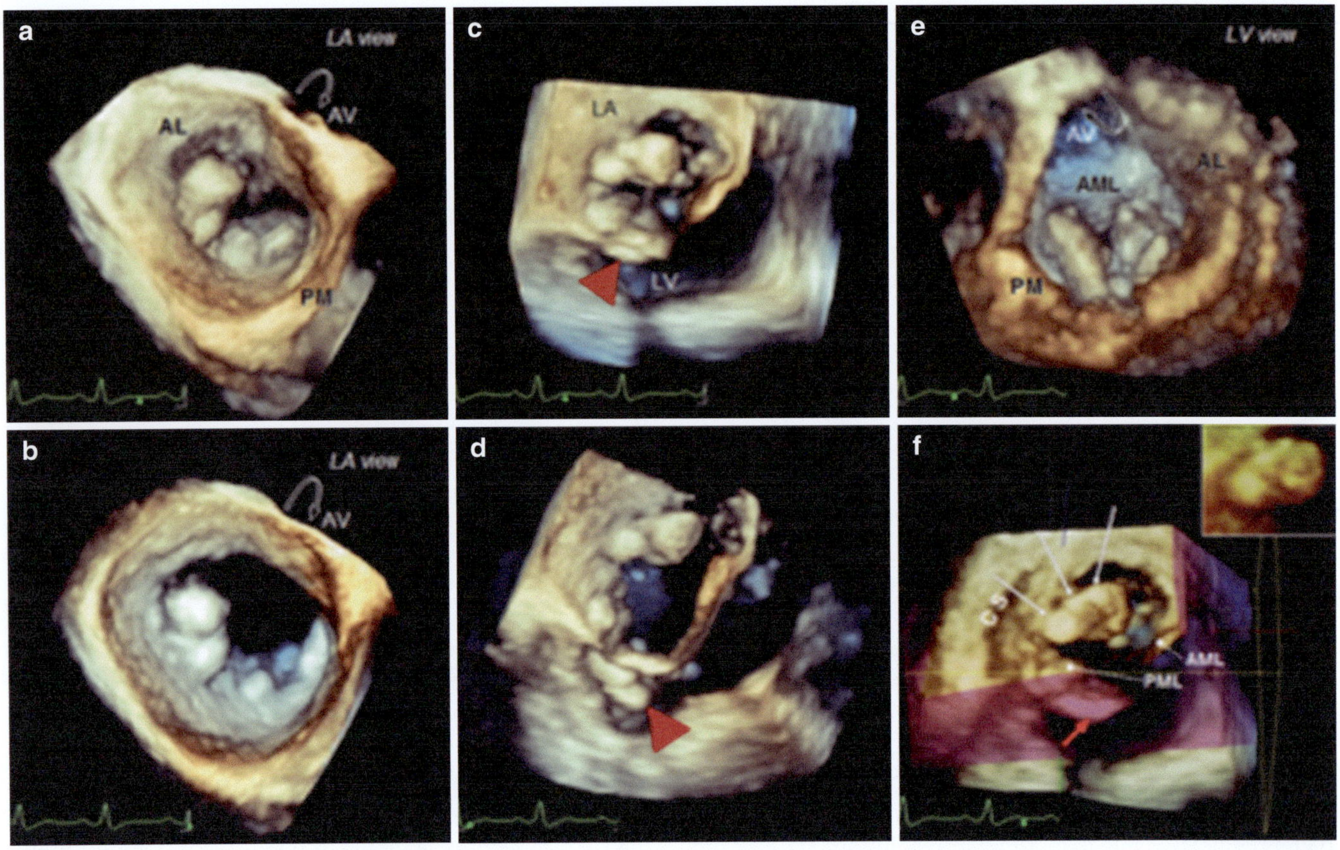

Fig. 26.1 Caseous Calcification of the Mitral Annulus. Live 3D zoom images show an en-face view of the mitral valve apparatus from the LA perspective in both end-systole (a) and end-diastole (**b**). The mitral annular calcification (arrow head) originating from the LV side of the posterior mitral annulus at end-systole (**c**) and end-diastole (**d**). Live 3D zoom en-face view of the mitral valve from the LV perspective reveals the extent of mitral annular calcification (**e**). Panel **f** with a rendering plate (purple plate) shows the interior texture of the caseous calcification. Used with permission of Mayo Foundation for Medical Education and Research. All rights reserved. LA, left atrium; LV, left ventricle; AV, aortic valve; AL, anterolateral; PM, posteromedial; CS, Coronary sinus; AML, anterior mitral leaflet; PML, posterior mitral leaflet

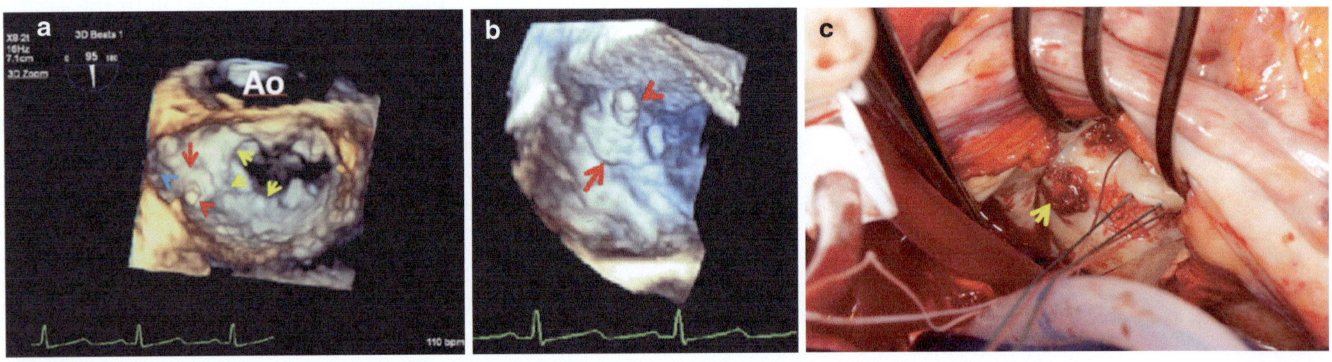

Fig. 26.2 Another patient with mobile mass on MAC. (**a**) Enface LA 3D TEE Zoom of MV showing MAC (yellow arrows) and a calcified nodule (red arrow) with a mobile component (red arrowhead) adjacent to ostium of LAA (blue arrowhead). (**b**) Focused 3D image of the calcified nodule (red arrow) and mobile component(red arrowhead). (**c**) Intraoperative image of the calcified nodule (yellow arrow). Pathology showed the mobile component to be semi solid calcium consistent with extruded MAC. Used with permission of Mayo Foundation for Medical Education and Research. All rights reserved. Ao, ascending aorta; LA, left atrium; LAA, left atrial appendage; MAC, mitral annular calcification; MV, mitral valve

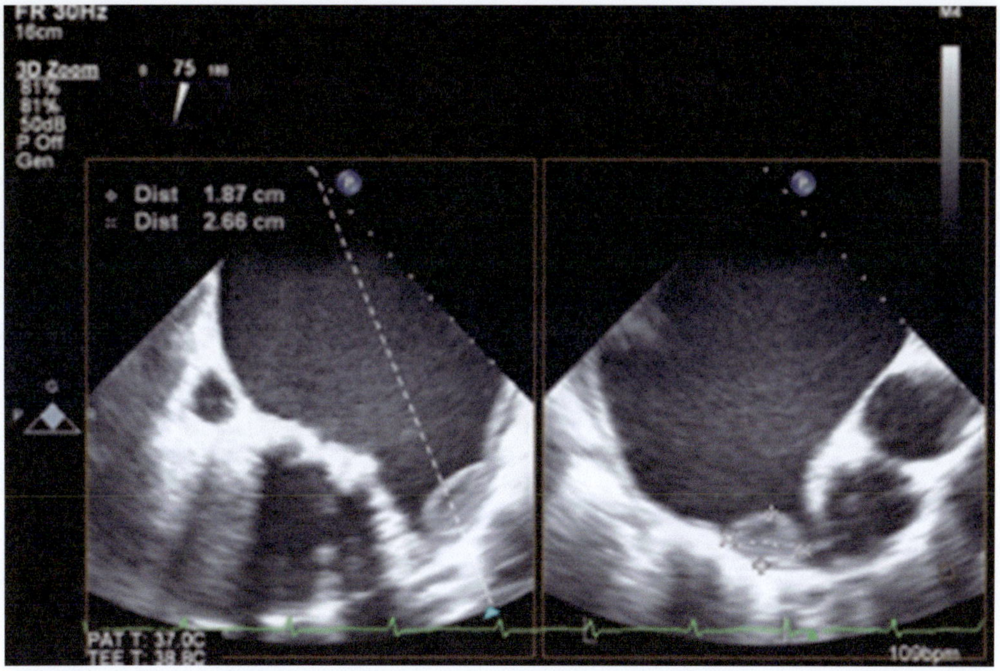

Fig. 26.3 Simultaneous biplane 3D TEE imaging reveals a left atrial appendage thrombus and markedly enlarged left atrial chamber with spontaneous echo contrast. Used with permission of Mayo Foundation for Medical Education and Research. All rights reserved

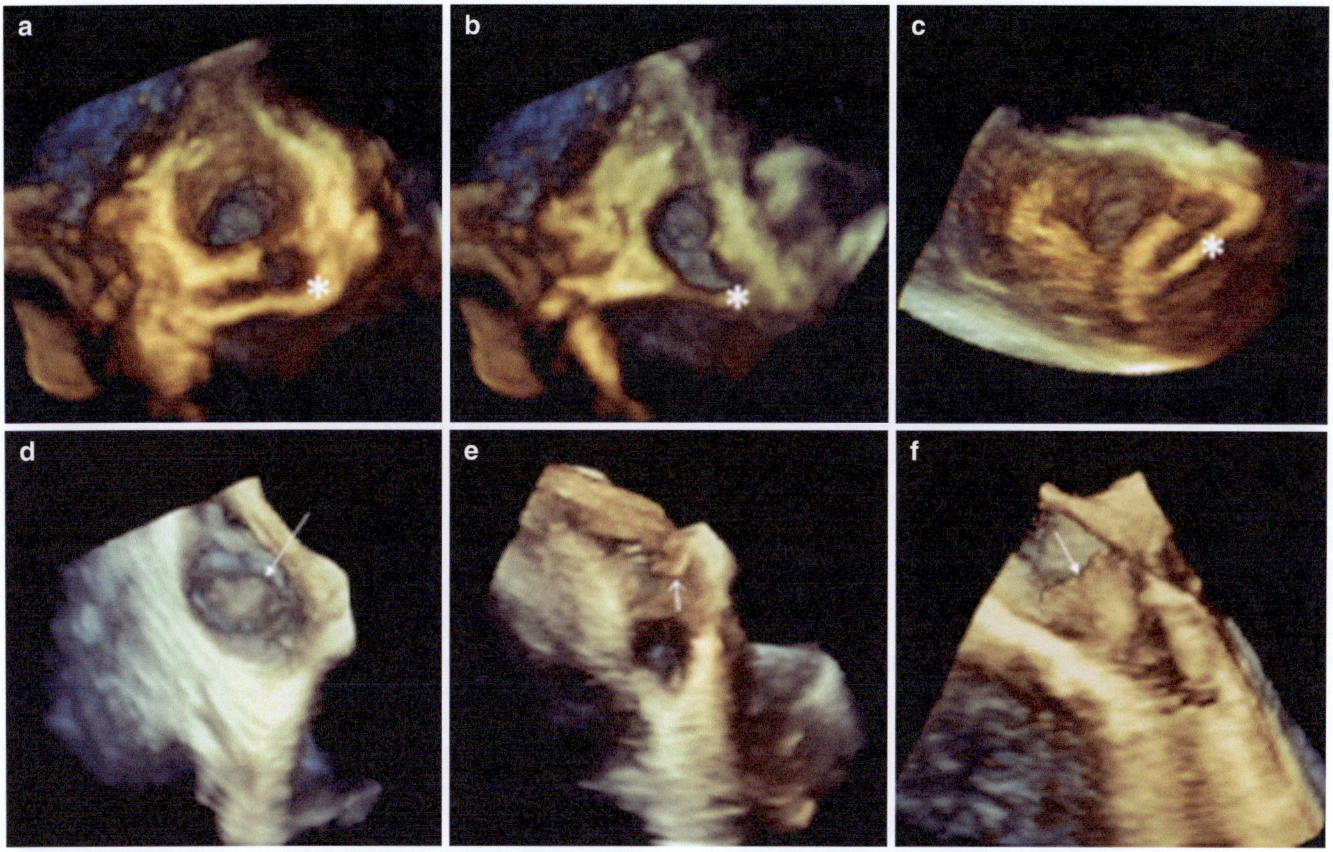

Fig. 26.4 The left atrial appendage shows an accessory lobe (asterisk) from the en-face view at upper (**a**) and mid (**b**) levels, as well as from the anterior approach (**c**). The bottom panels (**d**, **e**, and **f**) reveal the left atrial appendage thrombi (arrows). Used with permission of Mayo Foundation for Medical Education and Research. All rights reserved

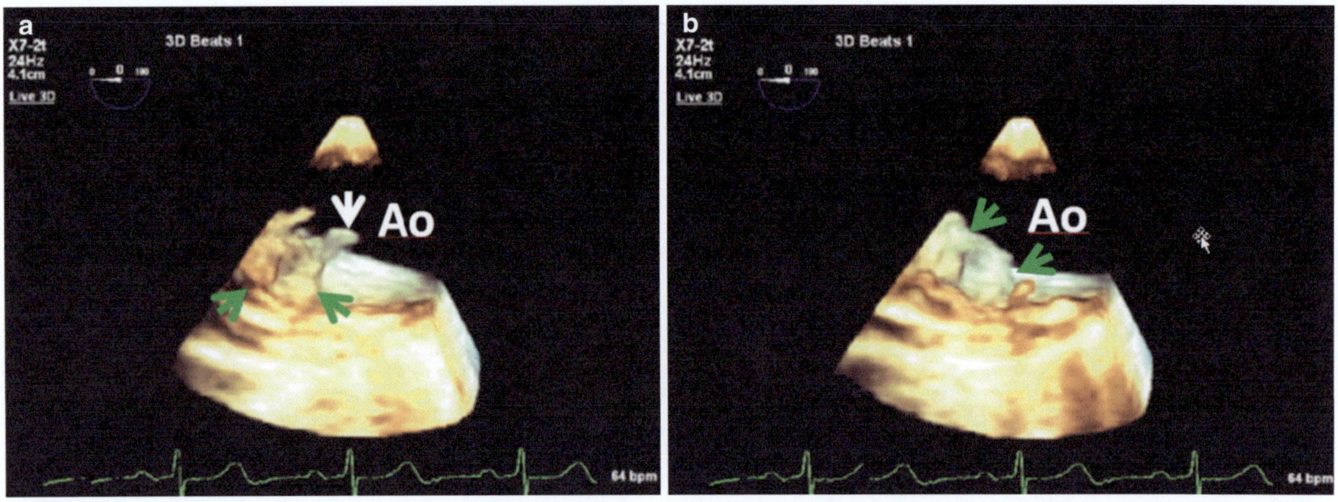

Fig. 26.5 Live 3D TEE in a patient with a descending thoracic aorta atheromatous plaque (green arrows) related mobile thrombus (**a**, white arrow) that moves out of the viewing plane in **b**. Used with permission of Mayo Foundation for Medical Education and Research. All rights reserved. Ao, aorta

Myxomas

About 80 percent of myxomas occur in the left atrium (LA) [5]. LA myxomas and thrombi can often be differentiated non-invasively with clinical and echocardiographic features. Myxomas are larger, with an average diameter of 5–6 cm, frequently arising from the endocardial surface of the LA with a stalk attached to the interatrial septum close to the fossa ovalis. In contrast, thrombi mostly originate from the LAA and often in combination with a stenotic mitral valve, spontaneous echo contrast, or atrial fibrillation. Grossly, cardiac myxomas show two morphologic subtypes: the solid type is lobular with a smooth surface, whereas the papillary type is friable with an irregular surface [6]. For evaluation of the mass in the LA, the following sequence generally is recommended: (1) biplane imaging and measuring the size of the mass (Fig. 26.6a and b), (2) Color flow imaging of the mitral inflow with continuous wave Doppler for assessing the mean pressure gradient if necessary (Fig. 26.6c and d), (3) focused live 3D or large volume /Full-Volume imaging and post-processing 3D rendering (Fig. 26.7). Finally, the specific details of the mass such as size, origin, shape, surface, mobility, prolapse, and whether there is significant mitral inflow interference can be assessed.

Papillary Fibroelastomas

Papillary fibroelastomas (PFE) are the second most common primary cardiac tumor in adults, often diagnosed incidentally by echocardiography, with a mean age of 60 years [7]. In one large study, 89 of 110 PFE seen by echocardiography were on the aortic (45%) or mitral valve (36%) with 72 PFE (81%) occurring on the downstream side of the aortic or mitral valves. A total of 48 out of the 110 PFE (44%) had a stalk and all were mobile, and in 85 patients (91%) the PFE was single, with nearly all PFE in the study <2 cm in size [8]. Two-dimensional (2D) echocardiography generally shows a well-demarcated, homogeneous, and round or oval appearance. Biplane and focused live 3D imaging with ROI on the mass including valves, gives the information of size, shape, attachment, and mobility—surgery is required in highly mobile or large (≥1 cm) tumors [7, 8] (Figs. 26.8 and 26.9, and see Figs. 12.24a and b and 12.25a–d Chap. 12).

Lipomas

Lipomas are rare cardiac primary tumors, occurring mainly in adults, typically presenting as well-circumscribed spherical or elliptical encapsulated fatty masses. Non-encapsulated lipomas within the heart are known as lipomatous hypertrophy, and lipomatous atrial septal hypertrophy (LASH) is defined by fatty deposits in the interatrial septum with a thickness of >2 cm [9] (see also Chap. 19). Often, LASH is found incidentally by 2D echocardiography via the characteristic features of a homogenous, dumbbell-shaped mass in the interatrial septum, sparing the fossa ovalis [10]. Focused live 3D imaging allows better discrimination between encapsulated lipoma from LASH in addition to providing information regarding spatial relationships, particularly a surrounding mass sparing fossa ovalis in en-face view from the right atrial perspective [10].

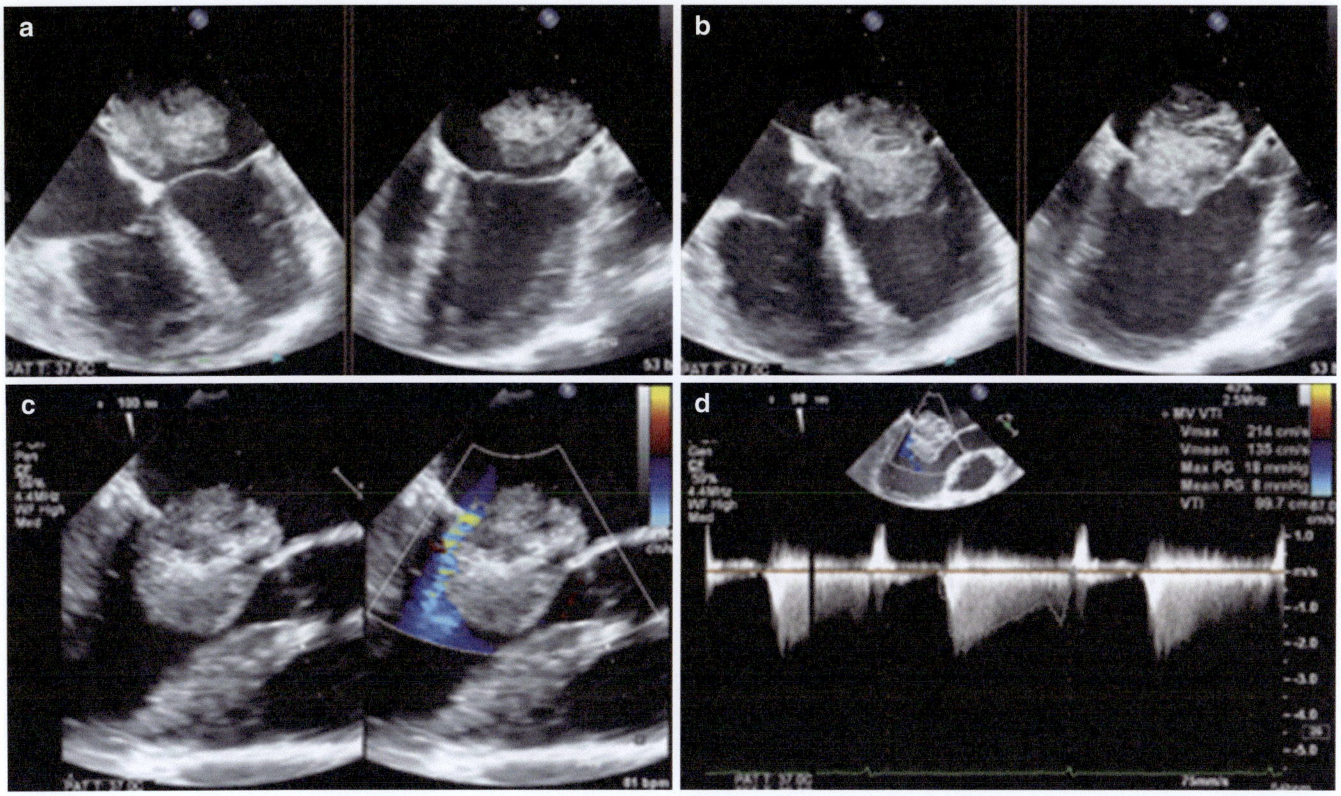

Fig. 26.6 A prolapsing left atrial myxoma attached at the interatrial septum. Evaluated by biplane imaging at systolic (**a**) and diastolic (**b**) phase. 2D Color Doppler imaging of the mitral inflow (**c**). The mean pressure gradient across the mitral valve measured 8 mm Hg (**d**). Used with permission of Mayo Foundation for Medical Education and Research. All rights reserved

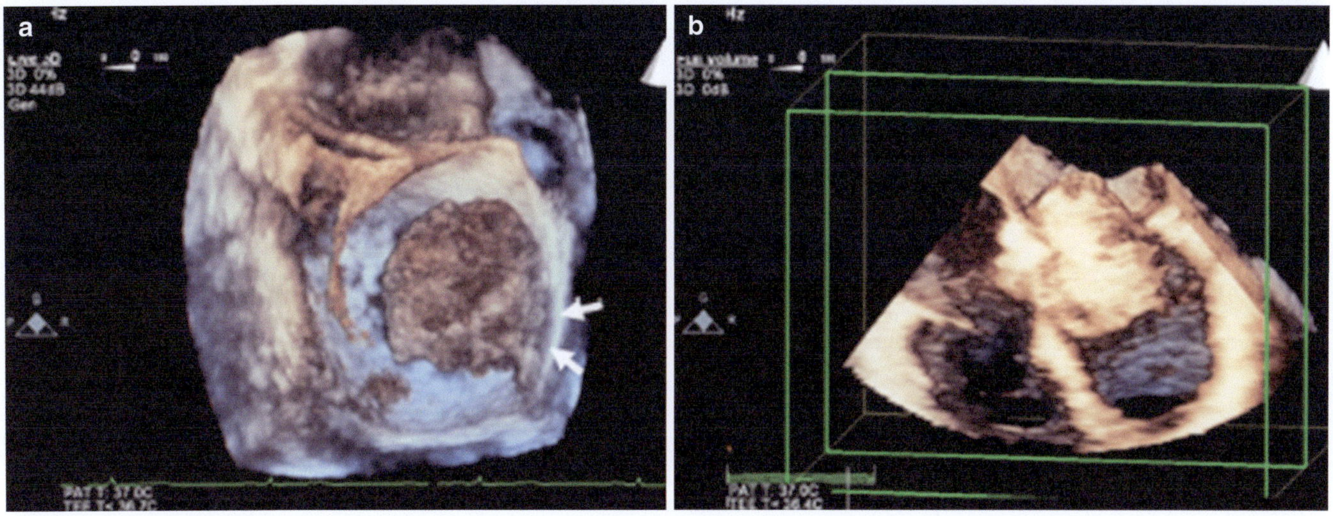

Fig. 26.7 Left atrial myxoma attached at the interatrial septum (arrows), acquired in live 3D mode (**a**) and an ECG-gated Full-Volume acquisition (**b**). Used with permission of Mayo Foundation for Medical Education and Research. All rights reserved

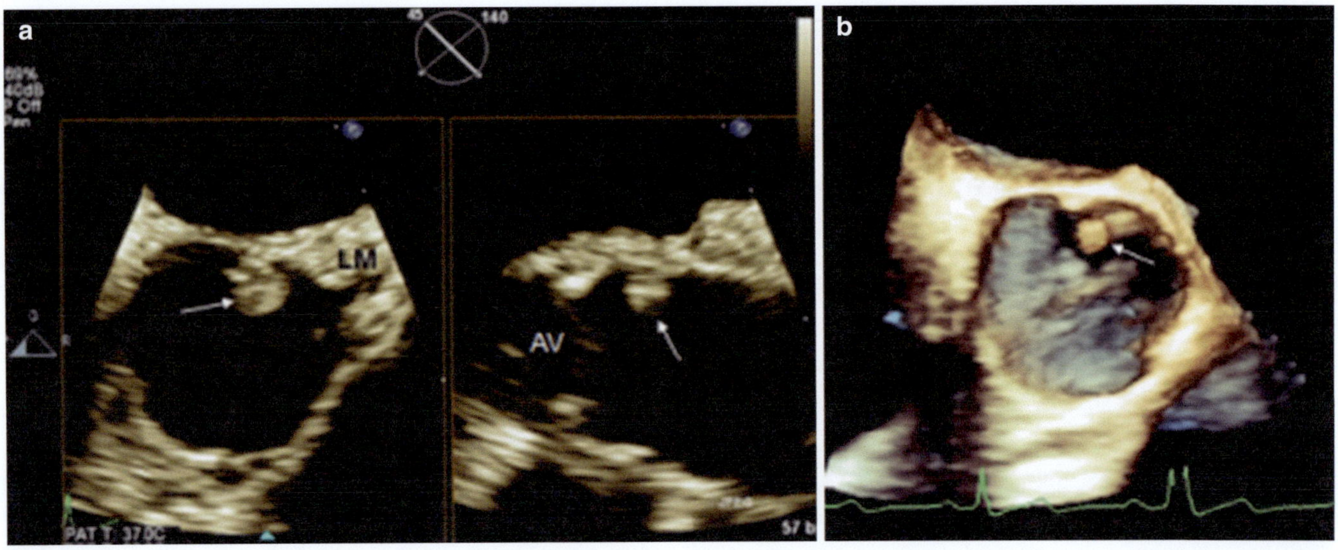

Fig. 26.8 Biplane (**a**) and live 3D zoom (**b**) Transesophageal echocardiography showing an aortic valve (AV) papillary fibroelastoma (arrows). It is a highly mobile, spherical, pedunculated mass 1.2 × 1.0 cm in size attached to the aortic root near the left main (LM) coronary artery ostia. Used with permission of Mayo Foundation for Medical Education and Research. All rights reserved

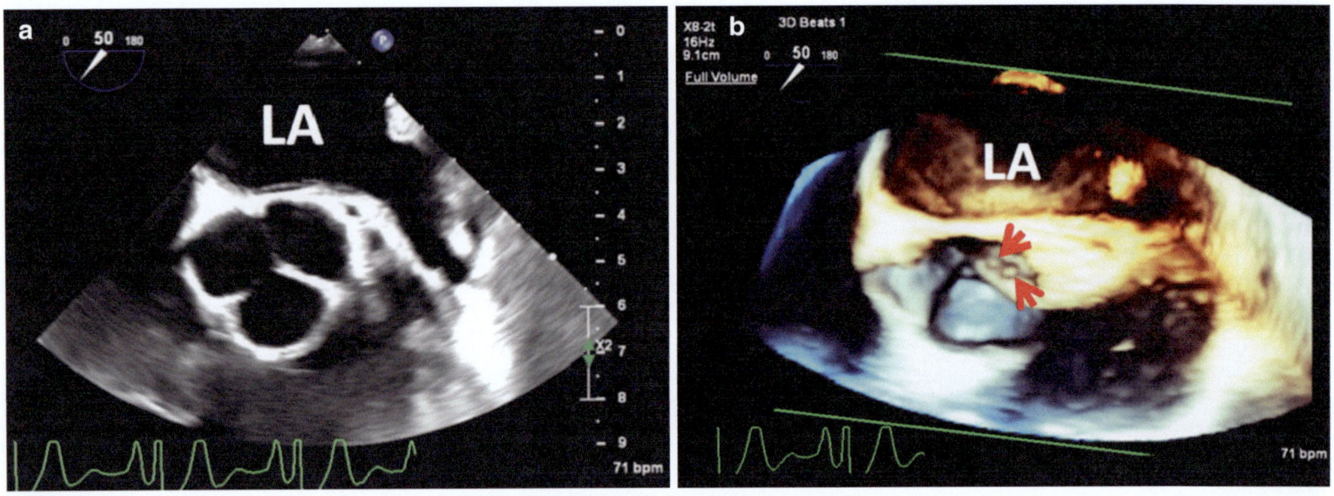

Fig. 26.9 (**a**) 2D TEE short-axis view of AV. There is no apparent pathology. (**b**) Live FV of same view showing two small mobile masses (red arrows) on aortic surface of left coronary cusp consistent with papillary fibroelastomas. The added depth provided by 3D imaging makes it possible to detect cusp pathology. Used with permission of Mayo Foundation for Medical Education and Research. All rights reserved. AV, aortic valve; FV, Full Volume

Fibromas

Cardiac fibromas are rare but still the second most common cardiac tumor, after rhabdomyomas, in the pediatric population, but rhabdomyomas often spontaneously regress while cardiac fibromas persist [11]. They mostly occur in the LV myocardium and are solitary, not distinctly capsulated, and vary in size between 4 and 7 cm. Due to the relatively large mass, biplane and focused live 3D imaging are important to measure the size and attachment, and to delineate the mass effect with respect to the surrounding structures [12] (Fig. 26.10).

Vegetations

The definition of vegetation is an abnormal outgrowth upon a body part, especially some warty excrescences on the cardiac valves, which are composed of fibrin and collagen, either infectious or sterile. The former (infective endocardi-

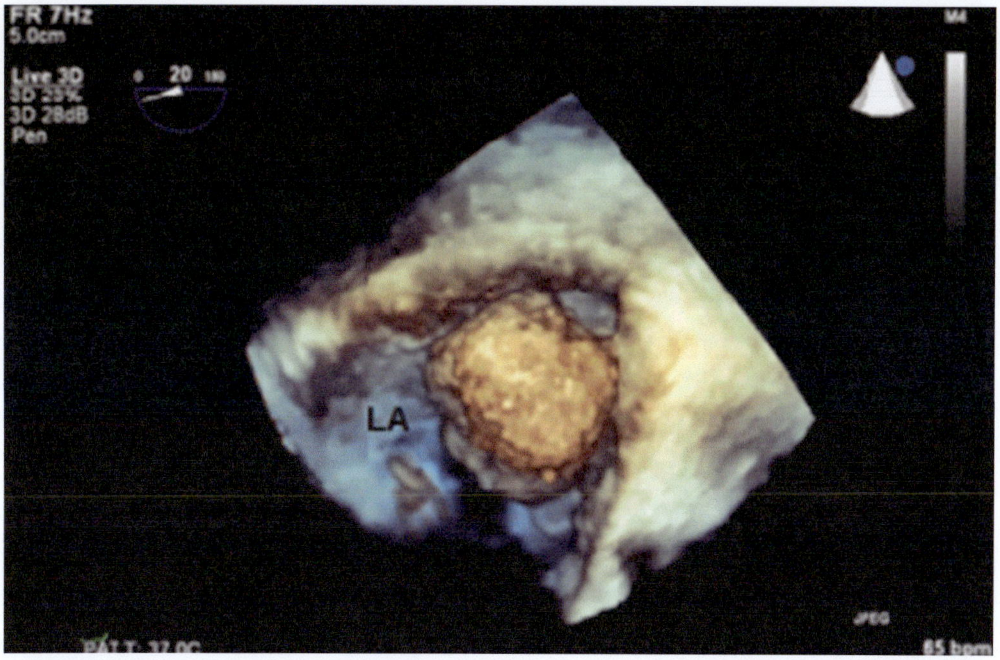

Fig. 26.10 Live 3D rendered image shows a fibroma attached to the superior and posterior wall of the left atrium (LA). Used with permission of Mayo Foundation for Medical Education and Research. All rights reserved

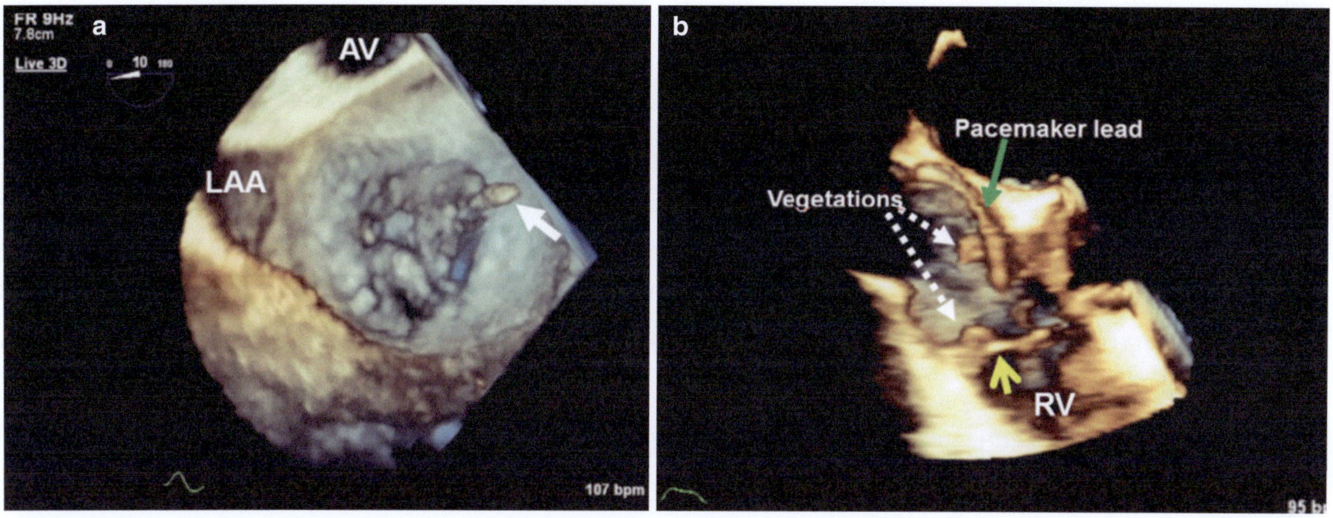

Fig. 26.11 (**a**) Live 3D image shows a highly mobile vegetation (arrow) attached to anterior mitral valve leaflet, presented as en-face view from the left atrial perspective, the same as a surgeon's view. (**b**) Live 3D image reveals a pacemaker lead through the right atrium and right ventricle (RV), and multiple vegetations following the pacemaker lead as well as the tricuspid valve (yellow arrow). Used with permission of Mayo Foundation for Medical Education and Research. All rights reserved. AV, aortic valve; LAA, left atrial appendage

tis, IE) contains clusters of bacteria and neutrophils, while the latter (nonbacterial thrombotic endocarditis, NBTE) contains adherent thrombi, platelets, lymphocytes or macrophages without microorganisms [13].

Infective Endocarditis (see also Chap. 17)

IE is defined by infection of the denuded endocardial surface, a native or prosthetic heart valve, or an indwelling cardiac device [14]. The diagnosis is based on clinical features, microbiologic evidence, and echocardiographic findings based on the modified Duke criteria [15]. Positive echocardiographic findings for IE include vegetations (oscillating intra-cardiac masses on valves or supporting structures, in the path of regurgitant jets, or on implanted materials), abscesses, or new dehiscence of prosthetic valves [15]. TTE is the first test for all patients with suspected IE; TEE is appropriate in patients having prosthetic valves or potential intra-cardiac complications. Biplane and live 3D imaging are useful supplements to standard 2D echocardiography (Figs. 26.11 and 26.12), offering two advantages: (1)

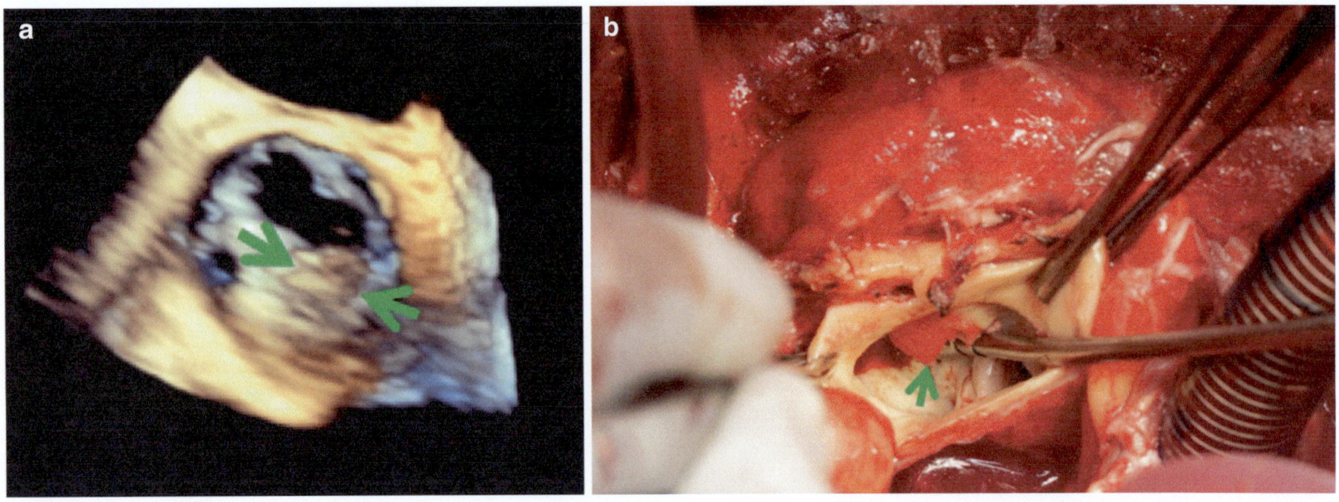

Fig. 26.12 (**a**) Live 3D in a patient with bicuspid aortic valve and large vegetation (green arrows). (**b**) Intraoperative view of the vegetation (arrow). Used with permission of Mayo Foundation for Medical Education and Research. All rights reserved

Localization or delineation of vegetations, especially in an en-face view of mitral valve vegetations from the LA perspective (Fig. 26.11a) or following the permanent pacemaker leads (Fig. 26.11b). (2) Detection of complications of IE such as paravalvular abscesses, paravalvular regurgitation, or prosthetic valve dehiscence [16, 17]. But, with a low frame rate it may be less sensitive in detection of smaller vegetation, so focused 3D echo is warranted as part of the routine echo imaging protocol [18].

Nonbacterial Thrombotic Endocarditis (NBTE)

NBTE is characterized by sterile vegetations on the cardiac valves, also known as marantic endocarditis to emphasize its association with wasting conditions such as cancer. NBTE is often associated with preexisting hypercoagulable states or malignant cancer [19], and is known as Libman-Sacks endocarditis when it occurs in the setting of systemic lupus erythematosus. Echocardiography is a good diagnostic choice to detect valvular vegetations, but it is not necessarily able to distinguish the vegetation in NBTE (aggregations of platelets and fibrin) from those in IE. Vegetations in NBTE, analogous to those of IE, are typically located on the atrial aspect of the mitral leaflets or ventricular aspect of the aortic leaflets, but may be located on either valve surface [19]. NBTE vegetations appear verrucous, rounded, with well-defined borders, which should be easily differentiated from Lambl's excrescences which are thinner (≤2 mm), elongated (>5 mm), independently hypermobile masses typically located at the valvular coaptation point [20]. Focused live 3D echocardiography has advantages over 2D for localization and delineation of vegetations (Figs. 26.13 and 26.14).

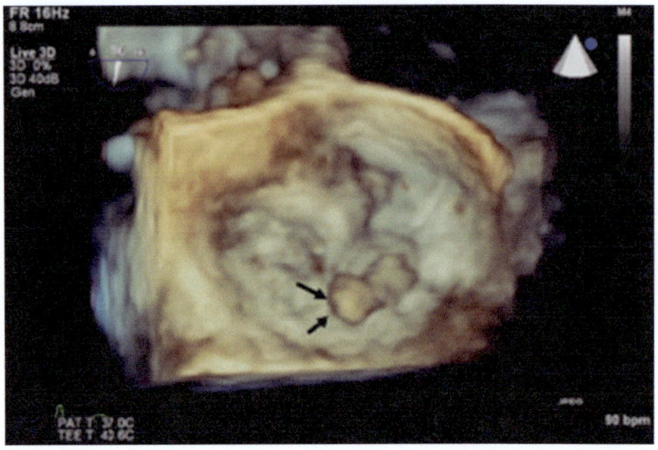

Fig. 26.13 Marantic endocarditis with multiple vegetations (arrows) on the posterior mitral valve leaflet in en-face view from the live 3D zoom rendered transesophageal echocardiography. Used with permission of Mayo Foundation for Medical Education and Research. All rights reserved

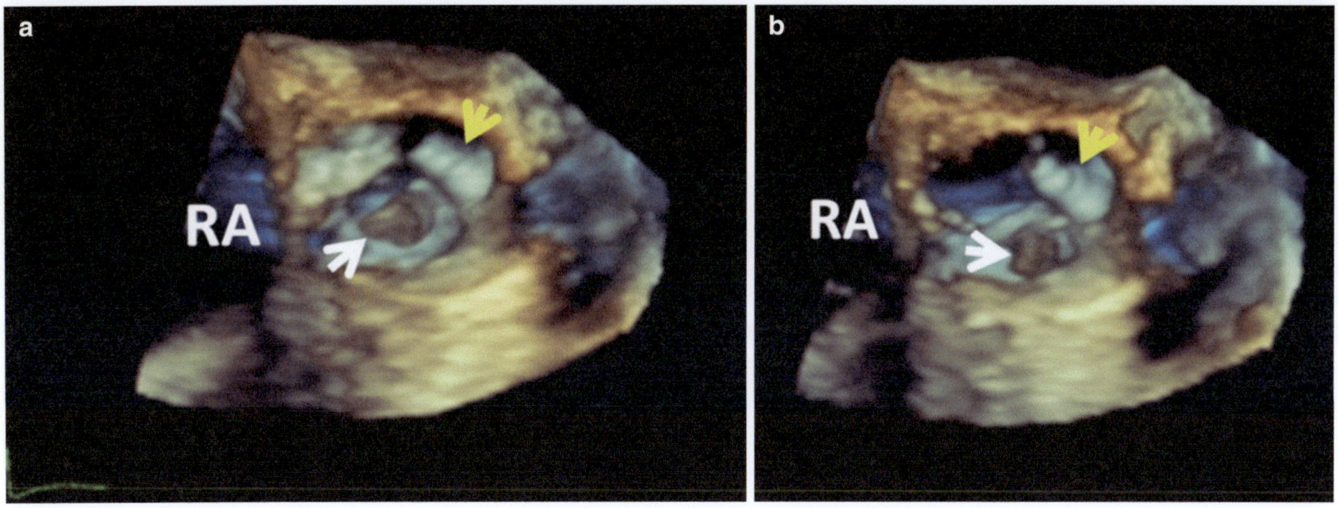

Fig. 26.14 3D TEE of Bicuspid AV in a 32 year old woman with breast cancer and history of recent acute inferior myocardial infarction. Patient did not have IE. (**a** and **b**) mobile vegetation seen on aortic side of anterior cusp (white arrows) consistent with NBTE. Yellow arrows point to calcified raphae. IE, infectious endocarditis; NBTE, non bacterial thrombotic endocarditis; RA, right atrium. Used with permission of Mayo Foundation for Medical Education and Research. All rights reserved

References

1. Lang RM, Badano LP, Tsang W, Adams DH, Agricola E, Buck T, et al. EAE/ASE recommendations for image acquisition and display using three-dimensional echocardiography. J Am Soc Echocardiogr. 2012;25:3–46.
2. Sommer M, Roehrich A, Boenner F, Aissa J, Kropil P, Antoch G, et al. Value of 3D TEE for LAA morphology. JACC Cardiovasc Imaging. 2015;8:1107–10.
3. Cresti A, Chiavarelli M, Glauber M, Tanganelli P, Scalese M, Cesareo F, et al. Incidence rate of primary cardiac tumors: a 14-year population study. J Cardiovasc Med (Hagerstown). 2016;17:37–43.
4. Vander Salm TJ. Unusual primary tumors of the heart. Semin Thorac Cardiovasc Surg. 2000;12:89–100.
5. Kuon E, Kreplin M, Weiss W, Dahm JB. The challenge presented by right atrial myxoma. Herz. 2004;29:702–9.
6. Jain D, Maleszewski JJ, Halushka MK. Benign cardiac tumors and tumorlike conditions. Ann Diagn Pathol. 2010;14:215–30.
7. Gowda RM, Khan IA, Nair CK, Mehta NJ, Vasavada BC, Sacchi TJ. Cardiac papillary fibroelastoma: a comprehensive analysis of 725 cases. Am Heart J. 2003;146:404–10.
8. Sun JP, Asher CR, Yang XS, Cheng GG, Scalia GM, Massed AG, et al. Clinical and echocardiographic characteristics of papillary fibroelastomas: a retrospective and prospective study in 162 patients. Circulation. 2001;103:2687–93.
9. Shirani J, Roberts WC. Clinical, electrocardiographic and morphologic features of massive fatty deposits ("lipomatous hypertrophy") in the atrial septum. J Am Coll Cardiol. 1993;22:226–38.
10. Laura DM, Donnino R, Kim EE, Benenstein R, Freedberg RS, Saric M. Lipomatous atrial septal hypertrophy: a review of its anatomy, pathophysiology, multimodality imaging, and relevance to percutaneous interventions. J Am Soc Echocardiogr. 2016;29:717–23.
11. Thomas-de-Montpreville V, Nottin R, Dulmet E, Serraf A. Heart tumors in children and adults: clinicopathological study of 59 patients from a surgical center. Cardiovasc Pathol. 2007;16:22–8.
12. Yang HS, Arabia FA, Chaliki HP, De Petris G, Khandheria BK, Chandrasekaran K. Images in cardiovascular medicine. Left atrial fibroma in Gardner syndrome: real-time 3-dimensional transesophageal echo imaging. Circulation. 2008;118:e692–6.
13. Lepidi H, Casalta JP, Fournier PE, Habib G, Collart F, Raoult D. Quantitative histological examination of bioprosthetic heart valves. Clin Infect Dis. 2006;42:590–6.
14. Cahill TJ, Prendergast BD. Infective endocarditis. Lancet. 2016;387:882–93.
15. Li JS, Sexton DJ, Mick N, Nettles R, Fowler VG Jr, Ryan T, et al. Proposed modifications to the Duke criteria for the diagnosis of infective endocarditis. Clin Infect Dis. 2000;30:633–8.
16. Bruun NE, Habib G, Thuny F, Sogaard P. Cardiac imaging in infectious endocarditis. Eur Heart J. 2014;35:624–32.
17. Afonso L, Kottam A, Reddy V, Penumetcha A. Echocardiography in infective endocarditis: state of the art. Curr Cardiol Rep. 2017;19:127.
18. Pfister R, Betton Y, Freyhaus HT, Jung N, Baldus S, Michels G. Three-dimensional compared to two-dimensional transesophageal echocardiography for diagnosis of infective endocarditis. Infection. 2016;44:725–31.
19. Liu J, Frishman WH. Nonbacterial thrombotic endocarditis: pathogenesis, diagnosis, and management. Cardiol Rev. 2016;24:244–7.
20. Roldan CA, Tolstrup K, Macias L, Qualls CR, Maynard D, Charlton G, et al. Libman-sacks endocarditis: detection, characterization, and clinical correlates by three-dimensional transesophageal echocardiography. J Am Soc Echocardiogr. 2015;28:770–9.

Part VI

Role of 3DE in Catheter-Based Structural Heart Disease Interventions

Atrial Interventions

27

Francesco F. Faletra, Laura A. Leo, Vera L. Paiocchi, Susanne A. Schlossbauer, Pedrazzini Giovanni, and Marco Valgimigli

Closure of PFO

Introduction

During fetal life, the presence of patent foramen ovale (PFO) is key to allow direct blood passage between the two atria. The unidirectional (right to left) oxygenated blood passes from inferior vena cava through the PFO into the left atrium (LA) bypassing the lungs and thereby reaching the fetal systemic circulation. At birth, the increase in pulmonary blood flow leads to a rise in LA pressure, and development of a pressure gradient between the LA and right atrium (RA), which pushes the septum primum (SP) against the septum secundum (SS). As a result, the PFO gets "functionally" sealed. A permanent "anatomic" fusion between SP and SS occurs only later throughout infancy. The contraction of atrial cavities may, in fact, produce a friction-induced injury on the two overlapping septa, generating an inflammatory response with formation of platelet/fibrin accumulation that eventually leads to a fibrotic fusion between SP and SS and to a definitive closure. However, in a sizable proportion of individuals this mechanism fails and SP and SS overlap each other leaving a slit-like gap at the superior margin of the two septa (Fig. 27.1). This kind of "flap valve" acts as a one-way door, opening towards the left atrial cavity when the RA pressure exceeds the LA pressure (as during coughing, sneezing or straining, actions that can be reproduced with a Valsalva maneuver) causing a flash of right-to-left shunt. Autoptic and contrast transesophageal echocardiography studies have shown that at least in one of every four adults the fusion between SP and SS is incomplete [1]. In such cases, because right atrial pressure is usually lower than that in the left atrium, the PFO remains functionally closed most of the time. Therefore, a PFO should be considered an anatomical variant rather than a pathological state, unless it is associated with other pathological conditions.

PFO and Cryptogenic Stroke

In the late 1980s, Lechat et al. demonstrated that in young and middle-aged patients (<55 years) who had suffered from cryptogenic stroke (CS), (i.e. stroke without any other recognizable cause), the prevalence of PFO was significantly higher than in normal individuals (40% vs 10–20%), suggesting a causal role for PFO [2]. Several other studies showed similar associations. In contrast, the first randomized clinical trial, designed to prevent recurrent CS among PFO patients, failed to show a clear clinical benefit from PFO closure [3–5]. The main reason was likely due to incorrect selection of patients in whom CS was PFO-related rather than caused by other etiologies. However, recent trials, using more advanced technological improvements in neuroimaging, adoption of prolonged ECG monitoring and extensive use of 2D/3D TEE, increased the likelihood of identifying PFO-related CS. As a result, other causes of stroke such as atrial fibrillation, mobile thrombi in the ascending aorta or aortic arch, left ventricular thrombi in acute myocardial infarction or other vascular causes including intracerebral vascular diseases were more effectively ruled-out [6, 7]. Thus, when only patients who truly had PFO-related CS were included, there is convincing evidence that PFO closure decreases the risk of recurrent stroke compared with medical therapy alone.

F. F. Faletra (✉)
Director of Cardiac Imaging Lab, Cardiocentro Ticino Institute, Lugano, Switzerland
e-mail: Francesco.Faletra@cardiocentro.org

L. A. Leo · V. L. Paiocchi · S. A. Schlossbauer
Cardiac Imaging Lab, Cardiocentro Ticino Institute, Lugano, Switzerland
e-mail: lauraanna.leo@cardiocentro.org; vera.paiocchi@cardiocentro.org; Susanne.schlossbauer@cardiocentro.org

P. Giovanni · M. Valgimigli
Professor, Division of Cardiology, Cardiocentro Ticino Institute, Lugano, Switzerland
e-mail: pedrazzini.giovanni@cardiocentro.org; marco.valgimigli@cardiocentro.org

J. F. Maalouf et al. (eds.), *Practical 3D Echocardiography*, https://doi.org/10.1007/978-3-030-72941-7_27

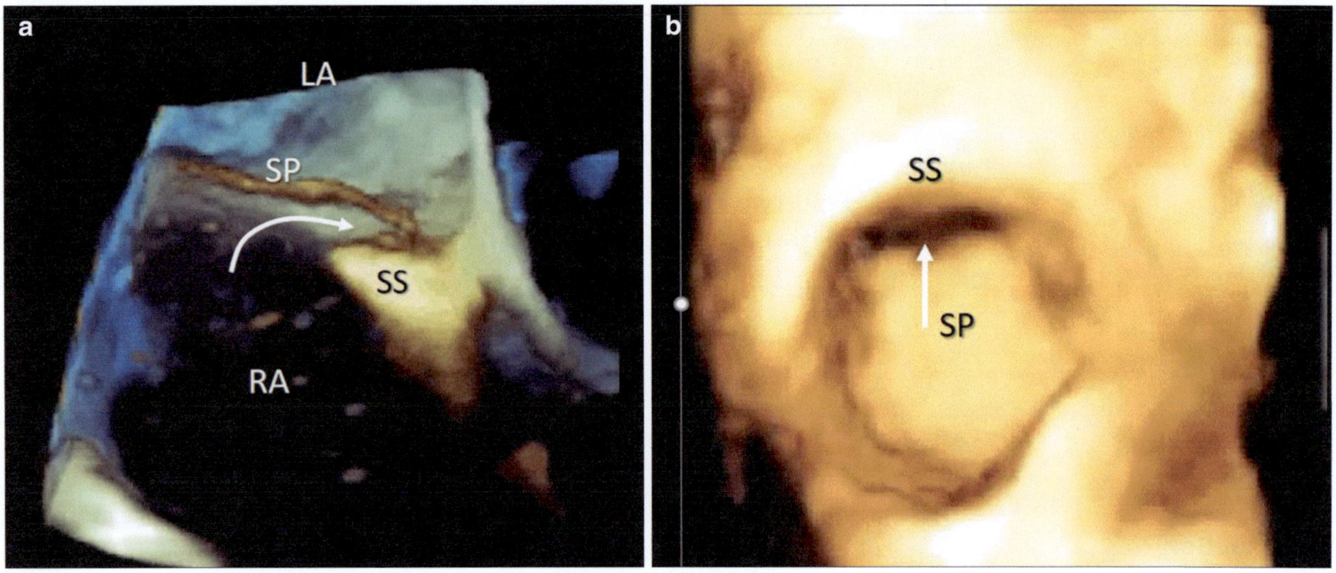

Fig. 27.1 (**a**) Cross-sectional cut of 3D TEE imaging showing the overlap between septum primum (SP) and septum secundum (SS) without fusion. Depending on the length of SP the opening may have a tunnel-shaped configuration (curved arrow). (**b**) PFO seen in "en face" view, from the right atrium perspective, showing a slit-like, crescent-shaped gap on the superior margin of the two septa (arrow). PFO, patent foramen ovale; RA, right atrium

Mechanism of Cryptogenic Stroke in Patients with PFO

Paradoxical embolism has been considered as the primary mechanism of PFO-related CS. Passage of venous thrombus to the arterial circulation occurs under hemodynamic conditions that increase the right atrial (RA) pressure. Transient increase in RA pressure during straining or coughing, may open a PFO and allow venous thrombus transit into the LA. Several case-reports showed images of serpiginous thrombus crossing a PFO [8, 9]. Because of the high prevalence of clinically latent venous thrombosis, paradoxical embolism through a PFO might be responsible for stroke more often than historically suspected. Moreover, it has been shown that in young or middle-aged patients with CS, the rate of pelvic vein thrombosis, or coagulation abnormalities are higher than in patients without CS [10, 11]. Another mechanism that may cause stroke is the "in situ" formation of thrombi in the setting of "long-channeled" PFO. This peculiar anatomical architecture may, in fact, be an "ideal milieu" for stasis and thrombi deposition especially when associated with hypercoagulable states [11, 12]. Finally, PFO closure appears more effective in preventing the recurrence of stroke in patients with large-size PFO (≥2 mm in height), long-tunnel PFO (≥10 mm in length), atrial septal aneurysm, prominent Eustachian valve or Chiari network [12]. Thus, patients with the above-mentioned morphological PFO characteristics should be considered at "high risk" of having PFO-related CS. The association between the presence of large PFO and persistence of a redundant, large Eustachian valve (EV), a remnant of the embryonic right valve of the sinus venosus, has been reported. During fetal life, the EV forms a kind of preferential path through which oxygenated blood from the inferior vena cava crosses the PFO reaching the systemic circulation. With the persistence of a large EV in adult life, blood from the inferior vena cava may continue to be directed towards the fossa ovalis (FO). Moreover, the pressure caused by the column of blood against the surface of the FO may favor the maintenance of large PFOs (Fig. 27.2).

Demonstration of Left to Right Shunt

Though some studies have shown that TTE is as good as TEE in diagnosing PFO [13, 14], there is no doubt that TEE is the gold standard for the diagnosis of a PFO and delineation of its morphologic characteristics. Sporadically spontaneous left-to-right shunt across a large PFO can be seen using color Doppler. However, a definitive diagnosis relies on 2D TEE and injection of agitated saline bubble with Valsalva maneuver. In patients with PFO, bubbles appear in the left atrium via a PFO immediately after Valsalva release (Fig. 27.3). If sparse bubbles appear in the left atrium after 5–6 beats and are not seen crossing the PFO, the passage occurs likely through a normal pulmonary vasculature or through a possible arteriovenous pulmonary shunt. False negative cases may occur especially in young patients, when the contrast injected via the antecubital vein is washed away by the contrast-free blood arriving from the inferior vena cava. When ruling out the presence of PFO is critical,

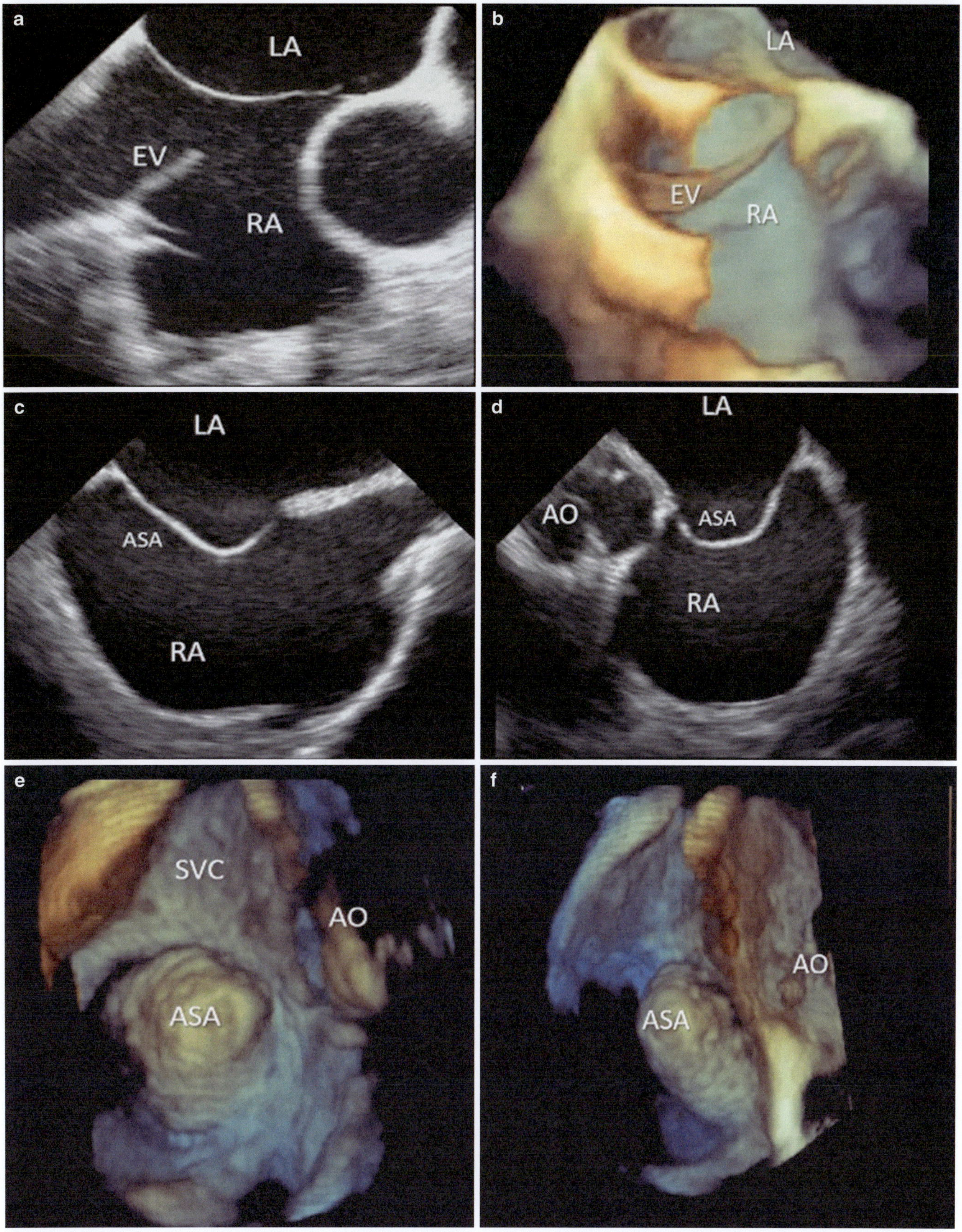

Fig. 27.2 (**a**, **b**) TEE showing the presence of a large Eustachian valve (EV) in 2D (**a**) and 3D (**b**) format. (**c**, **d**) 2D TEE shows an atrial septal aneurysm (ASA) in two orthogonal planes. (**e**) 3D TEE showing an ASA "en face" from a right atrial perspective. (**f**) Same ASA imaged from a lateral perspective. AO, aorta; LA left atrium; RA, right atrium; SVC, superior vena cava

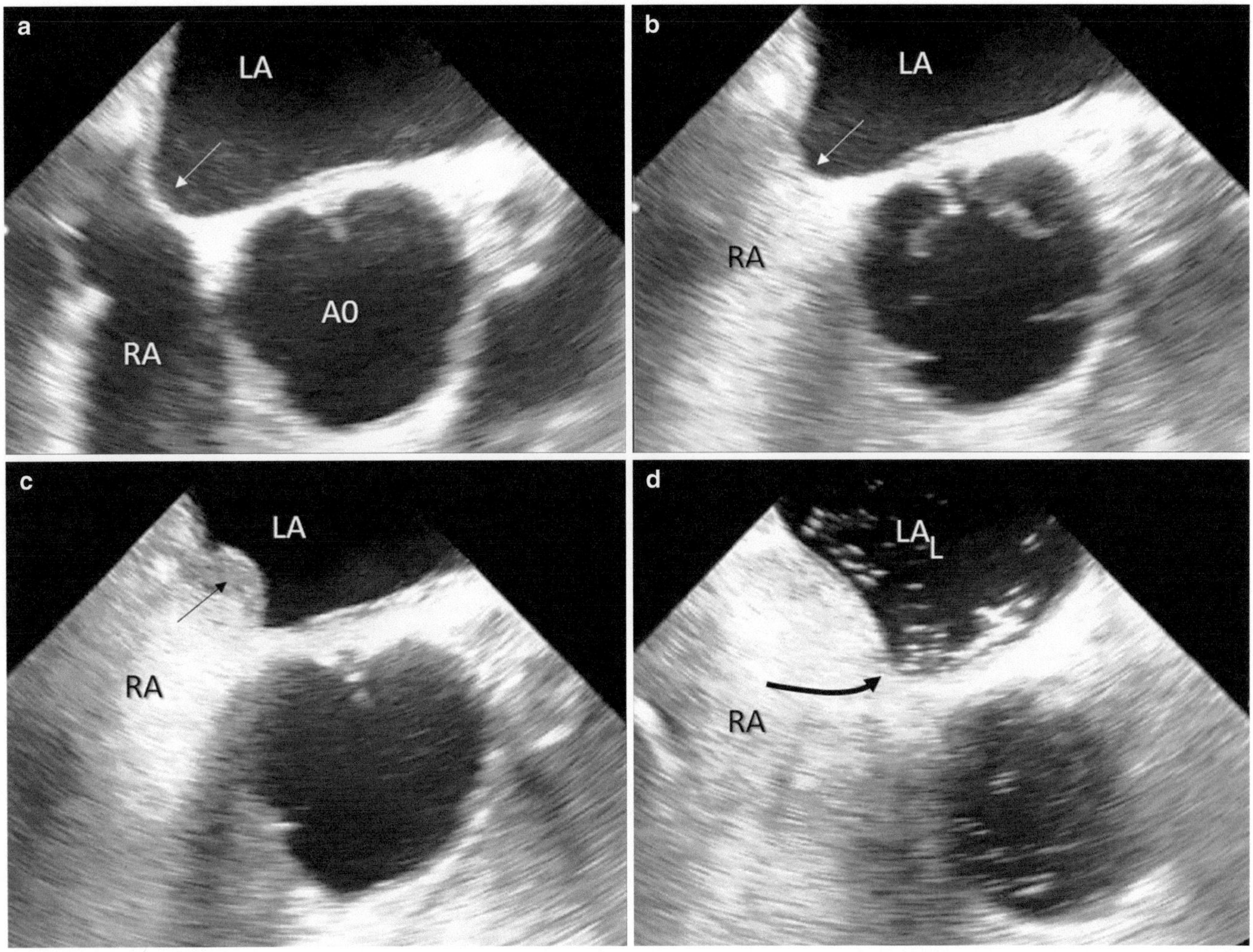

Fig. 27.3 Patient with PFO and ASA. (**a**) 2D TEE short axis view of the aorta (AO). During Valsalva maneuver, the RA pressure drops, the RA becomes smaller and the LA pressure exceeds that of the RA. As a consequence a redundant fossa ovalis (FO) is pushed towards the RA (white arrow). (**b**) the RA is filled by bubbles. (**c**) With Valsalva release, the RA pressure exceeds the LA pressure and the FO bulges towards the LA (black arrow) and (**d**) bubbles cross the FO into the LA through the PFO (curved black arrow). ASA, atrial septal aneurysm; LA, left atrium; PFO, patent foramen ovale; RA, right atrium

injection of contrast via the femoral vein may enhance the likelihood of detecting a right-to-left shunt.

The presence of PFO does not necessarily imply its closure. Before considering percutaneous closure, patients with suspected PFO-related CS should undergo evaluation by both a cardiologist and "stroke" neurologist. This "brain-heart team" is necessary to prevent inappropriate intervention in patients in whom the PFO plays a bystander rather than a causative role for CS.

PFO and Migraine

It has been observed that PFO closure in migraineurs who have suffered from CS may result in a dramatic reduction in migraine attack frequency. This has stimulated interest in a causal link between PFO and migraine. It has been speculated that subclinical emboli, as well as metabolites (e.g. serotonin) from the venous circulation may bypass the pulmonary circulation through the PFO and enter the systemic circulation, and thereby interact with the trigeminal nerve or brain vasculature triggering migraine [15]. However, it is still unclear if this is a *causal* relationship or simply coexistence of these two conditions. Thus, before performing PFO closure for migraine prevention, a clear evidence of safety and benefit associated with PFO closure must be demonstrated through large-scale trials. Unfortunately, at the present time, preliminary results of one such trial, the PREMIUM Trial (Prospective, Randomized Investigation to Evaluate Incidence of Headache Reduction in Subjects With Migraine and PFO Using the AMPLATZER PFO Occluder to Medical Management) failed to demonstrate that PFO closure significantly reduces migraine frequency among migraineurs refractory to multiple medications [16].

PFO and Scuba Diving

The notion that venous gas bubbles, common after diving and usually silent due to filtration by the pulmonary vasculature, could bypass the pulmonary filter through a PFO has alerted scuba divers. The Valsalva maneuver is known to facilitate right-to-left shunt. While climbing into boats and lifting heavy kit, divers may unconsciously perform Valsalva maneuver. Thus, PFO is thought to be a potential cause for decompression illness (DCI) which may lead to cerebral, spinal cord injury, certain types of skin bends and inner ear decompression sickness. However, while 20–30% of divers might be expected to have a PFO, DCI occurs in only 0.005–0.08% of dives. This figure is much lower than might be expected if every diver with a PFO and venous bubbles developed DCI. At this time, routine screening for PFO in divers is not recommended. However, it is reasonable to screen high-risk individuals such as those divers who had suffered from a migraine with aura or those who plan to participate in expedition-level dives involving extensive decompression [17].

The Left Atrial Pouch

Two pathologists, Krushnan and Salazar, in 2010, examined 94 autopsied hearts focusing on fusion patterns between SP and SS. As expected, 27% had a PFO. Among the remaining 68 hearts without PFO, 27 had complete fusion between SP and SS whereas in 41 the fusion was incomplete with a Kangaroo-like pocket opening into the left atrium in 37 (when the adhesion between SS and SP was only at the inferior limit of the zone of overlap) and into the right atrium in 4 (when the fusion occurred only at the superior limit of tissue overlap) [18]. They named this incomplete fusion as "*septal pouch*" which is how it appears in vivo when filled with blood. Whether the stagnant blood in this pocket may be, like the left atrial appendage, a source of thrombus formation and cerebral or systemic embolic events is still unclear. Anecdotal cases have shown thrombus within the pouch as well as in the setting of cryptogenic stroke [19–21]. Epidemiological studies remain largely inconclusive as the association between the presence of atrial septal pouch and embolic cerebral events could be shown in only a few cases. Moreover, the presence of a left-sided septal pouch is associated with a higher prevalence of atrial fibrillation, which may be the driver for systemic embolism [22] rather than atrial pouch *per se*. Thus, the clinical role of the septal pouch as a source of thromboembolism needs further investigations. Cross-section slices that transect this region provided by both CMR and CT may illustrate this particular anatomic feature. However, we believe that 2D/3D TEE remains the best technique to image the septal pouch (Figs. 27.4 and 19.3b Chap. 19).

Percutaneous Guidance of PFO Closure

Percutaneous closure of PFO may be guided by fluoroscopy and 2D/3D TEE. However, the use of TEE requires general anesthesia, thus some interventionalists prefer closing PFO with the use of fluoroscopic guidance alone or with intracardiac ultrasound. In our institution, PFO closure is usually accomplished with 2D and 3D TEE under general anesthesia. Amplatzer PFO Occluder (Abbott Structural, Santa Clara, CA) and the Gore Cardioform Septal Occluder (W.L. Gore and Associates, Inc., Newark, DE) are the only two US Food and Drug Administration (FDA)-approved devices for PFO closure. In our institution (and in most of European countries), the most widely used PFO device is the Amplatzer occluder. This device consists of 2 self-expanding discs composed of a nickel-titanium (Nitinol) wire mesh. The nitinol is a super-elastic material (when stretched inside a sheath, it assumes a cylindrical shape), but with a 'shape memory' which makes it self-expandable when free of constraints. The wire mesh contains a polyester fabric that enhances the device's ability to seal the PFO and eliminates interatrial shunting. The two discs are connected by a short and thin waist which is twisted around its long axis and hence, is extendable once it engages the PFO tunnel. The two disks are of different sizes. The right disk is larger than the left, and device sizing is based on the right disk diameter. Only the smallest device (18 mm) has two disks of equal size and is used for small PFOs without redundancy of the septum primum. Figure 27.5 shows a photograph of an Amplatzer PFO occluder and the corresponding 3D TEE image "in situ".

Percutaneous closure is usually performed through the right femoral vein. The septal crossing and the other steps of the procedure can be easily guided by 2D or 3D TEE using an oblique or lateral perspective of the interatrial septum which enhances visualization of disc deployment. The PFO is crossed using a standard exchange wire and multipurpose catheter. The multipurpose catheter is then exchanged for an 8–9 F trans-septal sheath which is advanced over the guidewire into the left atrium through the PFO. Once the guidewire is removed, the device is advanced within the sheath and, when out, the left disk assumes its original shape. The system is then pulled back until the left disc abuts against the atrial septum. By withdrawing the sheath and advancing the catheter, the right disk is then expanded. The whole process is fully reversible. At this point, 2D and/or 3D TEE confirm that the septum is clearly trapped between the two disks. Maneuvers of pulling and pushing the device ensure its firm engagement; then the device is released. Once the catheter is withdrawn, 2D/3D TEE and color Doppler provide final images of the correct position of the device (Fig. 27.6). With time, a fibrous and endothelial layer encapsulates the device leading to definitive closure of the PFO.

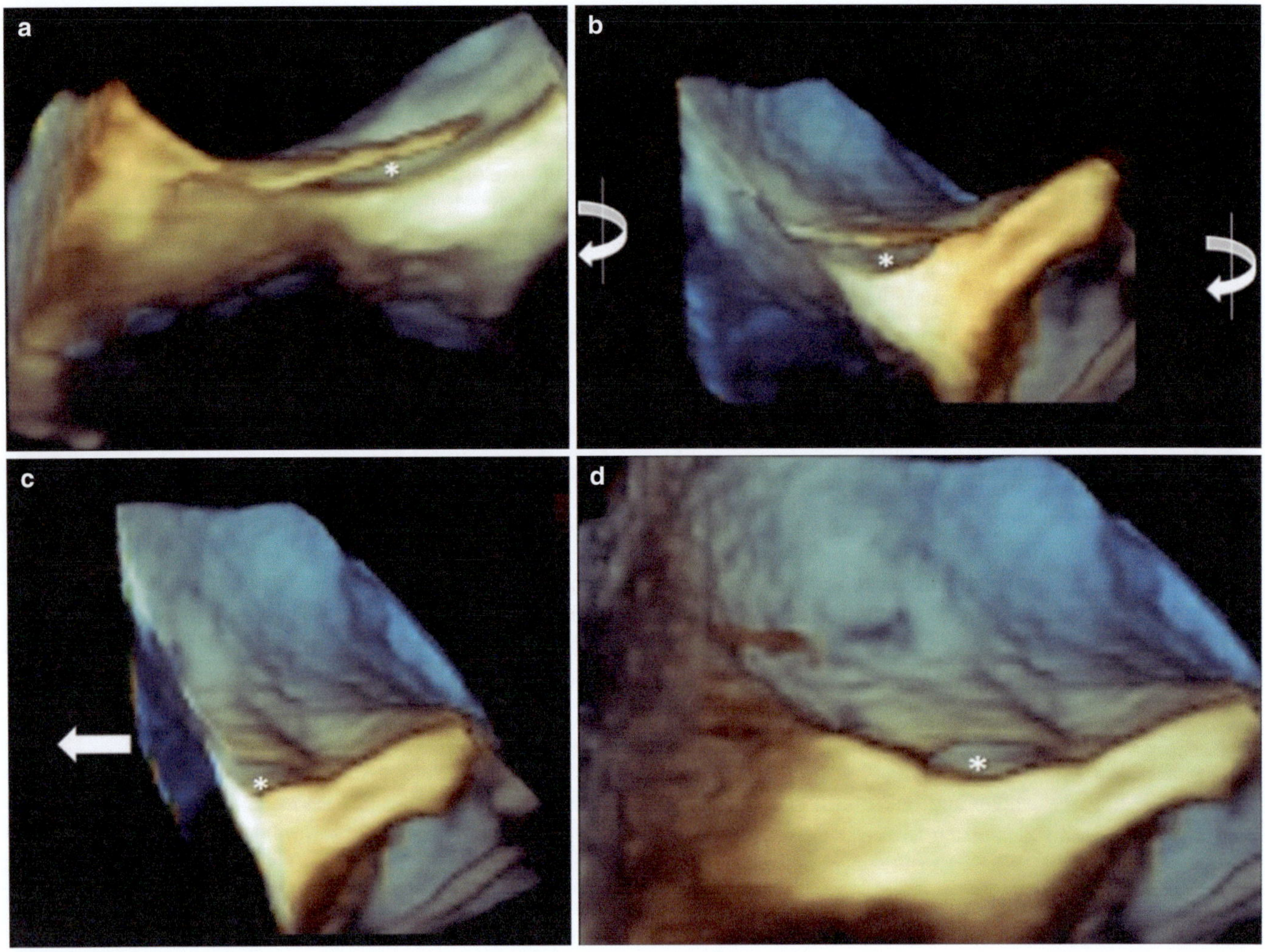

Fig. 27.4 (**a**) 3D TEE cross-section view, showing a left lateral pouch (asterisk) in its long axis orientation. Right-to-left rotation around the y-axis (curved arrow), leads to the image displayed in panel (**b**). Further right to left rotation is seen in panel (**c**). Cropping in the direction of the arrow leads to the image shown in panel (**d**). In this image the orifice of the pouch (asterisk) is seen in "en face" perspective

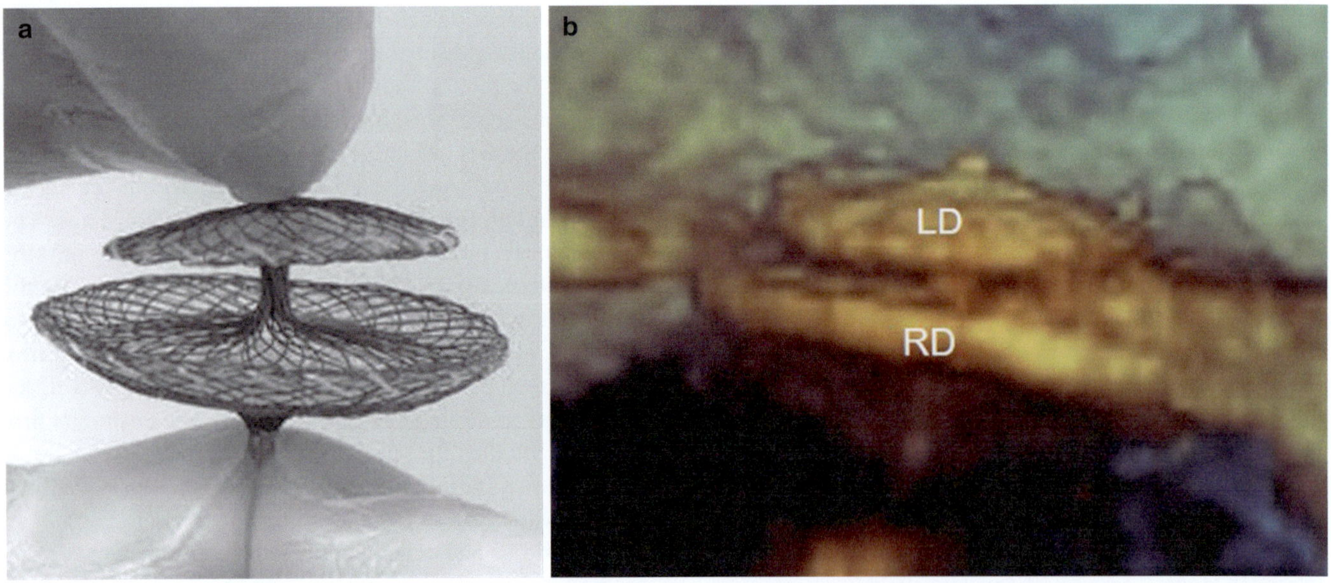

Fig. 27.5 Photograph of Amplatzer PFO occluder device and the corresponding 3D TEE image "in situ". LD, left disc; RD, right disc. Image from Francesco Faletra et al. in Real-time 3D interventional echocardiography. Springer-Verlag London 2014 page 35

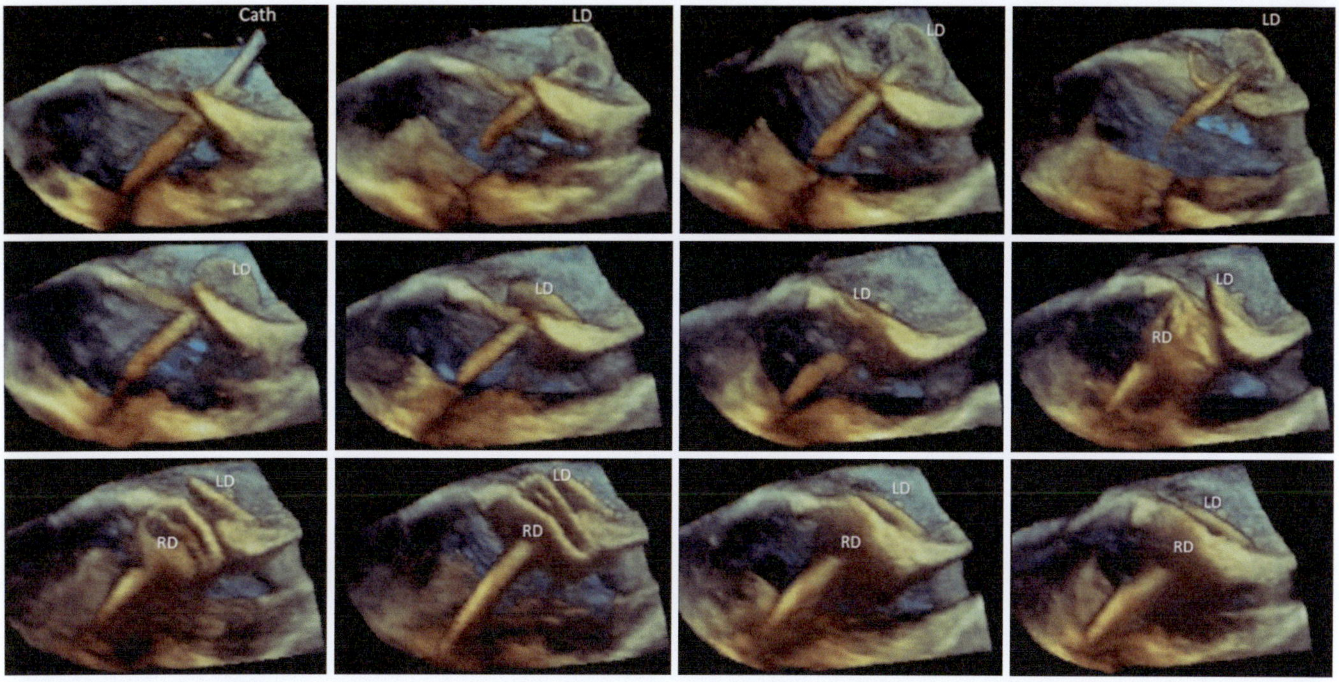

Fig. 27.6 Sequence of 3D TEE still frame images from a lateral perspective showing the opening of the left disc (LD) and the right disk (RD). Cath, catheter

A novel imaging technique (Echo-Navigator, Philips Medical System, Best, the Netherlands), is able to acquire patient-specific "real-time-data" from both fluoroscopy and 2D/3D TEE data set and to overlap them in the three-dimensional fluoroscopic space creating a sort of "hybrid image". This fused imaging has the unquestionable advantage of providing easy-to-interpret and reliable images for young interventional cardiologists, since soft tissues become "visible" and displayed within the standard fluoroscopic projections (Fig. 27.7a–d; see Chap. 35). A new volume rendering algorithm using a movable source of light, may enhance some specific structures. An illustration of an implanted PFO device is shown in Fig. 27.7 panels e and f, using the traditional (blue-bronze dual color) and new volume rendering algorithm. The light positioned beyond the volume data set enhances visualization of the septal tissue between the discs.

Percutaneous PFO closure is a safe procedure. Major complications, such as hemorrhage, perforation of left atrial appendage, cardiac tamponade, need for surgical intervention, pulmonary emboli and device embolization, are very uncommon with a total peri-procedural complication rate less than 1% [23]. Long term device-related complication risks, such as thrombus formation or erosion of cardiac structures, are also rare. Particularly harmful is the erosion of surrounding cardiac structures occurring with the Amplatzer device. This device has a relatively rigid structure which keeps it stable once implanted. However, when oversized, the device may erode and eventually penetrate the anterior atrial wall and the adjacent posterior aortic wall [24].

Closure of ASD

Introduction

Atrial septal defect (ASD) is a common congenital anomaly with an approximate birth prevalence of 1.6 out of 1000 individuals [25]. Although recognized as a relatively benign cardiac disease, large ASD, if untreated can eventually contribute to significant morbidity and mortality. Longstanding left-to-right shunt at atrial level, in fact, may cause right ventricular volume overload leading to right heart failure, elevated pulmonary vascular resistance, systemic embolism, and atrial arrhythmias. In addition, diastolic compression of the left ventricle (LV) by a dilated right ventricle reduces LV compliance, and this is responsible for the so called "masked LV diastolic disfunction". There are 4 main types of ASDs: secundum ASD, primum ASD, sinus venosus ASD, and unroofed coronary sinus (see also Chap. 20). *Secundum ASD* is the most common type accounting for about ¾ of all ASDs and is more common in females than males. Secundum ASD is caused by a deficiency of septum primum (SP) most likely due to an excessive resorption (via apoptosis) and therefore it is located within the borders of the FO. Its size varies from a few millimeters in diameter to more than 3 cm and its shape

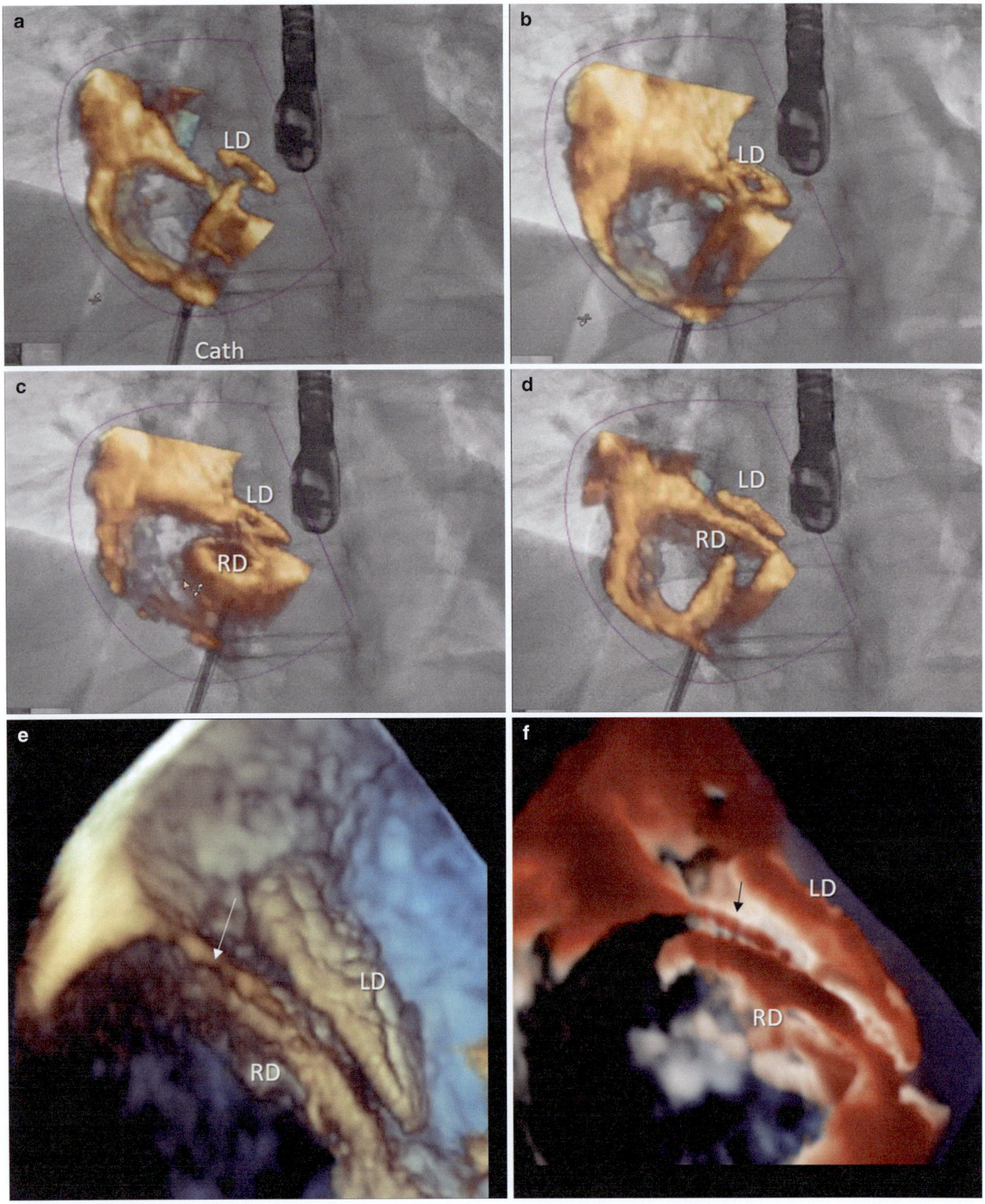

Fig. 27.7 (**a–d**) Fluoroscopic-3D TEE fused images during PFO closure. (**e**) Traditional and (**f**) new volume rendering display with movable source of light (TrueVue Philips Healthcare). The arrows points to the atrial tissue in between the two discs. Cath, catheter; LD, left disc; PFO, patent foramen ovale; RD, right disc

may be round, triangular, elliptic or irregular. Multiple secundum ASDs (Swiss cheese defect) represent a minority of all secundum ASD. Larger fenestrated ASD can be imaged easily with 2-dimensional transesophageal echocardiography and color-flow Doppler; however, smaller interatrial perforations, especially within a redundant FO, may not be appreciated.

Primum ASD is also called atrio-ventricular septal defect and accounts for about 15–20% of all ASDs. Rarely it may occur as an isolated lesion, being usually part of the atrioventricular septal defect's spectrum. *Sinus Venosus ASD* is relatively rare (5–10% of all ASDs) and is located at the interface between the right atrium and the embryologic sinus venosus. Such a defect may be located near the superior vena cava (SVC) or next to the inferior vena cava (IVC). The defect close to the SVC is typically associated with anomalous drainage of the right upper pulmonary vein into the right atrium or SVC.

The unroofed coronary sinus is the rarest form of ASD (<1% of all ASDs). Fenestrations in the roof of the coronary sinus allow for interatrial shunt.

With the exclusion of secundum ASD which is correctly labeled interatrial *septal* communication in that the left-to-right shunt occurs within the borders of the FO, the remaining ASDs should be labelled as interatrial *extra-septal* communications since the interatrial shunt occurs external to the "true" IAS [26]. All types of ASD can be repaired surgically. Although, very recently, transcatheter correction of sinus venous ASD with anomalous drainage, has been performed using a covered stent [27], at the time of this writing, the only ASD unanimously accepted for percutaneous closure remains the secundum ASD. Thus, this chapter will focus on the percutaneous closure of this type of ASD.

Percutaneous Closure

Surgical closure of atrial septal defect (ASD) has been the treatment of choice for decades, with excellent results, negligible mortality and limited morbidity. In 1974, King and Mills for the first time closed an ASD using a transcatheter approach guided only by fluoroscopy [28]. In 1980, Hellenbrand et al. described for the first time the use of 2D TEE in addition to fluoroscopy during percutaneous ASD closure [29]. In 2010, Perk et al. introduced the use of 3D TEE for guiding percutaneous procedures [30]. Following this seminal paper, 3D TEE was extensively used before and during ASD closure procedures. Intracardiac echocardiography (ICE) is purely an intraprocedural imaging tool, does not require general anesthesia and is particularly well suited for ASDs closure [31]. However, due to the high cost of ICE catheters, and the need of a dedicated machine and specific technical expertise by the interventional cardiologist, this technique is less frequently used than 2D/3D TEE. Percutaneous closure of ASD is associated with low complication rates, short anesthetic times, and short hospitalizations. Moreover, high-volume institutions have reported good long-term outcomes using this strategy.

Diagnosis of Secundum ASD

The diagnosis of secundum ASD is established by 2D/3D TTE and TEE. Transthoracic echocardiography assesses the type of ASD and its hemodynamic consequences (i.e. shunt direction, right heart dilatation, the degree of pulmonary hypertension and associated anomalies). However, detailed ASD anatomy (i.e. assessment of shape, size, number and extension of rims) requires 2D/3D TEE. In particular 3D TEE permits accurate visualization of ASDs using the unique "en face" perspective either from the left or right atrial perspective (Fig. 27.8).

ASD Size and Rims

Proper ASD sizing is essential for percutaneous closure. Accurate percutaneous device size selection avoids complications such as incomplete defect closure or device embolization (due to implantation of an undersized closure device) or disc erosion into surrounding cardiac structures (due to an oversized closure device). In general, the maximum diameter of a secundum ASD cannot exceed the device specific cutoff values. In the United States this cut-off is 38 mm, while in Europe it is 40-mm when using an Amplatzer atrial septal occluder (St Jude Medical, Inc., Little Canada, MN, USA). Large ASDs (>38 mm) and septal rim deficiencies remain challenging to treat percutaneously and are usually managed by surgery. It is important to distinguish between the 'unstretched diameter' and the 'stretched diameter' measured intra-procedurally using a balloon sizing technique. This technique consists of gradually inflating a sizing balloon placed across an ASD until no color Doppler flows across the ASD. Device selection is based on either the measured stretched diameter or by adding 6–8 mm to the unstretched diameter. It is also important to understand that the ASD orifice changes its shape and size throughout the cardiac cycle with the maximum ASD diameter occurring during ventricular systole. 3D TEE imaging allows for determination of a true maximum unstretched diameter. Sizing may be done directly on volume rendered 3D TEE images or

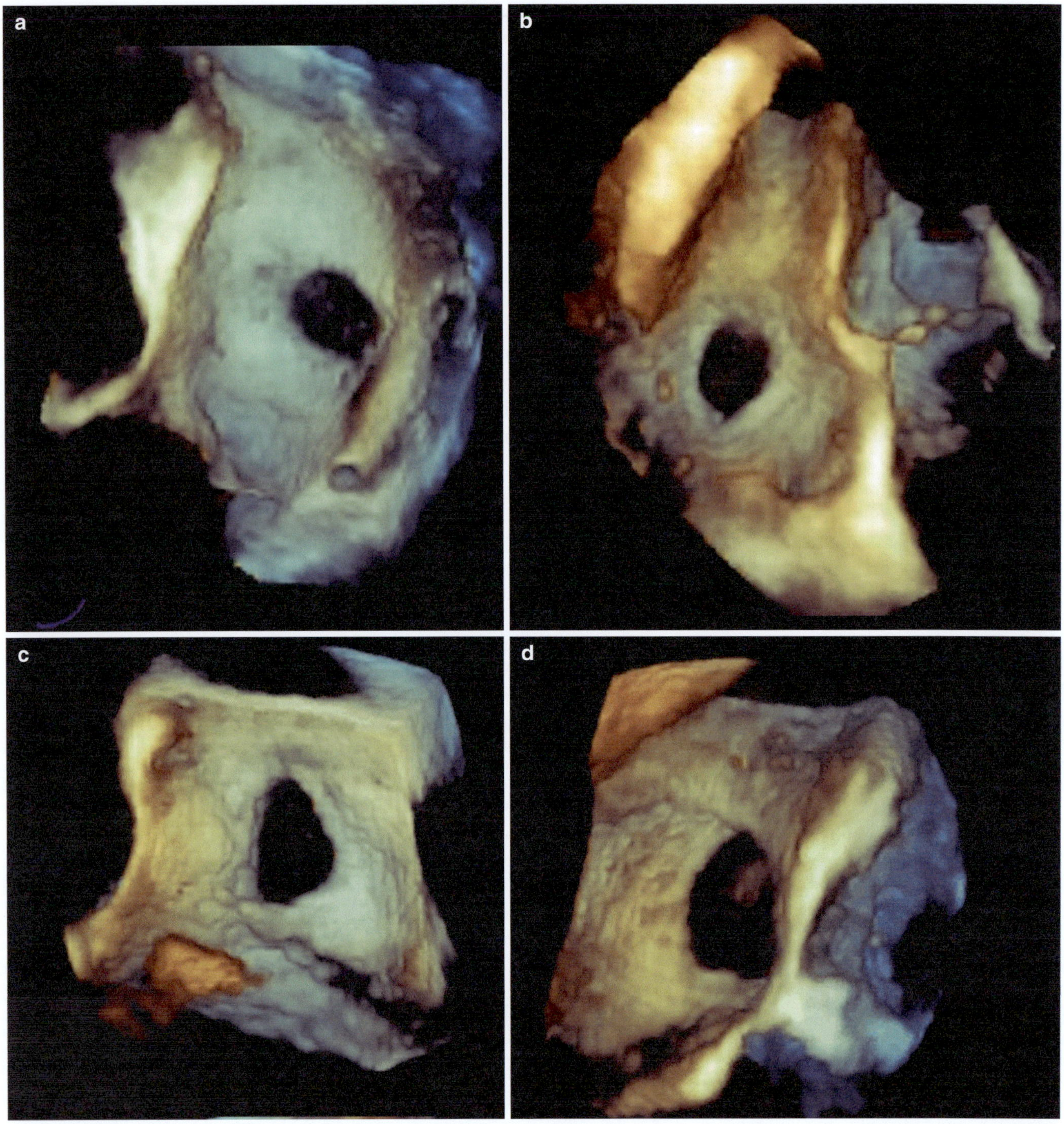

Fig. 27.8 3D TEE images of secundum atrial septal defect (ASD) of different sizes and shapes from left (**a**, **c**, **e**) and right (**b**, **d**, **f**) atrial perspectives

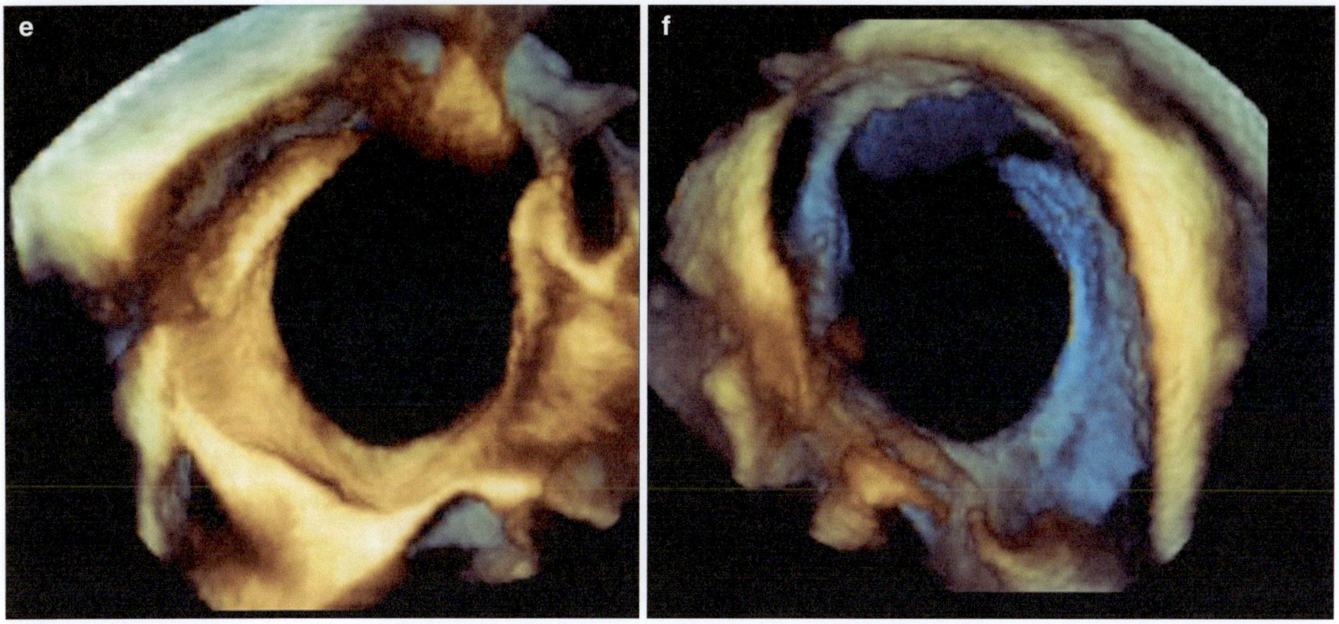

Fig. 27.8 (continued)

on multiplanar reconstruction images (Fig. 27.9). It must be emphasized that using a single diameter of the defect to choose the appropriate device size is not recommended because ASDs are usually not rounded structures. Thus, assessing at least two diameters is recommended for proper device sizing. In this respect, 3D TEE is the best imaging technique for clarifying the anatomic features of ASD.

ASD rims should be of sufficient length for secure anchoring of the closure device. Secundum ASDs have six distinct rims listed in a clockwise direction from a left atrial perspective as follows: Superior vena cava rim, posterior-superior rim (right upper pulmonary vein rim), posterior-inferior rim, inferior vena cava rim, atrioventricular rim and aortic (anterior) rim (Fig. 27.10). ASD devices require a rim length of at least 5 mm, with the exception for the aortic rim for which a length of 2 mm is sufficient for firm anchorage. Absence of inferior-posterior rim is considered a contraindication for percutaneous closure.

Devices and TEE Procedural Guiding

The most frequently implanted devices consist of a mesh covering opposable double discs (Amplatzer, AGA Medical Corporation, Plymouth, Minnesota), a helix spiral occluder (Helex, W. L. Gore & Associates, Inc., Flagstaff, Arizona), or 2 square umbrella-like spring frames (STARFlex, Inc., NMT Medical, Boston, Massachusetts). The Amplatzer was the first device used. A waist with a thickness of 3–4 mm (which roughly corresponds to the thickness of the atrial rims) connects the disks. The size of the device is determined by the diameter of the waist, which may range from 4 to 38–40 mm. The two discs extend radially, several mm (12 mm) beyond the diameter of the waist, to provide a firm anchorage. This was the first device approved by the FDA in 2001 followed by the helix spiral occluder in 2006.The use of 2D/3D TEE requires general anesthesia (although some institutions use TEE under propofol-induced deep sedation without endotracheal intubation). Traditionally, ASD closure requires the defect to be sized using a balloon catheter. The balloon catheter is advanced over the wire under fluoroscopy and TEE control and placed across the defect. The balloon is then inflated until the left-to-right shunt is blocked as observed by 2D TEE color Doppler (balloon stop-flow). ASD diameters are then measured by means of both echocardiography and fluoroscopy imaging, at the level of indentations made by the defect rims. Though balloon sizing is effective, in certain cases, it may overestimate the size of the ASD if the balloon is overstretched, which may lead to device oversizing. Device oversizing may increase the risk of erosion. Thus, it is not surprising that, in most institutions, a sizing balloon is no longer used, and measurements are made on the 3D TEE images. Once the device has been selected, the catheter with the device is advanced in the sheath into the mid left atrium.

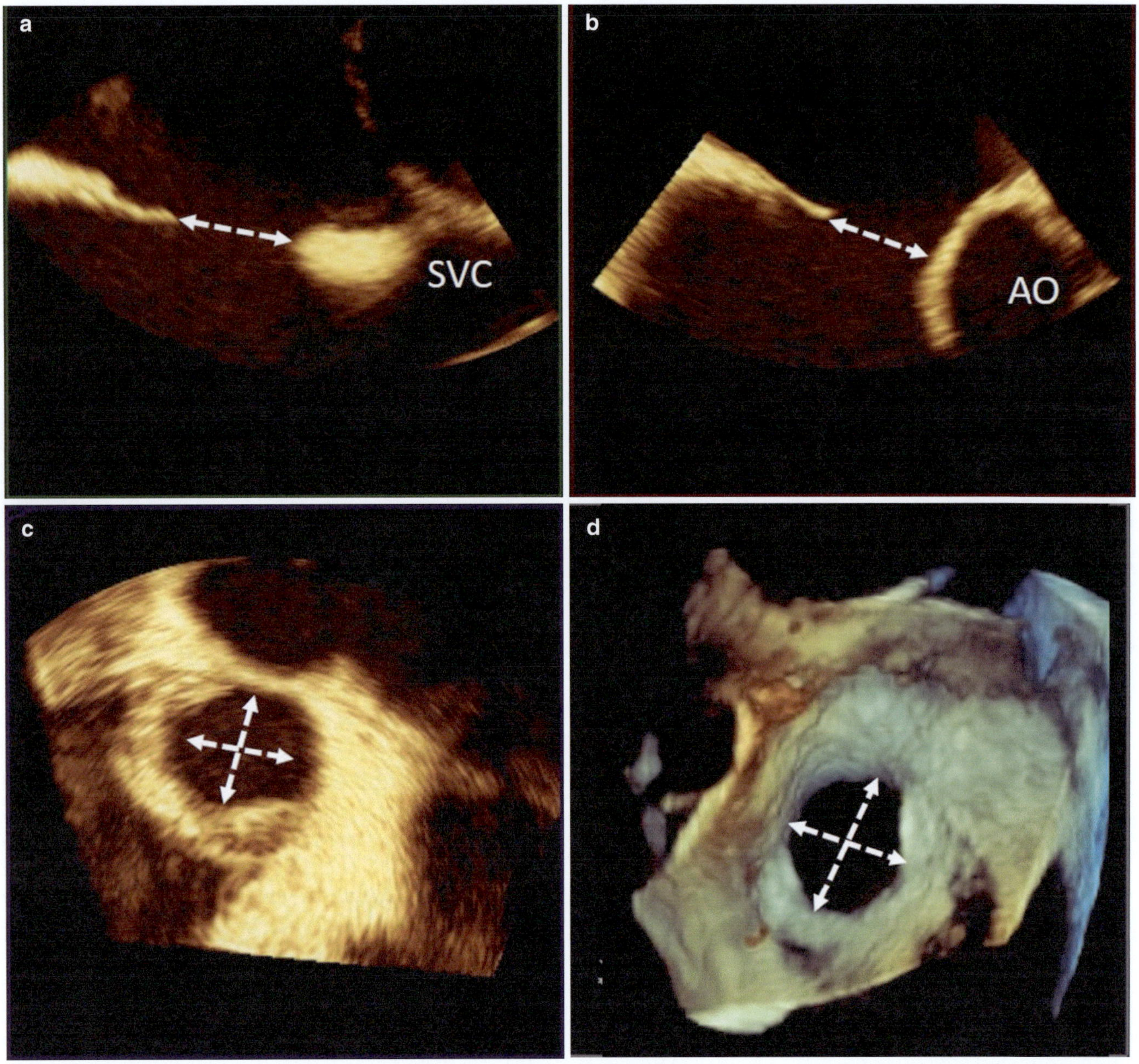

Fig. 27.9 Multiplanar reconstruction (MPR) showing (**a**) the bi-caval and aortic (**b**) diameters. (**c**) Same diameters measured from an "en face" perspectives using MPR (thick slices) and (**d**) 3D volume rendering format. AO, aorta; SVC, superior vena cava

The left disk is then expanded and pulled back to the left side of the septum (so that the connecting waist remains across the defect); at this point, the right disk is expanded in the right atrium, abutting the right side of the septum. After a pull-push maneuver that confirms that it is firmly anchored, the device is released (Fig. 27.11).

Complications

Transcatheter ASD closure is associated with all the risks inherent to any interventional cardiac catheterization procedure such as the risk of contrast dye reactions, vessel or cardiac perforation, and infections. Device embolization is the most frequent complication, occurring in 0.5% of the procedures [32]. Causative factors can be an undersized device, inadequate rim, malposition during the "push-pull" maneuver, or excessive tension on the delivery cable during device deployment [33]. In the majority of cases the device embolizes into the main pulmonary artery within the first 24 hours after the procedure and may be retrieved using a transcatheter approach in a majority of cases [34]. However, surgery is required when the transcatheter approach fails. Thus, although percutaneous closure of ASD appears as one of the simplest percutaneous procedures, with a short learning curve, operators must be prepared to retrieve the embolized device. Atrioventricular block, atrial fibrillation and

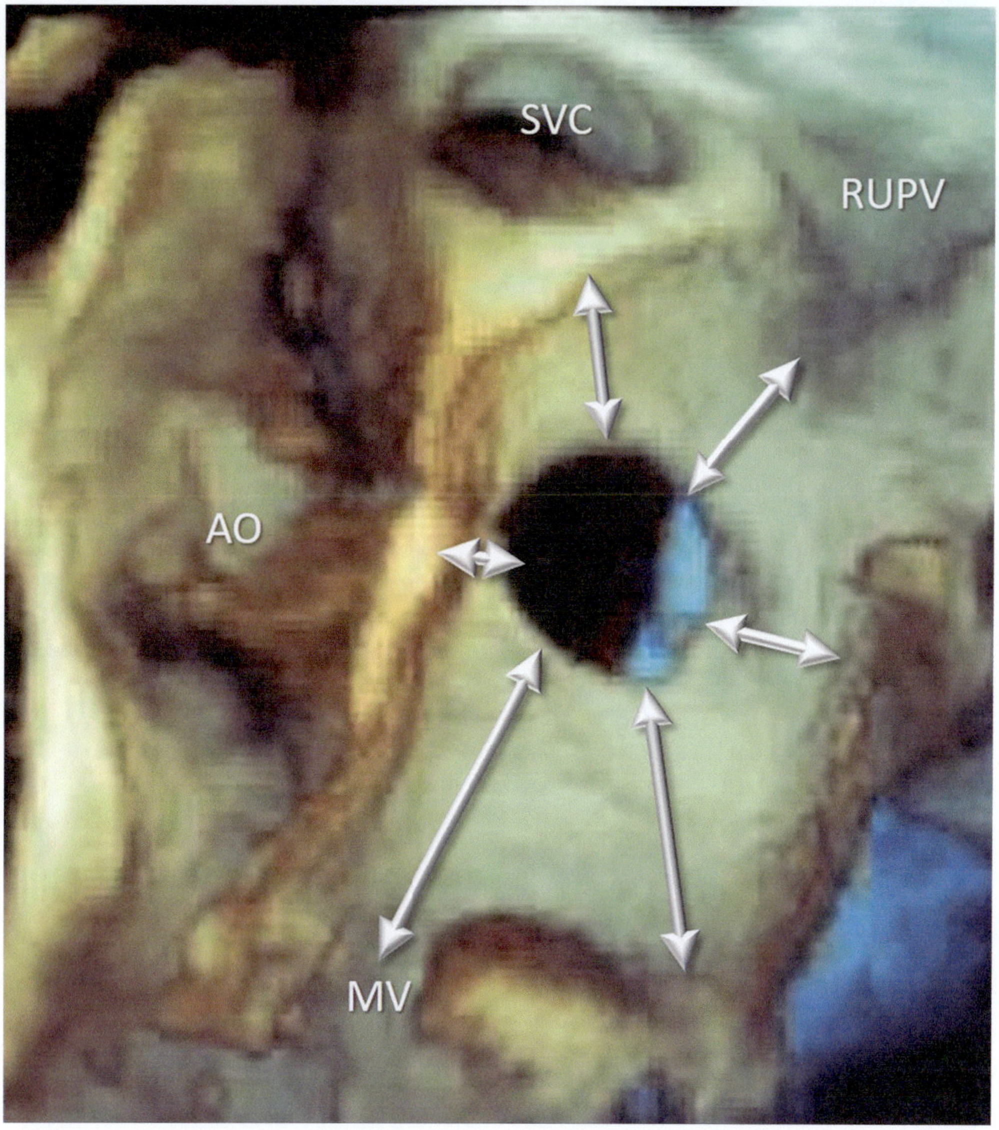

Fig. 27.10 3D TEE image of a secundum ASD showing the six distinct rims listed in a clockwise direction from a left perspective: SVC rim, posterior-superior rim (RUPV rim), posterior-inferior rim, IVC rim, atrioventricular rim and aortic (AO, anterior) rim (see text). AO, Aorta; IVC, inferior vena cava; SVC, superior vena cava; RUPV, right upper pulmonary vein; MV, mitral valve

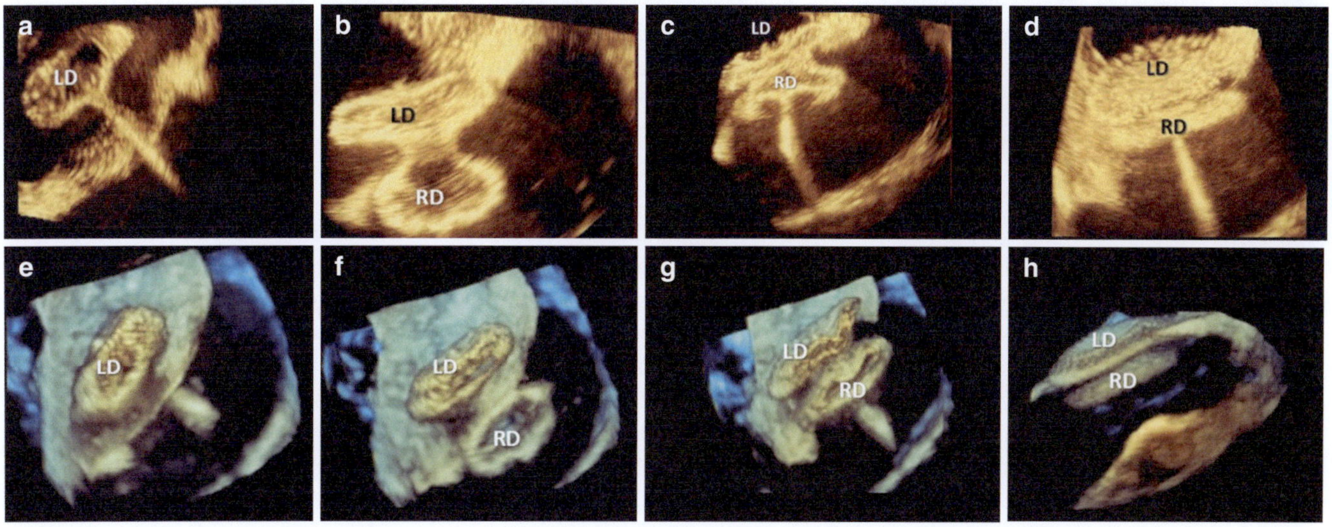

Fig. 27.11 (**a–d**) Sequential still images in multiplanar reconstruction (MPR) and in (**e–h**) volume rendering format showing percutaneous closure of an ASD. LD, left disk; RD, right disc

flutter may complicate ASD closure, especially in patients with history of previous arrhythmias and age >50 years at the time of ASD closure. While the incidence of AV block is low, occurring in 0.3% of patients, atrial arrhythmias, in particular atrial fibrillation, may increase post-closure [35]. In these patients, pulmonary vein isolation (PVI) or closure of the left atrial appendage (LAA) may be a necessary percutaneous treatment. However, the presence of a septal device makes septal crossing and/or subsequent catheter manipulation in the left atrium challenging. Although trans-device crossing is from time to time possible, enlarging the mesh of the device with an angioplasty balloon [36], device dislodgment or tearing of the interatrial septum tissue remain the major risks when performing this maneuver. The incidence of thrombus formation on the device is low, although significant differences between devices have been noted. The Amplatzer device seems to be the least thrombogenic. Atrial fibrillation and persistent atrial septal aneurysm after transcatheter closure are significant risk factors for thrombus formation. In most patients, the thrombus resolves on medical therapy without clinical consequences [37]. Device erosion through the atrial wall into the aorta or pericardial space (cardiac erosion) is a rare (0.1–0.3% of all Amplatzer device deployment world-wide) but serious adverse event. This complication may be fatal if not promptly recognized with a mortality rate as high as 20% [38]. Device-related erosion may, in fact, cause pericardial effusion /tamponade, atrial-aortic fistula and perforation of atrial wall. In the majority of cases, aortic erosion occurs within 24 h after device deployment although erosion years after atrial septal occluder implantation has been reported [39]. A particular concern arises from the fact that there are no definite identifiable risk factors and the etiology seems to be multifactorial including device size, rim deficiency, septal malalignment and patient factors. Recommendations include: (a) avoidance of overstretching the defect during balloon sizing; (b) avoidance of oversizing the device to avoid straddling of the aorta, and (c) identifying patients with a large aortic root [40]. In such patients, echocardiographic follow-up at 24 h, and 6 and 12 months is mandatory.

Closure of LAA

Introduction

Atrial fibrillation (AF) is among the most common arrhythmias, with a prevalence of 0.4–1% in adults <55 years old, 7.2% in patients up to 65 years, and 10.3% in octogenarians' [41]. AF is the second most common cause of stroke and the LAA the most common site of thrombus formation in patients with AF who have experienced stroke [42]. The combination of low flow LAA velocities, commonly seen in patients with AF, and the heavily trabeculated LAA morphology, generates a "perfect" milieu for blood stasis and thrombus formation. The risk of stroke is five time higher in patients with non-rheumatic AF and 17 times higher in patients with AF and mitral stenosis. Currently, oral anticoagulation with direct oral anticoagulants (or vitamin K antagonists if DOACs are contraindicated) are the treatment of choice for the prevention of systemic and cerebral thromboembolism in patients with non-rheumatic AF [43, 44]. Despite their proven efficacy, a significant percentage of patients with AF have absolute or relative contraindications to anticoagulant therapy such as high bleeding risk, poor drug compliance, drug interactions, and cost. The rationale for LAA surgical or percutaneous closure as non-pharmacological alternatives to anticoagulation is therefore based on the following four incontrovertible facts: (a) AF causes stroke; (b) thrombi are located in the LAA in the vast majority of cases; (c) the risk of thrombus embolization from the LAA is high and (d) patients with AF may have contraindications to anticoagulant therapy [45, 46]. In the ensuing paragraphs, we discuss in detail the physiology and the complex anatomy of the LAA, the LAA closure devices used, pre-procedural and intraprocedural assessment, and finally, procedural and post-procedural complications.

Physiology of LAA

Described as the most lethal appendix of our body, for a long time the LAA has been considered just a dormant embryological remnant and its role in hemodynamics and in volume homeostasis clinically and scientifically underappreciated [47]. Yet, the LAA is an active contractile chamber that augments left ventricular filling in late diastole. In sinus rhythm, it has a characteristic biphasic pattern of emptying (a first passive phase in protodiastole and a second active phase during left atrial contraction) and a prominent monophasic pattern of filling. Moreover, the LAA is a more compliant chamber than the body of the LA, and thus functions as an important reservoir or decompression chamber in case of high left atrial pressure or volume overload. Volume homeostasis is due to specialized endothelial cells within the LAA wall that produce and release either atrial natriuretic peptide (ANP) or B-type natriuretic peptide (BNP). In healthy hearts, the concentration of natriuretic hormones in the LAA is 40 times higher than in any other heart cavity. The secretion of these peptides is continuously modulated by means of stretch-sensitive receptors that respond to appropriate mechanical or neuroendocrine stimuli. Experimental studies in animals suggest that the LAA may also mediate thirst in a hypovolemic state. There are few data regarding the short and long-term effects of percutaneous LAA closure. Immediately after LAA occlusion, an increase in ANP and BNP levels (likely due to LAA stretching by introduction of the closure device) has been described with normalization within 24 hours. Other studies showed that after few months, ANP and BNP levels are comparable with those of normal individuals. The clinical utility of measuring ANP or BNP levels before or after LAA closure remains to be established, however.

Anatomy of Left Atrial Appendage

The LAA is the embryological left atrium (LA) and develops during the third week of gestation. The remaining smooth walls of the adult LA develop weeks later and are formed by an outgrowth of the pulmonary veins. The complete development of the LA occurs approximately at day 50 of the fetal life. The different embryology explains the morphological differences between the LAA and the remaining atrial structure: while the LAA is heavily trabeculated, (though the wall between trabeculae is remarkably thin having an average thickness of ~1 mm), the atrial body has a thicker wall with a smooth endocardial surface. Externally, the LAA extends between the anterior and lateral walls of the left atrium and its tip usually points antero-superiorly partially covering the right ventricular outflow tract (or the pulmonary trunk), and the left main coronary artery (or the circumflex artery). However, it is not uncommon to find the tip of the LAA directed laterally and backward. When viewed from an internal perspective, which is best obtained with 3D TEE (or observing an anatomic specimen from within the atrial cavity), the orifice of the LAA (i.e. the junction of LAA with the body of LA) is readily visible. In the normal adult heart, this orifice is almost oval-shaped, and it is located close to the left lateral ridge (LLR) also known as the Coumadin or warfarin ridge, the circumflex artery, the vestibule, (i.e. the outlet part of LA surrounding the mitral valve) and the right pulmonary artery (Fig. 27.12, panel a and b). The general aspect of the LAA is that of a relatively flat tubular "cul de sac" structure with an orifice, a body and peripheral lobes. However, its shape is extremely variable and this unique variability distinguishes each LAA from any other as a kind of fingerprint. Nevertheless, based on images provided by CT, the LAA may be roughly divided into four types creatively called: "cactus," "chicken wing," "windsock" and "cauliflower," [48]. The *cactus morphology* is composed of a dominant

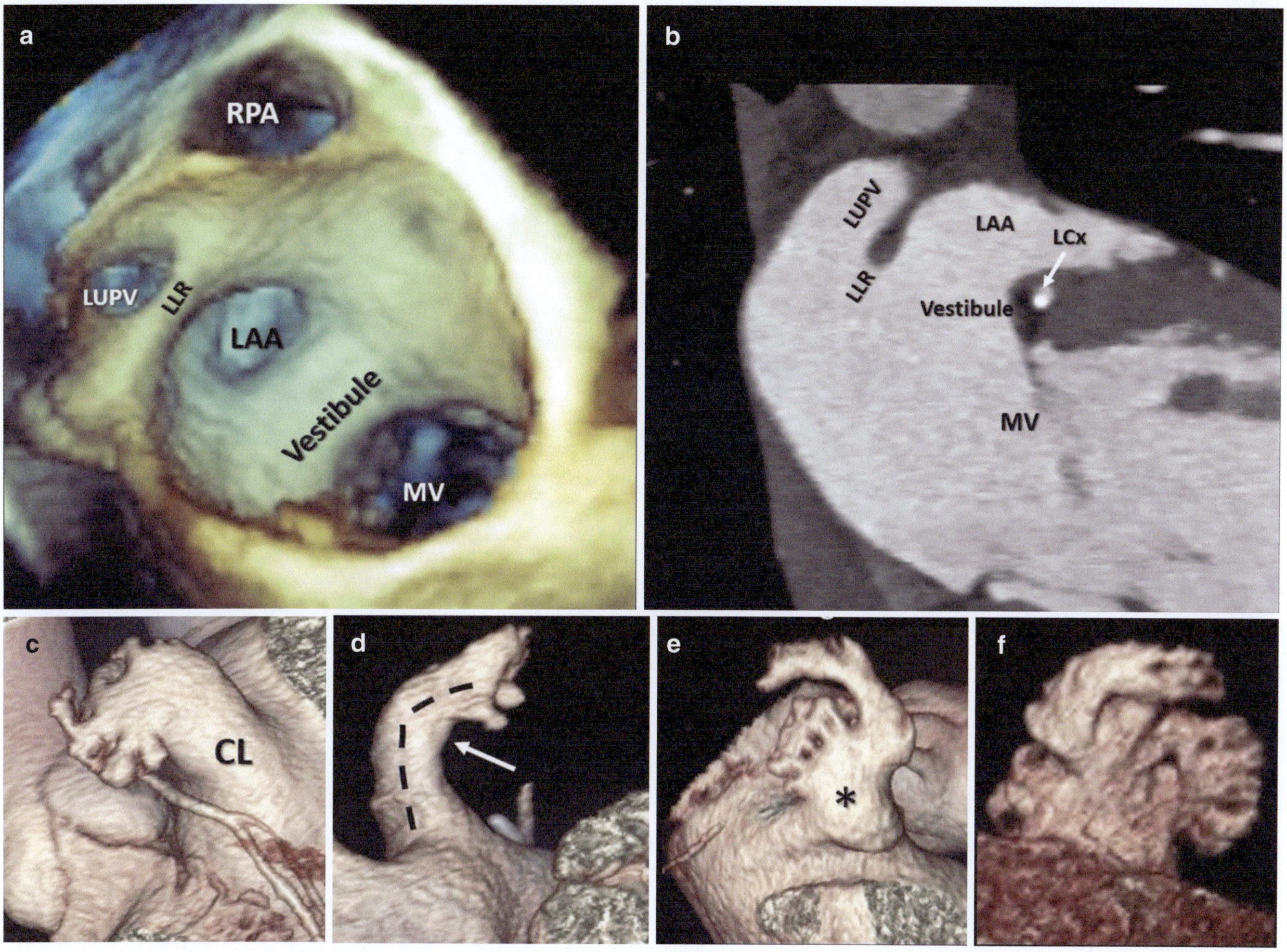

Fig. 27.12 (**a**) 3D TEE illustrating the internal surface of the left atrium and the spatial relationship of the left atrial appendage (LAA) to the left lateral ridge (LLR), left upper pulmonary vein (LUPV), right pulmonary artery (RPA), vestibule, and mitral valve (MV). (**b**) CT Multiplanar reconstruction showing the LAA and its spatial relationship to surrounding structures. (**c**) CT volume rendering showing the cactus morphology characterized by a dominant central lobe (CL) with secondary lobes extending from the CL in various directions. (**d**) The chicken wing morphology characterized by a sharp angulation within the body (black dotted line) with a thick and prominent pectinate in the middle of the LAA (arrow). (**e**) Windsock morphology with one dominant body (asterisk) and several secondary and tertiary lobes. (**f**) The cauliflower morphology has the most complex appearance, with many lobes and without a recognizable body. LCx, left circumflex coronary artery

central body with secondary lobes extending in both superior and inferior directions. The *chicken wing* morphology is characterized by a sharp angulation of the LAA body with a thick and prominent bend in the middle and absence of peripheral lobes. The *windsock morphology* presents one dominant body with several secondary and tertiary lobes. Finally, the *cauliflower morphology* is composed of many lobes without a central body. It has been suggested that patients with "non-chicken" wing morphology are significantly more likely to experience stroke than patients with chicken wing morphology [48], (Fig. 27.12, panel c–f). This is not surprising since LAAs with numerous lobes have lower LAA velocities, and, consequently, are more subject to blood stasis, thrombosis and eventually stroke.

In the most complex morphologies, the internal surface of the LAA is usually lined by a network of several ridges of muscular tissue, known as pectinate muscles (PMs) of different size, shape and thickness, often arranged in whorl-like fashion (Fig. 27.13a and b). Some PMs have a bizarre appearance that can be mistakenly diagnosed as

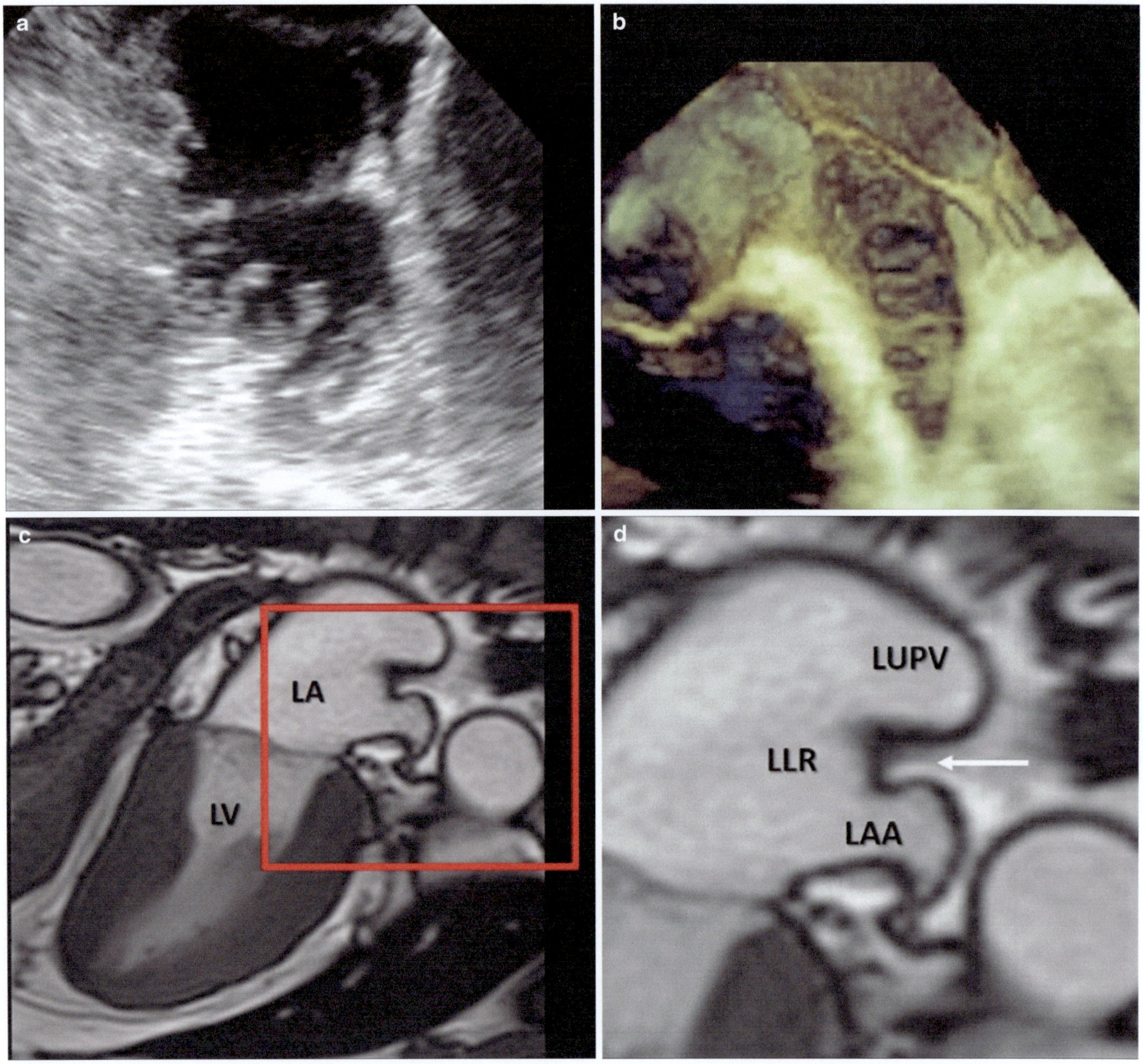

Fig. 27.13 (**a** and **b**) 2D and 3D TEE showing the complex morphology of the LAA with network of several ridges of muscular tissue (called pectinate muscles) of different size, shape and thickness. (**c** and **e**) Cardiac MRI cross section in two-chamber view, showing the particular anatomic arrangement of the left lateral ridge (LLR). (**d** and **f**) magnified images of the structure in the red box of panels **c** and **e**. In panel **d** it is evident that the LLR is actually an infolding of the atrial wall (arrow) separating the LAA from the left upper pulmonary vein (LUPV). (**d** and **f**) These images show the LLR ending with a bulbous (Q-tip sign or Coumadin ridge)

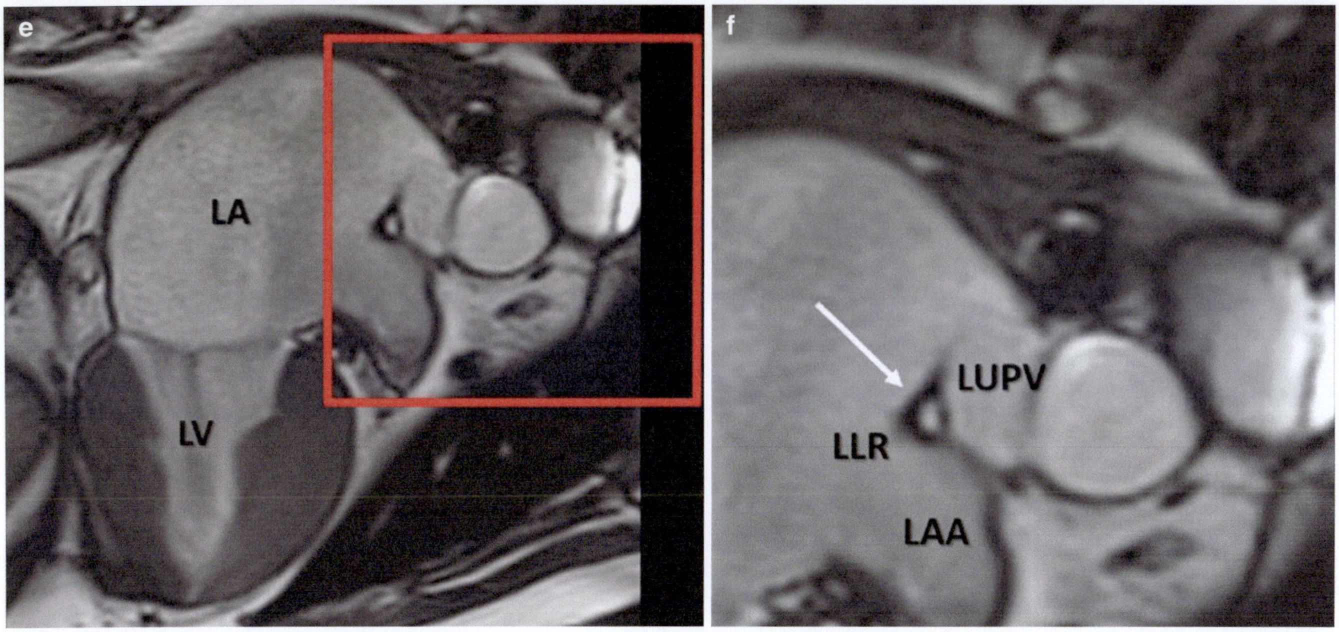

Fig. 27.13 (continued)

thrombi. The LLR is a band-like embryological remnant in the LA between the orifices of the LAA and left superior (upper) pulmonary vein. This protuberance is not a simple muscular ridge, as it might look at first glance, but rather an enfolding of the atrial wall, filled with epicardial adipose tissue, small vessels and nerves [49] (Fig. 27.13c–f). Among vessels, particularly relevant are: a) the artery to the sinus node that, when originating from the circumflex artery, runs through this enfolding, and b) the oblique vein, which is located on the epicardial surface of the LLR. This vein is the embryological remnant of the left superior vena cava which if persistent descends obliquely on the back of the left atrium and drains into the coronary sinus, but in some individuals it becomes a fibrous ligament. Of note, the oblique vein/ligament contains muscle bundles (Marshall bundles) that directly connect to atrial myocardium and coronary sinus muscle sleeves. These muscle structures may become a source of triggers for AF, and may form a substrate for reentry [50]. For this reason, electrophysiologists call the LLR the "ligament of Marshal". Frequently the enfolding is almost virtual, taking the appearance of a single ridge, but in some cases this folding of the atrial wall is relatively large and can be easily appreciated (especially by CMR, see Fig. 27.13c and d), and in others, the LLR ends with a bulbous filled with adipose tissue (see Fig. 27.13e and f). Because this bulbous morphology resembles a cotton-tip applicator, it is known as the "Q-tip sign", which was mistakenly diagnosed as a thrombus in the early days of TEE. This misdiagnosis explains the name of Coumadin ridge adopted by echocardiographers.

Preprocedural Assessment

The preprocedural assessment consists of (a) ruling out LAA thrombus; (b) providing detailed characterization of LAA anatomy and (c) measuring the LAA orifice and depth. Both TEE and CT are well suited for pre-procedural imaging.

Ruling Out Thrombus TEE is the current gold standard to rule-in/out LAA thrombus. Because TEE and fluoroscopy are the imaging techniques used for guiding the closure of LAA, it has been suggested that TEE can be performed directly in the cath-lab just before the procedure, avoiding preprocedural investigations with the associated costs. Although apparently cost-effective, the strategy of ruling-out "on the table" LAA thrombus and/or an unsuitable anatomy for closure could lead to *last minute* procedure cancellation, carrying the additional costs of general anesthesia, nursing coverage, and laboratory time. Using a specific protocol, (i.e. delayed imaging, dual-enhanced scan, prone positioning, dual energy source), CT is also utilized to rule-in/out thrombi. Advantages of CT, include noninvasive acquisition and high spatial resolution. Overall sensitivity ranges from 93 to 100% and specificity from 85 to 92%. Therefore, CT has an excellent negative predictive value for LAA thrombus detection and it is generally considered an ideal *ruling-out* technique. In addition, CT can help in selecting the most appropriate fluoroscopic projection during the procedure. Finally, whenever necessary CT may also be used to rule in/out coronary artery disease. Unfortunately contrast iodine administration, radiation exposure, restricted availability and costs still slow down its widespread use (Fig. 27.14).

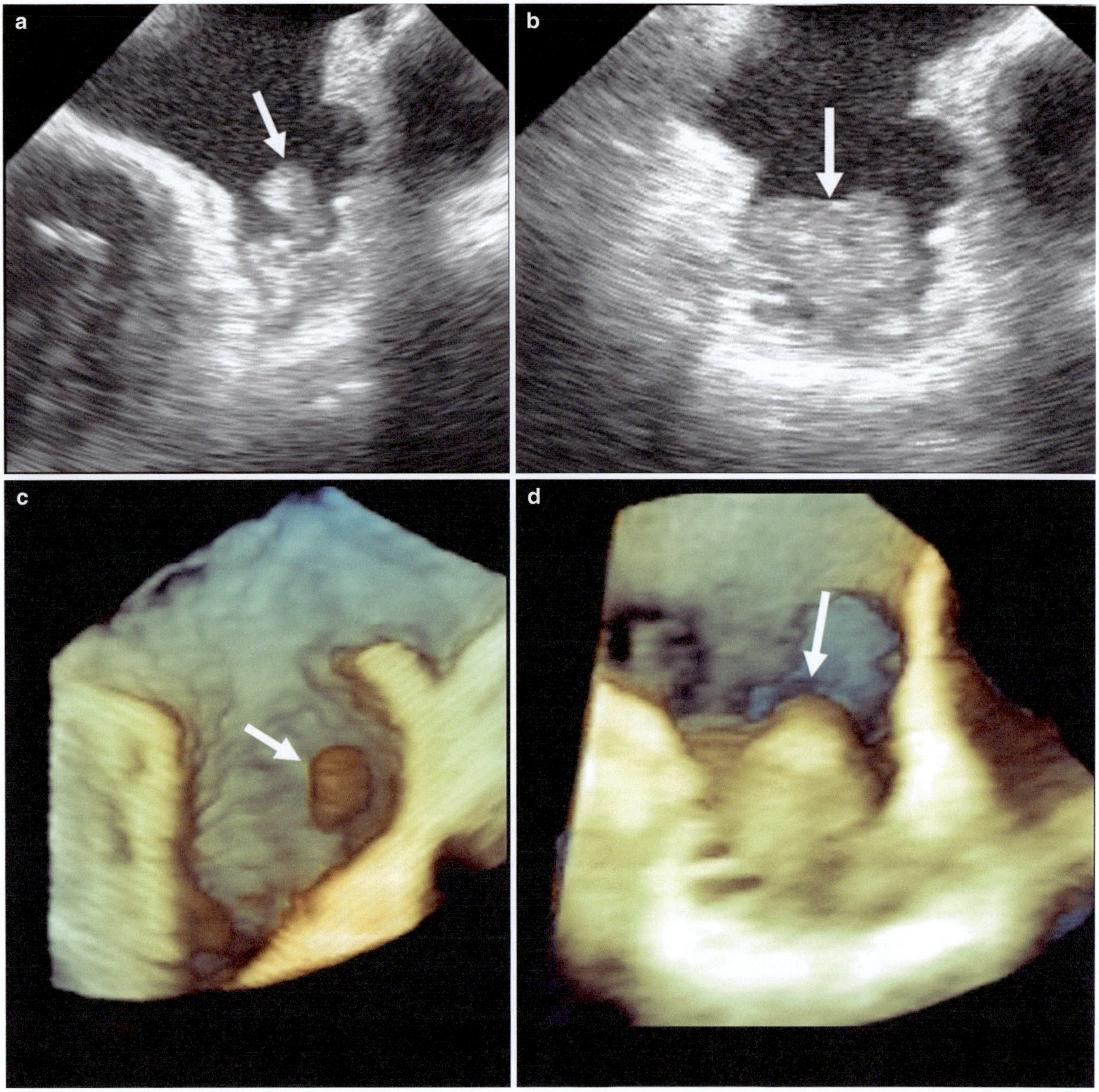

Fig. 27.14 (**a**, **b**) 2D TEE and (**c**, **d**) 3D TEE images of LAA showing a thrombus (arrow) in the LAA; (**e**, **f**) CT scan multiplanar reconstruction showing lack of complete filling of the LAA by contrast indicative of thrombus (asterisk). The curved dotted lines mark the wall of the LAA. LAA, left atrial appendage

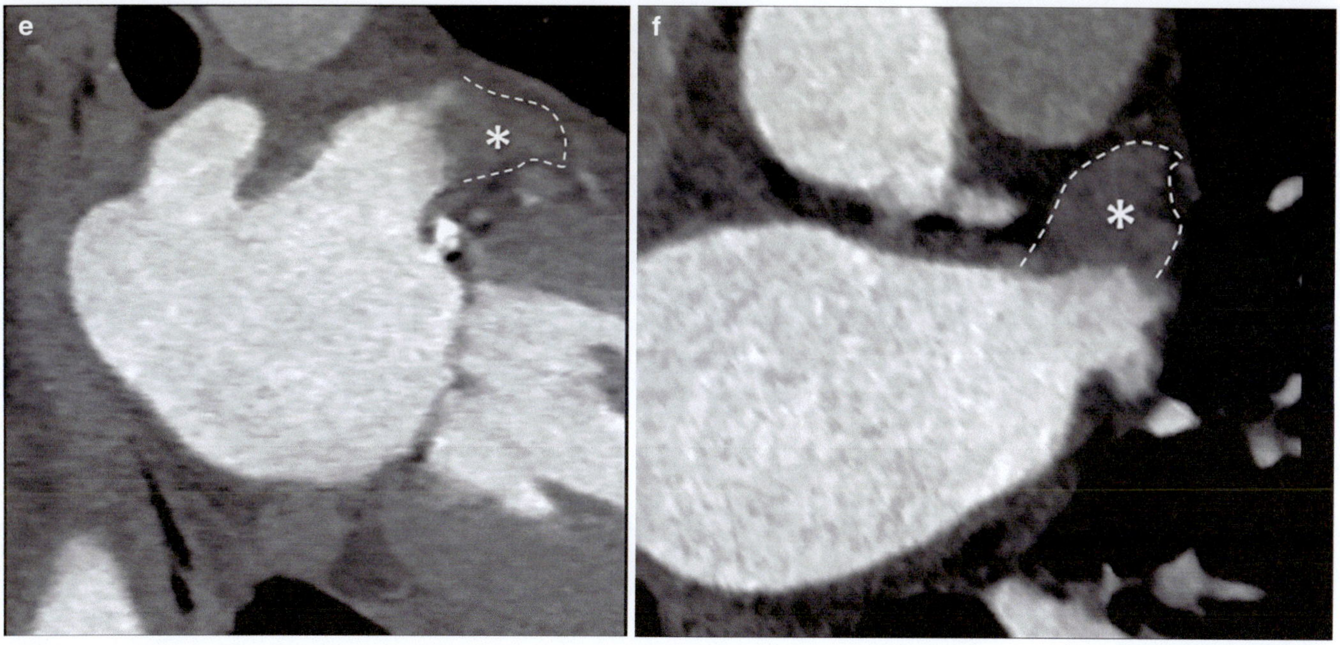

Fig. 27.14 (continued)

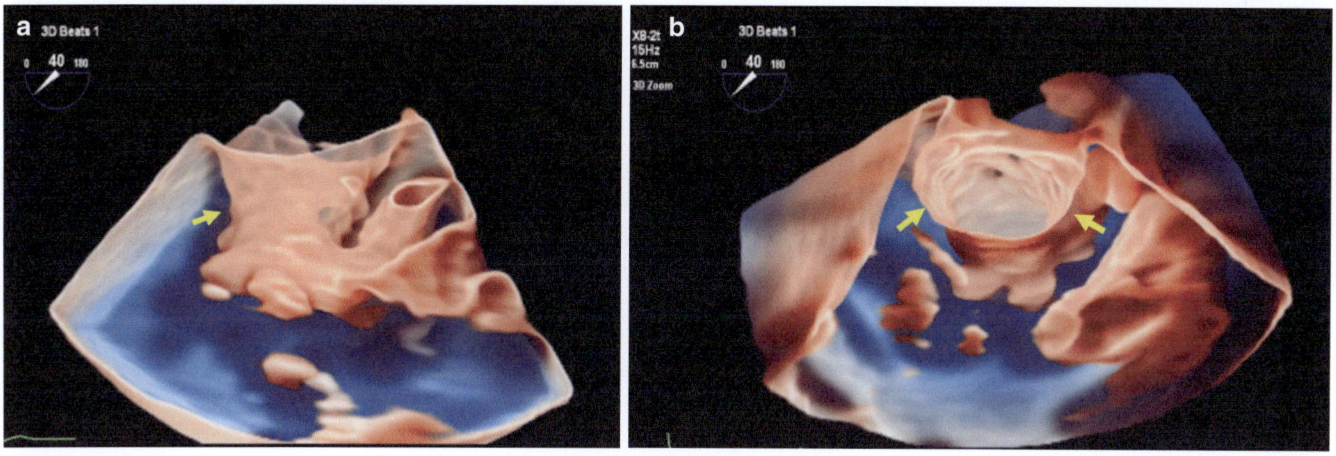

Fig. 27.15 (**a–b**) Two views of the left atrial appendage (arrows) using GlassVue (Philips Healthcare). Used with permission from Philips.

Detailed Characterization of LAA Anatomy

Detailed characterization of the shape of the LAA body and orifice is relevant for device selection. The presence and location of angulation, bifurcation into lobes, and thick pectinate ridges, can influence either the site of device implantation or device selection. Simulations of how the device fits within the LAA anatomy may help in choosing the optimal device. However, the effectiveness of an "envisioning fit" when a 3D structure is projected onto a 2D screen is questionable. Indeed, interventional cardiologists may have different visual spatial perceptions and a 3D image projected on a 2D screen might not be interpreted in the same way by different observers. A 3D-printed model of LAA anatomy, with its size, shape, length and lobulations, may help to simulate operative procedures prior to LAA occlusion, choosing the right size of the occluder and optimal depth for its release (see Chap. 36). A "personalized" 3D printed model may also assist in predicting the potential instability of the occluder and peri-device leaks. By allowing shapes and boundaries of structures to be more easily seen, recently introduced GlassVue (Philips Healthcare) may provide better insight into the anatomy of the LAA (Fig. 27.15).

LAA Measurements Correct sizing of the device requires accurate LAA measurements. When using 2D TEE, the probe should be positioned at the mid-esophagus and the

LAA scanned from 0–135°. Measurements should be taken in at least four angles (suggested angles in literature are 0°, 45°, 90° and 135°). However, the above-mentioned angles do not always correspond to a clear and measurable image of the LAA. 3D TEE, using multiplanar reconstruction (MPR), may provide a countless number of angles, from which the operator can choose the most informative images and angulations (Fig. 27.16a–f). Using CT, images of the LAA should be acquired with oblique MPR. Proximity to surrounding structures such as the LLR, the left upper(superior) pulmonary vein (LUPV) and the mitral annulus, should also be assessed. The measurements for the LAA ostium and LAA depth needed for proper device positioning are device-specific and should follow the manufacturer instructions. As a general rule the "landing zone" is the site within the LAA where the body of the device should be deployed. For the WATCHMAN device, appropriate device sizing is determined by the LAA landing zone diameter which is measured from the circumflex artery to 1–2 cm distal to the LA tip of the LLR while the LAA depth is measured from the landing zone to the apex (tip) of the LAA. For the Amplatzer Amulet device, the diameter of the landing zone is measured 10–12 mm inside the orifice (below the circumflex artery), to the LLR. Importantly, all measurements on 2D TEE should be taken at end of ventricular systole. 3D TEE can visualize the shape of the LAA ostium in an "en face" perspective. Our group demonstrated that measurements of LAA orifice area provided by 3D TEE closely matched the CT measurements (considered the Gold Standard), while 2D TEE significantly underestimated LAA dimensions and orifice size [51]. Measurements on CT should be performed during late atrial diastole when the LAA dimension is largest. Using MPR, an oblique view of the LAA ostium is selected where the circumflex artery, the LLR, and the LAA are well shown. Two co-axial cross-sectional orthogonal planes, and a third orthogonal "enface" view are used to measure dimensions of the LAA ostium. The depth of the LAA can be measured on MPR or using a maximal intensity projection. Of note, volume loading is critical to ensure proper measurements. Since the LAA is thin-walled and very distensible, measurements taken during the procedure under general anesthesia are smaller (up to 5 mm less) than those taken in conscious patients. As a general rule, the intra-procedural LAA morphology assessment for device sizing is performed only after verification that the left atrial pressure exceeds 12 mmHg. In cases in whom LA pressure is lower, a saline volume loading strategy of 500–1000 ml ensures proper measurements for device selection (Fig. 27.16). LAA orifice measurements can also be rapidly obtained using 3D Auto LAA (Philips Healthcare, Fig. 27.17) available on the most recent Philips 3D imaging platform.

Types of LAA Occlusion Devices and Procedural Imaging

Currently, two types of devices have been intensively studied and are available for LAA percutaneous closure [52]. The *Watchman* device (Boston Scientific, St. Paul, Minnesota, USA) consists of a self-expanding nitinol frame covered by a thin polyester membrane. Hooks are positioned around the mid-perimeter anchoring the device to the LAA. A second-generation device, the Watchman FLX, was developed and released in order to improve the efficacy and the feasibility of the previous device. This device was introduced in Europe in a limited fashion after it received CE Mark approval in November 2015. In 2016 the device was withdrawn from the market due to a higher than predicted device embolization rate (3.8%). At the beginning of 2019, Boston Scientific initiated a limited market release of a modified version which received CE mark in March 2019. The new generation Watchman FLX has a shorter device length (10–20%) and a less taper angle to simplify implantation and to fit a wider range of patients. Furthermore, the frame of the new device is designed to enhance sealing within the LAA and to reduce the risk of dislocation and embolization (12 "J" shaped fixation barbs arranged in two rows). The device typically has to be 10–20% larger than the LAA landing zone diameter to have sufficient radial forces for stable position. *The Amplatzer Cardiac Plug* is made up of a distal Lobe and a proximal Disk connected to each other by a flexible central waist. The Lobe has hooks to stabilize anchorage and should be fixed within the 'landing zone' (approximately 1 cm from LAA orifice). The disc fully covers the orifice. The second-generation of the Amplatzer (called Amulet) was redesigned to be more stable having a stiffer and wider lobe, more hooks, and more sizes available. Fluoroscopy and TEE are the preferred imaging modalities during LAA closure, although in some Institutions the LAA is closed under fluoroscopic/angiographic guidance alone to facilitate the logistics (less personnel and no sedation or intubation required). Angiography of the LAA is performed in right anterior oblique projection searching the best caudal and cranial angulations that typically outline the LAA, delineating size and lobes. Intracardiac echocardiography (ICE) is gaining popularity and has become standard in some institutions, given the convenience of minimal sedation and the ability to visualize some structures almost invisible to the traditional TEE (i.e. coronary sinus). However, for LAA occlusion, the main limitations to the widespread use of ICE are: (a) need for insertion of a second venous sheath (with an additional risk of vascular complications), (b) a limited field of view (particularly for 3D imaging), (c) catheter motion within cardiac chambers (which might provoke transient atrial arrhyth-

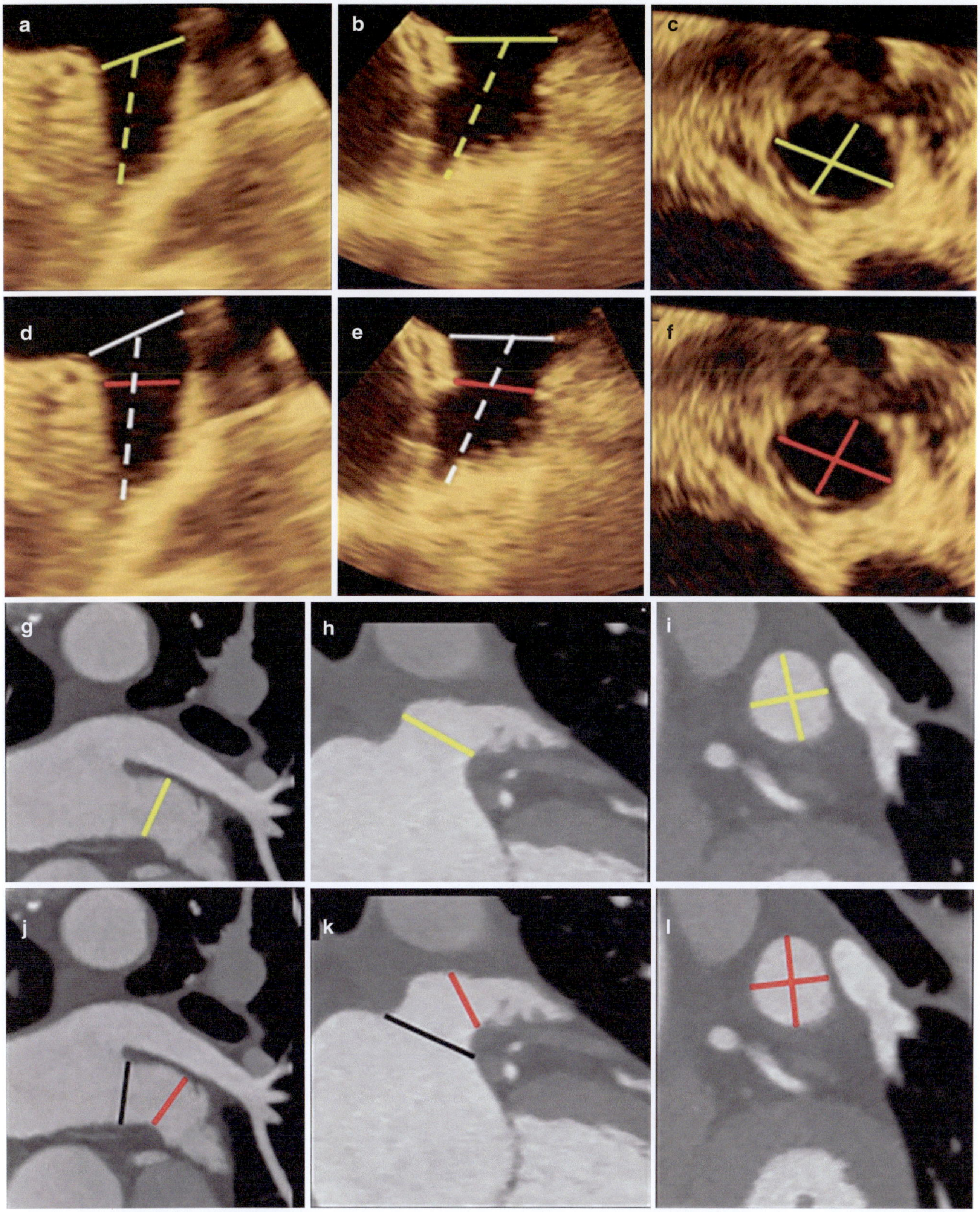

Fig. 27.16 (**a–c**) 3DTEEmultiplanar reconstruction showing the measurements of LAA for WATCHMAN device and (**d–f**) for the Amplatzer Amulet device. (**a–b**) The solid yellow line corresponds to the landing zone diameter for the Watchman device. (**d–e**) the grey line corresponds to the diameter of the LAA orifice, and the red line to the diameter of the"landing zone" for the Amplatzer Amulet device. (**g–h**) CT oblique multiplanar reconstruction showing the corresponding measurements for WATCHMAN device, and, (**j–k**) for the Amplatzer Amulet device. The black lines correspond to diameter of the LAA orifice (see text). (**c**, **f**, **i**, **l**) Diameters of the LAA orifice measured by 3D TEE multiplanar reconstruction (**c**, **f**) and CT oblique multiplanar reconstruction (**i**, **l**)

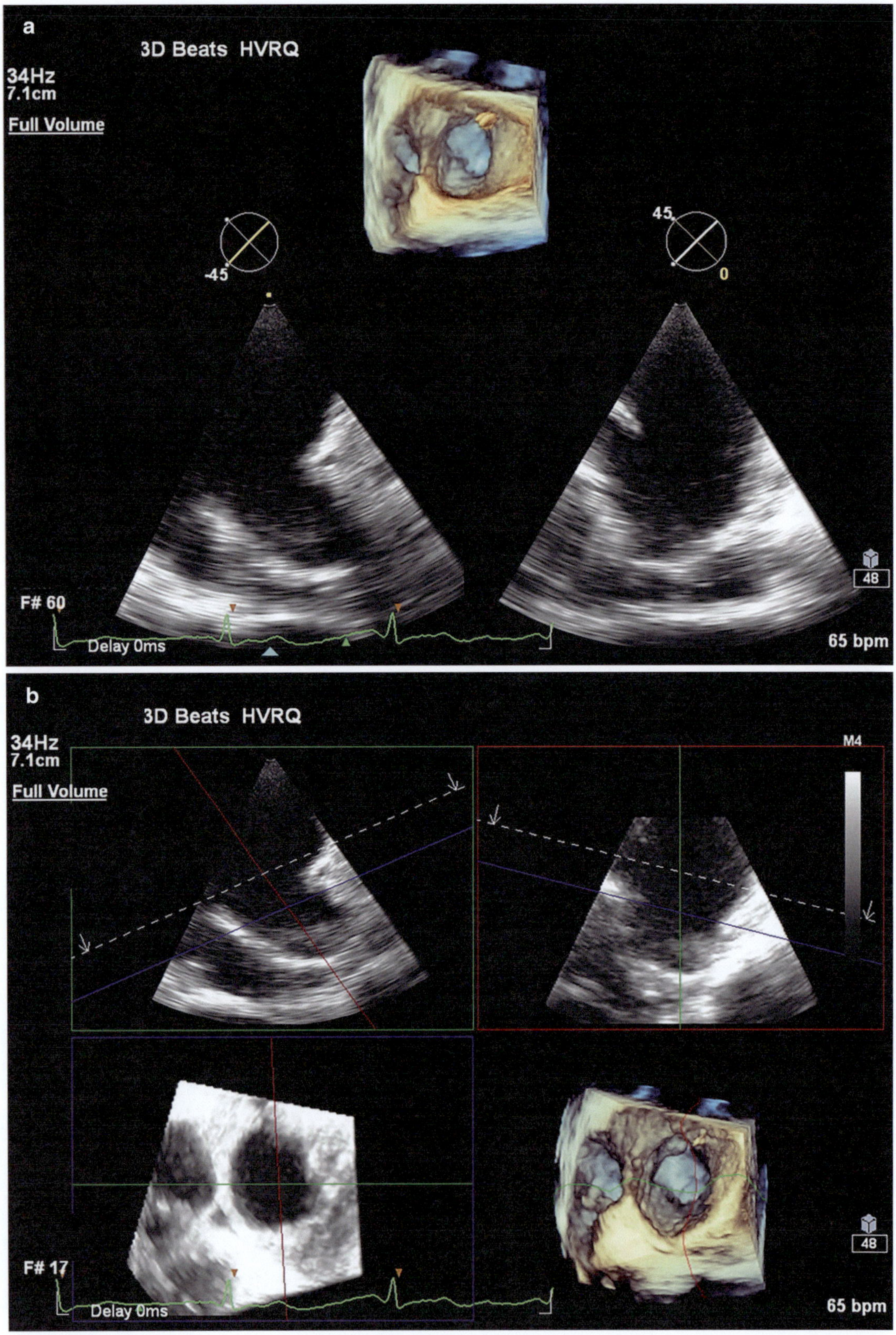

Fig. 27.17 LAA landing zone orifice measurement using 3D Auto LAA (Philips Healthcare). **Panel a**: 3D Full Volume (FV) of left atrial appendage (LAA) with component 2D images. **Panels b** and **c**: MultiVue of FV in panel a showing alignment of the blue plane with the landing zone (**b**) and landing zone orifice measurements (**c**). Images courtesy of Dr. Sari Padang. Used with permission of Mayo Foundation for Medical Education and Research. All rights reserved

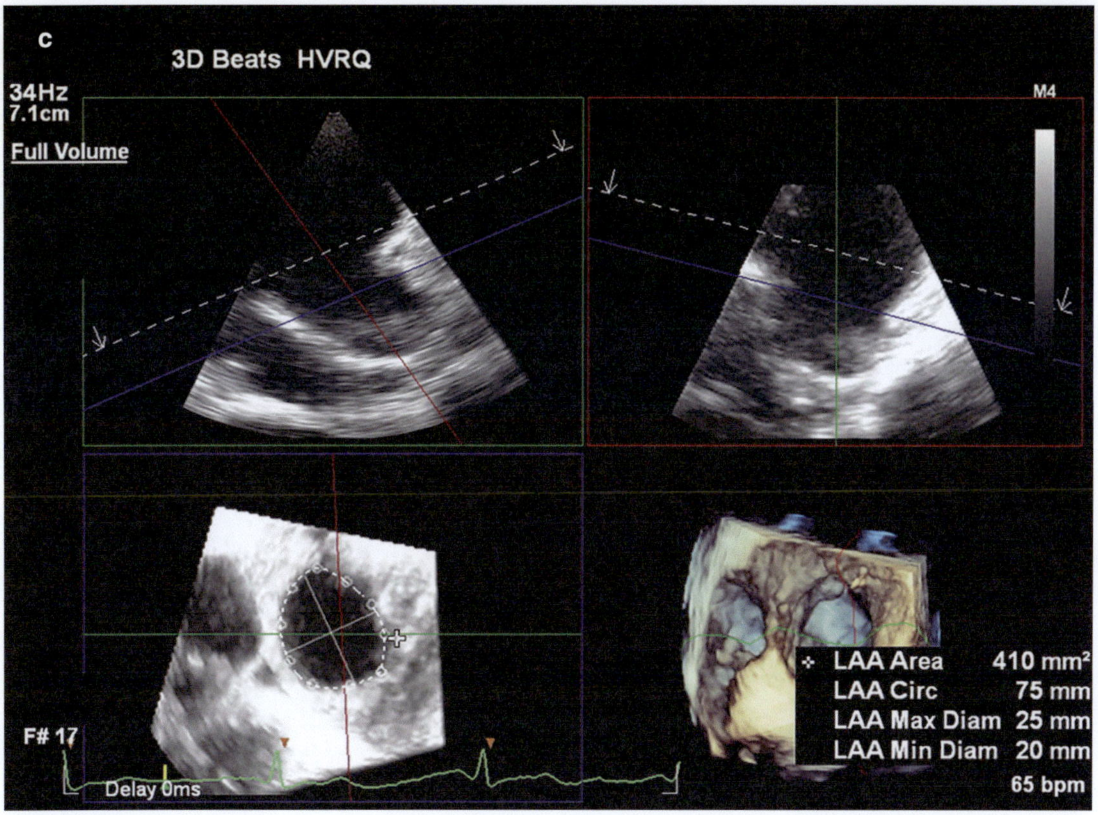

Fig. 27.17 (continued)

mias) (d) the need for supplemental training for interventionalists, who need to manipulate both the delivery catheter or the "imaging" catheter in order to obtain "working" ICE images, and, (e), a dedicated machine and the cost of the disposable ICE catheter [53].

The site-specific transseptal puncture for LAA closure is in the inferior-posterior portion of the fossa ovalis (FO), which permits a coaxial engagement of the main body, minimizing the risk of perforation. Once LA access is obtained, a guide catheter is advanced to engage the LAA. The deployment of the device, a pull-push maneuver (which assures that the device is firmly anchored) and the withdrawal of the delivery system are usually 2D/3D TEE guided (Fig. 27.18).

As described in the paragraph on PFO/ASD closure, fusion technology, that merges 2D/3D TEE images within the fluoroscopic silhouette in a kind of Hybrid image, should facilitate the navigation of catheter and device deployment, hopefully reducing the time of x-ray exposure and overall facilitating the procedure (Fig. 27.19).

Procedural and Post-Procedural Complications

There are four potential major procedural or post-procedural complications: pericardial effusion/tamponade (PE/PT), peri-device leak (PDL), device embolization (DE) and device-related thrombosis (DRT).

Pericardial Effusion (PE)/Pericardial Tamponade (PT) This is a rare but serious complication following left atrial appendage closure. The rate of PE/PT related to both devices is similar ranging from 2.0 to 5.0% of cases [53, 54]. Intra or periprocedural PE/PT typically occurs as a result of perforation of the right atrium, left atrium, and LAA due to manipulation of the cardiac delivery system or closure device. Cases of more delayed PE/PT may be due to penetration of device strut or engagements of the hooks into the tissue of the LAA which, as mentioned above, is particularly thin and friable between pectinate muscles. This mechanism may lead to micro-points bleeding. Although sinus rhythm was not identified as an indepen-

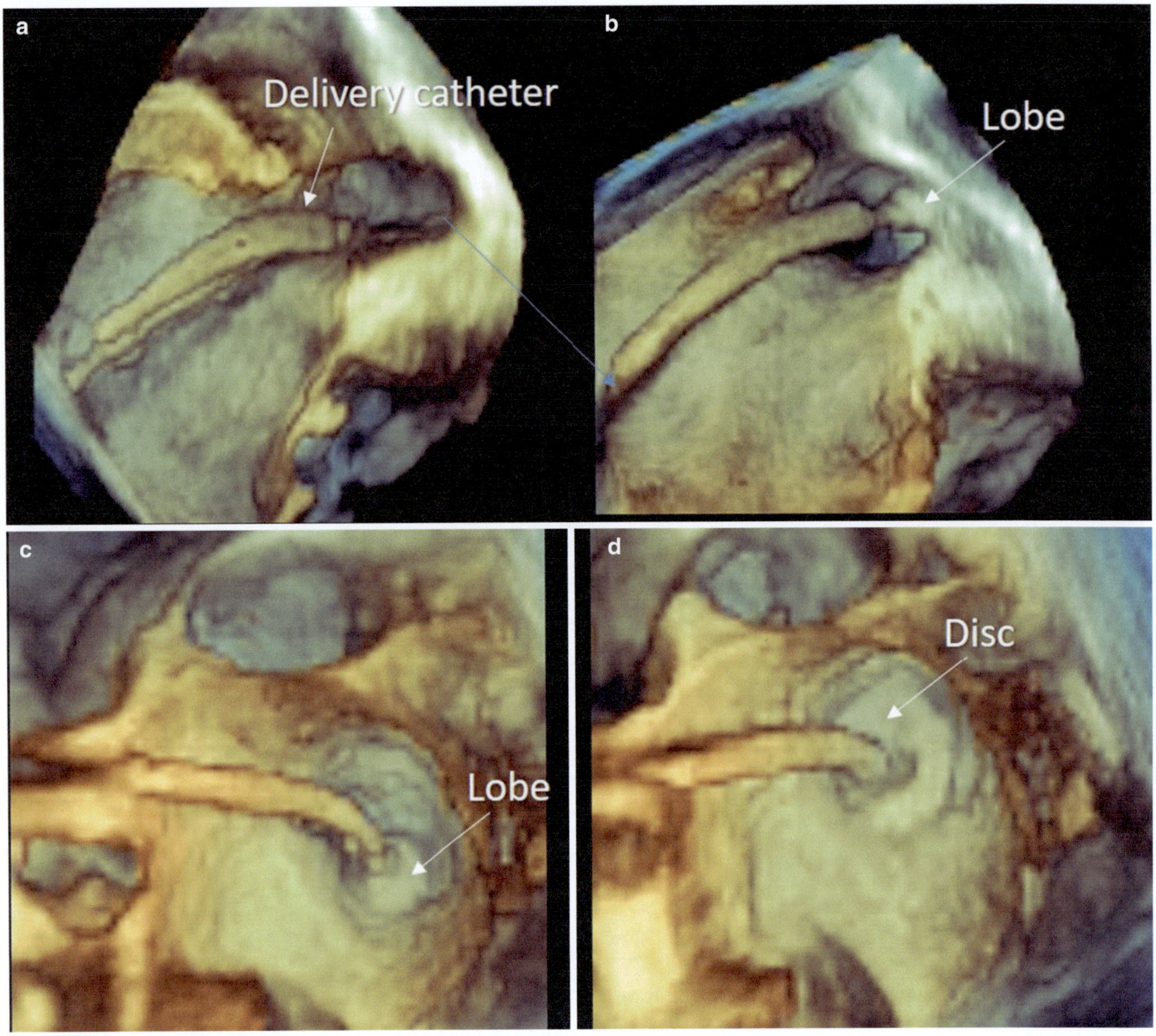

Fig. 27.18 Step-by-step 3D TEE images showing the deployment of the Amplatzer Amulet device

dent predictor of PE/PT, it may be speculated that the vigorous LAA contraction occurring in sinus rhythm may exert mechanical force on the device, exacerbating the bleeding.

Peri-Device Leak In complex LAA anatomies, a mismatch between device size and LAA ostium is not rare, and may cause incomplete LAA occlusion with residual *peri-device leak* (PDL) [55]. PDL may be confirmed and sized by measuring the vena contracta on 2D TEE color Doppler. More recently, CT has been found to be particularly effective in detecting and quantifying PDL. Saw et al. reported a case series of 45 patients treated with both ACP and Watchman, whose LAA post-procedure residual PDL rates were assessed by CT and/or TEE. This study observed higher sensitivity for CT as compared to TEE in the identification of residual LAA PDL [56]. TEE, using standard criteria, identified only half of the patients in whom LAA PDL was documented by CT. By measuring Hounsfield units (HU) in the LAA distal to the device and comparing the contrast density with sur-

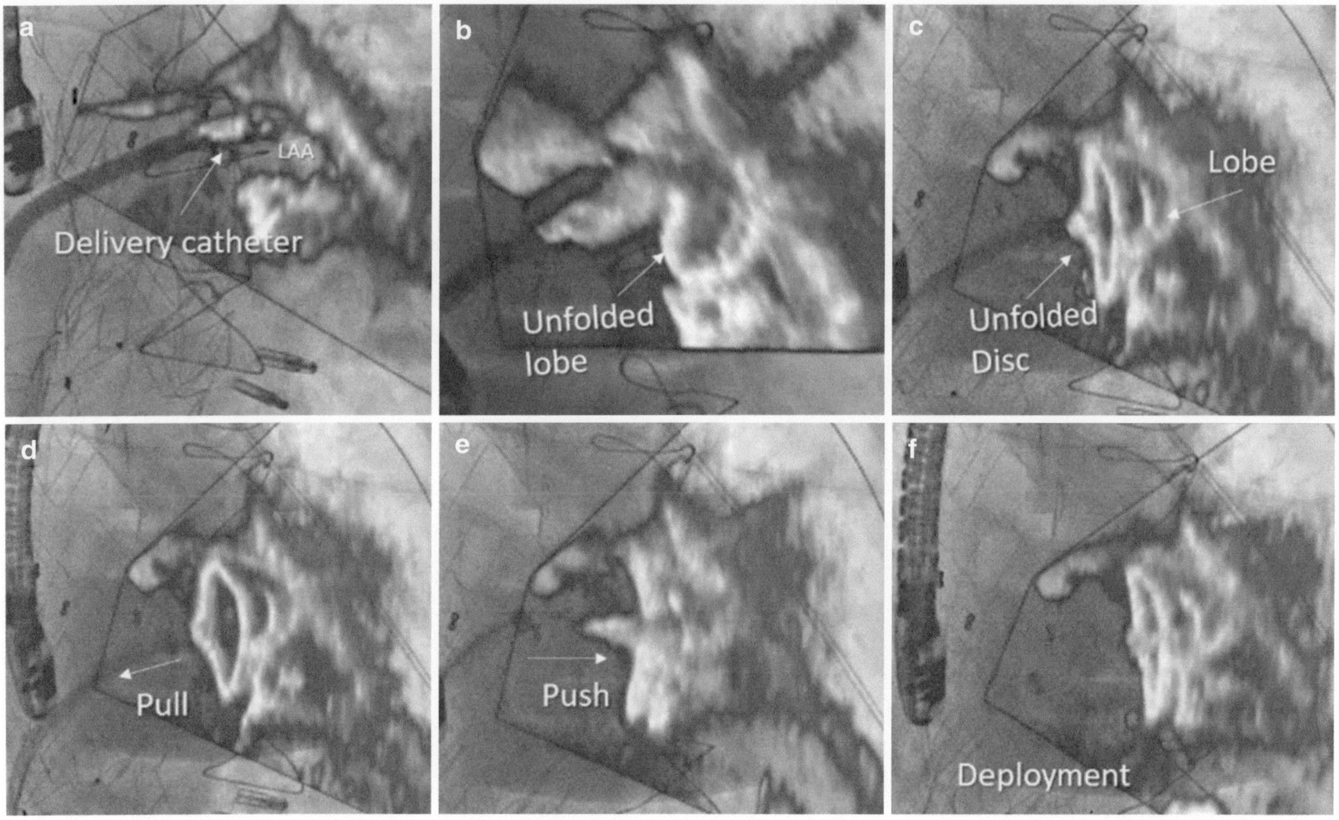

Fig. 27.19 Step-by-step "fused images" showing the deployment of the Amplatzer Amulet device. LAA, left atrial appendage

rounding cardiac chambers, a value <100 HU has been reported to suggest an occluded LAA on CT [57].

The prognostic significance of PDL remains a controversial issue, however. Criteria to classify the size of the residual leak vary according to the device used (<3 mm for the Watchman occluder and <5 mm for Amplatzer occluder) but they are still arbitrary. Indeed, the clinical significance of these cut-offs is poorly supported by evidence. Most of the published studies did not detect any association between the above-mentioned cut-offs and clinical events. Notably, study protocols have mandated the continuation or re-institution of OAC therapy in all cases where a PDL > 5 mm was observed at TEE, either at the end of the procedure or during follow-up. Therefore, it remains highly probable that the risk associated with the presence of a leak has been mitigated by concomitant OAC therapy. Furthermore, there is some evidence that PDL may be dynamic in nature, which can also, at least partially, explain why the assessment of leaks early after the procedure may not be entirely predictive of long-term success. Thus, the reasoning that complete sealing after percutaneous occlusion of the LAA is better than any degree of leak still remains only intuitive with lack of evidence. Consequently, closure of PDL with another device appears not to be justified, even if technically feasible.

Device Embolization Device embolization is rare ranging between 0.6 and 0.7% of cases, yet it may become a life-threatening complication [58]. Causes for device migration include incorrect sizing, suboptimal placement, and vigorous pull-push testing. Embolization occurs mainly in the periprocedural period but late embolization has been described. The location of the embolized device is a major determinant of recovery. Embolization into the aorta or the left atrium can be successfully managed by percutaneous techniques in most cases without surgical intervention [59]. Device embolization into the LV has a high risk of entrapment in the sub-valvular mitral apparatus and often requires surgical retrieval, increasing the procedure-related morbidity (Fig. 27.20).

Device Related Thrombosis (DRT) Incidence of DRT has been reported to be 3–7% with an average threefold increased

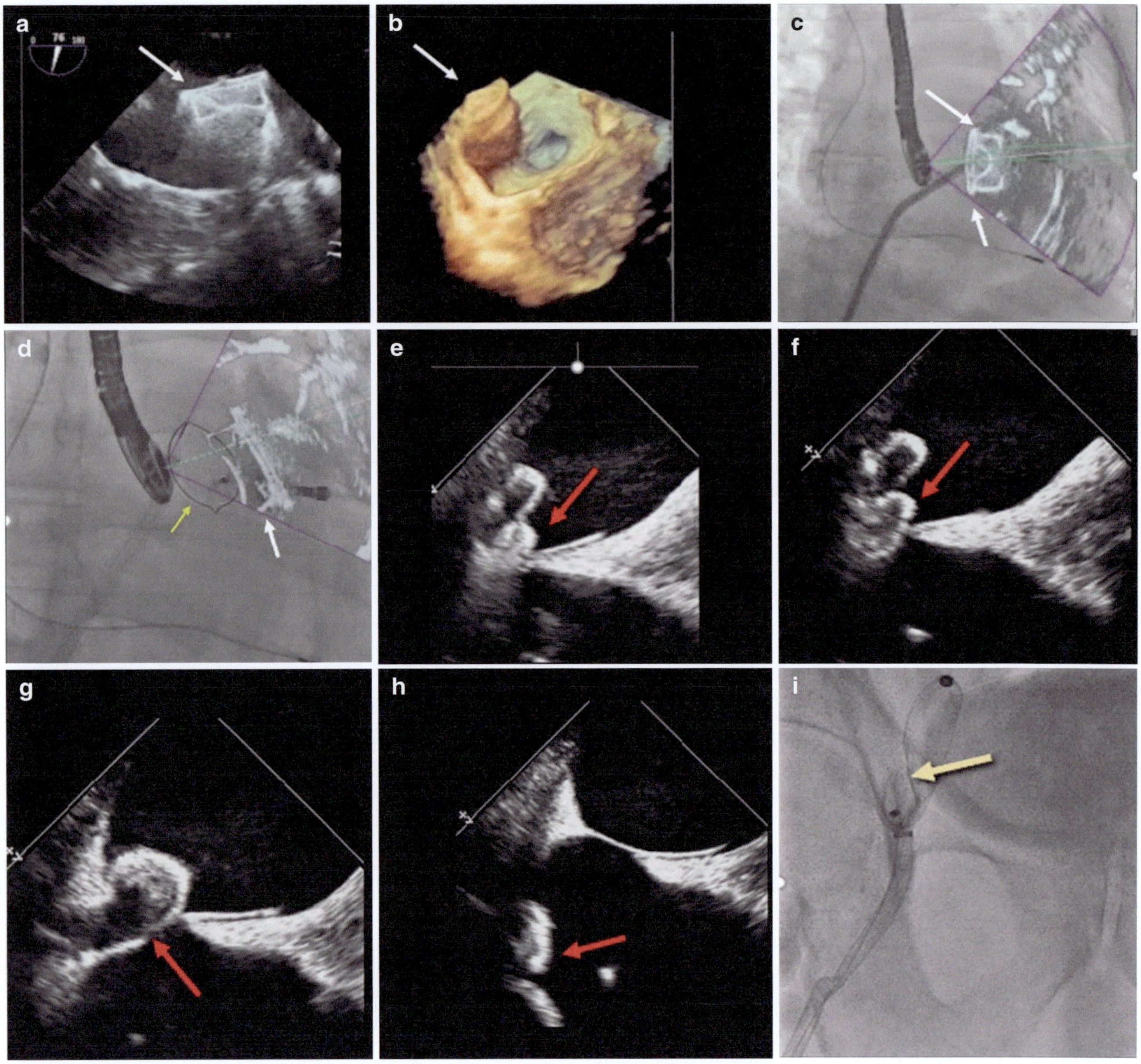

Fig. 27.20 (**a–c**) "Free" floating LAA occlusion device that embolized into the left atrium seen with 2D TEE, 3D TEE and fused imaging respectively (arrows). (**d**) Retrieval of the device (white arrow) with the snare endovascular catheter (yellow arrow). (**e–g**) Sequential still images of the passage of the LAA occlusion device (red arrow) through the atrial septum. (**i**) The LAA device in the iliac vein (yellow arrow) for retrival

risk of stroke or systemic embolism [60, 61]. The risk of DRT is higher among those patients with larger left atrial appendages, a history of stroke or transient ischemic attack, permanent AF, lower ejection fraction and vascular disease. Some cases may be also related to procedural characteristics such as deep implantation, that may leave an uncovered area of the LAA. In such a case, periodic transesophageal echocardiography should be considered, and effective anticoagulation should promptly be resumed until the thrombus disappears. Aggressive TEE surveillance and oral anticoagulant/antiplatelet strategies have not been shown to be associated with any proven clinical benefits, however. Therefore, implementation of dedicated strategies in these patients remains speculative and should be individualized (Fig. 27.21).

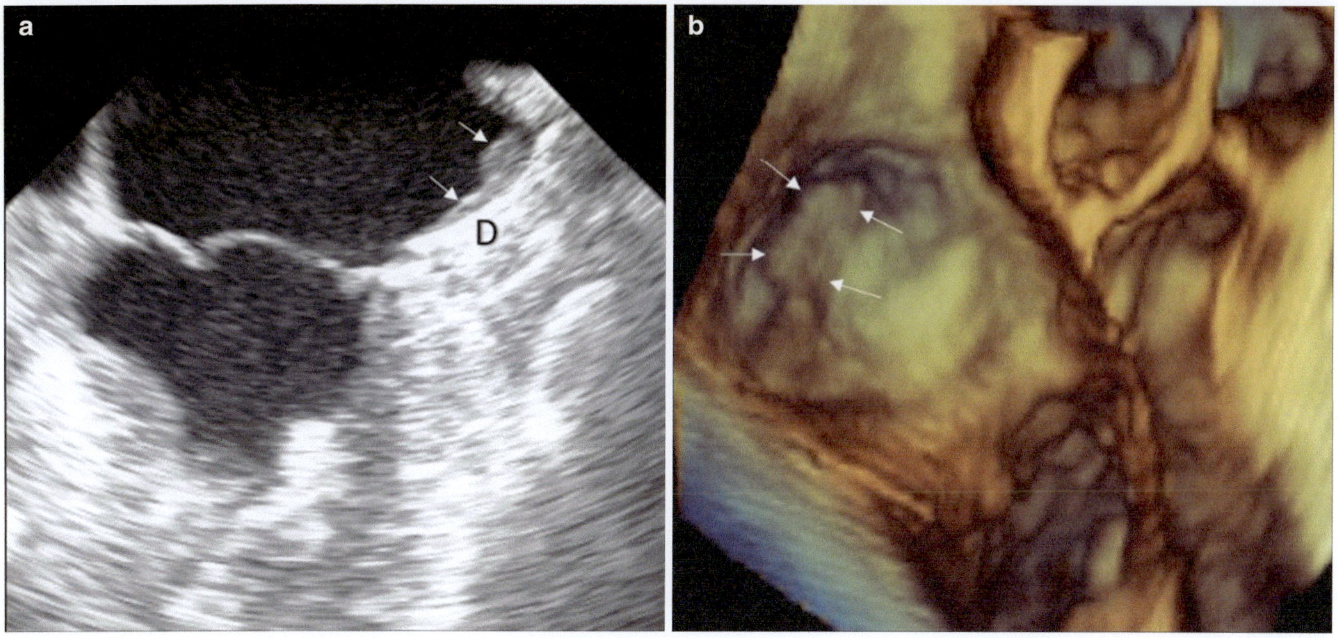

Fig. 27.21 Device (D) -related thrombus in 2D (**a**) and 3D (**b**) TEE (arrows)

References

1. Hagen PT, Scholz DG, Edwards WD. Incidence and size of patent foramen ovale during the first 10 decades of life: an autopsy study of 965 normal hearts. Mayo Clin Proc. 1984;59(1):17.
2. Lechat P, Mas JL, Lascault G, Loron P, Theard M, Klimczac M, Drobinski G, Thomas D, Grosgogeat Y. Prevalence of patent foramen ovale in patients with stroke. N Engl J Med. 1988 May 5;318(18):1148–52.
3. Furlan AJ, Reisman M, Massaro J, Mauri L, Adams H, Albers GW, et al. Closure or medical therapy for cryptogenic stroke with patent foramen Ovale. N Engl J Med. 2012;366:991–9.
4. Meier B, Kalesan B, Mattle HP, Khattab AA, Hildick-smith D, Dudek D, et al. Percutaneous closure of patent foramen Ovale in cryptogenic embolism. N Engl J Med. 2013;368:1083–91.
5. Saver JL, Carroll JD, Thaler DE, Smalling RW, MacDonald LA, et al. Long-term outcomes of patent foramen Ovale closure or medical therapy after stroke. N Engl J Med. 2017;377:1022–32.
6. Søndergaard L, Kasner SE, Rhodes JF, Andersen G, Helle K, et al. Patent foramen Ovale closure or antiplatelet therapy for cryptogenic stroke. N Engl J Med. 2017;377:1033–42.
7. Lee PH, Song JK, Kim JS, Heo R, Lee S, Kim DH, et al. Cryptogenic stroke and high-risk patent foramen ovale: the DEFENSE-PFO trial. J Am Coll Cardiol. 2018;71(20):2335–42.
8. Nellessen U, Daniel WG, Matheis G. Impending paradoxical embolism from atrial thrombus: correct diagnosis by transesophageal echocardiography and prevention by surgery. J Am Coll Cardiol. 1985;5(4):1002–4.
9. Myers PO, Bounameaux H, Panos A, Lerch R, Kalangos A. Impending paradoxical embolism: systematic review of prognostic factors and treatment. Chest. 2010;137(1):164–70.
10. Pezzini A, Del Zotto E, Magoni M, Costa A, Archetti S, Grassi M, Akkawi NM, Albertini A, Assanelli D, Vignolo LA, Padovani A. Inherited thrombophilic disorders in young adults with ischemic stroke and patent foramen ovale. Stroke. 2003;34:28–33.
11. Cramer SC, Rordorf G, Kaufman JA, Buonanno F, Koroshetz WJ, Schwamm L. Clinically occult pelvic-vein thrombosis in cryptogenic stroke. Lancet. 1998;351:1927–8.
12. Nakayama R, Takaya Y, Akagi T, Watanabe N, Ikeda M, Nakagawa K, et al. Identification of high-risk patent foramen Ovale associated with cryptogenic stroke: development of a scoring system. J Am Soc Echocardiogr. 2019 Jul;32(7):811–6.
13. Clarke NRA, Timperley J, Kelion AD, et al. Transthoracic echocardiography using second harmonic imaging with Valsalva manoueuvre for the detection of right to left shunts. Eur J Echocardiogr. 2004;5:176–81.
14. Pinto FJ. When and how to diagnose patent foramen ovale. Heart. 2005 Apr;91(4):438–40.
15. Nozari A, Dilekoz E, Sukhotinsky I, Stein T, Eikermann-Haerter K, Liu C, et al. Microemboli may link spreading depression, migraine aura, and patent foramen ovale. Ann Neurol. 2010;67:221–9.
16. Tobis JM, Charles A, Silberstein SD, Sorensen S, Maini B, Horwitz PA, et al. Percutaneous closure of patent foramen Ovale in patients with migraine: the PREMIUM trial. J Am Coll Cardiol. 2017 Dec 5;70(22):2766–277.
17. Sykes O, Clark EJ. Patent foramen ovale and scuba diving: a practical guide for physicians on when to refer for screening. Extrem Physiol Med. 2013;2:10.
18. Krishnan SC, Salazar M. Septal pouch in the left atrium: a new anatomical entity with potential for embolic complications. ACC Cardiovasc Interv. 2010;3:98–104.
19. Strachinaru M, Morissens M, Latifyan S, et al. Left atrial septal pouch thrombus assessed on three-dimensional transoesophageal echocardiography. Eur Hear J Cardiovasc Imaging. 2012;13:967.
20. Gurudevan SV, Shah H, Tolstrup K, et al. Septal thrombus in the left atrium: is the left atrial septal pouch the culprit? JACC Cardiovasc Imaging. 2010;3:1284–6.
21. Strachinaru M, Castro-Rodriguez J, Verbeet T, et al. The left atrial septal pouch as a risk factor for stroke: a systematic review. Arch Cardiovasc Dis. 2017;110:250–8.

22. Hołda MK, Koziej M, Wszołek K, et al. Left atrial accessory appendages, diverticula, and left-sided septal pouch in multi-slice computed tomography. Association with atrial fibrillation and cerebrovascular accidents. Int J Cardiol. 2017;244:163–8.
23. Luermans JGLM, Post MC, Plokker HWM, ten Berg JM, Suttorp MJ. Complications and mid-term outcome after percutaneous patent foramen ovale closure in patients with cryptogenic stroke. Neth Heart J. 2008 Oct;16(10):332–6.
24. Taggart NW, Reeder GS, Lennon RJ, Slusser JP, Freund MA, Cabalka AK, et al. Long-term follow-up after PFO device closure: outcomes and complications in a single-center experience. Catheter Cardiovasc Interv. 2017;89:124.
25. Van der Linde D, Konings EEM, Slager MA, et al. Birth prevalence of congenital heart disease worldwide: a systematic review and meta-analysis. J Am Coll Cardiol. 2011;58:2241–7.
26. Faletra FF, Leo LA, Paiocchi VL, Schlossbauer SA, Pedrazzini G, Moccetti T, Ho SY. Revisiting anatomy of the interatrial septum and its adjoining atrioventricular junction using noninvasive imaging techniques. J Am Soc Echocardiogr. 2019 May;32(5):580–92.
27. Garg G, Tyagi H, Radha AS. Transcatheter closure of sinus venosus atrial septal defect with anomalous drainage of right upper pulmonary vein into superior vena cava--an innovative technique. Catheter Cardiovasc Interv. 2014;84:473–7.
28. King TD, Mills ND. Nonoperative closure of atrial septal defects. Surgery. 1974;75:383–8.
29. Hellenbrand WE, Fahey JT, McGowan FX, Weltin GG, Kleinman CS. Transesophageal echocardiographic guidance of transcatheter closure of atrial septal defect. Am J Cardiol. 1990 Jul 15;66(2):207–13.
30. Perk G, Lang RM, Garcia-Fernandez MA, Lodato J, Sugeng L, Lopez J, et al. Use of real time three-dimensional transesophageal echocardiography in intracardiac catheter based interventions. J Am Soc Echocardiogr. 2009;22:865–82.
31. Mullen MJ, Dias BF, Walker F, et al. Intracardiac echocardiography guided device closure of atrial septal defects. J Am Coll Cardiol. 2003;41:285–92.
32. Moore J, Hegde S, El-Said H, Beekman R 3rd, Benson L, Bergersen L, Holzer R, Jenkins K, Ringel R, Rome J, Vincent R. Martin G; ACC IMPACT steering committee. Transcatheter device closure of atrial septal defects: a safety review.
33. Levi DS, Moore JW. Embolization and retrieval of the Amplatzer septal occluder. Catheter Cardiovasc Interv. 2004;61:543–7.
34. DiBardino DJ, McElhinney DB, Kaza AK, Mayer JE Jr. Analysis of the U.S. Food and Drug Administration Manufacturer and user facility device experience database for adverse events involving Amplatzer septal occluder devices and comparison with the society of thoracic surgery congenital cardiac surgery database. J Thorac Cardiovasc Surg. 2009;137:1334–41.
35. Johnson JN, Marquardt ML, Ackerman MJ, et al. Electrocardiographic changes and arrhythmias following percutaneous atrial septal defect and patent foramen ovale device closure. Catheter Cardiovasc Interv. 2011;78:254–61.
36. Zaker-Shahrak R, Fuhrer J, Meier B. Transseptal puncture for catheter ablation of atrial fibrillation after device closure of patent foramen ovale. Catheter Cardiovasc Interv. 2008;71:551–2.
37. Krumsdorf U, Ostermayer S, Billinger K, et al. Incidence and clinical course of thrombus formation on atrial septal defect and patient foramen ovale closure devices in 1,000 consecutive patients. J Am Coll Cardiol. 2004;43:302–9.
38. DiBardino DJ, McElhinney DB, Kaza AK, Mayer JE. Analysis of the US Food and Drug Administration manufacturer and user facility device experience database for adverse events involving Amplatzer septal Occluder devices and comparison with the Society of Thoracic Surgery Congenital Cardiac Surgery Databas. J Thorac Cardiovasc Surg. 2009;137:1334–41.
39. McElhinney DB, Quartermain MD, Kenny D, Alboliras E, Amin Z. Relative risk factors for cardiac erosion following transcatheter closure of atrial septal defects a case-control study. Circulation. 2016;133:1738–46.
40. Crawford G, Brindis RG, Krucoff MW, Mansalis BP, Carroll JD. Percutaneous atrial septal occluder devices and cardiac erosion: a review of the literature. Catheter Catheter Cardiovasc Interv. 2012 Aug 1;80(2):157–67.
41. Pritchett EL. Management of atrial fibrillation. N Engl J Med. 1992;326(19):1264.
42. Blackshear JL, Odell JA. Appendage obliteration to reduce stroke in cardiac surgical patients with atrial fibrillation. Ann Thorac Surg. 1996;61:755–9.
43. Hart RG, Pearce LA, Aguilar MI. Meta-analysis: antithrombotic therapy to prevent stroke in patients who have nonvalvular atrial fibrillation. Ann Intern Med. 2007;146:857–67.
44. Ruff CT, Giugliano RP, Braunwald E, et al. Comparison of the efficacy and safety of new oral anticoagulants with warfarin in patients with atrial fibrillation: a meta-analysis of randomised trials. Lancet. 2014;383:955–62.
45. Holmes DR, Reddy VY, Turi ZG, et al. Percutaneous closure of the left atrial appendage versus warfarin therapy for prevention of stroke in patients with atrial fibrillation: a randomized non-inferiority trial. Lancet. 2009;374(9689):534–42. PROTECT AF Investigators
46. Hanke T. Surgical management of the left atrial appendage: a must or a myth? Eur J Cardiothorac Surg. 2018;53(Suppl_1):i33–8.
47. Naksuk N, Padmanabhan D, Yogeswaran V, Asirvatham SJ. Left atrial appendage: embryology, anatomy, physiology, arrhythmia and therapeutic intervention. JACC Clin Electrophysiol. 2016 Aug;2(4):403–12.
48. Di Biase L, Santangeli P, Anselmino M, et al. Does the left atrial appendage morphology correlate with the risk of stroke in patients with atrial fibrillation? Results from a multicenter study. J Am Coll Cardiol. 2012;60(6):531–8.
49. Cabrera JA, Ho SY, Climent V, Sanchez-Quintana D. The architecture of the left lateral atrial wall: a particular anatomic region with implications for ablation of atrial fibrillation. Eur Heart J. 2008;29:356–62.
50. Kamanu S, Tan AY, Peter CT, Hwang C, Chen PS. Vein of Marshall activity during sustained atrial fibrillation. J Cardiovasc Electrophysiol. 2006;17:839–46.
51. Nucifora G, Faletra FF, Regoli F, Pasotti E, Pedrazzini G, Moccetti T, Auricchio A. Evaluation of the left atrial appendage with real-time 3-dimensional transoesophageal echocardiography: implications for catheter-based left atrial appendage closure. Circ Cardiovasc Imaging. 2011;4:514–23.
52. Cruz-Gonzalez I, Perez-Rivera A, Lopez-Jimenez R, et al. Significance of the learning curve in left atrial appendage occlusion with two different devices. Catheter Cardiovasc Interv. 2013;83:642–6.
53. Boersma LV, Schmidt B, Betts TR, Sievert H, Tamburino C, Teiger E, Pokushalov E, Kische S, Schmitz T, Stein KM, Bergmann MW. Implant success and safety of left atrial appendage closure with the WATCHMAN device: peri-procedural outcomes from the EWOLUTION registry. Eur Heart J. 2016;37:2465–74.
54. Tzikas A, Shakir S, Gafoor S. Left atrial appendage occlusion for stroke prevention in atrial fibrillation: multicentre experience with the AMPLATZER cardiac plug. EuroIntervention. 2016;11:1170–9.
55. Viles-Gonzalez JF, Kar S, Douglas P, et al. The clinical impact of incomplete left atrial appendage closure with the watchman device in patients with atrial fibrillation: a PROTECT AF (percutaneous closure of the left atrial appendage versus warfarin therapy for prevention of stroke in patients with atrial fibrillation) substudy. J Am Coll Cardiol. 2012;59(10):923–9.

56. Saw J, Fahmy P, DeJong P, et al. Cardiac CT angiography for device surveillance after endovascular left atrial appendage closure. Eur Heart J Cardiovasc Imaging. 2015;16(11):1198–206.
57. Angelillis M, Gargiulo G, Moschovitis A, et al. Computed tomography detection and quantification of left atrial appendage residual patency as collateral finding after percutaneous closure. Int J Cardiol. 2018;260:42–6.
58. Bajaj NS, Parashar A, Agarwal S, Sodhi N, Poddar KL, Garg A, Tuzcu EM, Kapadia SR. Percutaneous left atrial appendage occlusion for stroke prophylaxis in nonvalvular atrial fibrillation: A systematic review and analysis of observational studies. JACC Cardiovasc Interv. 2014;7(3):296–304.
59. Chan NY, Choy CC, Lau CL. Successful percutaneous retrieval of a dislodged left atrial appendage occlusion device with double transseptal sheaths and biopsy bioptome. Catheter Cardiovasc Interv. 2015;85:328–31.
60. Ren JF, Marchlinsky FE, Supple GE, Hutchinson MD, Garcia FC, Riley MP, Lin D, Zado ES, Callans DJ, Ferrari VA. Intracardiac echocardiographic diagnosis of thrombus formation in the left atrial appendage: a complementary role to transesophageal echocardiography. Echocardiography. 2013;30:72–80.
61. Dukkipati SR, Kar S, Holmes DR Jr, et al. Device-related thrombus after left atrial appendage closure: incidence, predictors, and outcomes. Circulation. 2018;138:874.

Ventricular Interventions

28

Joseph F. Maalouf, Krishnaswamy Chandrasekaran, and Francesco F. Faletra

Ventricular Septal Defects

The main indications for ventricular septal defect (VSD) closure are (1) a hemodynamically significant shunt (QP: QS > 1.5:1), (2) left ventricular (LV) volume overload, and (3) history of bacterial endocarditis. Surgical closure, remains the mainstay of treatment for most VSDs, but carries some risks such as, valve injury, bypass related myocardial injury, complications related to damage of the atrioventricular (AV) node or His bundle with complete AV block, and postoperative infections. Moreover, some defects cannot be adequately closed without a ventricular incision. In selected patients with suitable morphology, percutaneous catheter-based closure has emerged as an acceptable alternative to surgery for congenital (typically musclar or perimembranous), and traumatic or post infarction ventricular septal defects [1]. Indeed, when compared to surgery, transcatheter closure when feasible has (a) comparable success rate with lower risk of complications and infections, (b) avoids sternotomy and cardiopulmonary bypass, (c) is associated with less pain, and shorter hospital stay [1].

Supplementary Information The online version of this chapter (https://doi.org/10.1007/978-3-030-72941-7_28) contains supplementary material, which is available to authorized users.

J. F. Maalouf (✉)
Professor of Medicine, Mayo Clinic College of Medicine; Director, Interventional Echocardiography; Consultant, Department of Cardiovascular Medicine, Mayo Clinic, Rochester, MN, USA
e-mail: maalouf.joseph@mayo.edu

K. Chandrasekaran
Professor of Medicine, Mayo Clinic College of Medicine; Consultant, Department of Cardiovascular Medicine, Mayo Clinic, Rochester, MN, USA
e-mail: KChandra@mayo.edu

F. F. Faletra
Director of Cardiac Imaging Lab, Cardiocentro Ticino Institute, Lugano, Switzerland
e-mail: Francesco.Faletra@cardiocentro.org

Accurate assessment of defect size, location, and resultant ventricular changes therefore, is critical to the management of ventricular septal defects (VSD) including surgical versus percutaneous closure. A major limitation of 2D TEE is assessment of VSD size and morphology which is often irregular and that can assist in selection of the appropriate transcatheter occlusion device [3]. With 3D TEE, enface views of the entire VSD and surrounding structures from a single acoustic window is feasible [2] (Figs. 28.1, 28.2 and 28.3). Moreover, the VSD and its rims, critical for percutaneous closure considerations, can be viewed from both the left and right ventricular perspectives (Figs. 28.1, 28.2, and 28.6). Live 3D zoom mode with a biplane preview screen is useful to adjust sectors to include precisely the region of interest, and 3D volumetric data can be rotated and cropped until the VSD is in a proper en-face view (Fig. 28.1), and then the defect area (or long and short dimensions) can be manually traced in the 2D space using multiplanar reconstruction. In addition, live 3D color Doppler acquisition superimposes flow information on top of the 3D volumatric dataset which reveals the interventricular shunt flow direction and amount, though with a frame rate significantly lower than without color Doppler. Siemens' hemispheric 3D Color flow analysis package can be used for the measurement of flow volumes.

Assesment of adjacent vital structures can also provide invaluable information regarding feasiblity of VSD closure and potential complications. An important consideration for perimembraneous VSD is the minimal distance between the aortic valve leaflets and the defect so that the device does not compromise aortic valve function [4]. This measurement on 2DE is highly dependent on orientation of the tomographic slice and is facilitated on 3DE [4]. It is also important to show the relationship of the VSD to the tricuspid valve.

2D/3D TEE and fluoroscopy are the usual imaging techniques for guiding percutaneous VSD closure. Although early results showed that catheter-based closure was technically feasible, complications in the form of device embolization or residual shunt were not rare. The main reason was

J. F. Maalouf et al. (eds.), *Practical 3D Echocardiography*, https://doi.org/10.1007/978-3-030-72941-7_28

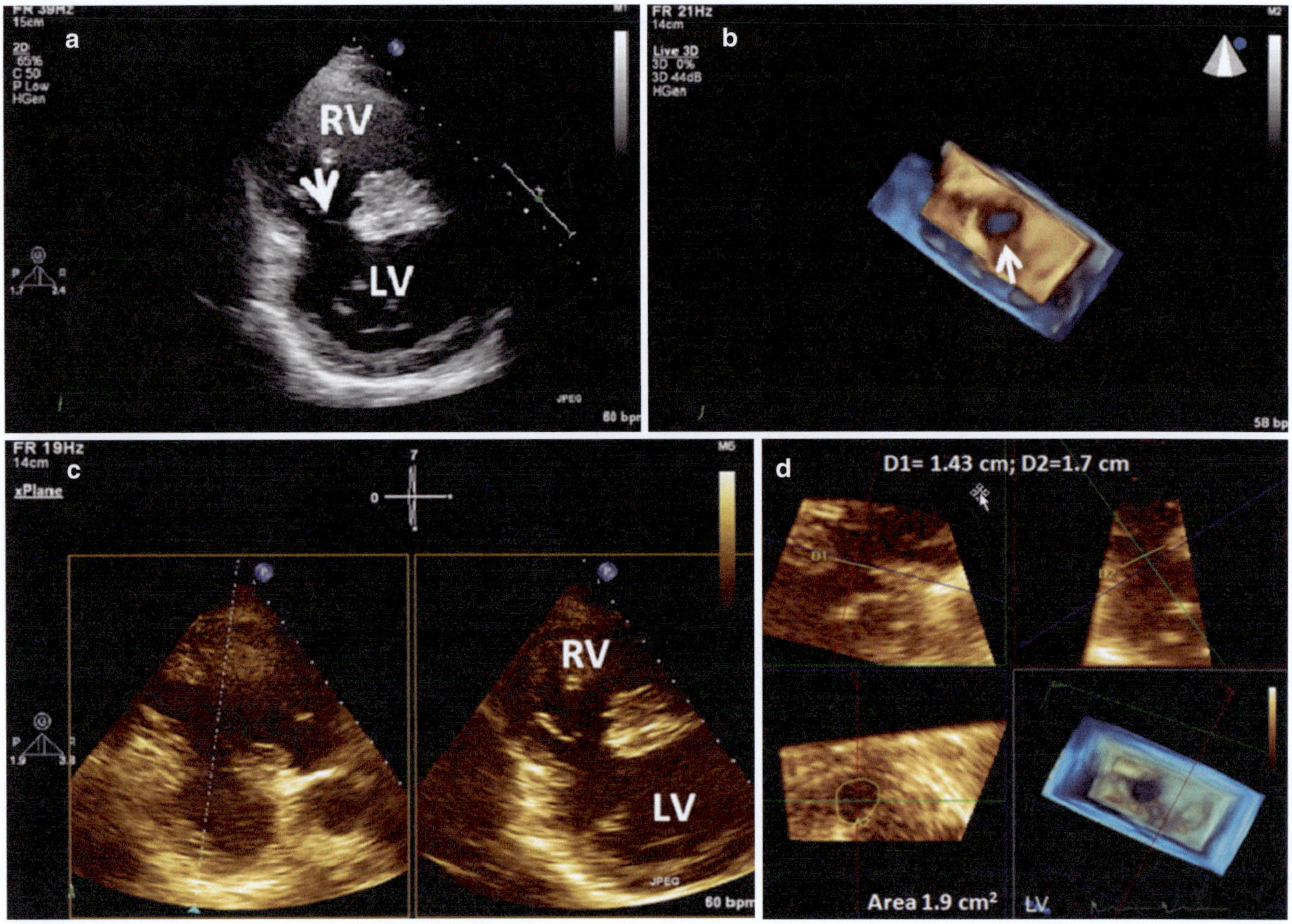

Fig. 28.1 A ventricular sepal defect (arrow) in 2D transthoracic short axis view (**a**), and in 3D rendered view from the right ventricle (RV) perspective (**b**). Biplane imaging (**c**) reveals two simultaneous orthogonal planes that are focused on the defect, (**d**) Measuring defect dimensions and tracing defect area using MPR. Used with permission of Mayo Foundation for Medical Education and Research. All rights reserved. LV, left ventricle; MPR, multiplanar reconstruction; RV, right ventricle

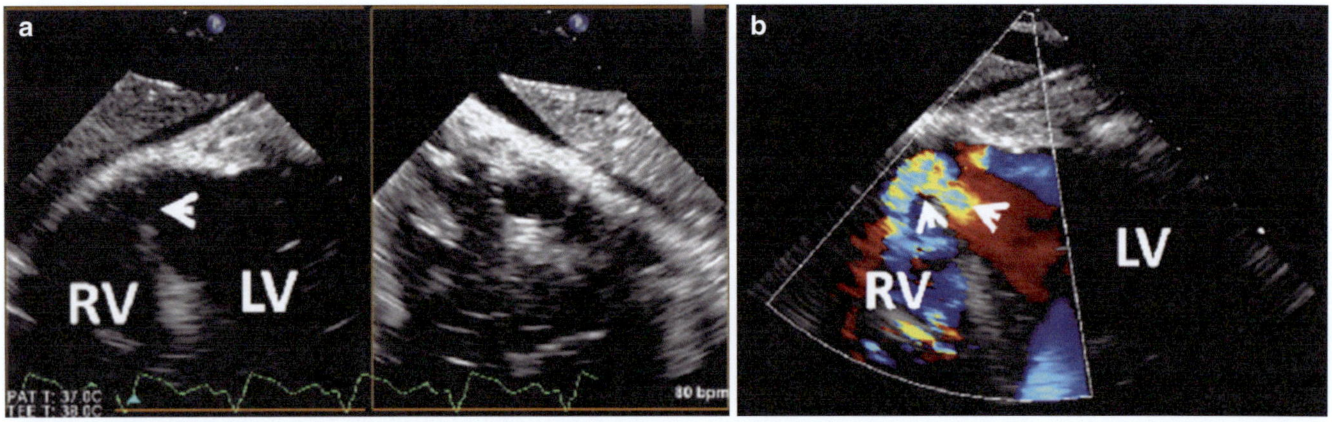

Fig. 28.2 3DE of post infarction VSD: (**a** and **b**): 2D TEE transgastric views showing an inferior septal defect (**a**, arrow) and left to right flow through the VSD on CFD (**b**, arrows). (**c** and **d**): 3D TTE views of same VSD from RV (**c**, arrows) and LV (**d**, arrows) perspectives. Yellow arrows point to parallel cropping of ventricular septum. Note that the shape and dimensions of the VSD are better appreciated on 3DE, and on line calipers can be used to measure the VSD dimensions. (**e**): Intraoperative 3D TEE view of the same VSD from RV perspective (white arrows). (**f** and **g**): Intravenous saline contrast injection shows opacification of the RV (**f**) followed by the LV (**g**, arrow). (**h**): Intraoperative image of the VSD from RV perspective (arrows). Used with permission of Mayo Foundation for Medical Education and Research. All rights reserved. CFD, color flow Doppler; LV, left ventricle; RV, right ventricle; VSD, ventricular septal defect

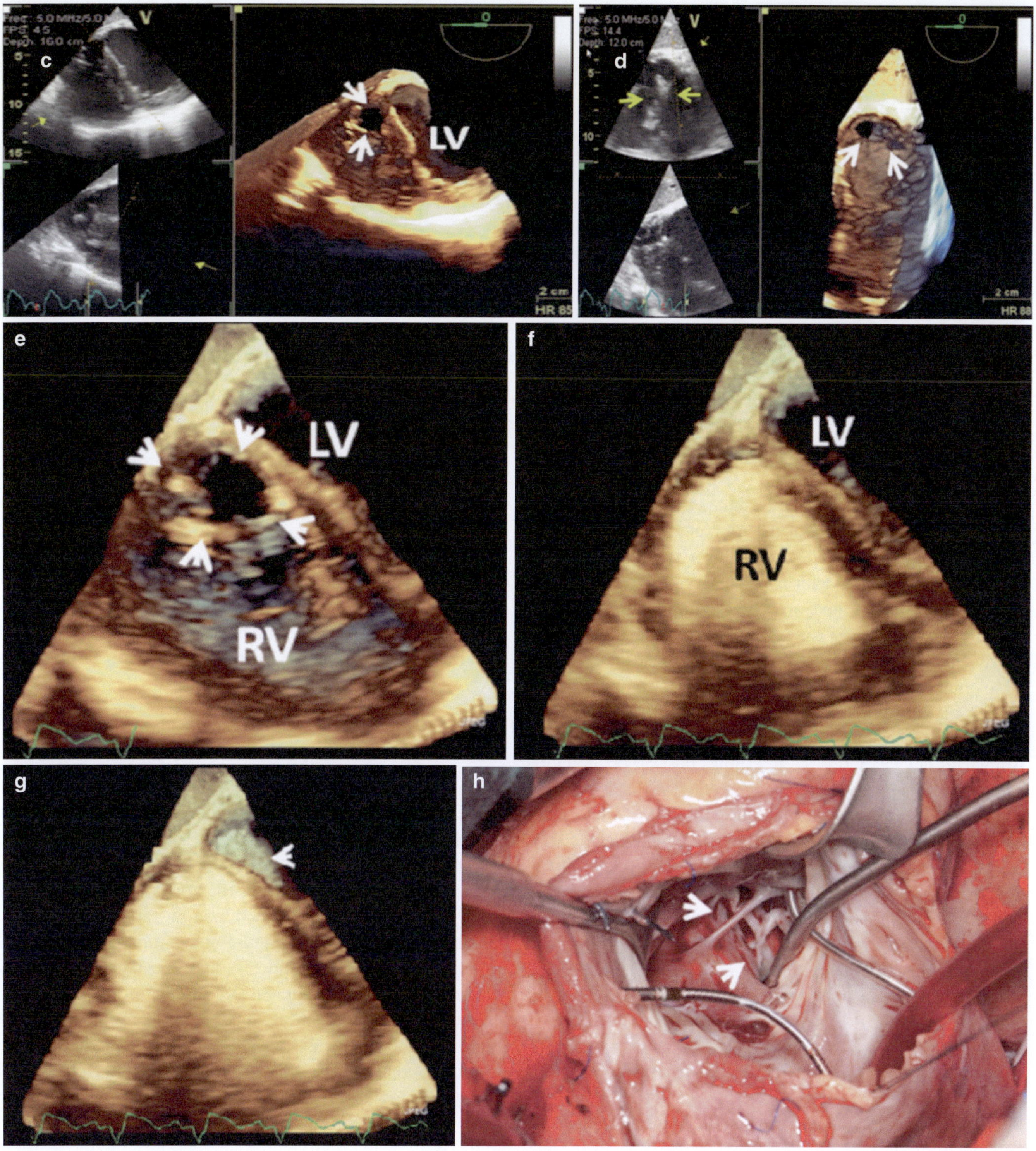

Fig. 28.2 (continued)

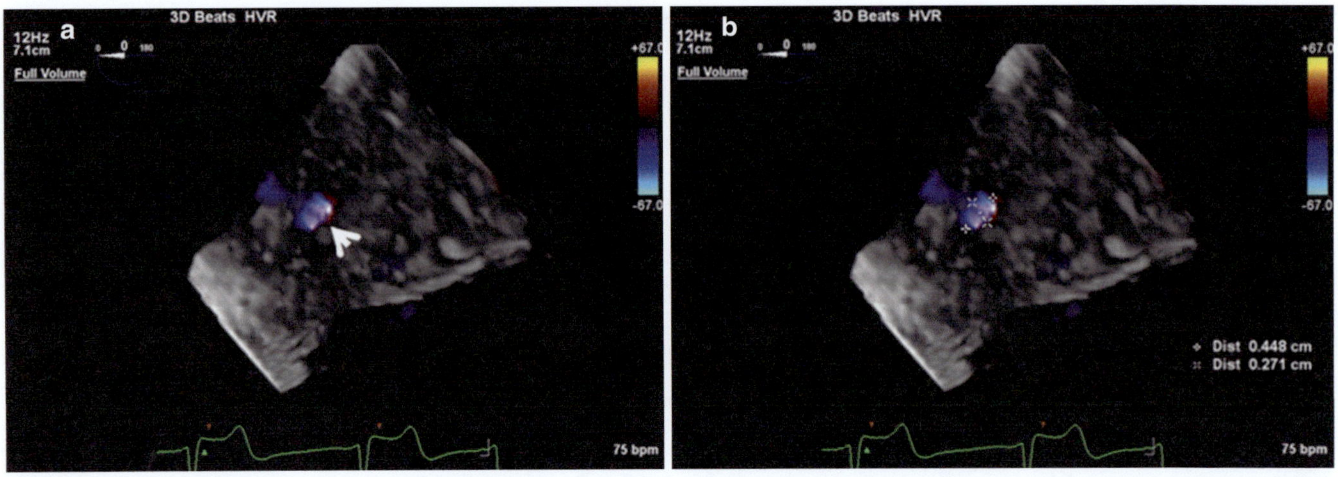

Fig. 28.3 (**a**): 3D TEE CFD of a congenital small muscular VSD (arrow). (**b**) VSD dimensions. Used with permission of Mayo Foundation for Medical Education and Research. All rights reserved. CFD, color flow Doppler; VSD, ventricular septal defect

absence of devices specifically designed for VSD closure . In fact, with the introduction of the Amplatzer device (St Jude Medical, Plymouth MN USA) which is made of nitinol wire, is self-expandable and with two flat discs linked through a central waist, results and outcome significantly improved. Current closure devices are designed to meet the wide variability in site, size and morphology of VSDs. Of note, for perimembranous VSD a device with asymmetric discs was specifically designed to minimize the incidence of heart block. Fig. 28.4 shows closure of a muscular VSD with an Amplatzer device, and Fig. 28.5 shows post-procedural closure of perimembranous VSD documented with CT scan.

Orientation of the occlusion device through the defect can be monitored on live 3D TEE (Fig. 28.6) thus obviating the need for frequent manupulations to obtain similar information using 2DTEE. It is important to show that the device once deployed does not interfere with surounding vital structures such as the aortic or tricuspid valves. Apposition of the left and right ventricular disc to the ventricular septum before device release can also be ascertained.

Intracardiac Fistulas and Pseudoaneurysms

Percutaneous transcatheter closure is now an option for patients with left ventricular (LV) psudoaneurysms and intracardiac fistulas particularly those at high surgical risk [5–7]. The latter includes fistulous communication between the left ventricle and left atrium, LV outflow tract and right atiurm (Gerbode type defect) and aorta to right atrium or right ventricle. 3D TEE allows appreciation of the spatial anatomy of pseudoaneurysms and/or intracardiac fistulas, and surrounding structures and is very useful in guiding and monitoring their closure [5–7] (Figs. 28.7, 28.8, 28.9, 28.10, 28.11, 28.12, and 28.13). Assessment of size and shape of the fistula entry and exit sites can be very useful to the interventional cardiologist. And, intraoperatively, pinpointing the origin of an intracardiac fistulous communication in complex cases may prove very difficult without use of 3D TEE (Fig. 28.13). There is typically a "garden hose" effect associated with fistula exit sites on color flow Doppler.

3D Echocardiography Guided Right Ventricular Biopsy

Right ventricular (RV) endomyocardial biopsy (EMB) is routinely used to rule out rejection in post cardiac transplant patients and to diagnose specific myocardial disorders such as myocarditis or amyloidosis, and the tissue sample is obtained from the ventricular septum. Transthoracic echocardiography (TTE) is increasingly used in conjunction with fluoroscopy to guide and position the bioptome on the ventricular septum, and to avoid perforation of the right ventricle by keeping the bioptome away from the right ventricular free wall and apex. Because of the added depth provided by 3DE (Fig. 28.14), the ventricular septum is better seen on 3DE compared with 2DE. 3D transthoracic echocardiography (TTE) therefore, has a role in guiding RV EMB particularly when the bioptome is not well seen on 2D TTE or if there are other intracavitary devices such as a pacemaker lead that may obscure visualization of the bioptome catheter on 2DE (Figs. 28.15, 28.16, and 28.17).

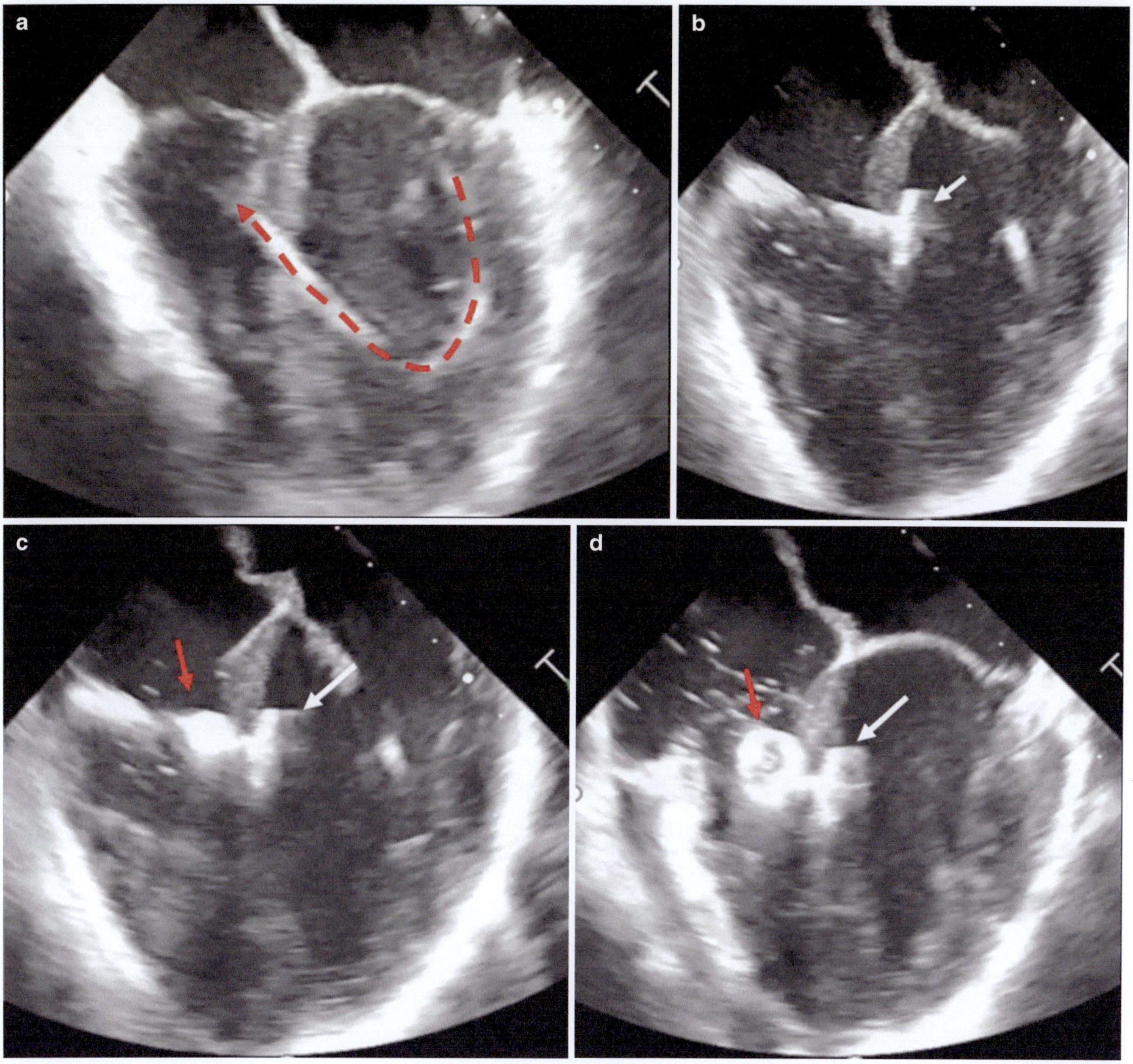

Fig. 28.4 2D TEE sequence of still frame images showing significant steps of percutaneous catheter-based muscular VSD closure with an Amplatzer device. (**a**) Image showing the catheter (red dotted line) crossing the defect. (**b**) opening the left disc (white arrow). (**c**, **d**) opening the right disc (red arrows), (**e**, **f**) the device does not restrict tricuspid leaflets opening (**e**) and closing (**f**)

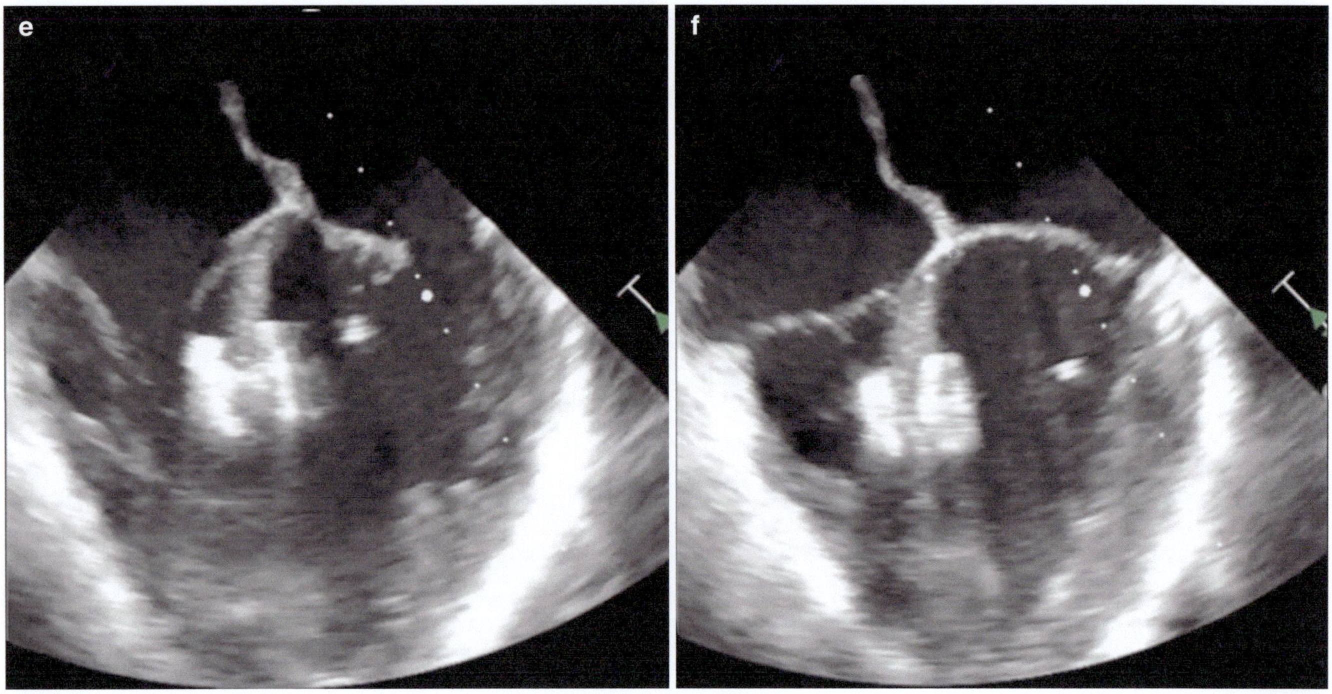

Fig. 28.4 (continued)

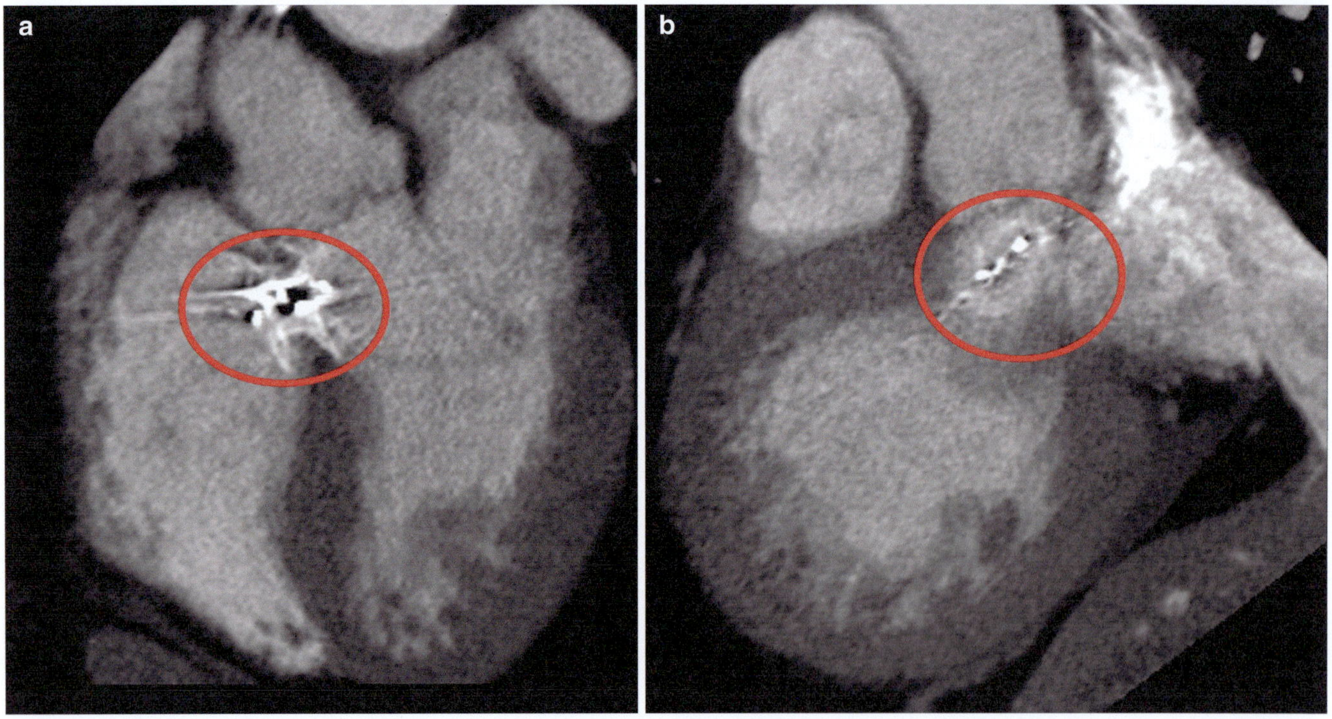

Fig. 28.5 CT scan of post-procedural percutaneous transcatheter closure of a perimebranous VSD with an asymmetric Amplatzer device. The device is seen in cross-section in panel **a** and in "en face"perspective in panel **b**. VSD, ventricular septal defect

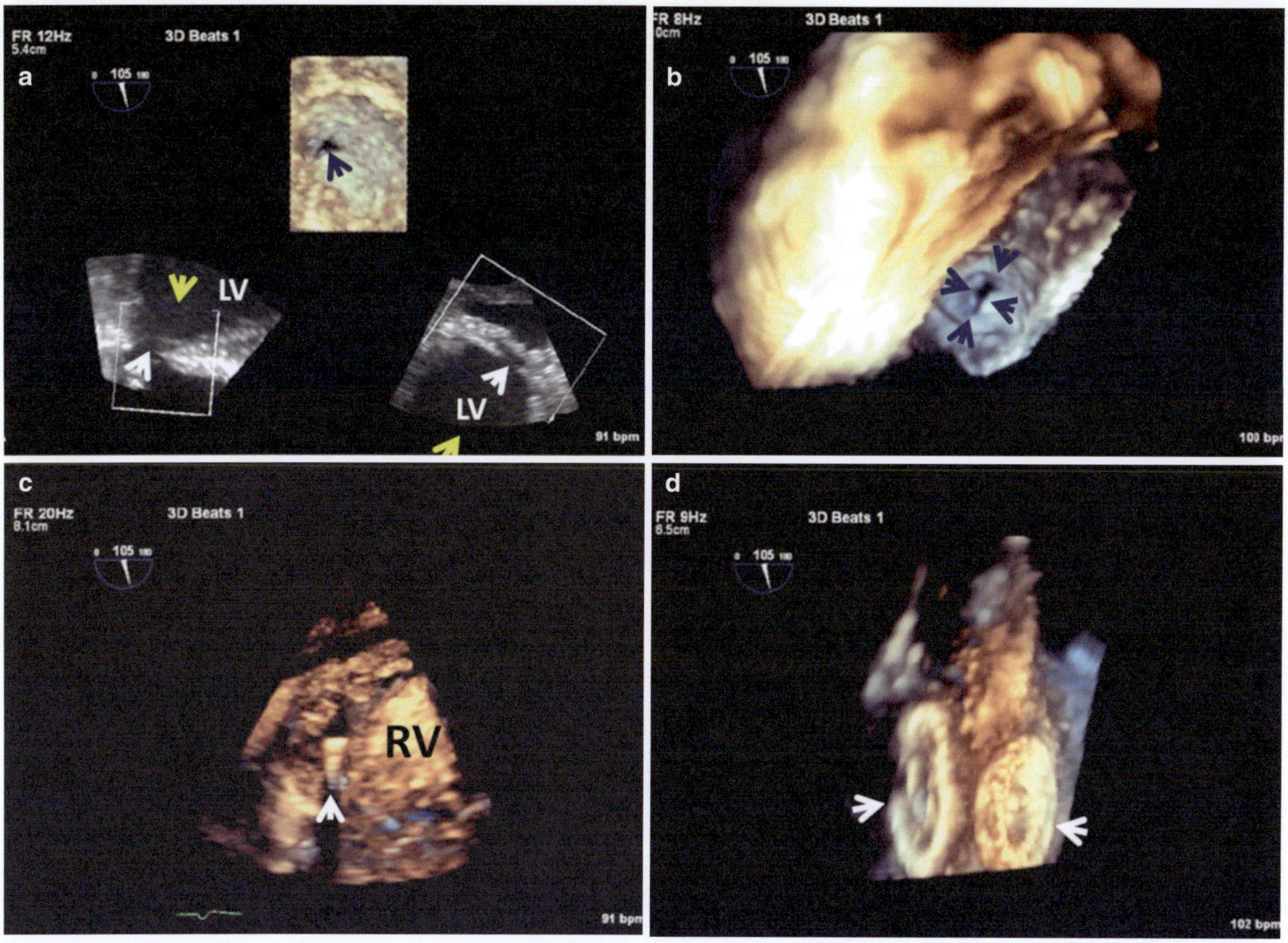

Fig. 28.6 3D TEE guidance of transcatheter closure of a post infarction VSD. **Top panel:** Enface views of the VSD from the LV (**a**, dark blue arrow) and RV (**b**, arrows) perspectives. Note the irregular shape of the defect. White arrows point to the VSD as seen on the orthogonal 2D views that make up the 3D image, and the yellow arrows point to direction from which the VSD is being viewed. **Bottom panel** (**c**): wire (arrow) in LV through the VSD and (**d**): LV and RV discs of a fully deployed 18 mm Amplatzer septal occluder device (arrows). Used with permission of Mayo Foundation for Medical Education and Research. All rights reserved. LV, left ventricle; RV, right ventricle; VSD, ventricular septal defect

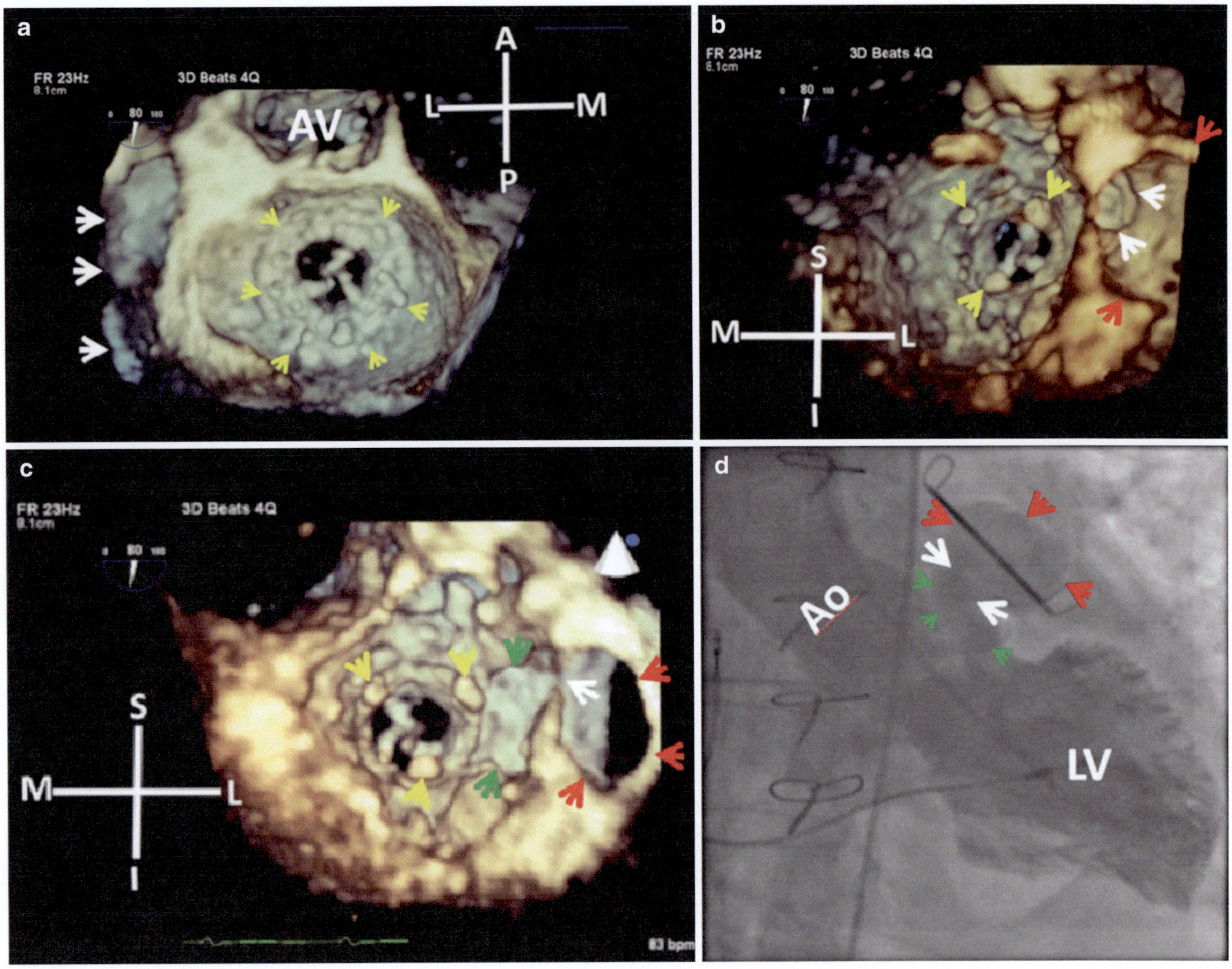

Fig. 28.7 LV pseudoaneurysm in a patient with history of MVR by a bioprosthesis. **Top panel** (**a**): enface 3D TEE LA view showing a large cavity adjacent to lateral wall of the LA (white arrows). Yellow arrows point to bioprosthesis SR. (**b**): Enface LV view showing the opening (white arrows) into the aneurysm (red arrows) from the LV. Yellow arrows point to the three bioprosthesis struts. **Bottom panel** (**c**): Same enface LV view after cropping. The narrow-necked channel (green arrows) that connects the LV with the aneurysm (red arrows) including opening into the aneurysmal sac (white arrow) can be appreciated. The findings are consistent with the diagnosis of a pseudoaneurysm. (**d**): LV gram confirming the morphology of the psuedoaneurysm as viewed on the 3D enface LV views. Used with permission of Mayo Foundation for Medical Education and Research. All rights reserved. A, anterior; Ao, aortic root; AV, aortic valve; I, inferior; L, lateral; LA, left atrium; LV, left ventricle; M, medial; MVR, mitral valve replacement; P, posterior; S, superior; SR, sewing ring

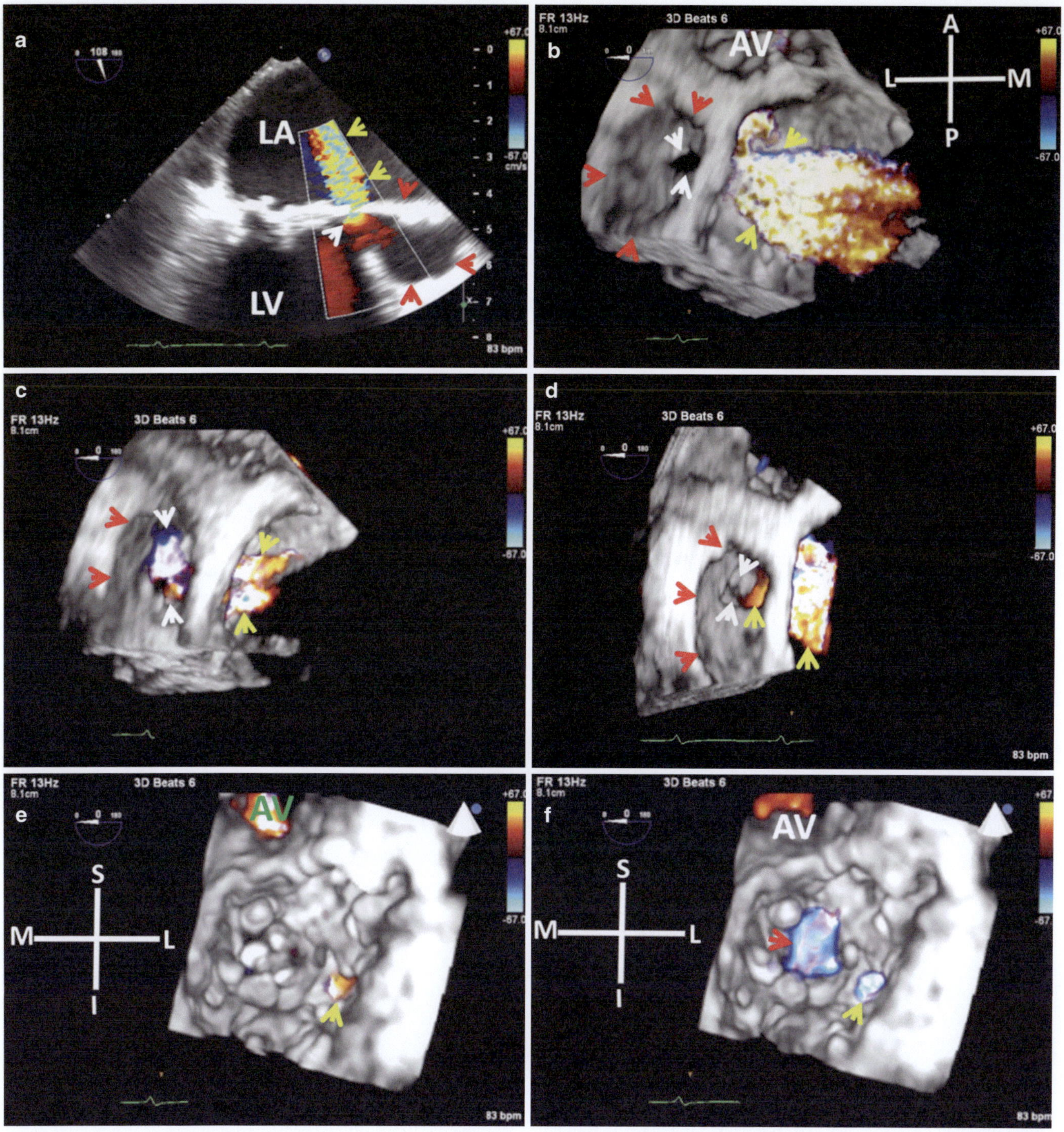

Fig. 28.8 Same patient as in Fig. 28.7: **Top panel**. (**a**): 2D TEE CFD showing the psuedoaneurysm (red arrows) with its LV connection (white arrow) and fistulous communication with the LA (yellow arrows). The morphology of this complex pathology is not well defined, however. (**b**): Multibeat 3D CFD TEE showing the pesudoaneurysm (red arrows) with narrow opening from LV (white arrows) and fistulous communication with LA (yellow arrows). **Middle panel**: Multibeat 3D TEE CFD enface LA sequential systolic frames showing the fistulous communication from LV (white arrows) through the psudoaneurym (red arrows) into the LA (yellow arrows) in early systole (**c**) and late systole (**d**). **Bottom panel.** Multibeat 3D CFD TEE enface LV views in late systole (**e**) and diastole (**f**) demonstrating flow into the narrow pseudoaneurysm neck in systole and back into the LV in diastole (yellow arrows). Red arrow points to diastolic flow through the prosthesis orifice. Used with permission of Mayo Foundation for Medical Education and Research. All rights reserved. A, anterior; AV, aortic valve; CFD, color flow Doppler; I, inferior; L, lateral; LA, left atrium; LV, left ventricle; M, medial; P, posterior; S, superior

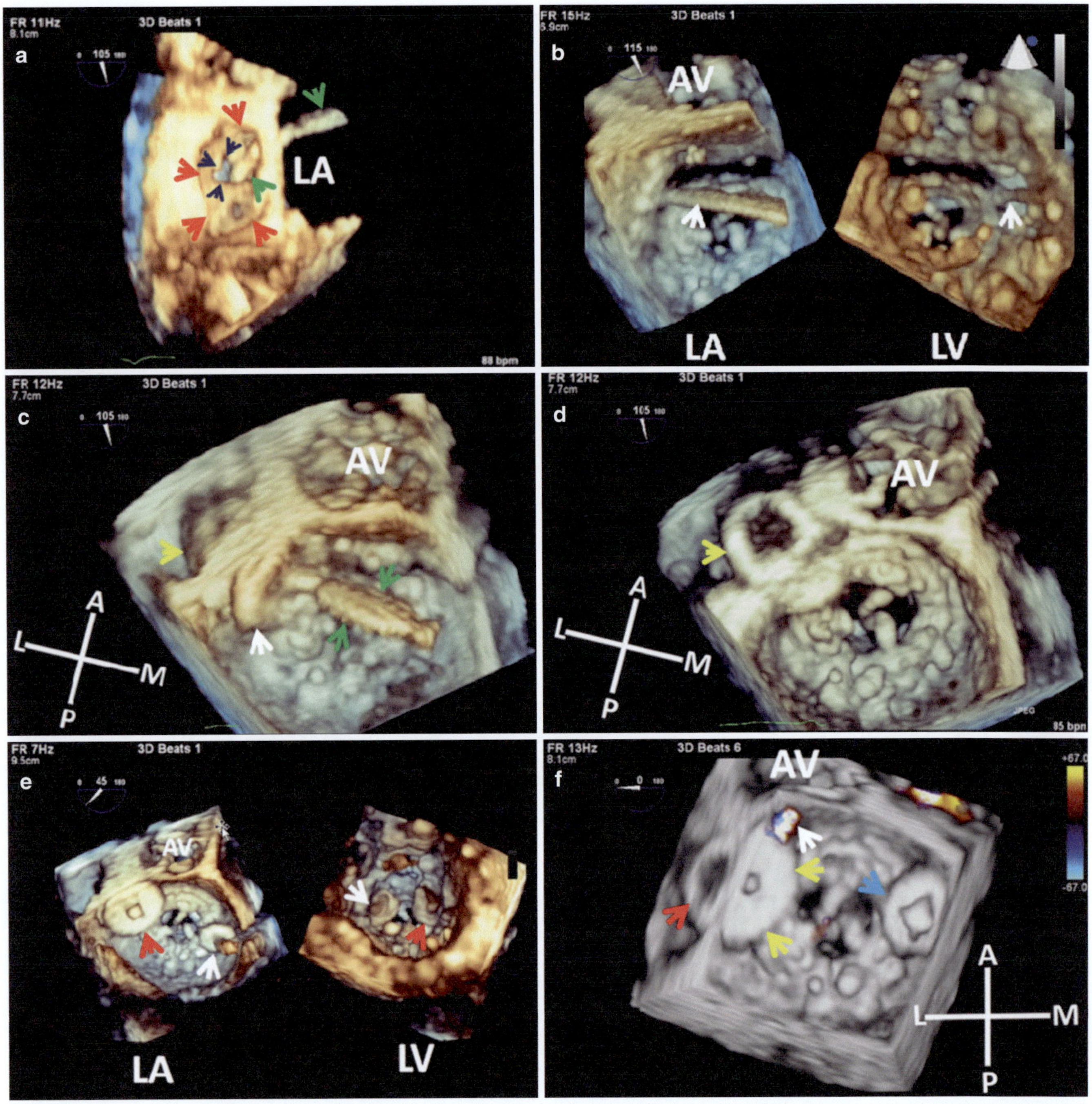

Fig. 28.9 3D TEE transcatheter guidance of closure of the LV to LA fistula shown in Figs. 28.7 and 28.8. **Top panel** (**a**): Enface view of the psuedoaneursm (red arrows) showing a catheter (green arrows) being advanced through the LA into the fistulous opening (dark blue arrows) between the psudoaneurysm and LV. (**b**): Dual layout view showing simultaneously the LA and LV segments of the catheter (arrows). **Middle panel** (**c** and **d**): Deployment of a 20 mm AVP II beginning with the ventricular side of the defect and extended into the left atrial side (white arrow) with the body of the device (yellow arrows) within the pseudoaneurysm. Green arrows point to the AVP delivery sheath. **Bottom panel** (**e**): Dual layout showing the LA and LV ends of the 20 mm AVP (red arrows). Another 12 mm AVP II (white arrows) was used to close a medial PPL. (**f**): 3D LA view CFD showing mild residual flow into LA (white arrow) from LV to LA fistula following AVP deployment. Blue arrow points to the smaller medial AVP. Red arrow points to body of the AVP device within the pseudoaneurysm. Used with permission of Mayo Foundation for Medical Education and Research. A, anterior; AV, aortic valve; AVP, Amplatzer Vascular Plug; CFD, color flow Doppler; L, lateral; LA, left atrium; LV, left ventricle; M, medial; P, posterior; PPL, periprosthetic leak

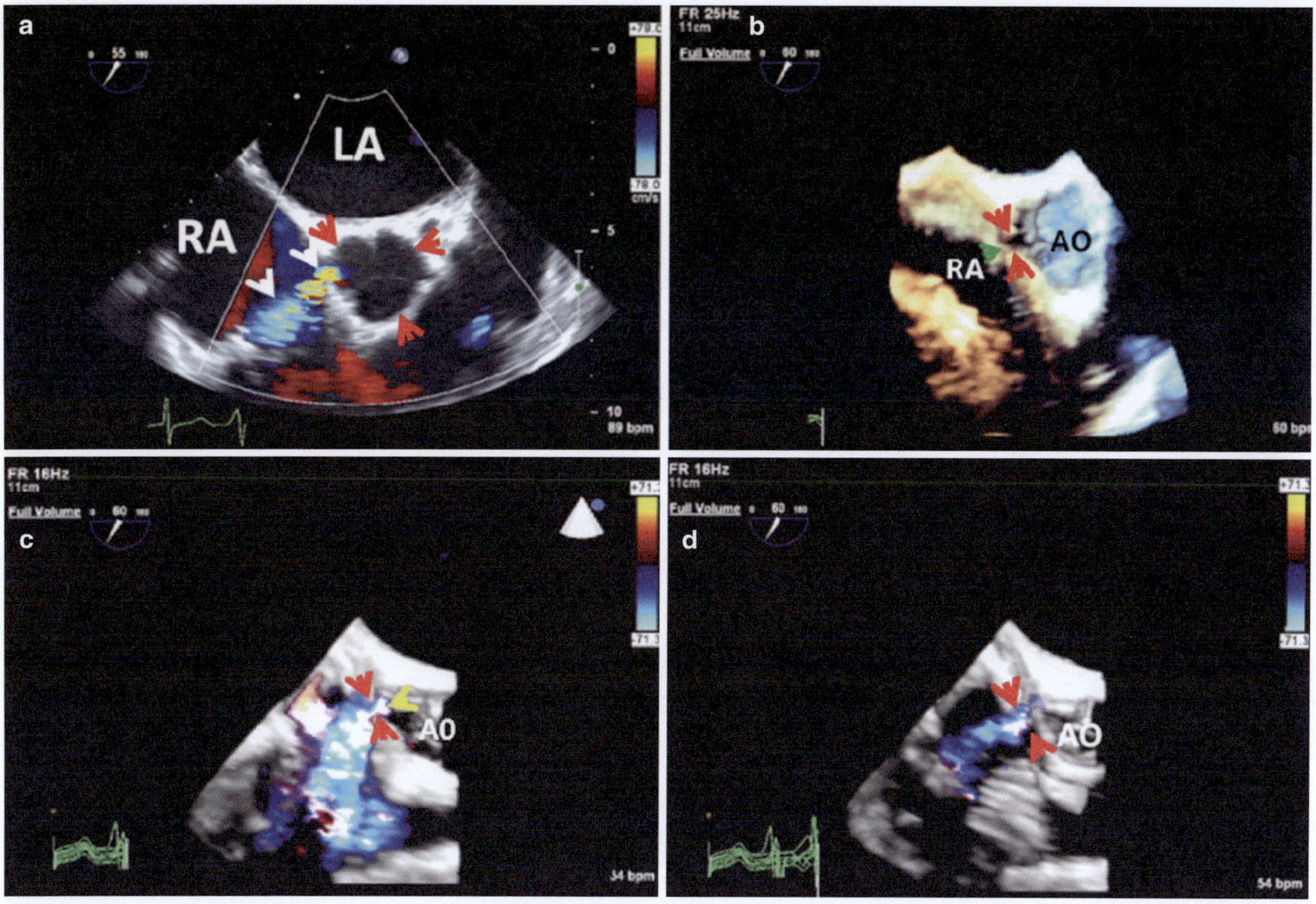

Fig. 28.10 Aorto to RA fistula. **Top panel** (**a**): 2D TEE CFD showing fistulous drainage into RA (white arrows). Red arrows point to aortic root. (**b**): 3D TEE FV showing the opening (green arrow) of the fistula from the aortic root (red arrows) into the RA. **Bottom panel:** 3D TEE CFD showing continous aorto to RA flow (red arrows) in systole (**c**) and diastole (**d**). Yellow arrow points to origin of the fistula. Used with permission of Mayo Foundation for Medical Education and Research. All rights reserved. AO, aortic root; CFD, color flow Doppler; FV, Full Volume; LA, left atrium; RA, right atrium

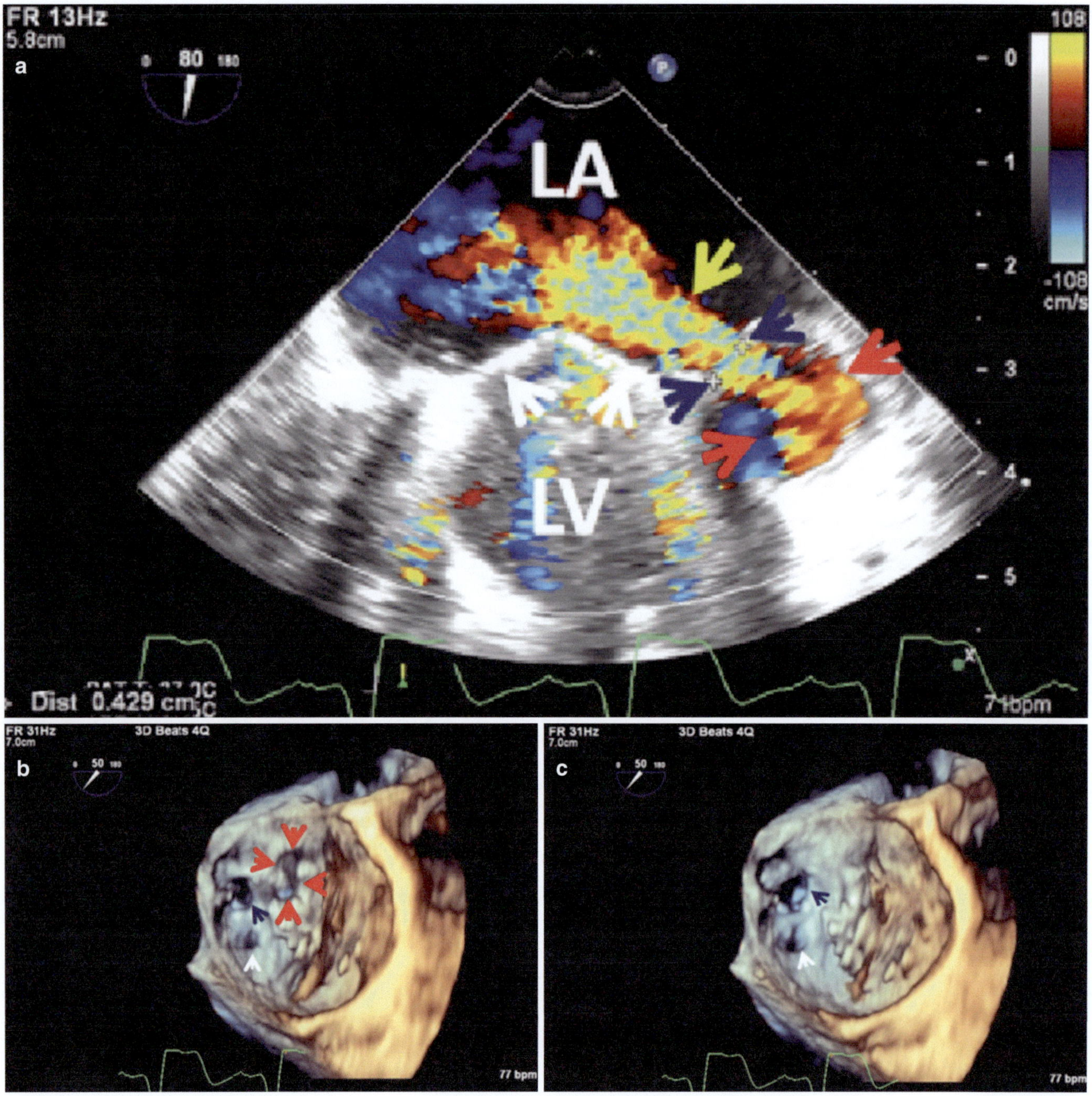

Fig. 28.11 LV to LA fistulous communication through a pseudoaneyrsm of the basal inferior wall in a patient with a mechanical bileaflet prosthesis. (**a**): 2D CFD showing site of fistulous communication (dark blue arrows) between the psudoaneurysm (red arrows) and LA. Yellow arrow points to this fistulous flow in the LA. White arrows point to the two mechanical prosthesis leaflets. (**b** and **c**): 3D TEE showing opening of the fistulous communication from the pseudoaneyrsm into the LA in systole (**b**, red arrows) and closure of this fistulous communication in diastole (**c**). Note the irregular oblong shape of the fistula opening. Also note the adjacent LAA ostium that had been partially surgically ligated (dark blue arrow). White arrow points to a pulmonary vein. Used with permission of Mayo Foundation for Medical Education and Research. All rights reserved. CFD, color flow Doppler; LA, left atrium; LAA, left atrial appendage; LV, left ventricle

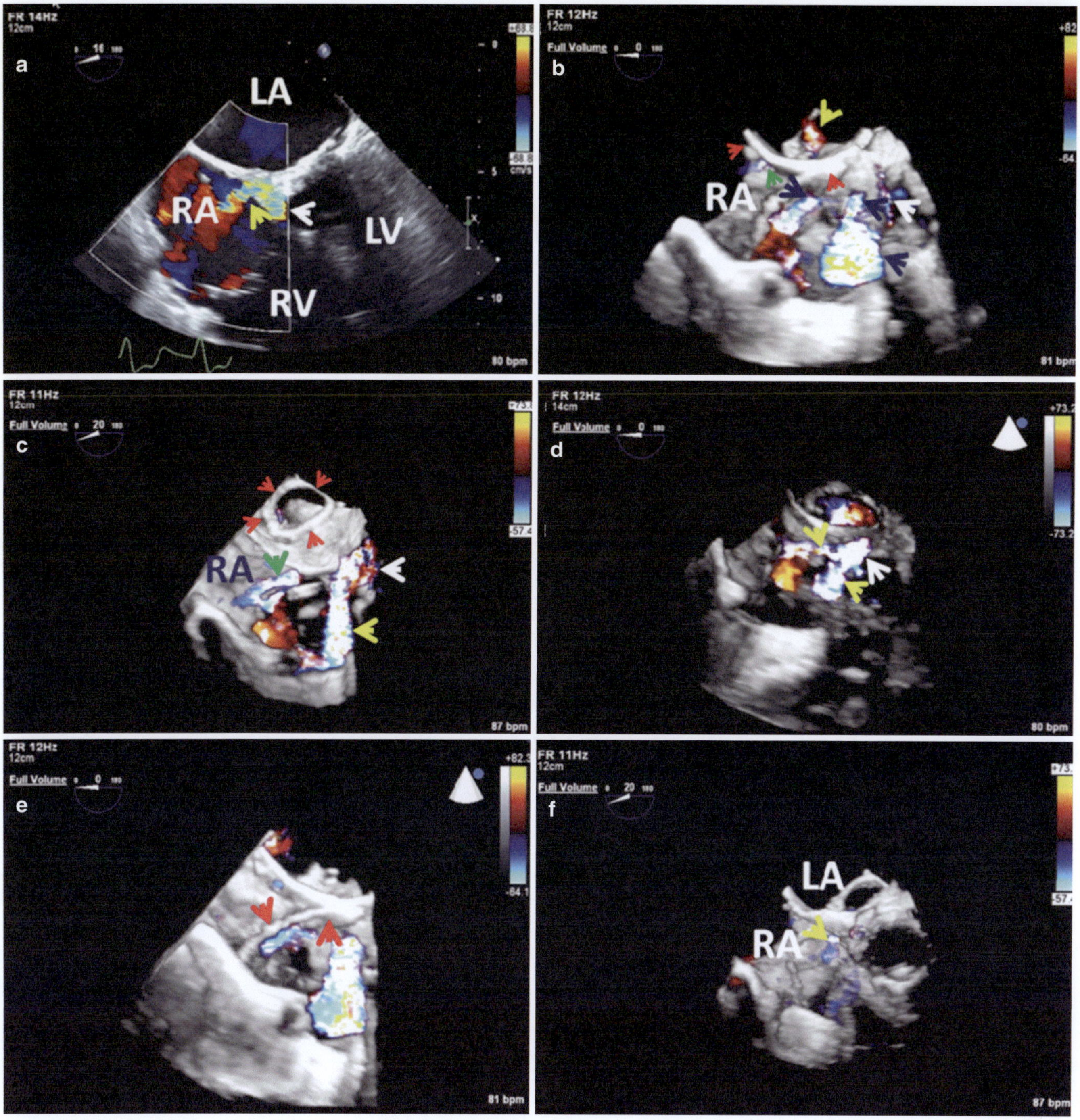

Fig. 28.12 LV to RA fistula (Gerbode) in a patient status post AVR. **Top panel** (**a**): 2D CFD shows flow in systole from the LVOT (white arrow) to RA (yellow arrow). (**b**): 3D TEE CFD showing two jets (dark blue arrows) in the RA. White arrow points to LVOT and green arrow points to a small PFO. Yellow arrow points to mild mitral regurgitation and red arrows point to mitral annuloplasty ring. **Middle panel** (**c**): Cropping confirms the LVOT origin (white arrow) of the fistulous tract into the RA (yellow arrow). Green arrow points to the other jet in RA but its origin is not yet clear. Red arrows point to MV complete annuloplasty ring. (**d**): Further cropping confirms the LVOT origin (white arrow) of both fistulous communications with the RA (yellow arrows). **Bottom panel** (**e**): catheter in RA (red arrows) negotiating the fisulous tract. (**f**): Trivial residual flow (yellow arrow) into RA from the LVOT after percutaneous closure of the fistula with a vascular plug. Used with permission of Mayo Foundation for Medical Education and Research. All rights reserved. AVR, aortic valve replacement; CFD, color flow Doppler; LA, left atrium; LV, left ventricle; LVOT, left ventricular outflow tract; MV, mitral valve; PFO, patent foramen ovale; RA, right atrium; RV, right ventricle

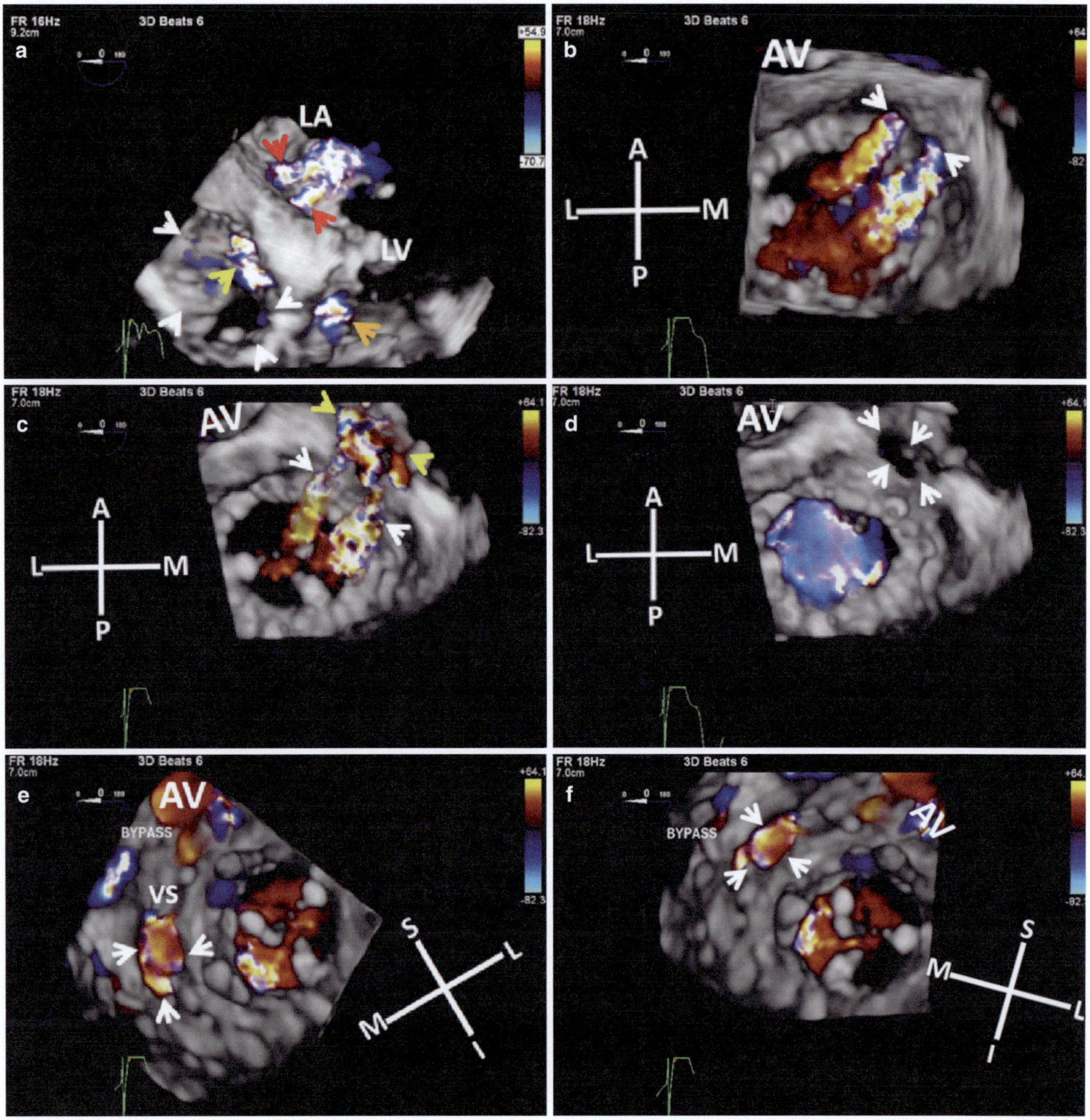

Fig. 28.13 Intraoperative 3D TEE in a patient post surgical repair of Gerbode-type VSD, aorto to LV fistula, MAIVF pseudoaneyrsm, AV perforation, and MVR with a bioprosthesis, secondary to complex endocarditis. A residual shunt into the LA was seen on the post bypass 2D CFD images but the origin of the shunt could not be ascertained. **Top panel** (**a**): Flow from LV (orange arrow) into LA (red arrows) through a pseudoaneurysm (white arrows). Yellow arrow points to LA exit site of this complex fistulous communication. (**b**): 3D TEE CFD enface LA view showing the two systolic fistula exit jets (white arrows) above the plane of the mitral bioprosthesis SR. **Second panel** (**c**): Cropping of view in **b** brings out the pseudoanueyrsm (yellow arrows) and fistula exit jets into LA (white arrows). (**d**): Same image in diastole showing the pseudoaneurysm (white arrows). **Third panel** (**e** and **f**): 3D TEE CFD enface LV views showing that the origin of this complex fistulous communication is the VS (white arrows). **Bottom panel:** 3D TEE CFD enface LV (**g**) and LA (**h**) views showing a tiny residual shunt (white arrows) following closure of the fistula at its origin. Yellow arrows point to bioprosthesis SR. Used with permission of Mayo Foundation for Medical Education and Research. All rights reserved. A, anterior; AV, aortic valve; CFD, color flow Doppler; I, inferior; L, lateral; LA, left atrium; LV, left ventricle; LVOT, left ventricular outflow tract; M, medial; MAIVF, mitral aortic intervalve fibrosa; MV, mitral valve; MVR, mitral valve replacement; P, posterior; RA, right atrium; RV, right ventricle; S, superior; SR, sewing ring; VS, ventricular septum; VSD, ventricular septal defect

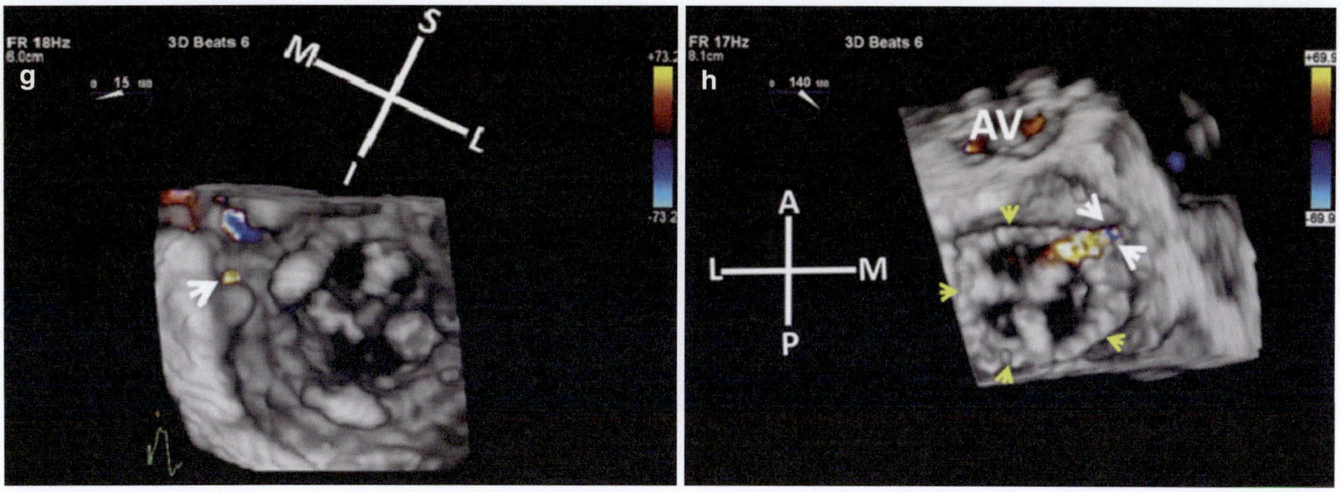

Fig. 28.13 (continued)

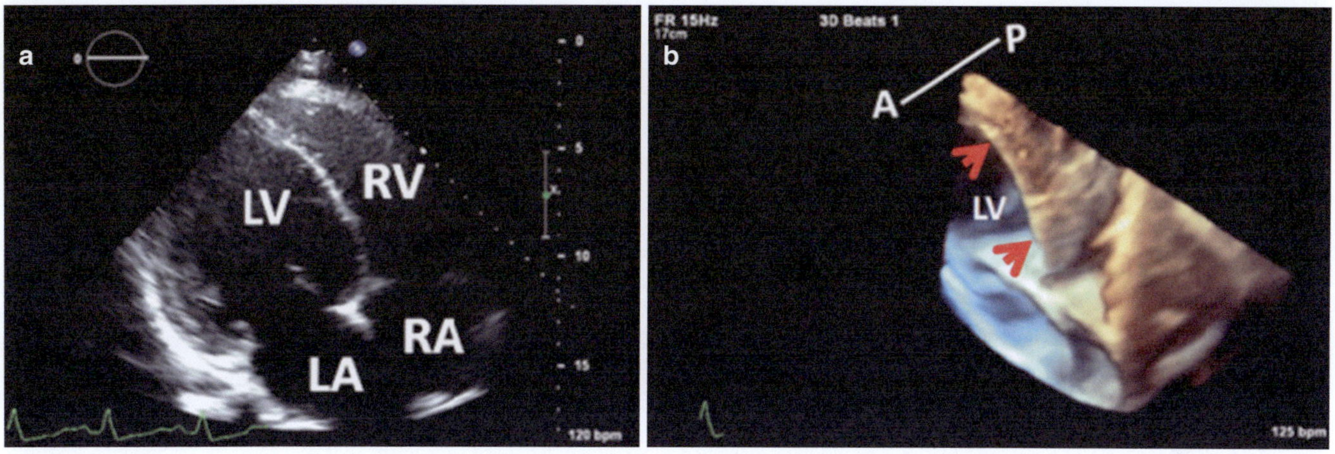

Fig. 28.14 (**a**). Apical four chamber view in a patient with dilated cardiomyopathy showing a thin ventricular septum. (**b**). 3D transthoracic echocardiogram of same 2D view shown in panel **a**. The entire anteroposterior (A-P) depth of the ventricular septum (arrows) can be appreciated. Used with permission of Mayo Foundation for Medical Education and Research. All rights reserved. LA, left atrium; LV, left ventricle; RA, right atrium; RV, right ventricle

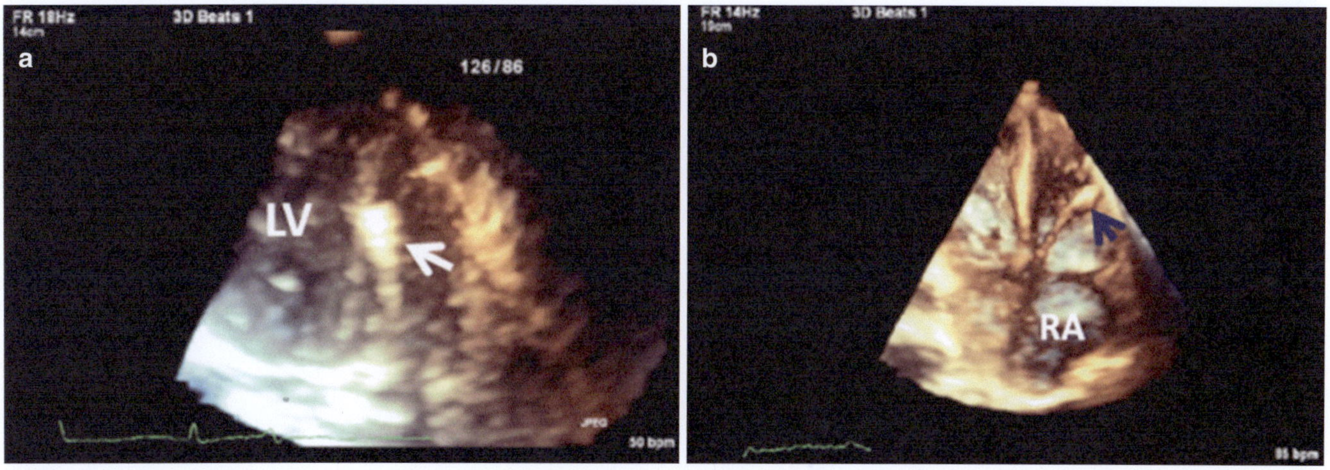

Fig. 28.15 Real time 3D TTE guided RV EMB in a post cardiac transplant patient. (**a**): Bioptome (arrow) at the basal VS. (**b**): Bioptome (arrow) abutting the RV free wall. EMB, endomyocardial biopsy; LV, left ventricle; RV, right ventricle; TTE, transthoracic echocardiography; VS, ventricular septum. Used with permission of Mayo Foundation for Medical Education and Research. All rights reserved

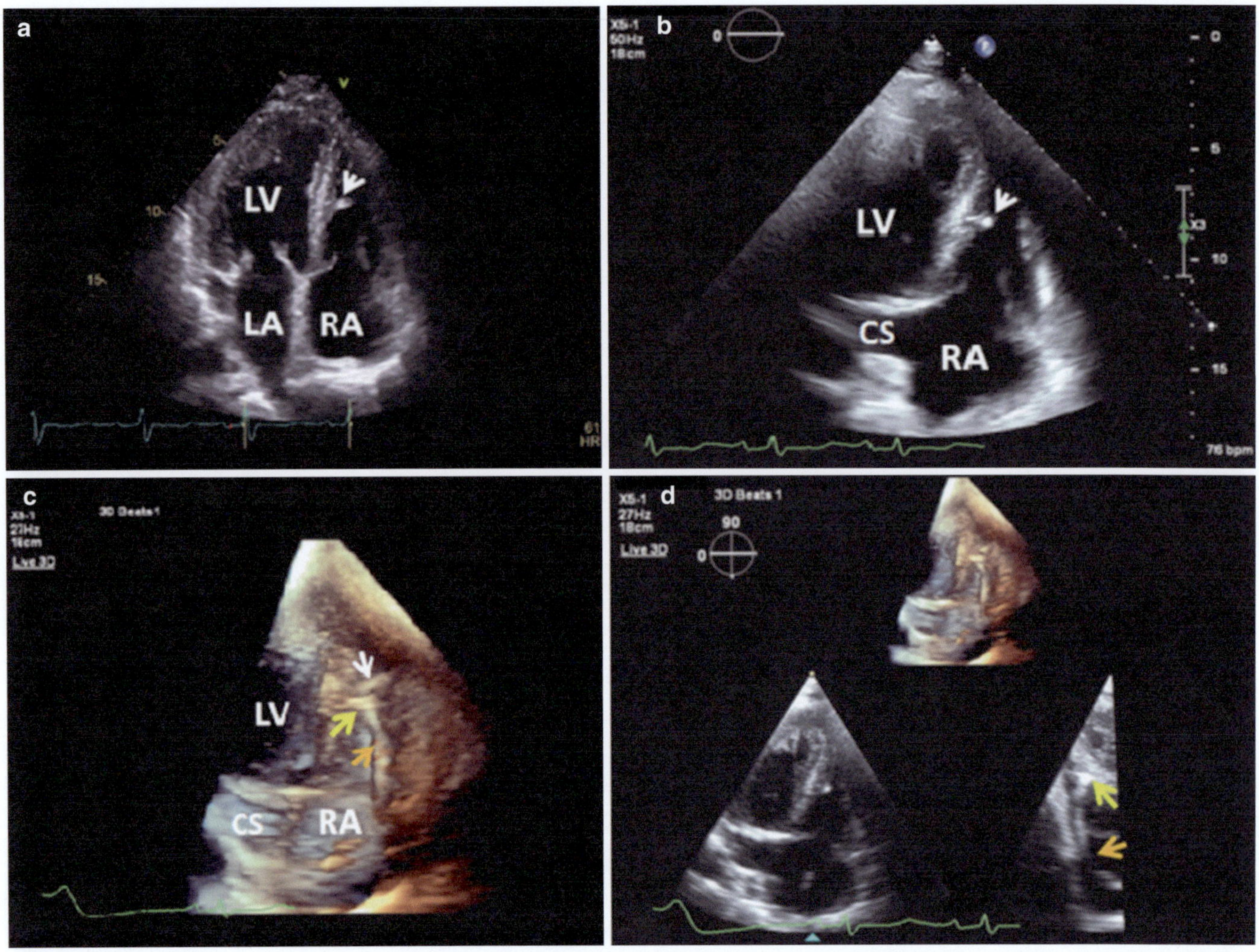

Fig. 28.16 Real time 3D TTE guided EMB in a patient with suspected cardiac amyloidosis. **Top panel** (**a** and **b**): 2D apical views showing an echogenic moderator band (white arrows) consistent with focal calcification. **Bottom panel**: (**c**): 3D view of **b** showing the moderator band (white arrow), and bioptome catheter (orange arrow) in RV with its tip (yellow arrow) abutting the mid VS. (**d**): Same 3D in **c** with component orthogonal 2D biplane . Note that the bioptome is not seen in the conventional 2D space (left lower) but is seen in the orthogonal 2D tomographic plane (right lower). Used with permission of Mayo Foundation for Medical Education and Research. All rights reserved. EMB, endomyocardial biopsy; CS, coronary sinus; LA, left atrium; LV, left ventricle; RA, right atrium; RV, right ventricle; TTE, transthoracic echocardiography; VS, ventricular septum

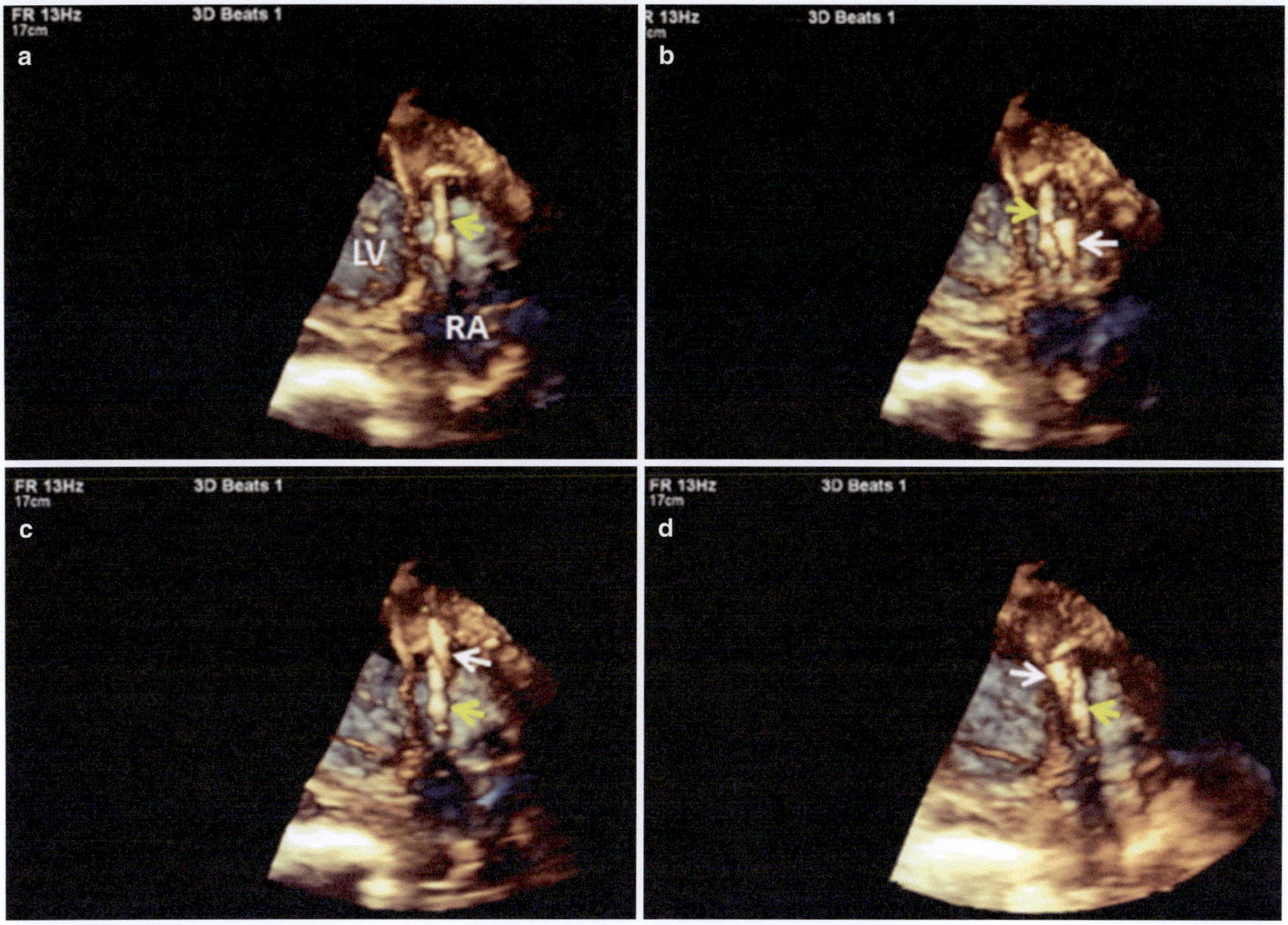

Fig. 28.17 Collage of real time 3D TTE during RV biopsy in a patient with a ventricular pacemaker lead. (**a**). Pre procedure image showing pacemaker lead (yellow arrow). (**b**). bioptome (white arrow) is advanced into the RV and is anterior to the pacemaker lead (yellow arrow). (**c**). Bioptome (white arrow) is too apical and overlies the pacemaker lead (yellow arrow). (**d**). bioptome (white arrow) is in contact with mid VS. Note the proximity to the pacemaker lead (yellow arrow). LV, left ventricle; RA, right atrium; RV, right ventricle; VS, ventricular septum. Used with permission of Mayo Foundation for Medical Education and Research. All rights reserved

References

1. Saurav A, Kaushik M, Mahesh Alla V, et al. Comparison of percutaneous device closure versus surgical closure of peri-membranous ventricular septal defects: a systematic review and meta-analysis. Catheter Cardiovasc Interv. 2015;86(6):1048–56.
2. Cossor W, Wei Cui V, Roberson DA. Three-dimensional echocardiographic en face views of ventricular Septal defects: feasibility, accuracy, imaging protocols and reference image collection. JASE. 2015;28:1020–9.
3. Charakida M, Qureshi S, Simpson JM. 3D echocardiography for planning and guidance of interventional closure of VSD. J Am Coll Cardiol Img. 2013;6(1):PP120–3.
4. Hoch M, Roemer U, Kozlik-Feldmann R, Fuchs A, Netz H. Three-dimensional echocardiography of ventricular septal defects. Images Paediatr Cardiol. 2002 Jul–Sep;4(3):4–20.
5. Arat N, Ozbulbul NI. Three-dimensional echocardiography is a useful tool in the diagnosis of left ventricular pseudoaneurysm. Eur J Cardio-Thoracic Surg. July 2007;32(1):164.
6. Dudiy Y, Jelinin V, Einhorn BN, Kronzon I, Cohen HA, Ruiz CE. Percutaneous closure of left ventricular pseudoaneurysm. Circulation Cardiovasc Interv. 2011;4:322–6.
7. Taskesen T, Goldberg SL, Gill EA. Role of three-dimensional echocardiography in management of acquired intracardiac shunts Echocardiography. 2014 Sep;31(8):E250–E253.

29 Edge-to-Edge Mitral Valve Repair

Joseph F. Maalouf and Francesco F. Faletra

Introduction

Percutaneous transcatheter mitral valve repair (TMVR) involves grasping the *free* edges of the anterior and posterior leaflets at site of mitral regurgitation (MR), and is used to treat severe symptomatic functional MR or high surgical risk patients with degenerative MR. Currently, the only FDA approved device for TMVR is the MitraClip which will be the focus of this chapter (for the PASCAL device see Chap. 34). 3D TEE is very useful in localizing the site of MR and for providing accurate assessment of the wide spectrum of degenerative mitral valve (MV) disease pathology (see Chap. 6). 3D TEE is also superior to 2D TEE for detecting mitral "clefts" (see Chap. 9), which if associated with significant mitral regurgitation (MR) may preclude successful TMVR, and for recognizing commissural or paracommissural MR (Fig. 29.1; see Chap. 9) generally considered a contraindication to TMVR because of high risk of entanglement of the MitraClip by the sub commissural chordae. Multibeat full volume or 3D zoom acquisition (typically 6 beats) may be necessary to obtain optimal 3D color flow Doppler (CFD) of the entire left atrial (LA) or left ventricular (LV) surface of the MV at an adequate frame rate (at least 10 volumes/second). Single beat real time high volume rate (HVR) full volume CFD can be useful in patients with irregular heart rhythm, or intra procedurally when time to obtain 3D CFD is limited and real time imaging is preferred (see Chap. 3). *The newest 3D platforms frequently provide adequate single beat real time MV CFD volume rates.*

Supplementary Information The online version of this chapter (https://doi.org/10.1007/978-3-030-72941-7_29) contains supplementary material, which is available to authorized users.

J. F. Maalouf (✉)
Professor of Medicine, Mayo Clinic College of Medicine; Director, Interventional Echocardiography; Consultant, Department of Cardiovascular Medicine, Mayo Clinic, Rochester, MN, USA
e-mail: maalouf.joseph@mayo.edu

F. F. Faletra
Director of Cardiac Imaging Lab, Cardiocentro Ticino Institute, Lugano, Switzerland
e-mail: Francesco.Faletra@cardiocentro.org

Pre Procedural Planning [1, 2]

A distinct advantage of 3D TEE over conventional 2D TEE is the ability to visualize the entire MV and surrounding structures from a single transducer position and in real time with minimal or no probe manipulation. The images obtained reliably reflect actual anatomy in a format that is readily appreciated by non-imaging cardiologists. Moreover, because the MR jet tends to fan-out in the LA, enface 3D views of the MV from the left ventricle (LV) are very useful in pinpointing the exact origin of MR, and the shape, width, and number of MR jet(s), which may help determine the number of clips needed (Fig. 29.2).

In addition to delineating MV anatomy and assessing the mechanism of regurgitation, an important objective of 3D TEE during the pre-procedural phase of TMVR is to perform an imaging "dry-run" in preparation for the actual procedure. This serves the dual purpose of choosing the most appropriate image planes to guide the various steps of the procedure including optimal views for perpendicular orientation of the MitraClip arms to site of leaflet malcoaptation.

Important left atrial (LA) anatomic landmarks during the first stages of procedural guidance include the left atrial appendage (LAA) and left superior (upper) pulmonary vein (LSPV) ostia, and both the free wall and dome of the LA because the LSPV serves as a wire anchor, and instrumentation of the LA by stiff wires and bulky catheters can perforate the LA or its thin walled appendage. Imaging of the atrial septum and LA with 3D TEE to guide these initial steps of the procedure after septal puncture is best achieved from the bicaval 2D window using real time single beat full volume (FV) or 3D zoom. An advantage of FV over 3D zoom is that it minimizes the number of steps needed to achieve the desired images. This is particularly important because of the need for

J. F. Maalouf et al. (eds.), *Practical 3D Echocardiography*, https://doi.org/10.1007/978-3-030-72941-7_29

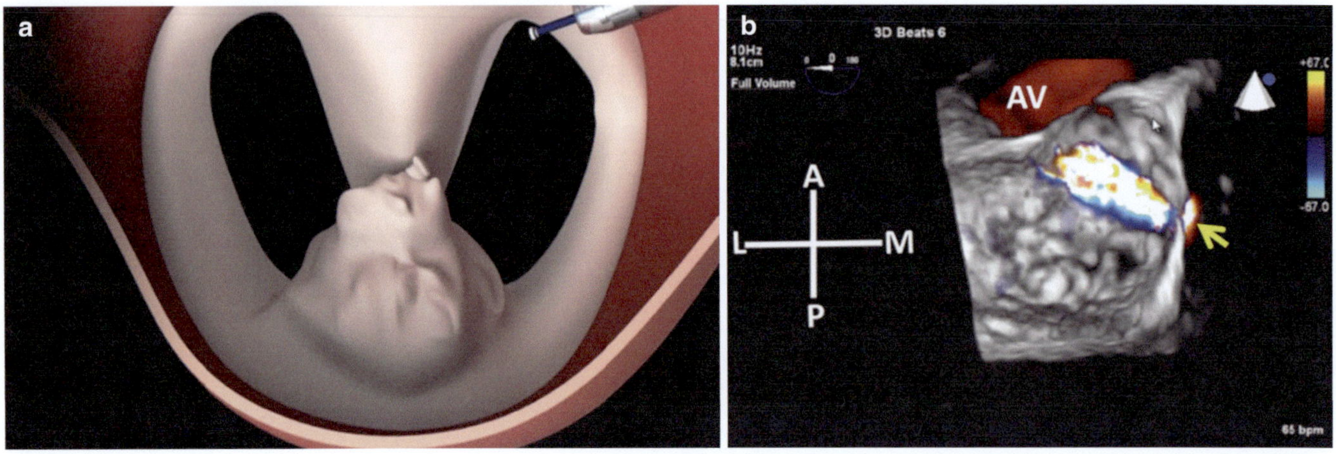

Fig. 29.1 (**a**): Schematic of edge to edge MV repair; (**b**): En face 3D LA view of paracommissural MR (yellow arrow). Used with permission of Mayo Foundation for Medical Education and Research. All rights reserved. A, anterior; AV, aortic valve; L, lateral; M, medial; P, posterior

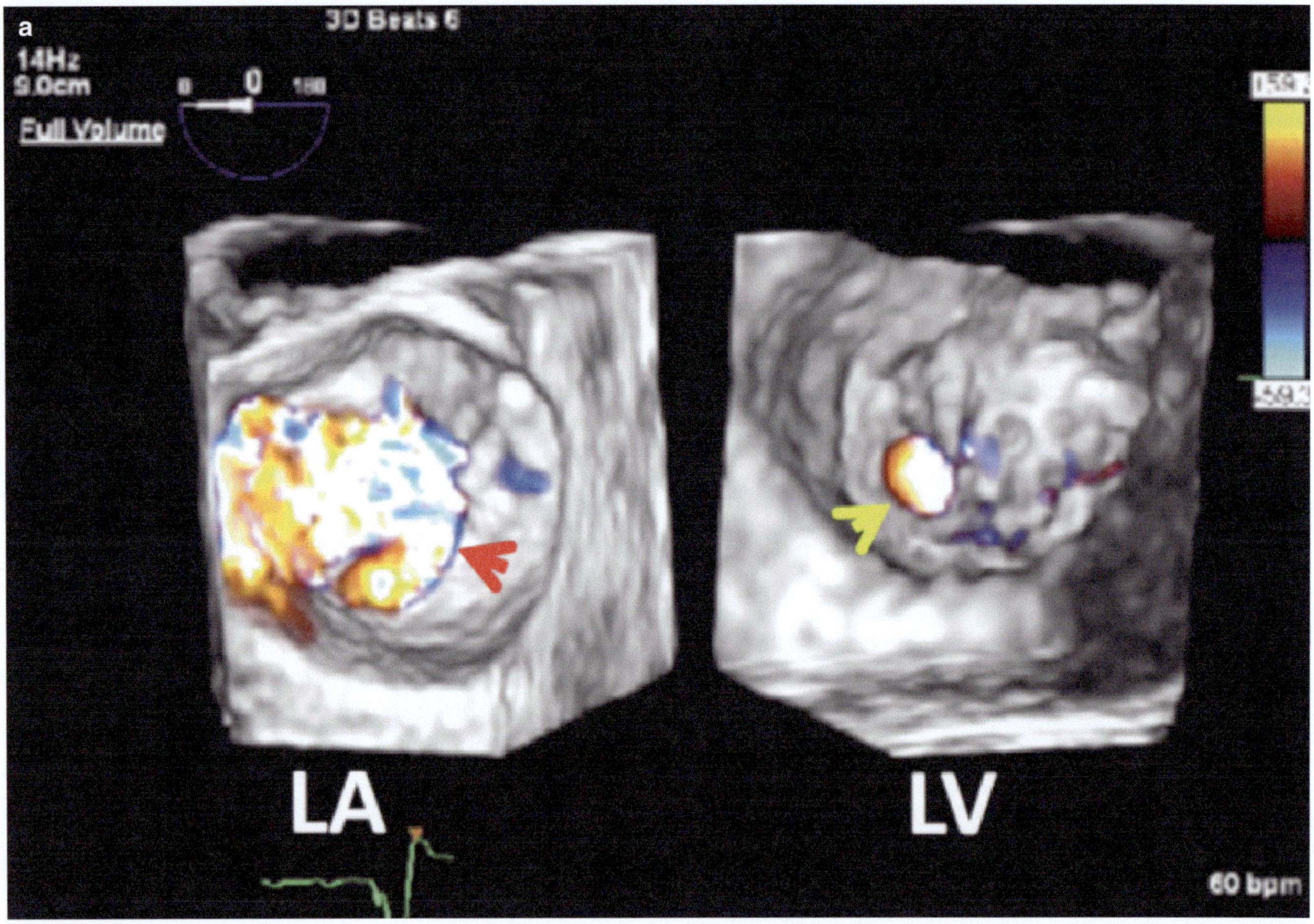

Fig. 29.2 3D FV multibeat CFD of MR (**a**): Dual layout enface LA and LV views. Note that the MR jet has a discrete origin (yellow arrow) when viewed from the LV perspective, but fans out in the LA (red arrow). **Second and third panels:** LV views; (**b**): Discrete central MR jet (arrow) in a patient with flail P2 segment. (**c**): Broad based MR jet (arrows) that spans the entire MV coaptation surface in a patient with severe FMR. (**d**): Two separate MR jets (arrows). (**e**): medial paracommissural MR jet (arrow). Used with permission of Mayo Foundation for Medical Education and Research. All rights reserved. CFD, color flow Doppler; FMR, functional mitral regurgitation; FV, Full Volume; I, inferior; L, lateral; LA, left atrium; LV, left ventricle; M, medial; MR, mitral regurgitation; MV, mitral valve; S, superior

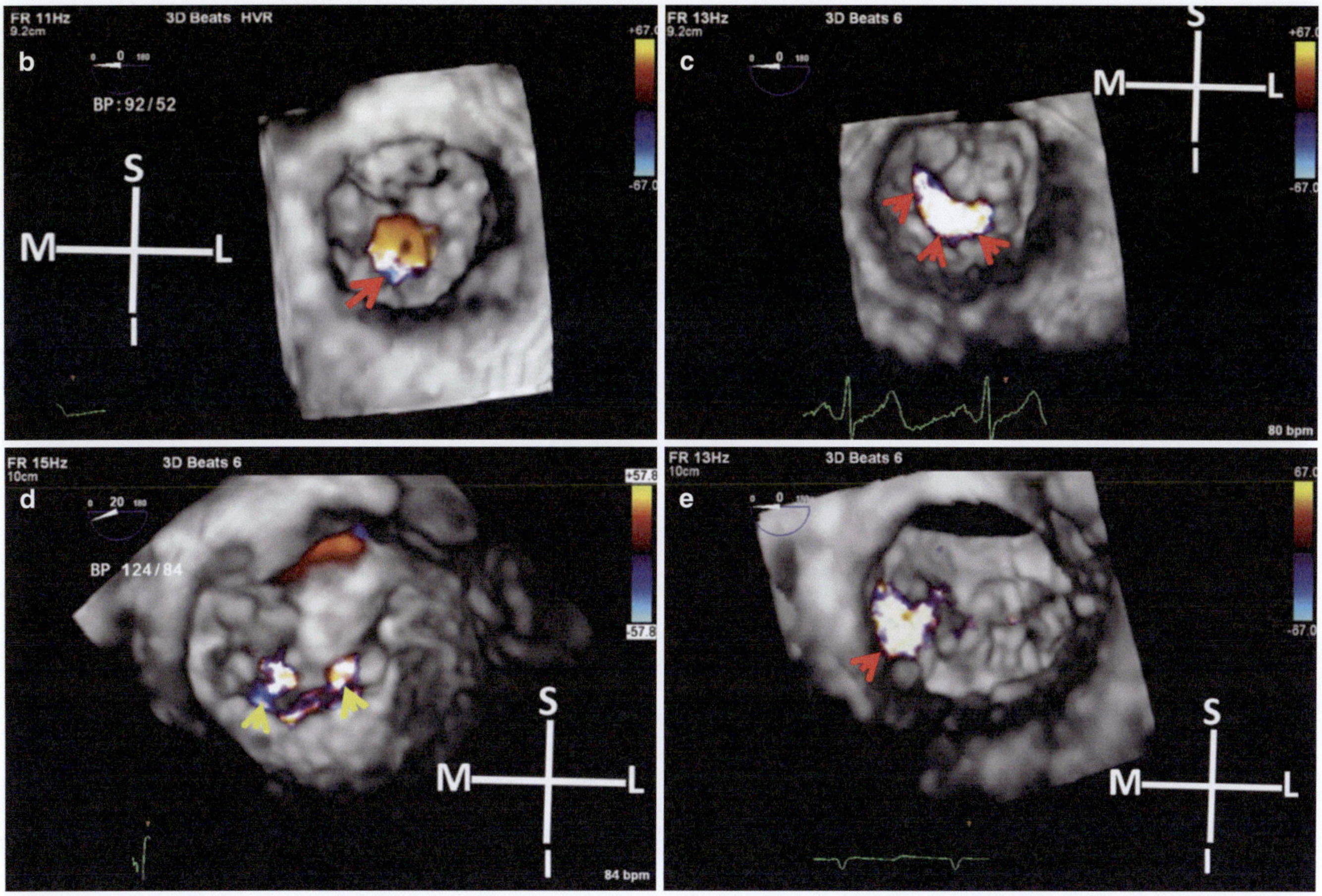

Fig. 29.2 (continued)

rapid switching from 3D to 2D and vice versa intraprocedurally. A 3D image of the atrial septum is first optimized by using the lateral width button to include most of the superior and inferior septal rims (Fig. 29.3). Enface view of the MV and its adjacent structures including the atrial septum and aortic valve is then obtained by leftward (usually counterclockwise) rotation of the transducer (Fig. 29.3). The ostia of the LAA and LSPV can be viewed simultaneously on further leftward rotation of the transducer (Figs. 29.3 and 29.7). With rightward (usually clockwise) rotation of the transducer from the mitral plane the entire atrial septum including fossa ovalis can be seen (Fig. 29.3). Further rightward rotation of the transducer tip reveals the most superior aspect (dome) of the LA including the right superior pulmonary vein (RSPV) (Fig. 29.5). Standard 3D image optimization techniques (lowest compression and gain settings and use of appropriate cropping tools to crop out additional noise artifacts) are used to enhance 3D image quality always keeping in mind that optimal 3D images require optimal 2D images.

Intraprocedural Guidance

The first step in TMVR is the transseptal puncture (TSP) and biplane or xPlane (Philips Healthcare) is the imaging tool of choice to guide this step (Fig. 29.4). The TSP site should generally be posterior and mid superior-inferior or slightly inferior. And, utilizing the newer generation longer clip delivery system (CDS), the TSP should be approximately 4.5 cm posterior to the plane of the mitral annulus in systole (or 4–6 cm to the leaflets in systole) as viewed from the mid-esophageal four chamber window regardless of whether the MR is functional or degenerative in etiology in order to provide adequate room to maneuver the device within the left atrium; major variation from this measurement will pose procedural challenges due to CDS being too high or too low relative to the MV plane.

3D TEE may be a useful adjunctive imaging modality to guide TSP particularly when the transseptal needle is not

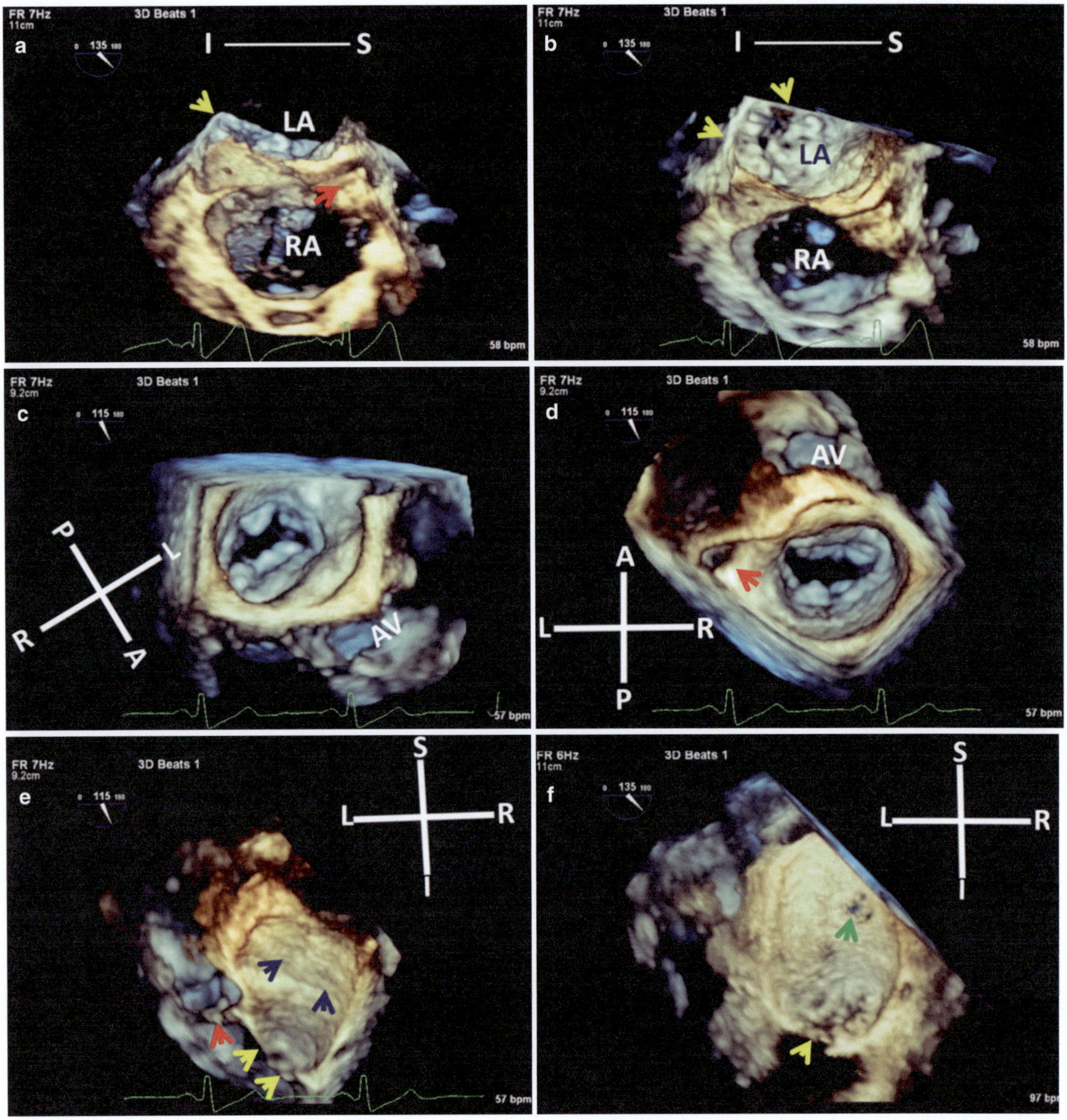

Fig. 29.3 Technique for 3D FV acquisition of the MV from a 2D bicaval view. (**a**): The MV is partially seen (yellow arrow) on 3D FV of a standard 2D bicaval view. Red arrow points to SVC. (**b**): with leftward (counterclockwise) rotation of the probe, the MV (arrows) is better exposed. (**c**): further counterclockwise rotation exposes the entire MV. (**d**): The image is rotated such that the aortic valve is at the top. The ostium of the LAA is partially seen (red arrow). (**e**): with progressive clockwise rotation of the probe from the MV view, the entire wall of the atrial septum (dark blue arrows) is exposed and there is corresponding counterclockise rotation in position of the aortic valve (red arrow). (**f**): The entire thin fossa ovalis (green arrow) can be seen with this maneuver. Yellow arrows point to MV. Used with permission of Mayo Foundation for Medical Education and Research. All rights reserved. A, anterior; AV, aortic valve; FV, Full Volume; I, inferior; L, left; LA, left atrium; LAA, left atrial appendage; M, medial; MV, mitral valve; P, posterior; R, right; RA, right atrium; S, superior; SVC, superior vena cava

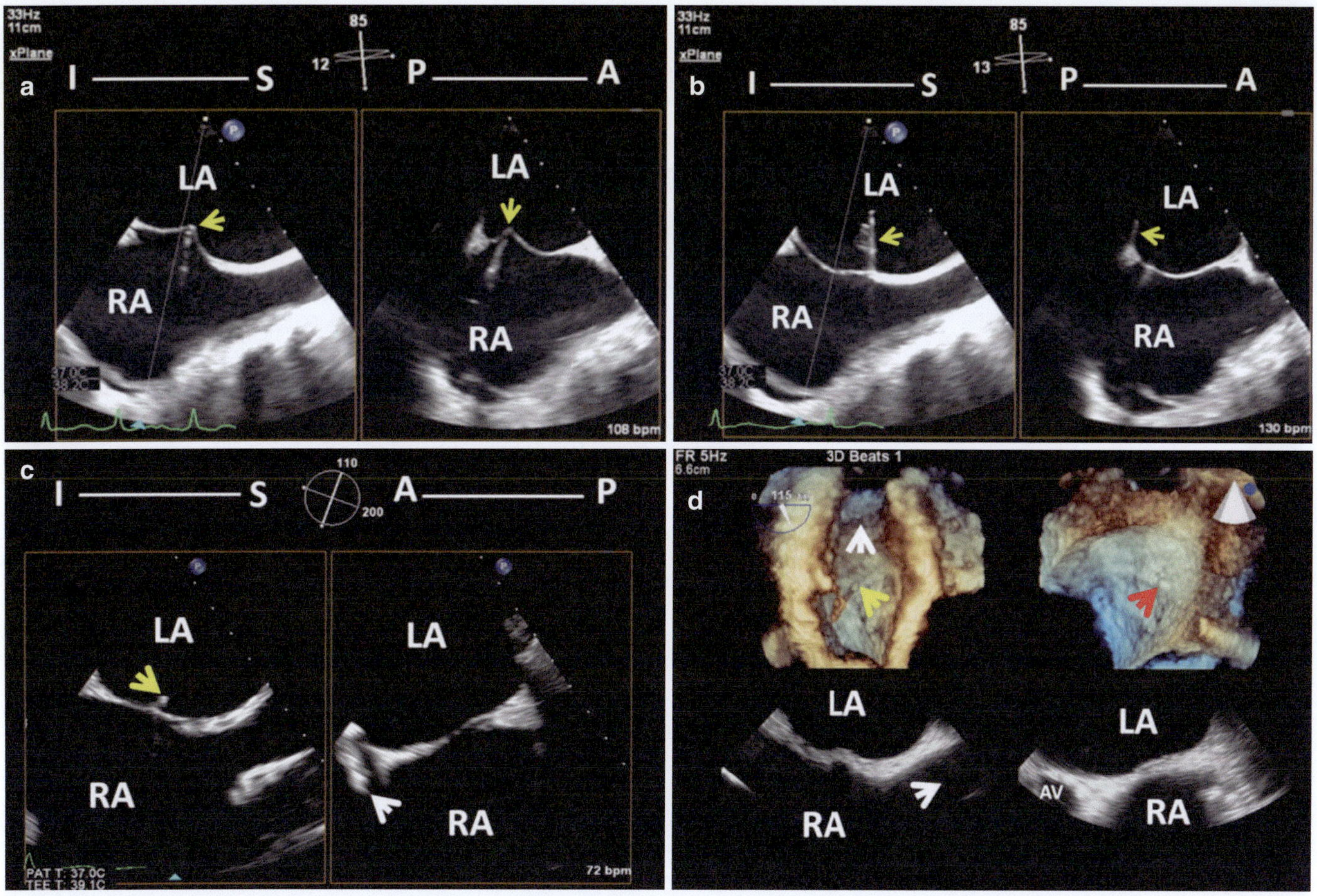

Fig. 29.4 Top panel: TSP using xPlane (Philips Healthcare). Mid superior-inferior and posterior tenting of atrial septum by transseptal needle (**a**, arrows) and corresponding images (**b**) following TSP. **Bottom** (**c**): Transseptal needle is seen in S-I plane (yellow arrow) but not A-P plane. White arrow points to AV. (**d**): Real time 3D zoom dual RA and LA layout during TSP. Yellow arrow points to TS needle in RA, and red arrow points to tenting of atrial septum as viewed from the LA (red arrow). White arrows point to superior vena cava. Note that the transseptal needle is not seen in the corresponding 2D images. Used with permission of Mayo Foundation for Medical Education and Research. All rights reserved. A, anterior; AV, aortic valve; I, inferior; LA, left atrium; P, posterior; RA, right atrium; S, superior; TS, transseptal; TSP, transseptal puncture

well seen on xPlane (Fig. 29.4). And, when the desired puncture site is too posterior, visualization may be difficult by 2D TEE, whereas 3D TEE may enhance ease of visualization. The optimal TSP site can be imaged on 3D TEE of the right atrial surface of the atrial septum, and simultaneous 3D of the left atrial surface shows tenting of the atrial septum (Fig. 29.5). The distance from transseptal needle tenting site to plane of the MV is crucial in determining the optimal transseptal puncture site. This can be measured from the enface left atrial view of atrial septum and plane of the MV(Fig. 29.5).

Following the TSP, 2D and 3D TEE are used to help position the guidewire, guide catheter, and ultimately the MitraClip and delivery system in the left atrium.

3D TEE has been shown to be superior to 2D TEE in guiding many of the steps involved in TMVR [1–3] particularly when the MR is not central [4]. Moreover, real time enface imaging of the MV and adjoining structures provides contextual anatomical guidance during transcatheter interventions. As with any catheter-based intervention, a major prerequisite for use of 3DTEE to guide TMVR is thorough knowledge of all types of catheters/sheaths/wires and dilators that are used during the procedure as they may have a unique 3D "finger print".

The actual transseptal puncture can next be viewed (Fig. 29.6). Following TSP, a Mullins sheath and dilator are advanced over the Brockenbrough needle into the left atrium and the needle and dilator are removed (Fig. 29.6).

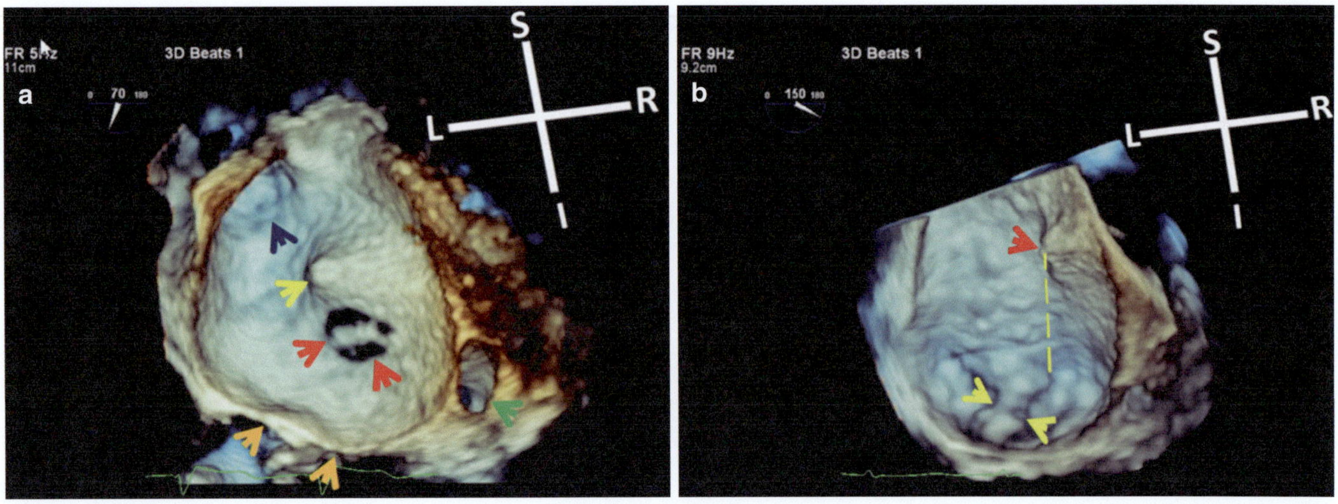

Fig. 29.5 Real time single beat 3D views of left side of atrial septum. (**a**): Brockenbrough needle tenting of the atrial septum (yellow arrow) is seen superior to the fossa ovalis (red arrows). Dark blue arrow points to RSPV and orange arrows point to MV. Green arrow points to CS. (**b**): Distance (dashed yellow line) from site of tenting (red arrow) to plane of MV. Yellow arrows point to flail AML. Used with permission of Mayo Foundation for Medical Education and Research. All rights reserved. AML, anterior mitral leaflet; CS, coronary sinus; I, inferior; L, left; MV, mitral valve; R, right; RSPV, right superior pulmonary vein; S, superior

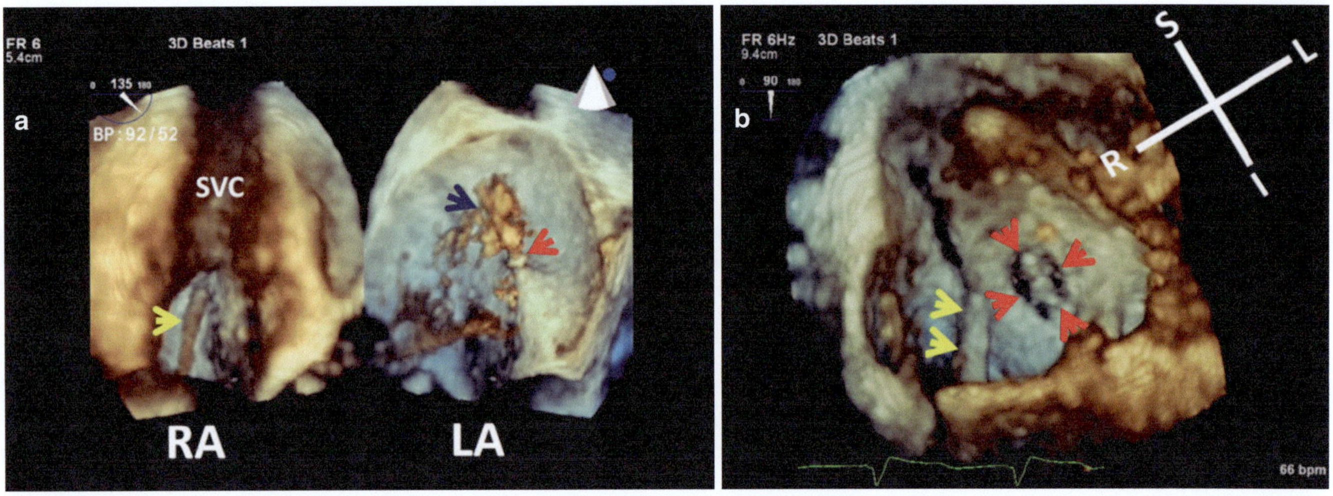

Fig. 29.6 (**a**): Real time 3D zoom dual layout of atrial septum showing actual TSP. Red arrow points to tip of Brockenbrough needle and the dark blue arrow points to contrast injected into LA. Yellow arrow points to Brockenbrough needle delivery system in RA. (**b**): Real time 3D zoom RA: Mullins assembly (yellow arrows) is seen behind fossa ovalis (red arrows). Used with permission of Mayo Foundation for Medical Education and Research. All rights reserved. I, inferior; L, left; LA, left atrium; R, right; RA, right atrium; S, superior; SVC, superior vena cava; TSP, transseptal puncture

One or two Amplatz wires are next advanced through the Mullins sheath and anchored in the LSPV (Fig. 29.7). Next, the Mullins sheath is removed over the Amplatz wire and may be replaced by an Inoue septal dilator (see Fig. 29.4, Chap. 31) to facilitate delivery of the steerable guide cathether (SGC) and clip delivery system (CDS) through the atrial septum. A 4F multipurpose catheter may be advanced over an Amplatz wire for continuous LA pressure monitoring (Figs. 29.8, 29.10, and 29.11). 3D TEE is an invaluable tool to guide all these steps from a single window and without the need for excessive probe manipulation. *Unsuitable sites for transseptal access include patent foramen ovale because of its far anterior location, and atrial septal defects because the MitraClip delivery sheath cannot be stabilized in the defect and there is increased risk of atrial septal tear.*

The SGC is a large sized (24F) sheath with its own dilator through which the clip delivery system (CDS) is advanced into the left atrium. On 3D imaging it may appear as a tubular structure with a clear center that is flanked by two linear echoes due to railroad-shaped artifact (see Fig. 29.13a, Chap. 3), and an echo bright radio opaque double ring characterizes its tip (Fig. 29.8).

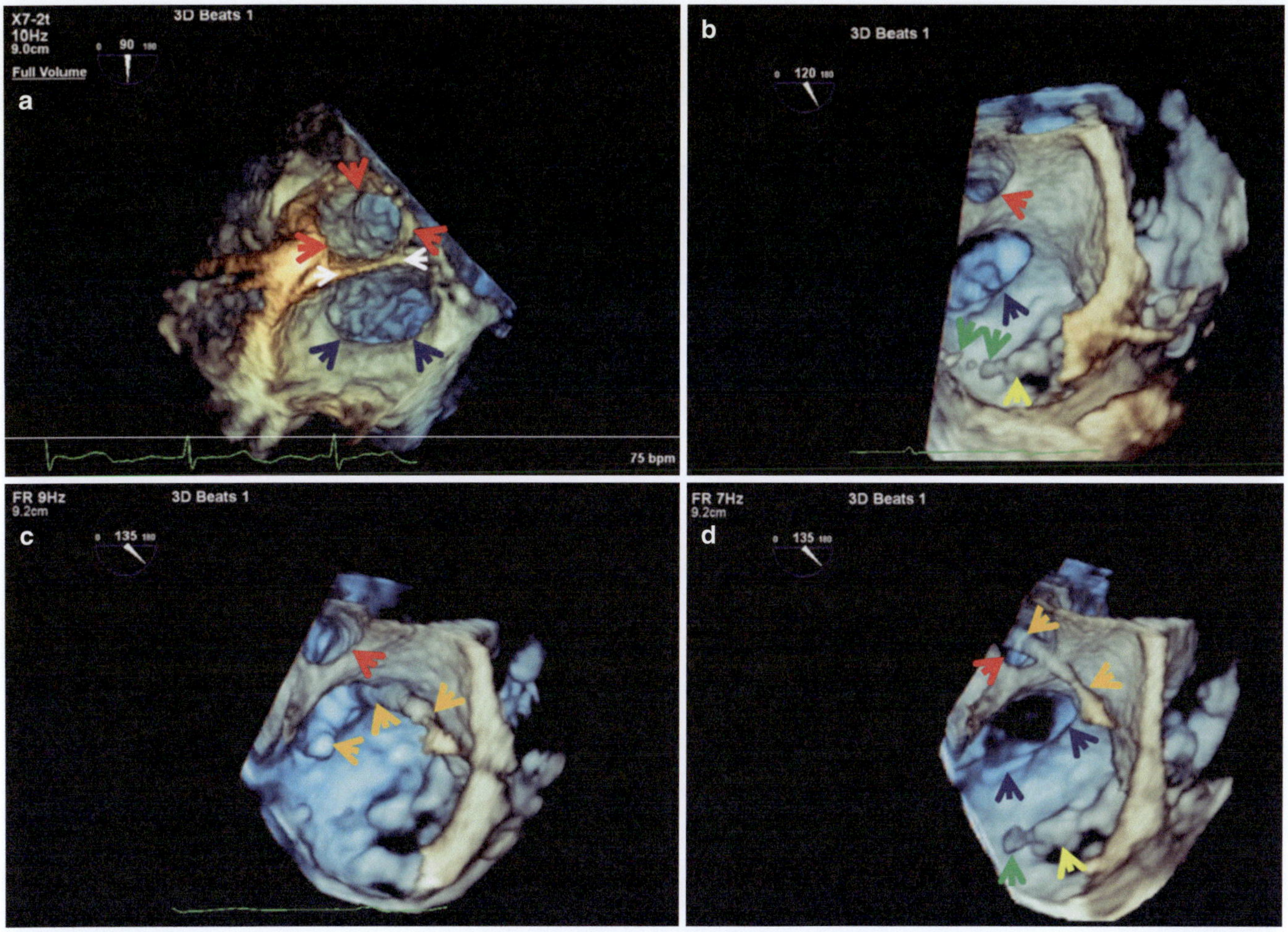

Fig. 29.7 (**a** and **b**): Real time enface LA views of ostia of LAA (dark blue arrows) and LSPV (red arrows). White arrows point to the left lateral ridge also known as the Coumadin ridge. (**c**): Amplatz extra stiff wire (orange arrows) curling at ostium of LAA. (**d**): Amplatz extra stiff wire (orange arrows) parked inside LSPV (red arrows, **c** and **d**). Yellow arrows points to AML and green arrows point to ruptured chordae (**b** and **d**). Used with permission of Mayo Foundation for Medical Education and Research. All rights reserved. AML, anterior mitral leaflet; LAA, left atrial appendage; LSPV, left superior pulmonary vein

The SGC is advanced into the left atrium over the Amplatz wire that was anchored in the LSPV (Fig. 29.7). Advancement of the SGC within the LA can be continuously monitored using 3D TEE and distance of SGC tip from septum can be quantified (Fig. 29.8). This avoids inadvertent puncturing of the LA free wall. After the SGC is safely placed in the LA, its dilator is retrieved first, followed by the Amplatz wire.

The MitraClip device consists of two arms, and two grippers used to grasp the opposing free edges of the anterior and posterior leaflet, and are readily seen on 3D TEE (Fig. 29.9). Both arms and grippers are covered with polyester fabric to enhance endothelialization. *MitraClip XTR has a 3 mm wider arm span than MitraClip NTR intended to improve grasping and reach (*Fig. 29.9*), and both have an improved clip delivery system compared with the first generation MitraClip.*

The CDS is advanced into the left atrium through the SGC under continuous fluoroscopic and TEE guidance (Fig. 29.10). It is necessary during this step to ensure that the tip of the SGC remains across the atrial septum (Figs. 29.8 and 29.10), and to continuously track the CDS as it is advanced within the left atrium to ensure that it remains away from the LA free wall and LAA. Whereas with 2D TEE this step requires multiple views in different planes and multiple probe manipulations, with 3D TEE enface imaging permits visualization and tracking of the SGC and CDS within the left atrium. The MitraClip can be seen in real time as it advances through and exits the SGC.

In order to position the CDS above the MV, the SGC is angled down towards the mitral leaflets using several maneuvers (Figs. 29.10 and 29.11). Instead of the frequent probe manipulations and multiple views necessary with 2D TEE guidance during this step, real time live 3D using either FV or

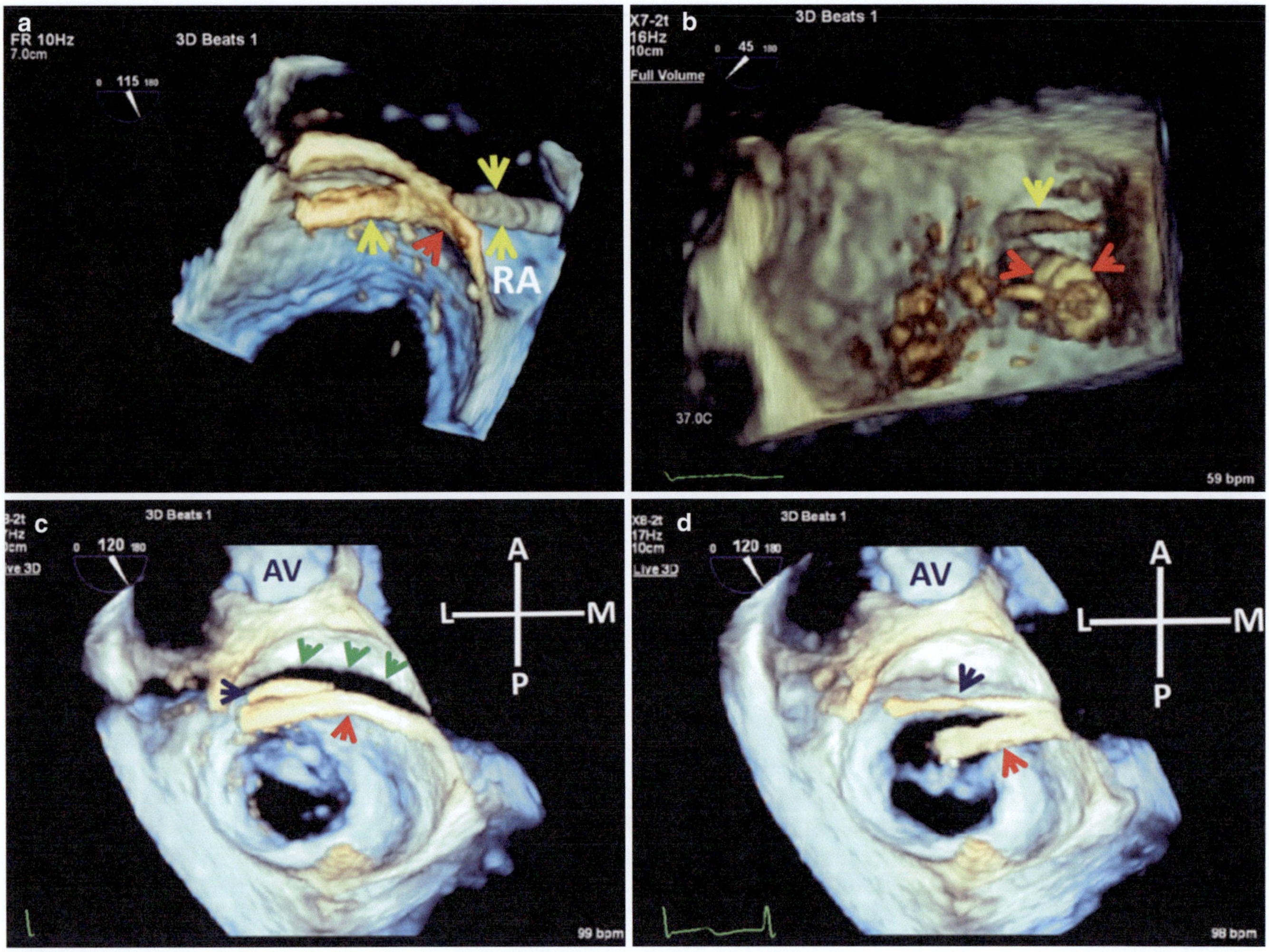

Fig. 29.8 **Top panel**. (**a**): SGC (yellow arrows) crossing atrial septum (red arrow) from RA. (**b**): Enface view of SGC with its distinctive double ring tip (red arrows), and multipurpose LA pressure monitoring catheter (yellow arrow). **Bottom panel** (**c** and **d**): SGC (red arrow) being advanced into LA (**c**) and pulled back towards the atrial septum (**d**). Dark blue arrow points to multipurpose LA pressure monitoring catheter. Green arrows point to acoustic shadow artifact caused by the catheters. Used with permission of Mayo Foundation for Medical Education and Research. All rights reserved. A, anterior; AV, aortic valve; L, lateral; LA, left atrium; M, medial; P, posterior; RA, right atrium; SGC, steerable guide catheter

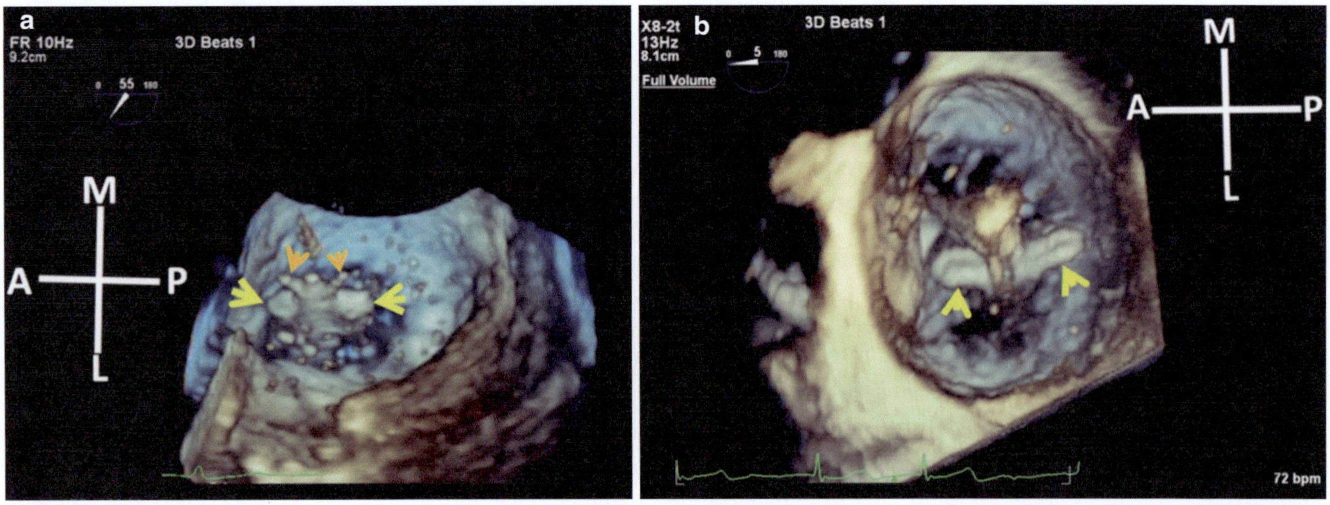

Fig. 29.9 Enface LA views of the MitraClip. (**a**): NTR clip with its open arms (yellow arrows) and two grippers (orange arrows) in a semi open position. (**b**): XTR clip with its wider arm span (yellow arrows). Used with permission of Mayo Foundation for Medical Education and Research. All rights reserved. A, anterior; L, lateral; LA, left atrium; M, medial; P, posterior

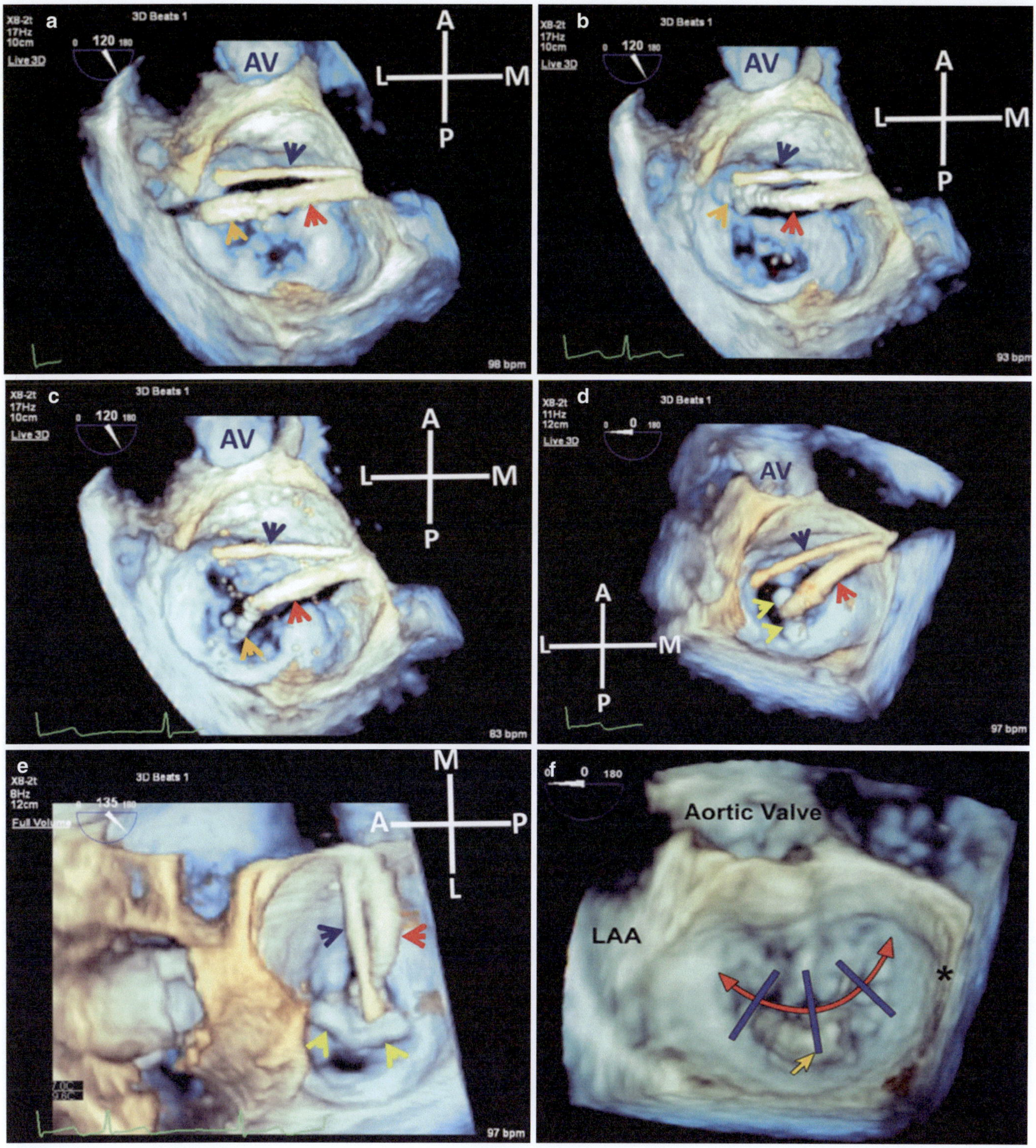

Fig. 29.10 (**a–d**): Sequential collage of enface real time 3D LA views showing angulation of the SGC (red arrow) and MitraClip (orange arrow) towards plane of the mitral valve. Yellow arrows point to open Mitraclip arms. (**e**): open Mitraclip arms (yellow arrows) perpendicular to A2-P2 as viewed enface from LAA. Red arrow points to SGC. (**f**): 3D TEE MV LA view demonstrating schematic of perpendicular orientation of the MitraClip arms (blue lines) relative to the curvilinear relationship of the anterior and posterior leaflets from medial to lateral (curved double arrowed red line with the arrows pointing to the medial and lateral commissures); orange arrow points to flail P2. * marks the IAS. Dark blue arrow in all images points to a multipurpose LA pressure catheter. Used with permission of Mayo Foundation for Medical Education and Research. All rights reserved. A, anterior; AV, aortic valve; IAS, interatrial septum; L, lateral; LA, left atrium; LAA, left atrial appendage; M, medial; P, posterior

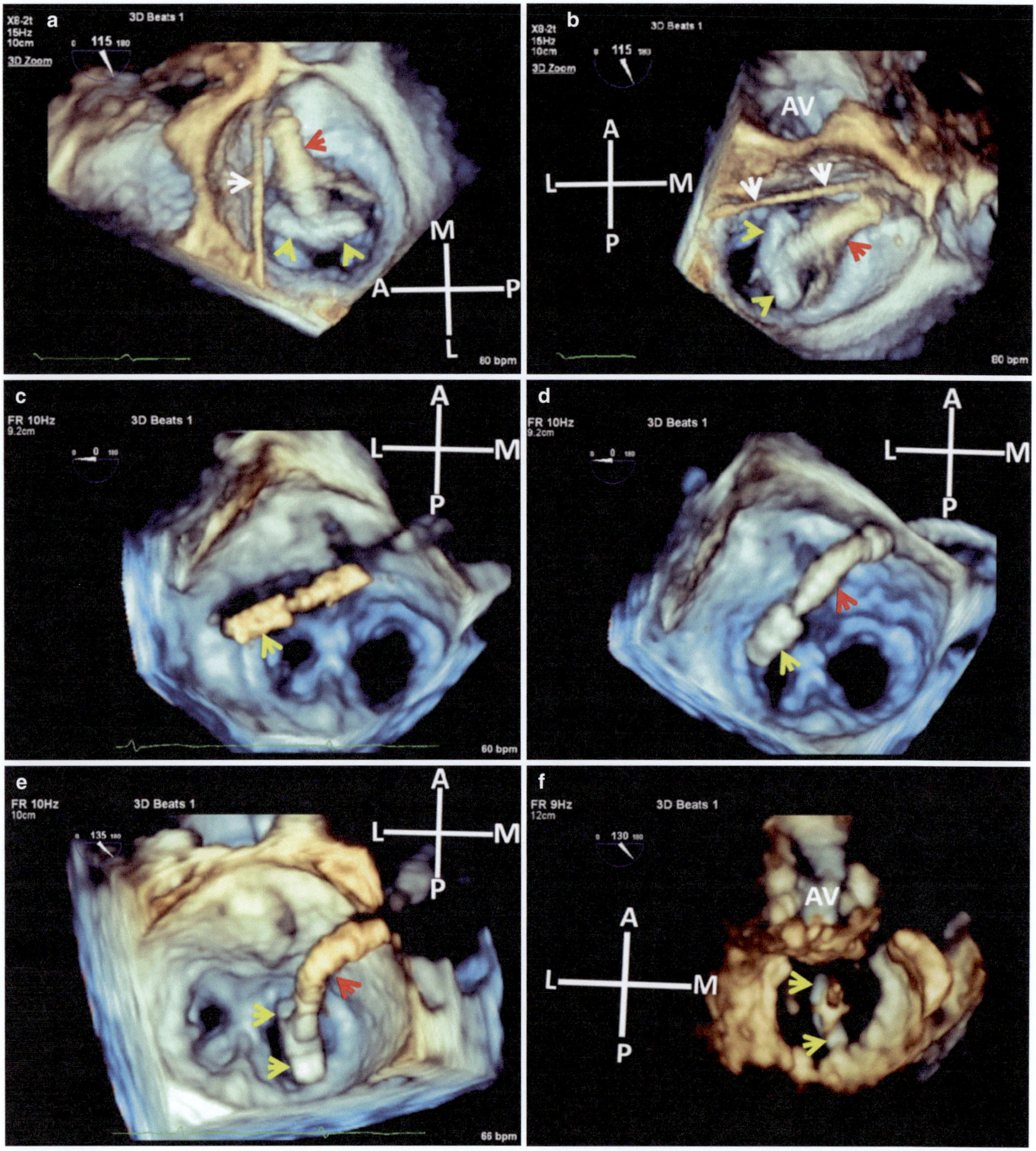

Fig. 29.11 (**a** and **b**): Perpendicular alignment of XTR MitraClip arms (yellow arrows) in a patient with central MR. Red arrow points to SGC and white arrows point to a multipurpose pressure catheter. (**c** and **d**): Maneuvering a second NTR Mitraclip (yellow arrow) into position in a different patient. Red arrow points to SGC. (**e**): perpendicular alignment of second Mitraclip arms (yellow arrows) medial to first Mitraclip. Red arrow points to SGC. (**f**): Ensuring continued perpendicular arms (arrows) alignment when MitraClip is advanced into LV by lowering overall gain setting. Used with permission of Mayo Foundation for Medical Education and Research. All rights reserved. A, anterior; AV, aortic valve; L, lateral; M, medial; MR, mitral regurgitation; P, posterior; SGC, steerable guide catheter

3D zoom with wide angle acquisition can greatly facilitate this part of the procedure as it provides an intuitive en-face view (surgeon's view) of the mitral leaflets and approaching clip. Assuring perpendicularity of the open arms of the advancing MitraClip to line of malcoaptation is of paramount importance and is challenging with 2DTEE, particularly in patients with non-central MR (either medial or lateral to A2-P2 scallops or paracommissural) [4] because of the curvilinear relationship of the anterior and posterior leaflets from medial to lateral commissure, but relatively easy with 3D TEE (Fig. 29.10f).

Enface 3D color flow Doppler (CFD) imaging from the LA and LV surfaces of the MV using appropriate filter settings can assist in localizing the jet origin, thus facilitating proper alignment of the clip arms. 3D TEE can guide medial/lateral, anterior/posterior repositioning and clockwise or counter clockwise rotation of the MitraClip as it is being advanced towards the plane of the MV (Figs. 29.10 and 29.11). Live 3D is also invaluable in guiding placement of additional clips when necessary (Fig. 29.11).

Advancing the MitraClip into the left ventricle remains primarily 2D TEE guided. 3D TEE is used to ensure continued perpendicularity of the open arms to the line of leaflet malcoaptation (Fig. 29.11f) because the MitraClip device may rotate as it is advanced from the LA to the LVin preparation for leaflet grasping. Lowering the overall gain provides a good view of the open arms of the MitraClip in the left ventricle and their orientation relative to the line of coaptation (Fig. 29.11f). 3D TEE color flow Doppler enface views of the MV from the LV may also help confirm splitting of the MR jet by the MitraClip. Pull back from the LV towards the LA and grasping of the MV leaflets remains exclusively a 2D TEE guided step with no role for 3D TEE except when proper orientation of the clip arms is in question. xPlane can be helpful, however (Fig. 29.12).

Adequacy of tissue grasp is best judged by 2D imaging of the partially closed clip but can also be appreciated on 3D imaging (Fig. 29.13). Leaflet tissue must be seen between the clip arms and the grippers. Restricted motion of both leaflets must be seen as well, to indicate adequate approximation of leaflet edges by the MitraClip. x-Plane/biplane imaging is very useful during this step. After full closure of the MitraClip, it is necessary to assess the morphology of the mitral valve and to determine the severity of residual regurgitation and stenosis prior to release of the MitraClip. Echocardiographic grading of residual MR after MitraClip deployment is very challenging. The presence of multiple or eccentric jets can lead to underestimation of MR severity by 2D echocardiography (2DE) based techniques [5]. This is compounded by the fact that the newly distorted mitral valve anatomy can not be assumed to fit the geometric assumptions that support measurements using the proximal isovelocity surface acceleration or venacontracta width methods [5]. With 3D TEE color Doppler, the number, location, and extent of MR jets may be better appreciated (Fig. 29.14). It may also be possible to quantify severity of residual MR after a MitraClip procedure by measureing the 3D vena contracta area [5] (Fig. 29.15).

Final orifice size and geometry can be evaluated best on 3D using either either FV or 3D zoom formats. The MV should be imaged enface from both the LA and LV projections (Fig. 29.16). The enface LV 3D view is particularly helpful when more than one MitraClip is deployed to verify

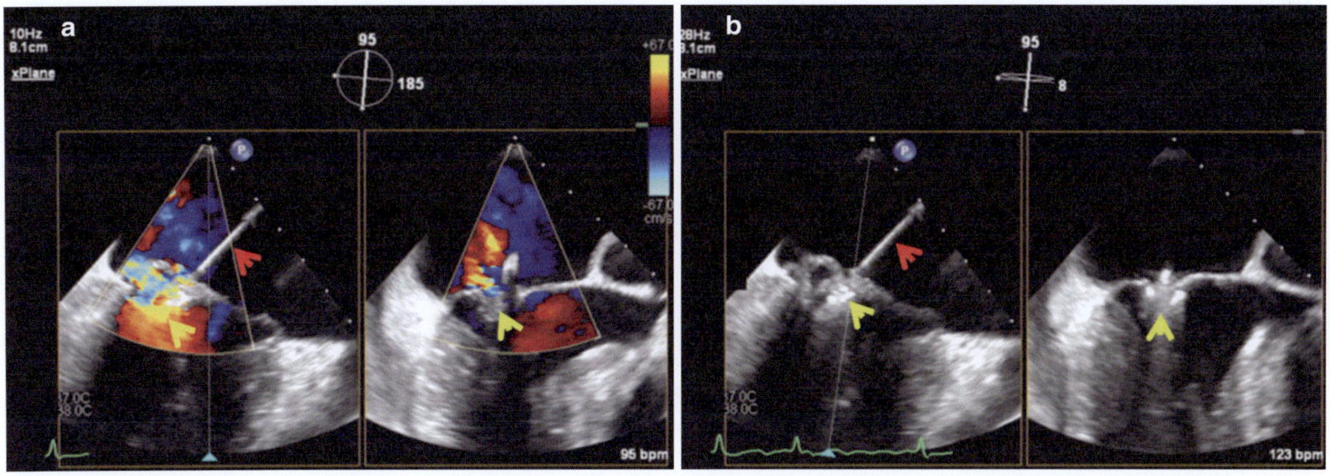

Fig. 29.12 (**a** and **b**): xPlane (Philips Healthcare) guidance of Mitraclip (yellow arrows) positioning with respect to origin of MR jet prior to leaflet grasping. Red arrow points to the lock line of the CDS. Used with permission of Mayo Foundation for Medical Education and Research. All rights reserved. CDS, clip delivery system

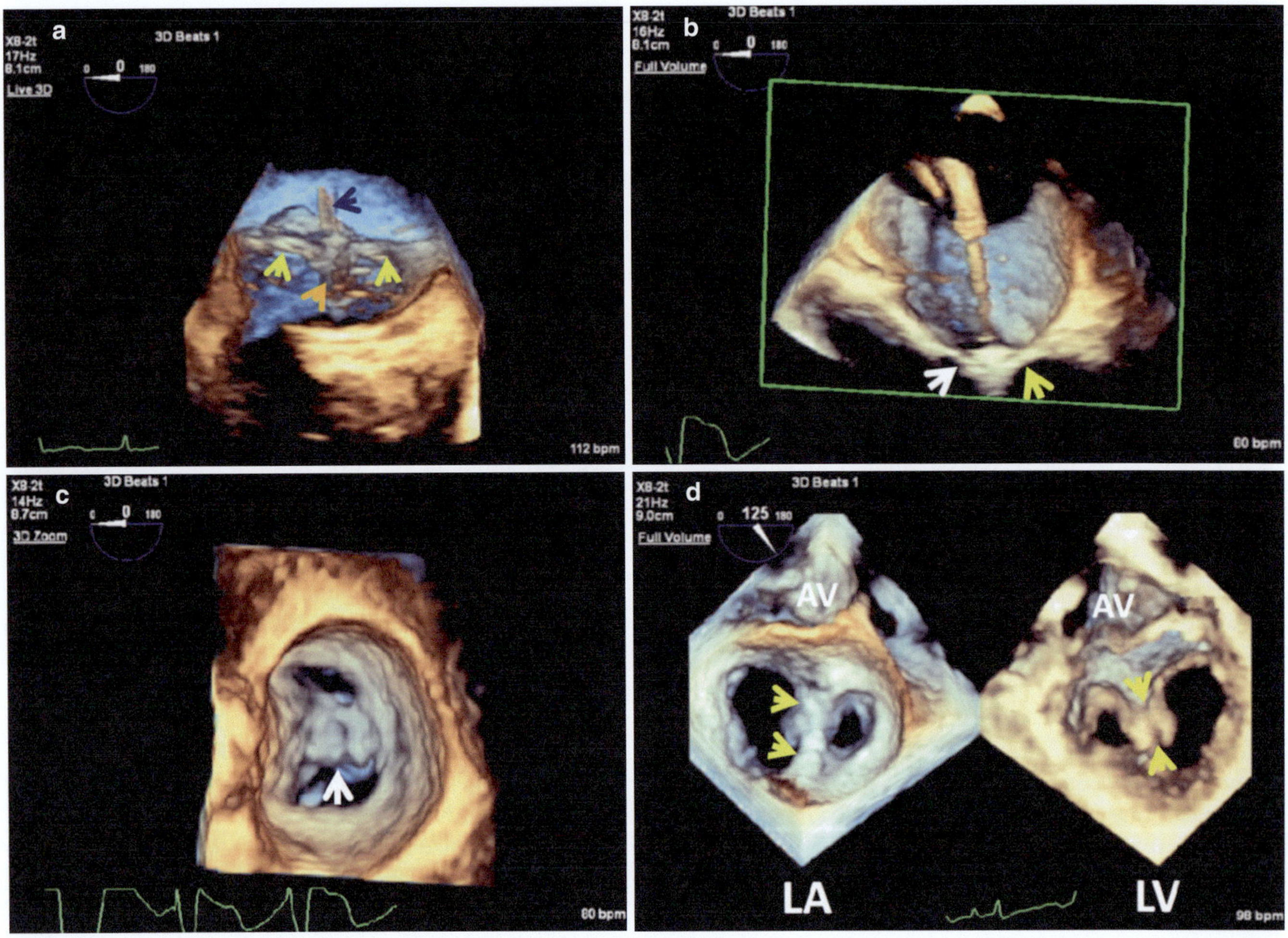

Fig. 29.13 Tissue bridge: (**a**): Live 3D TEE enface view of XTR MitraClip arms (yellow arrows) showing an excellent tissue bridge prior to release of MitraClip. Orange arrow points to leading edge of the Mitraclip device in the LV and dark blue arrow points to lock line of the CDS. (**b**): Live auto-cropped FV 3D of NTR MitraClip prior to being released showing good grasping of the AML (white arrow) and PML (yellow arrow) between the Mitraclip arms and grippers. (**c**): Live 3D Zoom of post NTR MitraClip release tissue bridge (white arrow) between AML and PML. The MV is viewed from its side. (**d**): Live 3DTEE enface FV dual layout (LA and LV) views of the MV post release of XTR MitraClip showing an excellent tissue bridge (yellow arrows). Note the unequal double orifice. Used with permission of Mayo Foundation for Medical Education and Research. AML, anterior mitral leaflet; AV, aortic valve; CDS, clip delivery system; FV, Full Volume; LA, left atrium; LV, left ventricle; MV, mitral valve; PML, posterior mitral leaflet

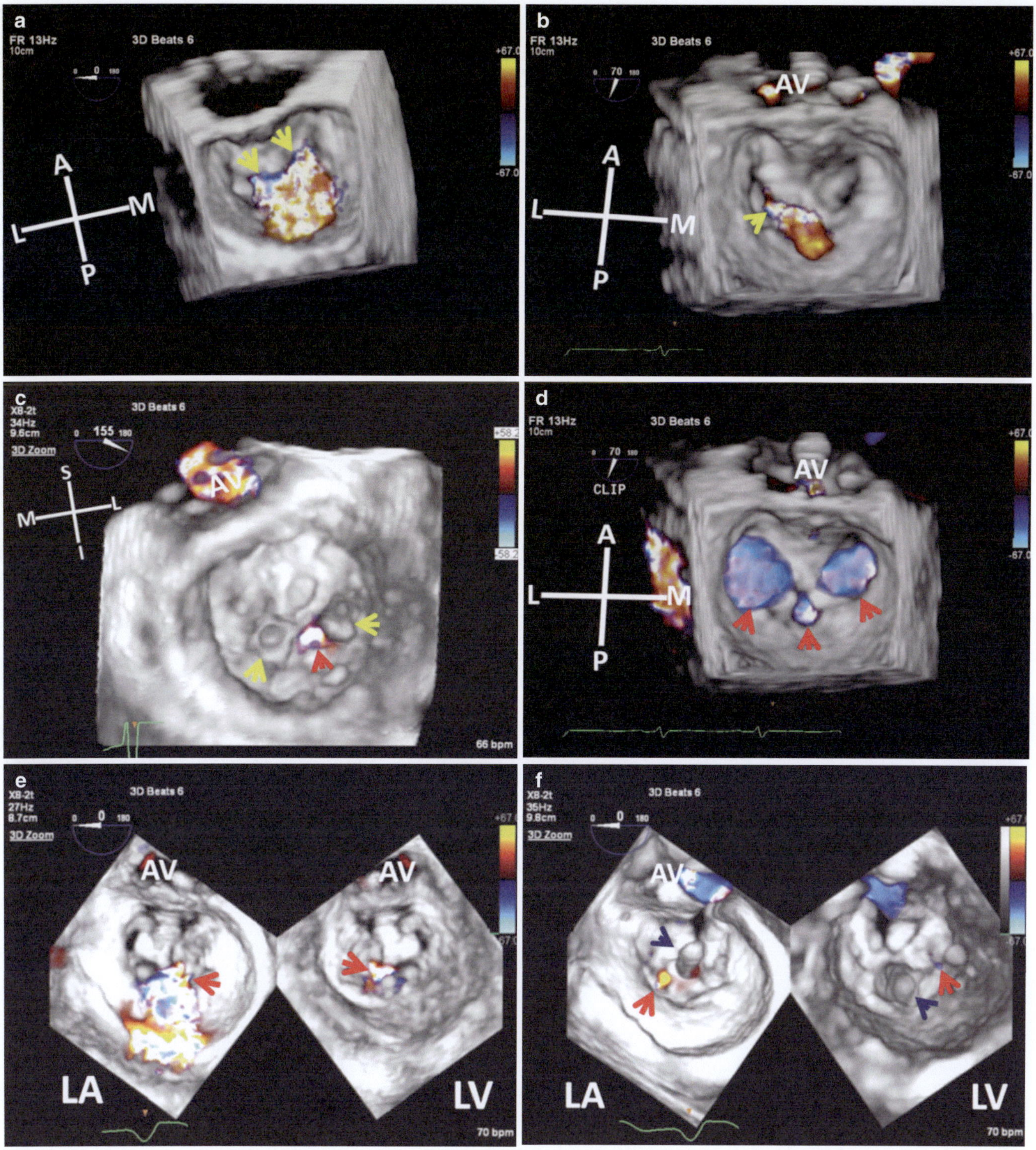

Fig. 29.14 3D TEE multibeat CFD. **Top panel**: Enface LA views of the MV showing MR before (**a**, arrows) and after Mitraclip deployment (**b**, arrow) **Middle panel**. (**c**): Enface LV view of residual central MR (red arrow) following deployment of two Mitraclips (yellow arrows). (**d**): LA view post MitraClip deployment diastolic frame showing two large orifices, and a smaller orifice (red arrows). **Bottom panel**: Enface dual layout LA and LV views before (**e**) and after deployment of a single Mitraclip (**f**, dark blue arrows) showing marked reduction in MR jet (red arrows). Used with permission of Mayo Foundation for Medical Education and Research. All rights reserved. A, anterior; AV, aortic valve; CFD, color flow Doppler; I, inferior; L, lateral; LA, left atrium; LV, left ventricle; M, medial; MR, mitral regurgitation; MV, mitral valve; P, posterior; S, superior

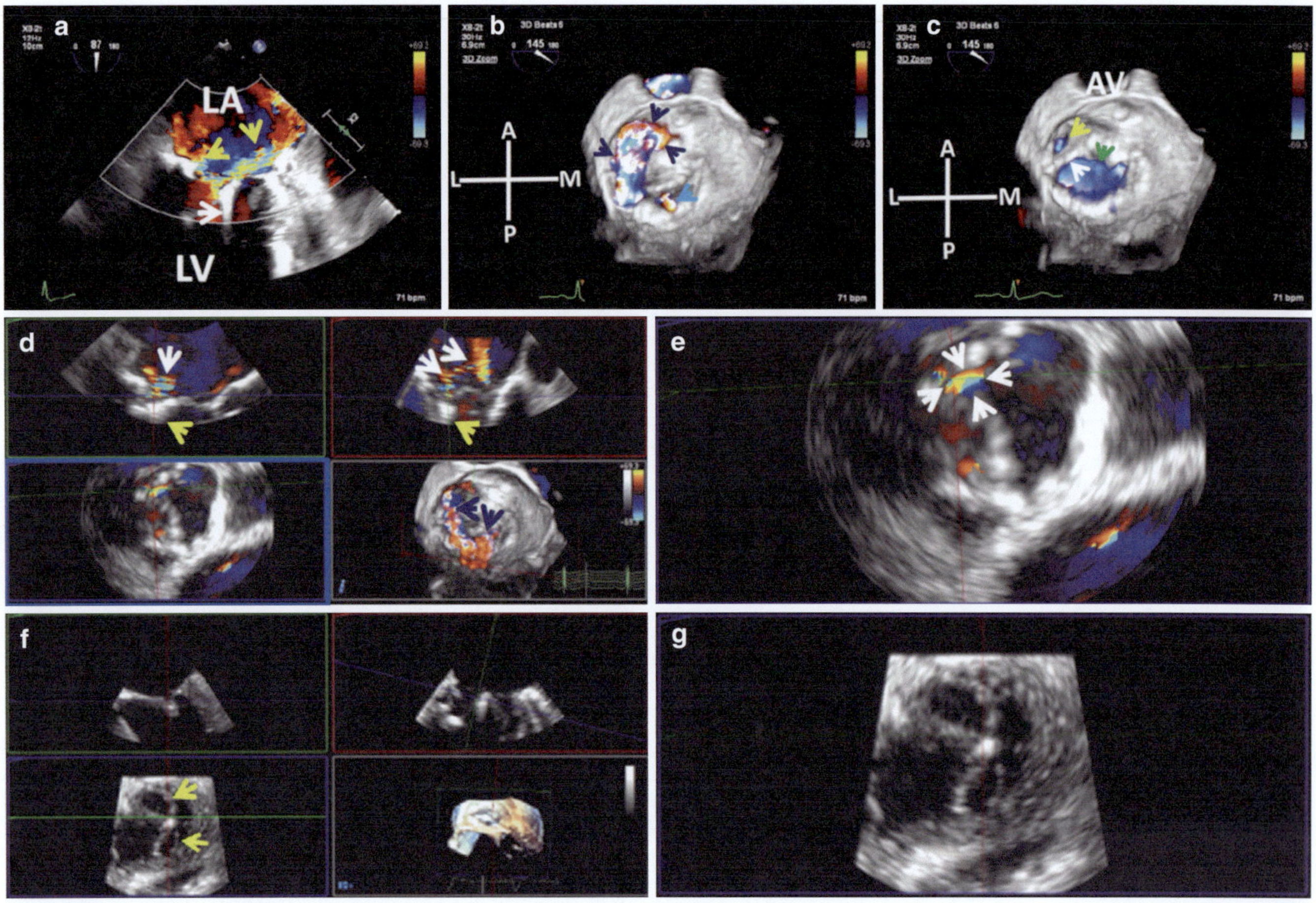

Fig. 29.15 (**a–e**). Quantifying severity of post MitraClip MR. (**a**): 2D color Doppler shows the MitraClip (white arrow) and MR jet (yellow arrows) that splits in LA and is eccentric in its trajectory. (**b** and **c**): 3DTEE CFD enface LA views of the MV post MitraClip deployment in systole (**b**) and diastole (**c**). The Mitraclip (white arrow) is seen. Note the asymmetric double orifice (green and yellow arrows) and eccentric MR (dark blue arrows). Light blue arrow points to a second trivial MR jet. (**d**): MPR of same MR (white arrows on MPR and dark blue arrows on 3D volume lower right) with delineation of the VC area in the transverse plane (blue box, left lower quadrant). Yellow arrows point to MitraClip. (**E**): Enlarged image of the VC in the transverse plane (arrows). The VC area or EROA measured 0.28 cm.sq. on planimetry. (**f** and **g**): Post A2-P2 MitraClip deployment. The two residual mitral orifices (yellow arrows in **f** and same image enlarged in **g**) are delineated using MPR and can be planimetered. Used with permission of Mayo Foundation for Medical Education and Research. All rights reserved. A, anterior; AV, aortic valve; CFD, color flow Doppler; EROA, effective regurgitant orifice area; L, lateral; LA, left atrium; LV, left ventricle; M, medial; MPR, multiplanar reconstruction; MR, mitral regurgitation; P, posterior; VC, vena contracta

the side by side positioning of the clips, hence correct deployment, prior to their release (Fig. 29.16). Whereas with central jets, a symmetric double orifice MV is created (Firgure 16), paracentral jets are typically associated with the creation of a large and smaller orifice (Fig. 29.16). The residual mitral orifice(s) area(s) can be planimetered using the 3D measurement software (Fig. 29.15f and g).

When the mitral regurgitation is paracentral and is associated with commissural MR, optimal transcatheter treatment of MR may require placement of an Amplatzer vascular plug

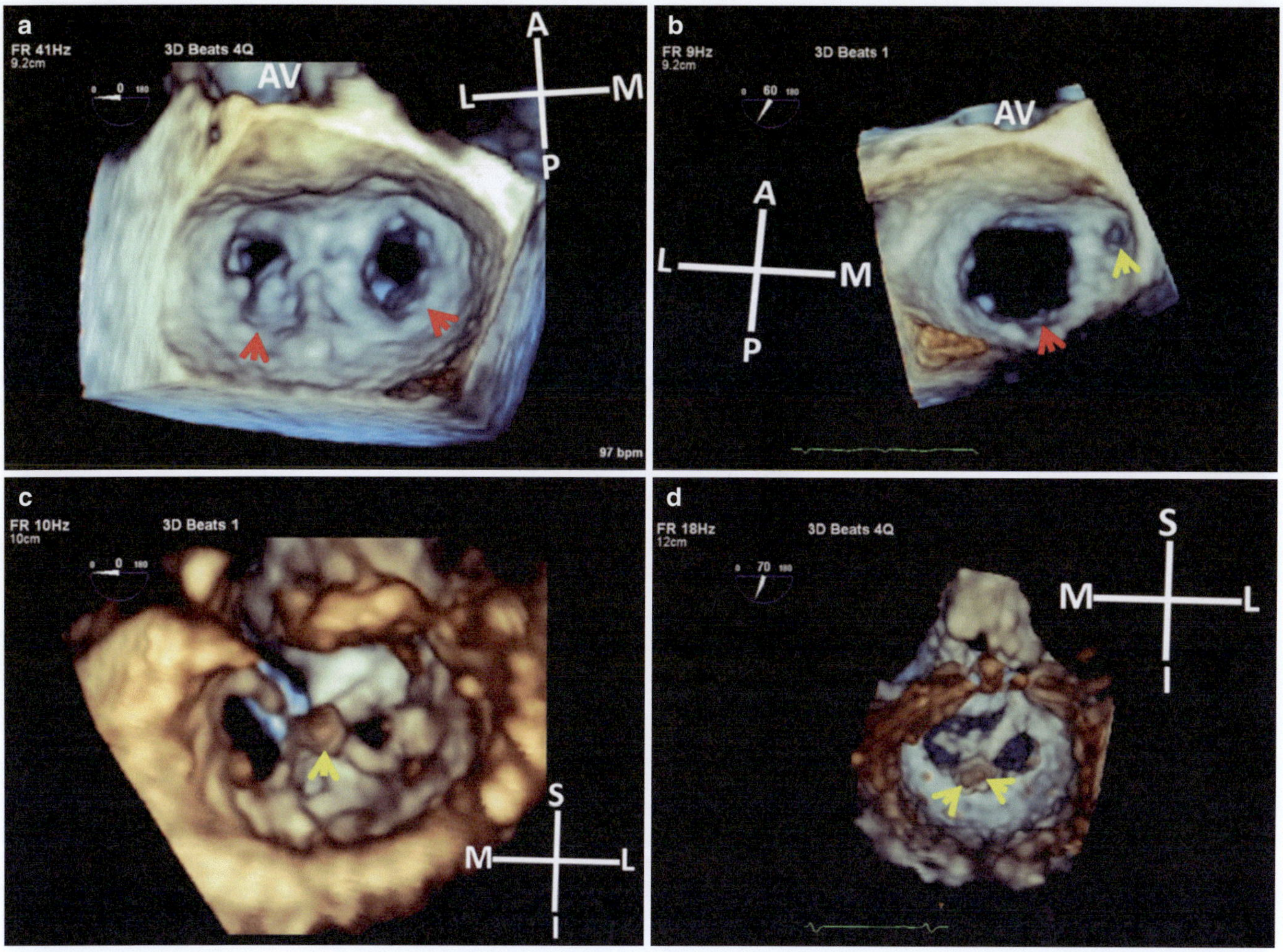

Fig. 29.16 Post Mitraclip deployment. **Top panel**: Enface 3D LA views of MV. (**a**): Double orifice (arrows). (**b**): large single orifice (red arrow) and rudimentary medial orifice (yellow arrow). **Bottom panel**: Enface 3D LV views of MV. (**c**): Single MitraClip (arrow). (**d**): two MitraClips (arrows). Note that the clips are aligned side by side. Used with permission of Mayo Foundation for Medical Education and Research. All rights reserved. A, anterior; AV, aortic valve; I, inferior; L, lateral; LA, left atrium; LV, left ventricle; M, medial; MR, mitral regurgitation; MV, mitral valve; P, posterior; S, superior

occluder between the commissure and MitraClip [6, 7] (Fig. 29.17).

Finally, complications related to MitraClip deployment are fortunately rare, but include leaflet damage or tear, clip embolization, thrombus formation on the clip, and single leaflet device attachment [8]. These complications are usually detected on 2DTEE, but 3D TEE can also be useful (Fig. 29.18).

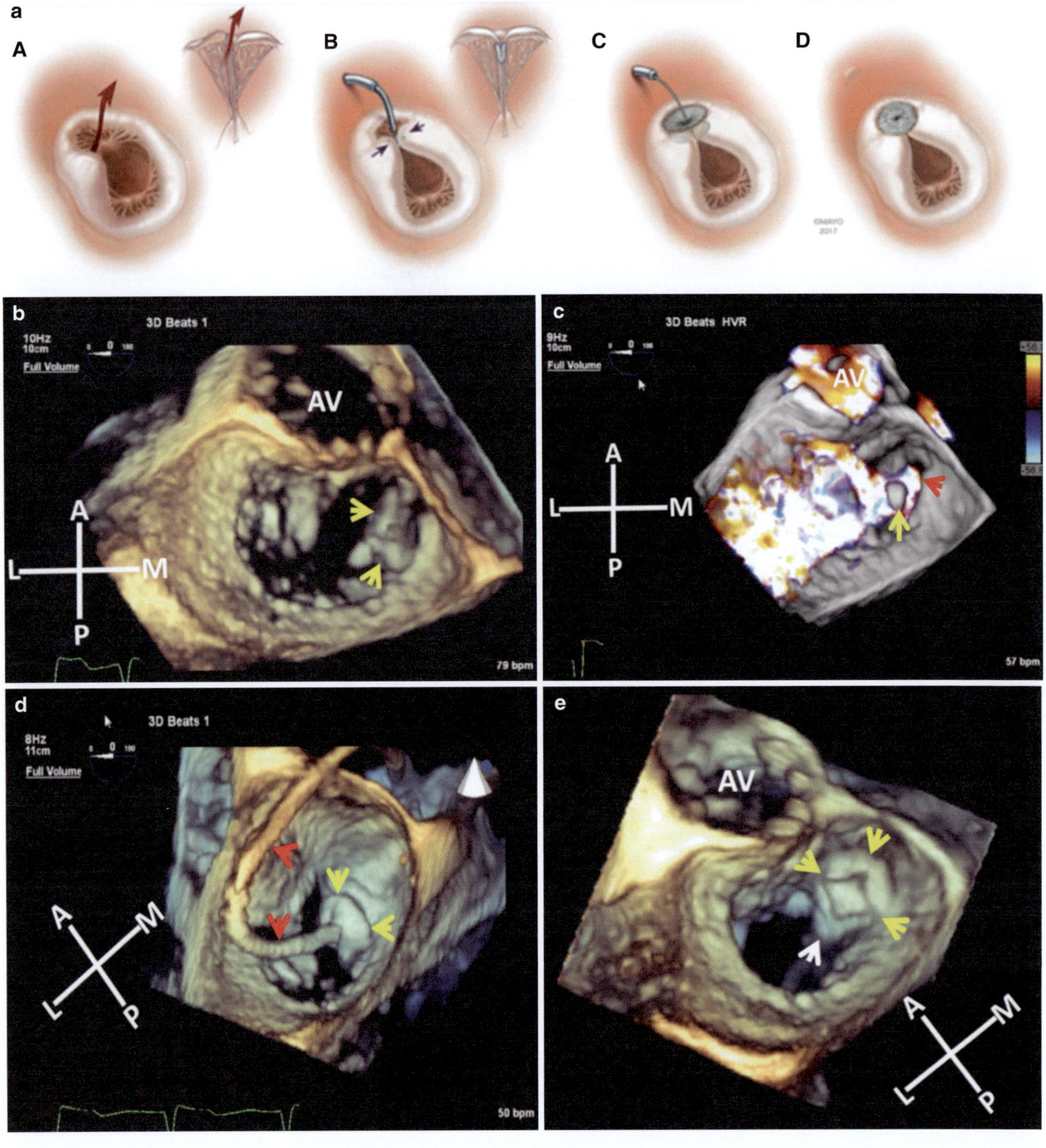

Fig. 29.17 (**a**): Illustration of use of a hybrid MitraClip-AVP II occluder approach for the treatment of associated commissural MR (with permission from Raphael et al.: A hybrid technique for treatment of commissural primary mitral regurgitation. Catheter Cardiovasc Interv. 2019 Mar 1;93(4):692–698). Example case shows MR secondary to A3 prolapse and concomitant commissural MR (**A**). A MitraClip is placed toward A3/P3 (**B**) and released. Next an AVP II occluder is inserted between the MitraClip and the commissure (**C**) and then released (**D**). (**b** and **c**): RT 3D TEE enface LA views post MitraClip deployment (yellow arrows) in a patient with A3-P3 MR and residual medial commissural MR(**c**, red arrow). (**d** and **e**): RT enface LA views of deployment of an AVP II occluder (yellow arrows) between the MitraClip (white arrow) and medial commissure. Red arrows point to AVP delivery catheter. Images B-E are used with permission from Mayo Foundation for Medical Education and Research. All rights reserved. A, anterior; AV, aortic valve; AVP, Amplatzer Vascular Plug; L, lateral; LA, left atrium; M, medial; MR, mitral regurgitation; P, posterior; RT, real time

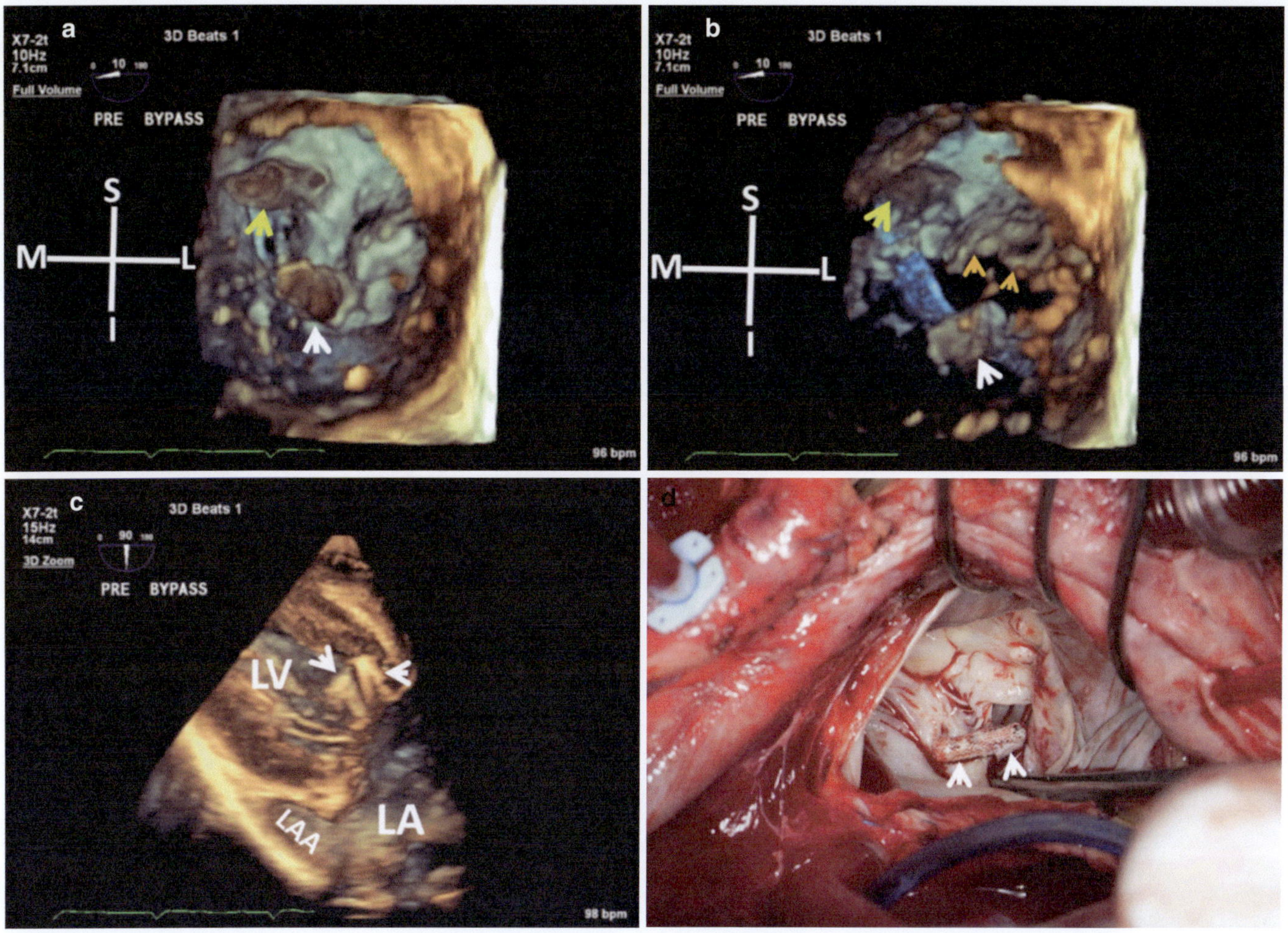

Fig. 29.18 Dislodged MitraClips. (**a** and **b**): Intraoperative pre-bypass live FV enface LV views showing two dislodged MitraClips. An A2/P2 MitraClip (white arrows) is attached to the tip of the posterior leaflet only, and the other MitraClip (yellow arrows) is partially attached to the anterior mitral leaflet at the medial commissure. Orange arrows point to AML. (**c**): TG view of the two dislodged MitraClips (arrows). (**d**): One of the dislodged MitraClips as seen by the surgeon (arrows). Used with permission of Mayo Foundation for Medical Education and Research. All rights reserved. AML, anterior mitral leaflet; FV, Full Volume; I, inferior; L, lateral; LA, left atrium; LAA, left atrial appendage; LV, left ventricle; M, medial; S, superior; TG, transgastric

Referrences

1. Bushari LI, Reeder GS, Eleid MF, Chandrasekaran K, Eriquez-Sarano M, Rihal CS, Maalouf JF. Percutaneous transcatheter edge-to-edge mitraclip technique: a practical "step-by-step" 3-dimensional transesophageal echocardiography guide. Mayo Clinic Proceedings. 94(1):89–102.
2. Faletra FF, Berrebi A, Pedrazzini G, Leo LA, Paiocchi VL, Cautilli G, Casso G, Cassina T, Moccetti T, Malouf JF. 3D transesophageal echocardiography: A new imaging tool for assessment of mitral regurgitation and for guiding percutaneous edge-to-edge mitral valve repair. Prog Cardiovasc Dis. 2017 Nov–Dec;60(3):305–21.
3. Faletra FF, Pedrazzini G, Pasotti E, Muzzarelli S, Dequarti MC, Murzilli R, Schlossbauer SA, Slater IP, Moccetti T. 3D TEE during catheter-based interventions. JACC: Cardiovasc Imag. 2014, March;7(3):292–308.
4. Estévez-Loureiro R, Franzen O, Winter R, Sondergaard L, Jacobsen P, Cheung G, Moat N, Ihlemann N, Ghione M, Price S, Duncan A, Rosenberg TS, Barker S, Di Mario C, Settergren M. Echocardiographic and clinical outcomes of central versus non-central percutaneous edge-to-edge repair of degenerative mitral regurgitation. J Am Coll Cardiol. 2013 December;62(25):2370–7.
5. Eleonora A, Burkhard Mackensen G, El-Tallawi KC, Reisman M, Gruye L, Barker CM, Little SH. Diagnostic value of 3-dimensional vena contracta area for the quantification of residual mitral regurgitation after MitraClip procedure. JACC: Cardiovasc Interv. 2019, March;12(6):582–91.
6. Alkhouli M, El Sabbagh A, Vilarraga HR, Hagler DJ, Rihal C, Eleid M. Novel treatment of residual peri-mitraclip regurgitation with an amplatzer vascular plug II. JACC: Cardiovasc Intervent. 9(17):e171–5.
7. Raphael CE, Malouf JF, Maor E, Panaich SS, Pollak PM, Reeder GS, Rihal CS, Eleid MF. A hybrid technique for treatment of commissural primary mitral regurgitation. Catheter Cardiovasc Interv. 2019 Mar 1;93(4):692–8.
8. Gheorghe L, Ielasi A, Rensing BJWM, Eefting FD, Timmers L, Latib A, Swaans MJ. Complications following percutaneous mitral valve repair. Front Cardiovasc Med. 2019, October;18:1–13.

Periprosthetic Leak Repair

30

Joseph F. Maalouf, Sushil Allen Luis, Jeremy J. Thaden, and Krishnaswamy Chandrasekaran

Introduction

Paravalvular regurgitation also known as periprosthetic leak (PPL) affects 5% to 17% of all surgically implanted prosthetic heart valves [1]. Because reoperation for PPL is associated with a high likelihood of recurrence as well as increased surgical morbidity and mortality, there has been significant growth in percutaneous transcatheter PPL closure, and various devices have been used to close these defects [1–3]. The most commonly used devices are from the Amplatzer family of septal, ductal and vascular occluders (St. Jude Medical, St. Paul, MN) [1–3] (Fig. 30.1). 3D transesophageal echocardiography (3D TEE) is a very useful tool for guiding closure of periprosthetic leaks and for communicating the location and size of periprosthetic defects to the interventional cardiologist (see chap. 15). Additionally, this technique (Fig. 30.2) offers the opportunity to visualize catheters in real-time to guide percutaneous interventions. 3D TEE can also help guide the transseptal puncture when the tip of the transseptal needle is not well seen on 2D TEE (see Fig. 29.4 Chap. 29).

Supplementary Information The online version of this chapter (https://doi.org/10.1007/978-3-030-72941-7_30) contains supplementary material, which is available to authorized users.

J. F. Maalouf (✉)
Professor of Medicine, Mayo Clinic College of Medicine; Director, Interventional Echocardiography; Consultant, Department of Cardiovascular Medicine, Mayo Clinic, Rochester, MN, USA
e-mail: maalouf.joseph@mayo.edu

S. A. Luis
Associate Professor of Medicine, Mayo Clinic College of Medicine; Consultant, Rochester, MN, USA
e-mail: Luis.S@mayo.edu

Role of 3D TEE in Guiding Closure of Mitral PPL

3D TEE is critical to guide closure of mitral PPL. Defect size, shape, number and location (Fig. 30.3; see Chap. 15) need to be effectively communicated to the interventionalist. This is a key element of procedural success and establishing a common language is fundamental. *If the PPL defect exceeds 25% of the sewing ring circumference, device closure may not be possible and risk of device embolization is increased (see* Fig. 15.5 *Chap. 15). If the dehiscence is large multiple devices will be necessary to achieve satisfactory closure.*

Real time 3D TEE enface left atrial views of the mitral prosthesis play a pivotal role in guiding catheter defect cannulation and positioning of the vascular occluder device(s) (Figs. 30.4, 30.5, 30.6, and 30.7). This includes confirming that the guide wire has crossed the defect rather than inadvertently being advanced through the prosthestic valve orifice, and to monitor for interference with prosthesis leaflet function by the vascular device(s) deployed (Fig. 30.9). In the case of mechanical mitral prostheses, only 3D TEE can localize the periprosthetic defect in relation to the fluroscopically visible prosthesis lealfelts and hinges which may prove invaluable in guiding the procedure (Figs. 30.5 and 30.8). *Mitral PPL involving the undersurface of the prosthesis sewing ring or in very close proximity to it (see Figs. 30.4 and 30.5) may be more difficult to close and in the case of mechanical prostheses, a major concern is interference of the vascular plug with motion of the prosthesis leaflets.*

J. J. Thaden
Assistant Professor of Medicine, Mayo Clinic College of Medicine; Co-Chair for Clinical Practice and Quality, Division of Cardiovascular Ultrasound; Consultant, Department of Cardiovascular Medicine, Mayo Clinic, Rochester, MN, USA
e-mail: Thaden.Jeremy@mayo.edu

K. Chandrasekaran
Professor of Medicine, Mayo Clinic College of Medicine; Consultant, Department of Cardiovascular Medicine, Mayo Clinic, Rochester, MN, USA
e-mail: KChandra@mayo.edu

J. F. Maalouf et al. (eds.), *Practical 3D Echocardiography*, https://doi.org/10.1007/978-3-030-72941-7_30

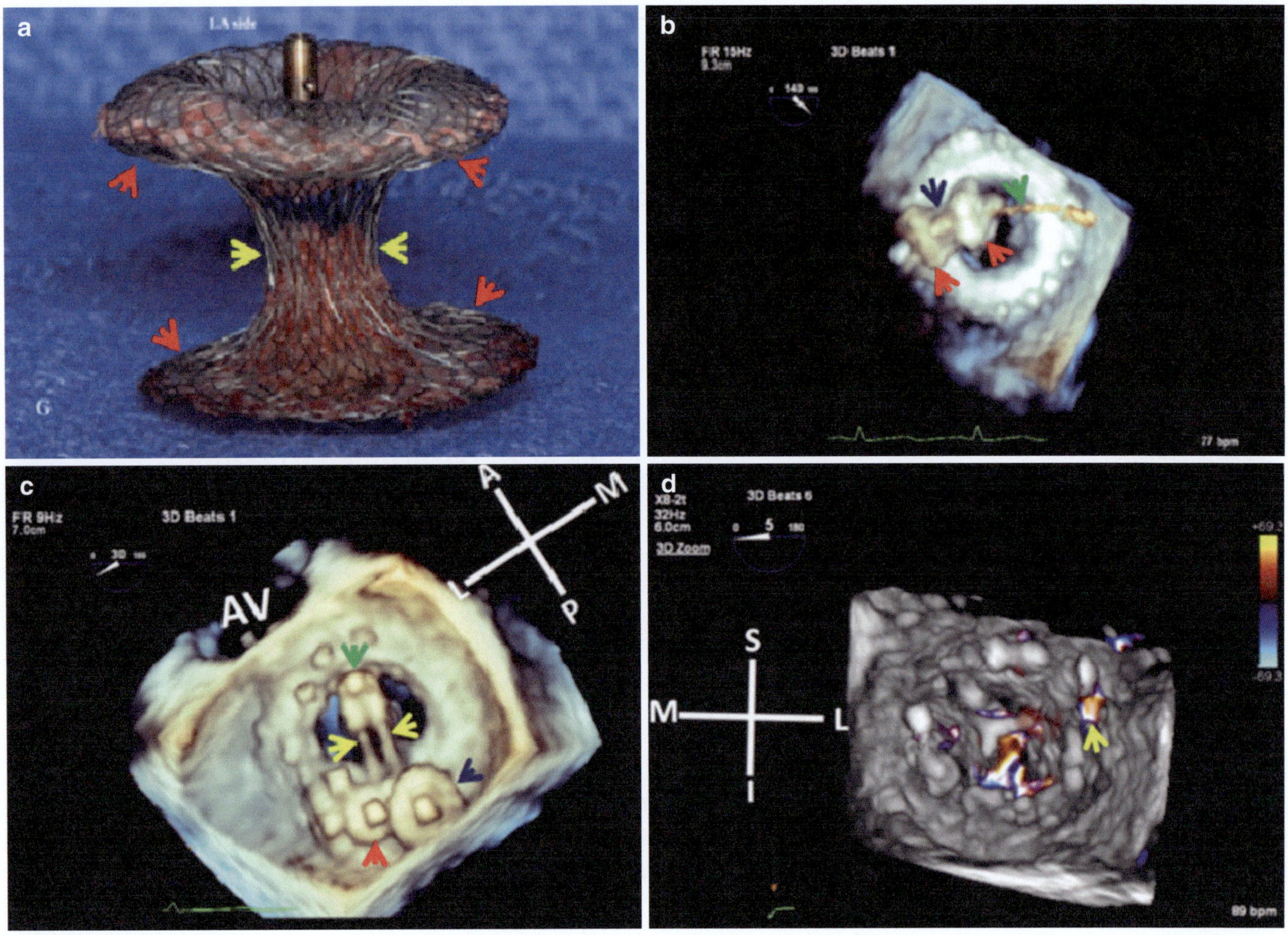

Fig. 30.1 **Top panel**. (**a**): AVP. (**b**): 3D TEE view of AVP. Note the dumbbell like shape, narrower in the middle which appears tubular (**a**: yellow arrows and **b**: dark blue arrow) than on either end that is circular in shape (red arrows). Green arrow points to delivery wire. **Bottom panel**. (**c**): 3DTEE enface LA view of mitral mechanical bileaflet prosthesis post deployment of two AVPs of unequal size (dark blue and red arrows) adjacent to posterior occluder hinge. Green arrow points to anterior hinge and yellow arrows to the bileaflet occluders. (**d**): Multibeat 3D TEE CFD enface LV view of lateral PPL (arrow). This view may help determine the number and size of AVP needed to close the periprosthetic defect. Used with permission of Mayo Foundation for Medical Education and Research. A, anterior; AV, aortic valve; AVP, Amplatzer Vascular Plug; CFD, color flow Doppler; I, inferior; L, lateral; LA, left atrium; M, medial; P, posterior; PPL, periprosthetic leak, S, superior

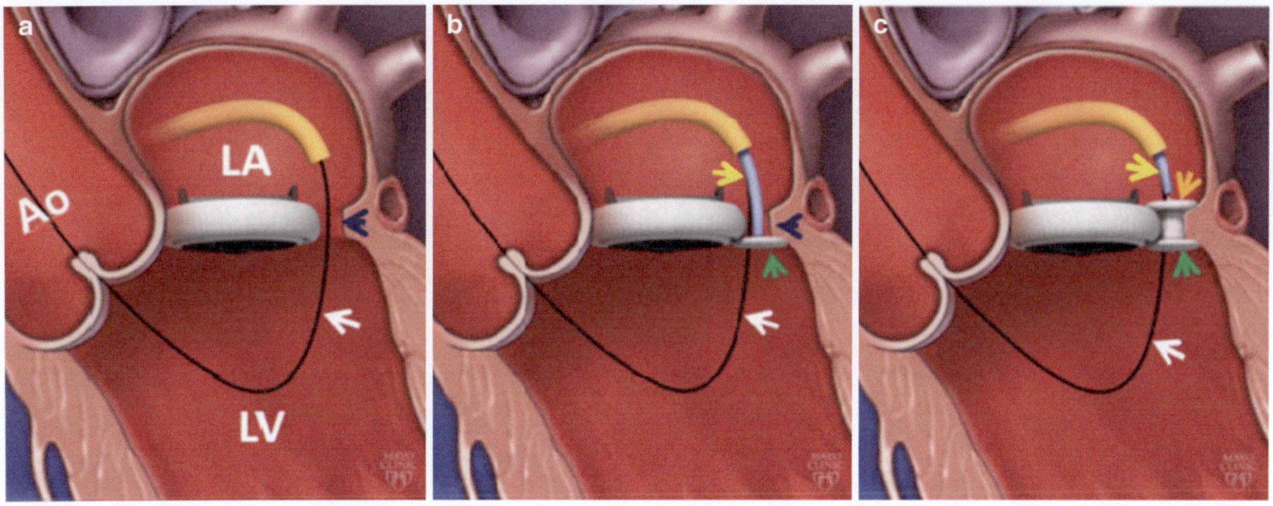

Fig. 30.2 (**a–c**): Animation of AVP deployment to close a periprosthetic defect (dark blue arrow) following TSP. In this illustration, a guide wire (white arrow) is passed through the defect into the LV and out through the aortic valve into the aorta to create an arterio-venous rail. An AVP on a shuttle sheath (yellow arrow) is advanced into the defect over the guide wire (white arrow). The ventricular end of the AVP (green arrow) is deployed first followed by the atrial end (orange arrow). Used with permission of Mayo Foundation for Medical Education and Research. All rights reserved. Ao, ascending aorta; AVP, Amplatzer Vascular Plug; LA, left atrium; LV, left ventricle; TSP, transseptal puncture

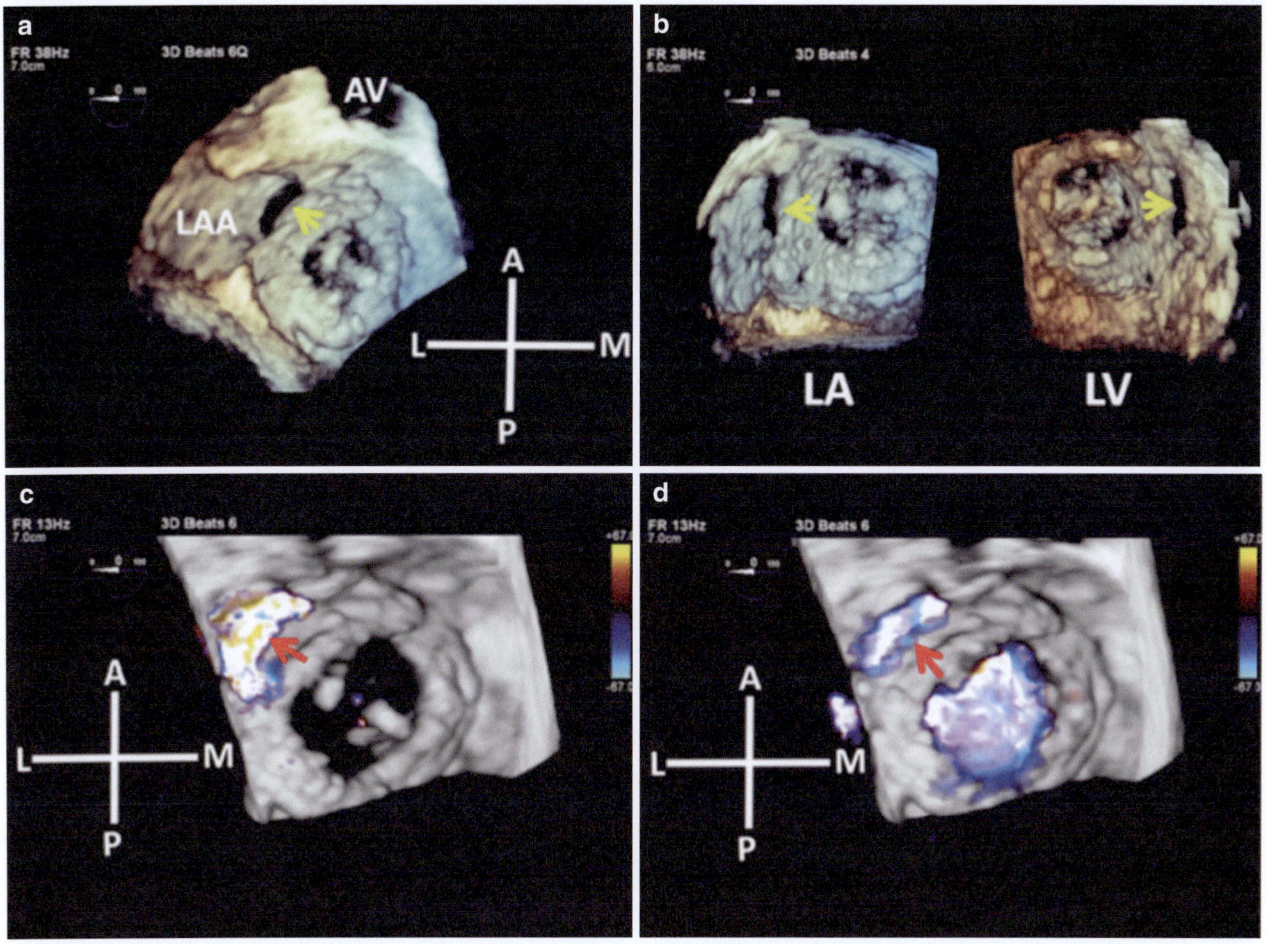

Fig. 30.3 Multibeat 3D TEE prior to closure of a lateral mitral bioprosthesis PPL. **Top panel**. (**a**): Enface LA view of periprosthetic defect adjacent to ostium of LAA (yellow arrow). (**b**): Dual LA and LV layout of the defect (arrows). Note that the enface LV perspective simulates the fluoroscopic view used by interventional cardiologists. **Bottom panel**: Enface LA CFD views of the PPL showing regurgitation into LA in systole (**c**, arrow) and diastolic flow through the periprosthetic defect and prosthesis orifice (**d**). Used with permission of Mayo Foundation for Medical Education and Research. All rights reserved. A, anterior; AV, aortic valve; CFD, color flow Doppler; L, lateral; LA, left atrium; LAA, left atrial appendage; LV, left ventricle; M, medial; P, posterior; PPL, periprosthetic leak

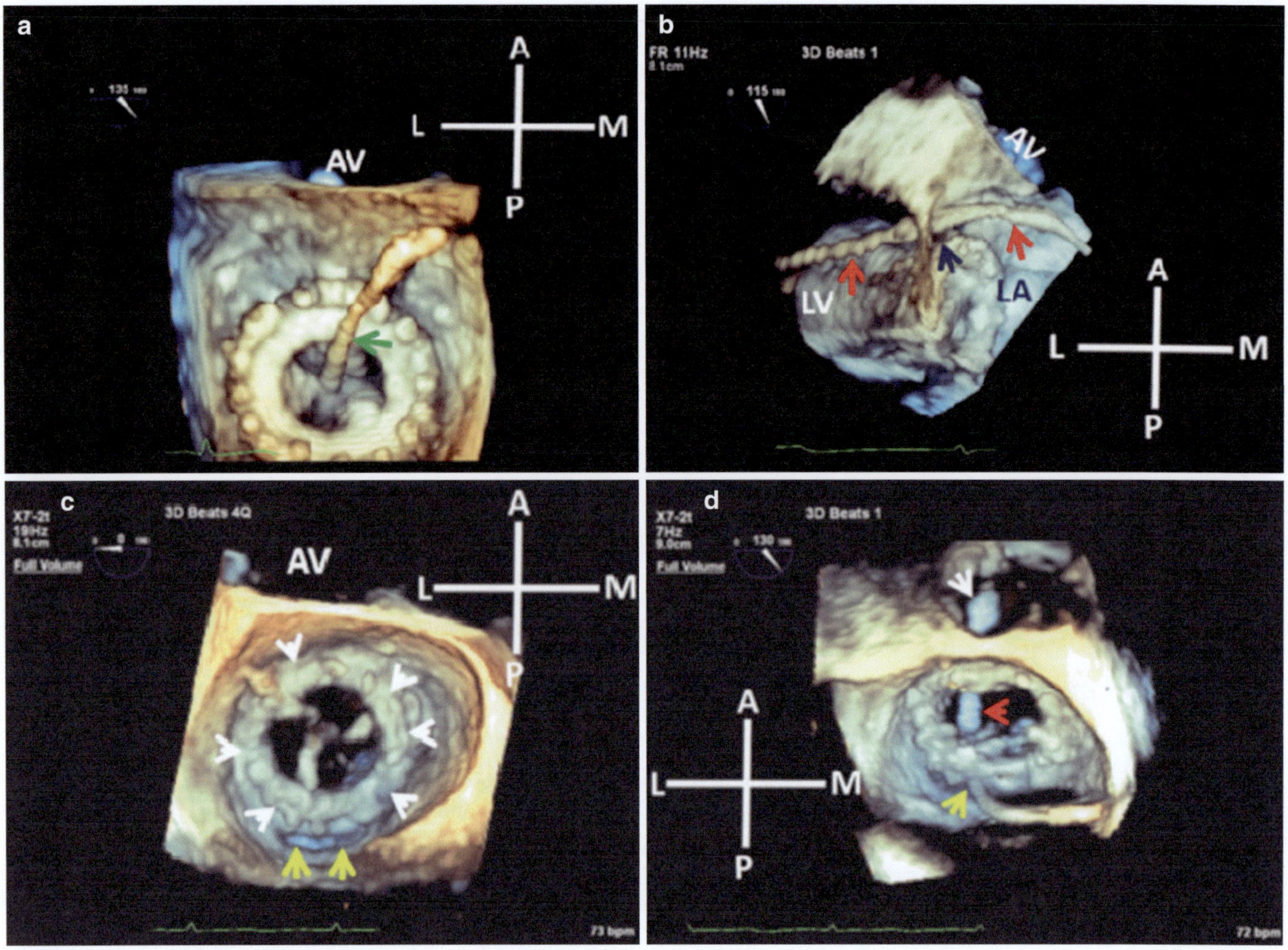

Fig. 30.4 **Top panel:** Real time 3D TEE enface views during transcatheter closure of a PPLfollowing transseptal puncture. (**a**): Guide wire inside prosthesis lumen (arrow). (**b**): Guide wire (red arrows) through a lateral defect (dark blue arrow) into the LV. **Bottom panel**. (**c**): Enface LA view of mitral bioprosthesis with cresent shaped posterior periprosthetic defect (yellow arrows). White arrows point to prosthesis SR. (**d**): Guide wire through the defect (yellow arrow) into the LV (red arrow) and out of the aortic valve (white arrow) to create an arteriovenous rail. Note that on 3D TEE wires can appear thick due to blooming artifacts and distinguishing wires from catheters therefore, may not be possible. Used with permission of Mayo Foundation for Medical Education and Research. All rights reserved. A, anterior; AV, aortic valve; L, lateral; LA, left atrium; LV, left ventricle; M, medial; P, posterior; PPL, periprosthetic leak; SR, sewing ring

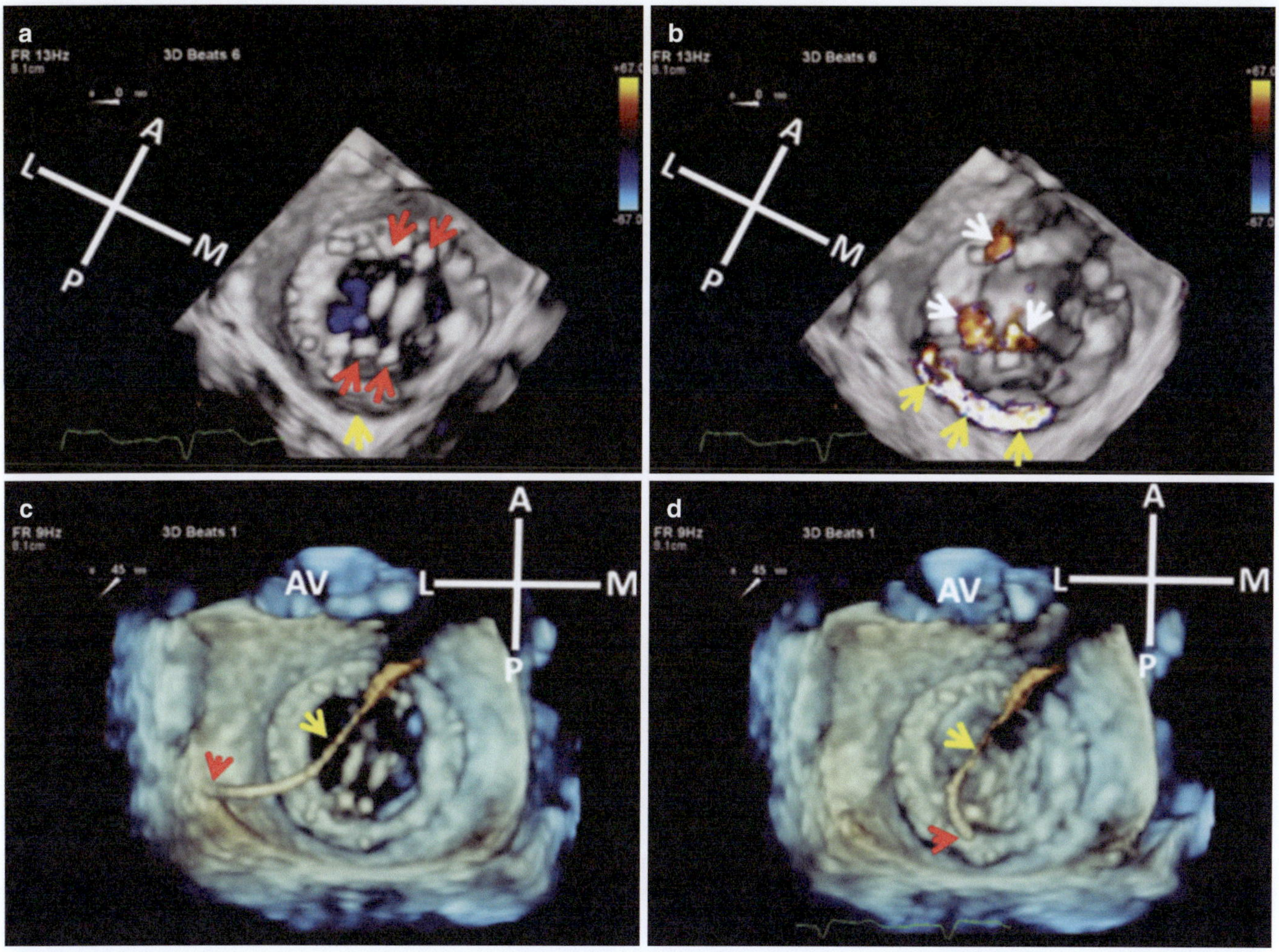

Fig. 30.5 3D TEE enface LA views during closure of a posterior PPL in a patient with a mechanical mitral bileaflet prosthesis. **Top panel:** Multibeat acquisition. The posterior defect (**a**, yellow arrow) is in very close proximity to the prosthesis SR undersurface, and is best appreciated on CFD (**b**, yellow arrows). Red arrows point to the prosthesis bileaflet occluders. Note that the occluder hinges can serve as fluoroscopic beacons to guide closure of mechanical bileaflet PPLs. The white arrows point to built-in prosthesis regurgitation. **Bottom panel:** Intraprocedural live 3D. (**c**): The tip of the guide wire (red arrow) is away from the PPL defect and abuts the LA free wall. (**d**): The tip of the guide wire (red arrow) is inside the defect. Yellow arrows point to proximal segment of the guide wire. Used with permission of Mayo Foundation for Medical Education and Research. All rights reserved. A, anterior; AV, aortic valve; CFD, color flow Doppler; L, lateral; LA, left atrium; M, medial; P, posterior; PPL, periprosthetic leak; SR, sewing ring

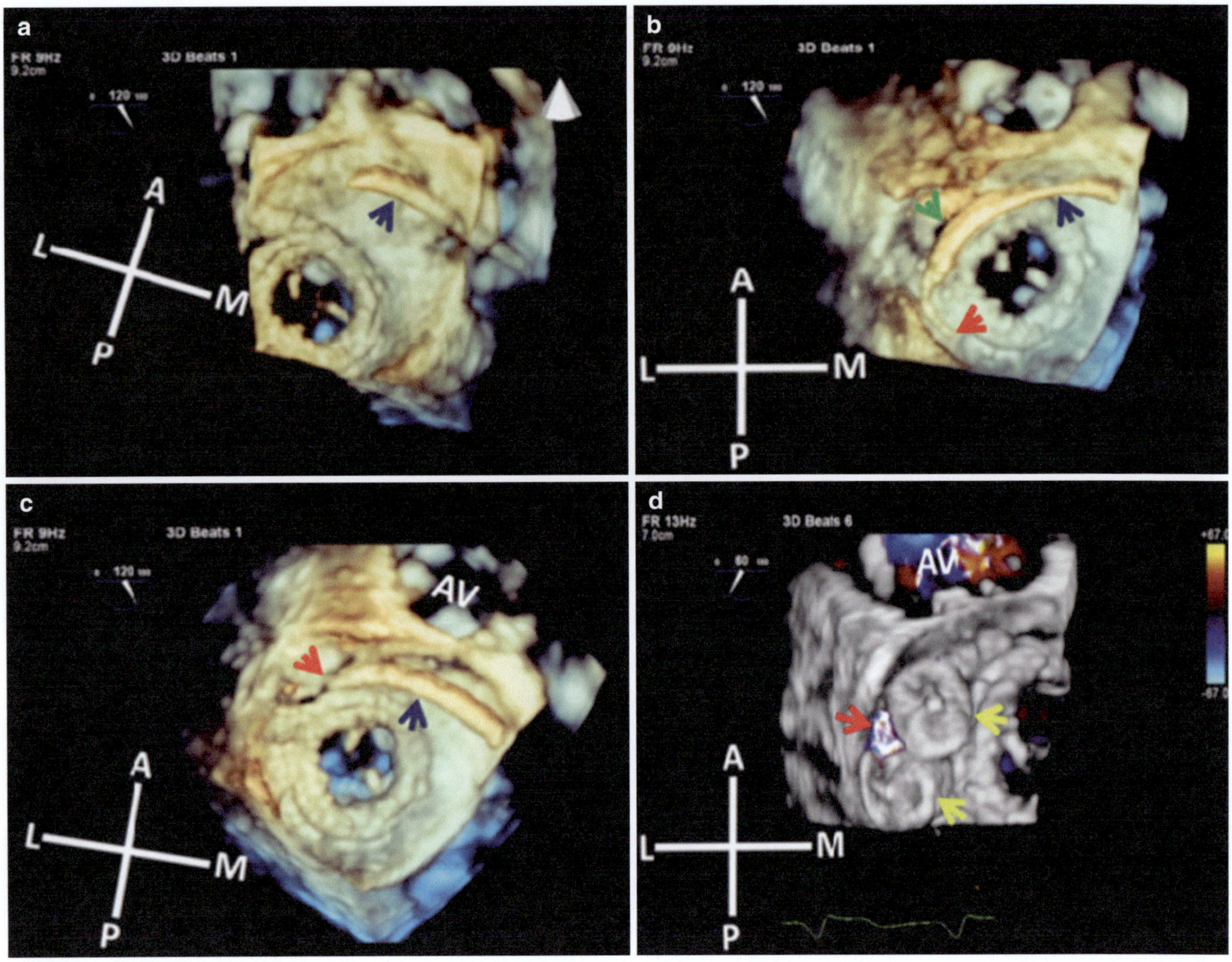

Fig. 30.6 Enface LA 3D TEE during closure of the lateral PPL shown in Fig. 30.3. **Top panel**. (**a** and **b**): Live (real time) 3D of guide wire (dark blue arrow) as it enters the LA (**a**) and during an attempt (**b**) at guide wire (dark blue arrow) negotiation of the defect with its tip (red arrow) away from the defect (green arrow). **Bottom panel**. (**c**): Live 3D showing tip of guide wire (red arrow) inside the lateral defect. Dark blue arrow points to proximal segment of the wire. (**d**): Multibeat CFD acquisition following deployment of two AVPs (yellow arrows) showing mild residual PPL (red arrow) between the two AVPs. Used with permission of Mayo Foundation for Medical Education and Research. All rights reserved. A, anterior; AV, aortic valve; AVP, Amplatzer Vascular Plug; CFD, color flow Doppler; L, lateral; LA, left atrium; M, medial; P, posterior; PPL, periprosthetic leak

The vascular device(s) should not be released until proper prosthetic valve leaflet motion and device stability is confirmed. Findings on 3D TEE suggestive of device impingement on leaflet motion include immobile or partial opening of the leaflet during device deployment (Fig. 30.9) or abrupt increase in valvular regurgitation due to device interference with proper leaflet closure in systole. Rarely, a device may tilt after deployment obstructing leaflet motion or may get dislodged [4] (Fig. 30.9). After device release, evaluation of residual PPL is undertaken (Figs. 30.6d and 30.10c). 3D TEE is also very useful for the evaluation of the iatrogenic post procedure atrial septal defect and for guiding its closure if need be (see Fig. 31.9 Chap. 31). 3D echocardiography has a role in assessment of aortic paravalvular defects (see Chap. 16), but not yet in guiding closure of these defects.

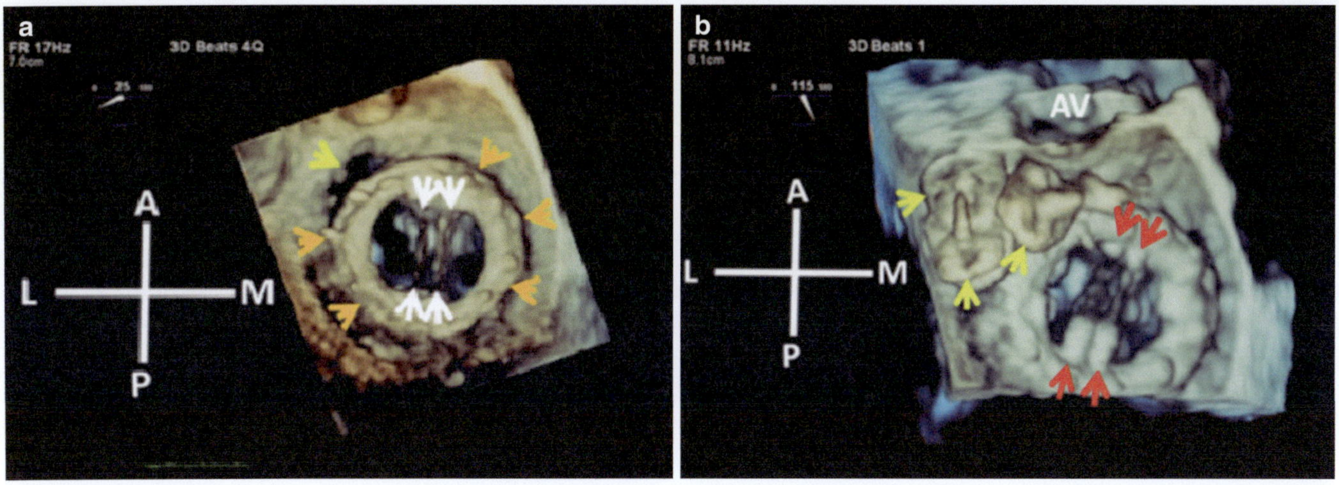

Fig. 30.7 3D TEE enface LA views of mechanical bileaflet mitral prosthesis with a lateral periprosthetic defect. (**a**): pre procedure image showing a cresent shaped periprosthetic defect (yellow arrow). White arrows point to the bileaflet occluders and orange arrows point to prosthesis SR. (**b**): post closure of periprosthetic defect with 3AVPs (yellow arrows). Note that the AVPs do not impinge on the prosthesis orifice. Also note the thickened appearance of the bileaflet occluders due to blooming artifacts (red arrows). Used with permission of Mayo Foundation for Medical Education and Research. All rights reserved. A, anterior; AV, aortic valve; AVP, Amplatzer Vascular Plug; L, lateral; LA, left atrium; M, medial; P, posterior; SR, sewing ring

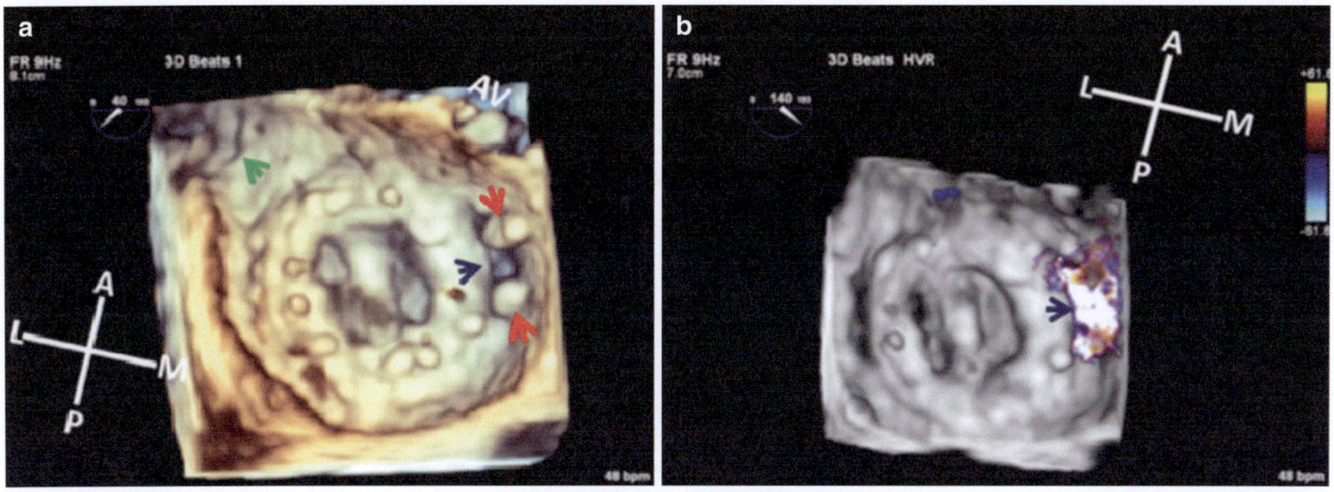

Fig. 30.8 3D TEE enface LA views of transcatheter closure of a Carbomedics mechanical bileaflet periprosthetic defect. (**a**): Live 3D of medial PPL defect (dark blue arrow) that is straddled by calcified ridges (red arrows). Green arrow points to LAA. (**b**): Live 3D HVR CFD showing flow through the defect (arrow). (**c–f**): Sequential real time 3D imaging of deployment of first AVP. White arrows point to delivery sheath inside the defect. Note the various stages of deployment of the AVP (red arrows). (**g–h**): Real time deployment of second AVP (dark blue arrows). Orange arrow points to AVP delivery wire and yellow arrows point to prosthesis SR. Red arrow points to first AVP. (**I**): fully deployed second AVP (dark blue arrow) overlapping with first AVP (red arrow). (**j**): Post deployment of a total of 3 AVPs (arrows). Used with permission of Mayo Foundation for Medical Education and Research. All rights reserved. A, anterior; AV, aortic valve; AVP, Amplatzer Vascular Plug; CFD, color flow Doppler; HVR, High Volume Rate; L, lateral; LA, left atrium; LAA, left atrial appendage; M, medial; P, posterior; PPL, periprosthetic leak; SR, sewing ring

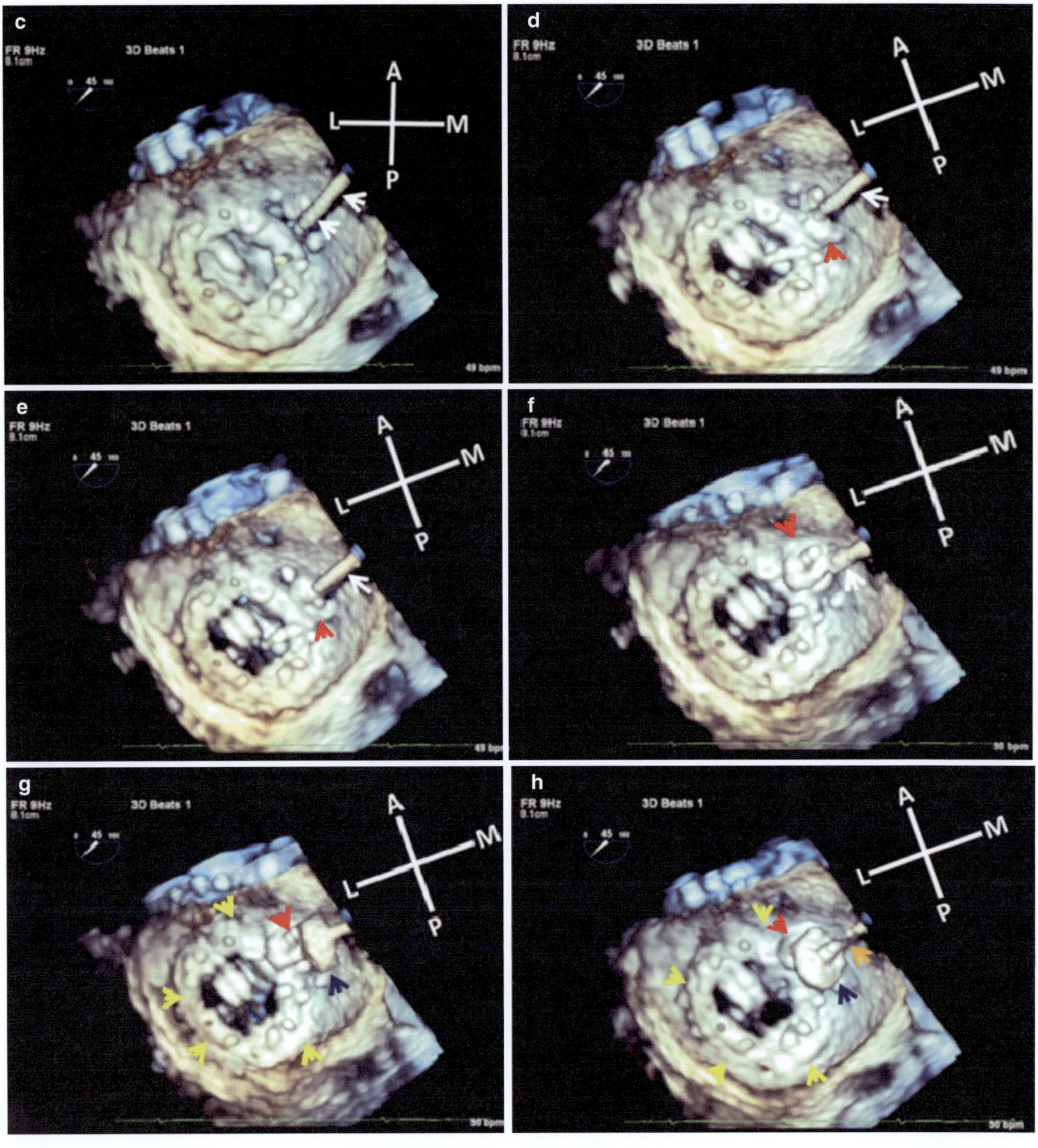

Fig. 30.8 (continued)

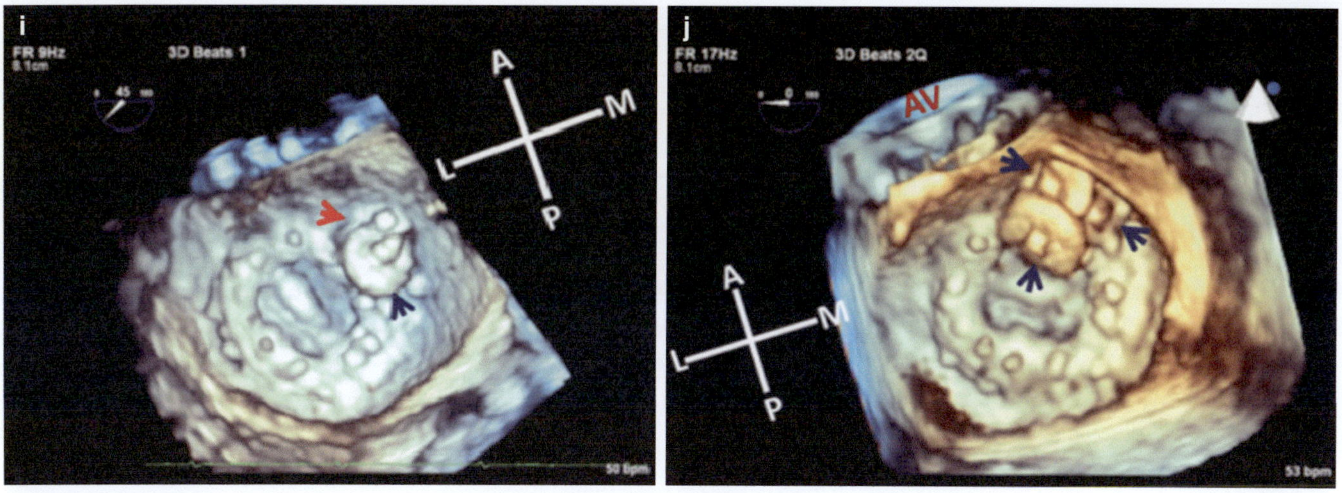

Fig. 30.8 (continued)

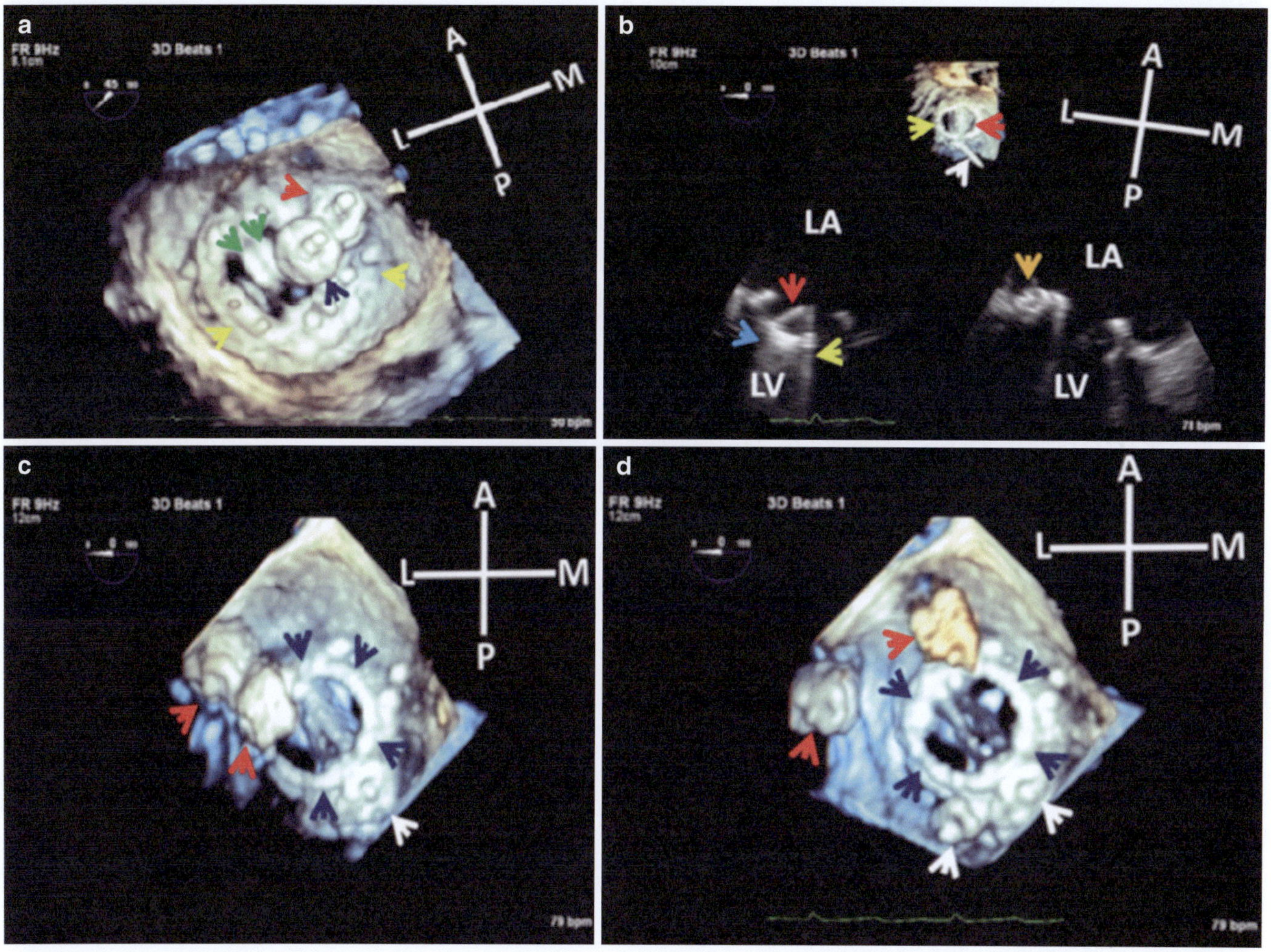

Fig. 30.9 Live 3D TEE enface LA views during deployment of AVPs in patients with mechanical mitral bileaflet prostheses. **Top panel**. (**a**): One of the AVPs (dark blue arrow) is impinging on the prosthesis orifice and leaflets (green arrows). Yellow arrows point to prosthesis SR and red arrow points to a correctly deployed AVP. (**b**): Live 3D with biplane layout. There is interference with opening of the medial prosthesis leaflet (red arrows) by the ventricular surface of the AVP (blue arrow). There is normal opening of the lateral prosthesis leaflet (yellow arrows). Orange arrow points to atrial component of the AVP, and white arrow points to AVP delivery sheath. **Bottom panel** (**c** and **d**): Dislodged AVPs (red arrows) floating feely in the LA. Dark blue arrows point to prosthesis SR and white arrows point to well seated fully deployed AVPs. Used with permission of Mayo Foundation for Medical Education and Research. All rights reserved. A, anterior; AVP, Amplatzer Vascular Plug; L, lateral; LA, left atrium; LV, left ventricle; M, medial; P, posterior; SR, sewing ring

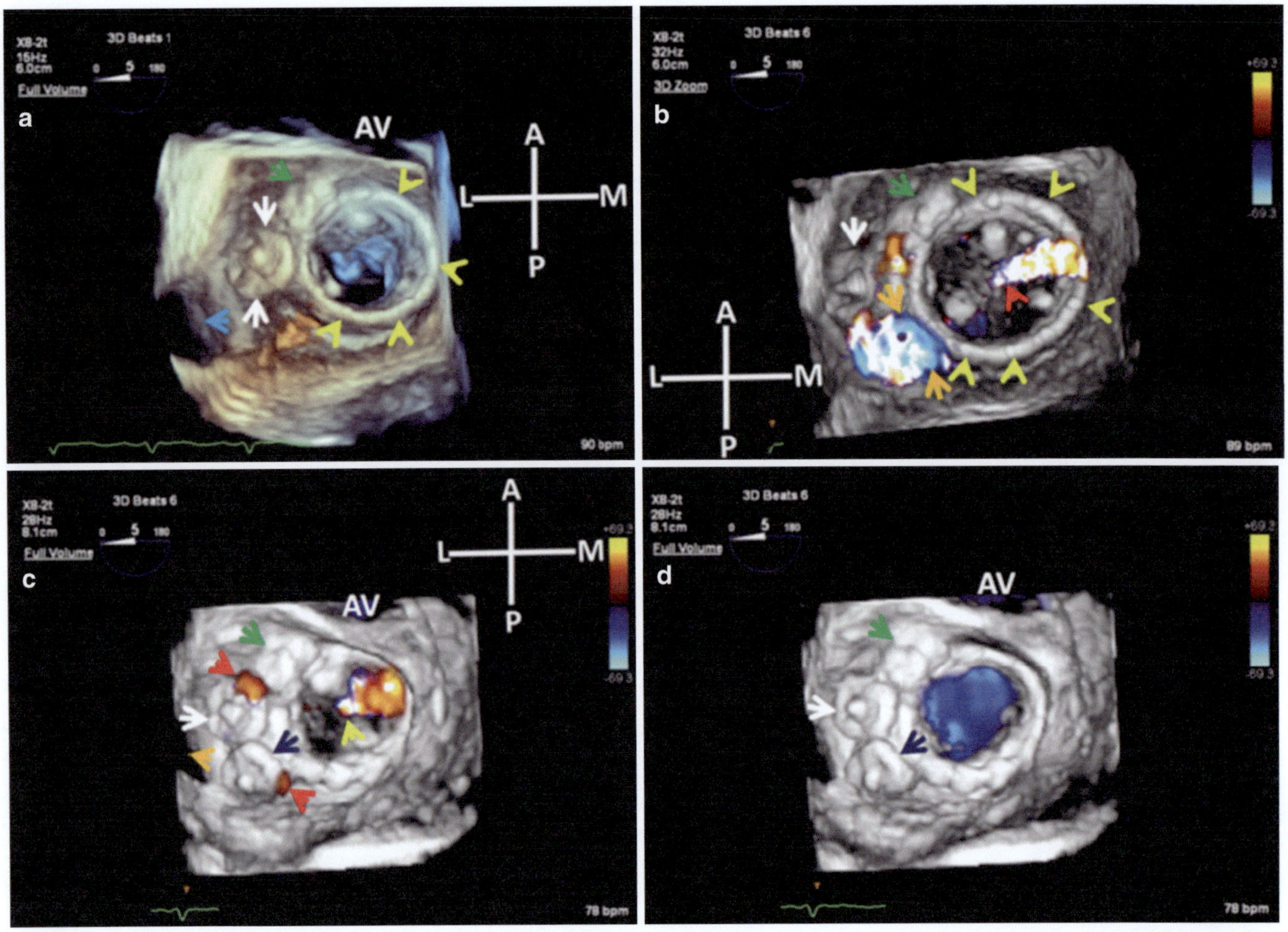

Fig. 30.10 **Top panel:** 3D TEE enface LA views of post mitral valve-in-valve implantation of a SAPIEN THV and deployment of a single AVP to close a PPL. Patient had severe MS due to MAC. (**a**): Diastolic frame showing the deployed AVP (white arrows) adjacent to ostium of LAA (light blue arrow). (**b**): CFD of same image in systole showing residual PPL (orange arrows) posterior to AVP (white arrow) and mild central prosthesis regurgitation (red arrow head). Yellow arrowheads point to SAPIEN THV stent-frame. **Bottom panel:** Multibeat 3D CFD acquisitions in systole (**c**) and diastole (**d**) showing trivial residual PPL (red arrowheads) following deployment of a second AVP (dark blue arrows). White arrows point to first AVP, orange arrowhead points to ostium of LAA, and yellow arrowhead points to central prosthesis regurgitation. Green arrows in all images points to a MAC nodule just anterior to first AVP. Used with permission of Mayo Foundation for Medical Education and Research. All rights reserved. A, anterior; AV, aortic valve; AVP, Amplatzer Vascular Plug; CFD, color flow Doppler; L, lateral; LA, left atrium; LAA, left atrial appendage; M, medial; MAC, mitral annular calcification; MS, mitral stenosis; P, posterior; PPL, periprosthetic leak; THV, transcatheter heart valve

References

1. Rihal CS, Sorajja P, Booker JD, Hagler DJ, Cabalka AK. Principles of percutaneous paravalvular leak closure. J Am Coll Cardiol Intv. February 2012;5(2):121–30.
2. Eleid MF, Cabalka AK, Malouf JF, Sanon S, Hagler DJ, Rihal CS. Techniques and outcomes for the treatment of paravalvular leak. Circ Cardiovasc Interv. 2015;8(8):e001945.
3. Alkhouli M, Rihal CS, Zack CJ, Eleid MF, Maor E, Sarraf M, Cabalka AK, Reeder GS, Hagler DJ, Maalouf JF, Nkomo VT, Schaff HV, Said SM. Transcatheter and surgical management of mitral paravalvular leak: long-term outcomes. JACC: Cardiovasc Interv. 2017 October;10(19):1946–56.
4. Alkhouli M, Sievert H, Rihal CS. Device embolization in structural heart interventions: incidence, outcomes, and retrieval techniques. JACC Cardiovasc Interv. 2019 Jan 28;12(2):113–26.

Valve-in-Valve/Ring Implantation

31

Joseph F. Maalouf, Jeremy J. Thaden, and Sushil Allen Luis

Valve-in-Valve for Failed Bioprostheses or Valve Repair

Catheter based TEE guided treatment of degenerated bioprosthetic valves in the mitral and tricuspid positions is now feasible in high-risk surgical patients [1–5]. A balloon expandable valve (typically a Melody valve or Edwards SAPIEN valve) is implanted inside the degenerated bioprosthesis. 3D TEE has an important role in patient selection, assessment of the degeneratd bioprosthesis, and intraprocedurally [6–8]. Because the sewing ring of the degenerated bioprosthesis acts as a docking station for the transcatheter valve, the internal diameter of the degenerated bioprosthesis is key to determining patient eligibility, and the *external* diameter of the transcatheter valve should match or slightly exceed the *internal* diameter of the failed bioprosthesis in order to allow for secure fixation and sealing. *Regurgitant bioprostheses may have relatively larger internal diameters compared with stenotic bioprostheses.* With 2D TEE, the sewing ring is carefully scanned from 0 to approximately 140 degrees in order to obtain the optimal internal diameter measurement. With 3D TEE, measurement of both the internal and external diameters using vendor provided "online" calipers can be readily made from a single view (Fig. 31.1), but although this"online" measurement has been validated using a phantom model, we prefer multiplanar reconstruction of the 3D data set for making any measurments (Fig. 31.1). Valve-in-ring implantation for failed mitral or tricupid valve repair is also feasible using the same TEE guided approach provided the ring is a complete one [9] (Fig. 31.2).

Valve-in–valve implanations can be performed via a transapical or transseptal access [1–3]. Successful valve-in-valve implantation is contingent on ensuring coaxial alignment of the transcatheter heart valve (THV) (Figs. 31.3 and 31.4), particularly with the transseptal approach, in order to avoid tilting the THV towards the left ventricular outflow tract [2]. This is especially important with valve-in-ring deployment which is more challenging.

All steps of valve-in-valve implantation begining with the transeptal puncture and septal balloon dilatation (Figs. 31.5, 31.6, 31.7, and 31.8) can be captured on real time 3D TEE imaging and the results can be readily assessed. A critically important step is identifying the optimal orientation of the annular plane that would ensure coaxial positioning of the transcather valve. With real time (live) 3D TEE, enface views of the annular plane and degenerated bioprosthesis can be viewed from both the left atrial and left ventricular perspectives for mitral bioprotheses and right atrial and right ventricular perspectives for tricuspid bioprostheses. The sheaths/catheters and guide wires used to advance the transcather valve delivery system can be viewed as they cross the orifice of the degenerated bioprosthetic valve into the ventricle (Fig. 31.4) and maintaining coaxial positioning of the distal wire in the right or left ventricle can be ascertained from the live 3D enface ventricular views (Fig. 31.10). Live 3D can also be useful in guiding positioning and deployment of the transcatheter valve. After deployment, 3D TEE can verify adequate positioning, normal cusp mobilty of the implanted

Supplementary Information The online version of this chapter (https://doi.org/10.1007/978-3-030-72941-7_31) contains supplementary material, which is available to authorized users.

J. F. Maalouf (✉)
Professor of Medicine, Mayo Clinic College of Medicine; Director, Interventional Echocardiography; Consultant, Department of Cardiovascular Medicine, Mayo Clinic, Rochester, MN, USA
e-mail: maalouf.joseph@mayo.edu

J. J. Thaden
Assistant Professor of Medicine, Mayo Clinic College of Medicine; Co-Chair for Clinical Practice and Quality, Division of Cardiovascular Ultrasound; Consultant, Department of Cardiovascular Medicine, Mayo Clinic, Rochester, MN, USA
e-mail: Thaden.Jeremy@mayo.edu

S. A. Luis
Associate Professor of Medicine, Mayo Clinic College of Medicine; Consultant, Rochester, MN, USA
e-mail: Luis.S@mayo.edu

J. F. Maalouf et al. (eds.), *Practical 3D Echocardiography*, https://doi.org/10.1007/978-3-030-72941-7_31

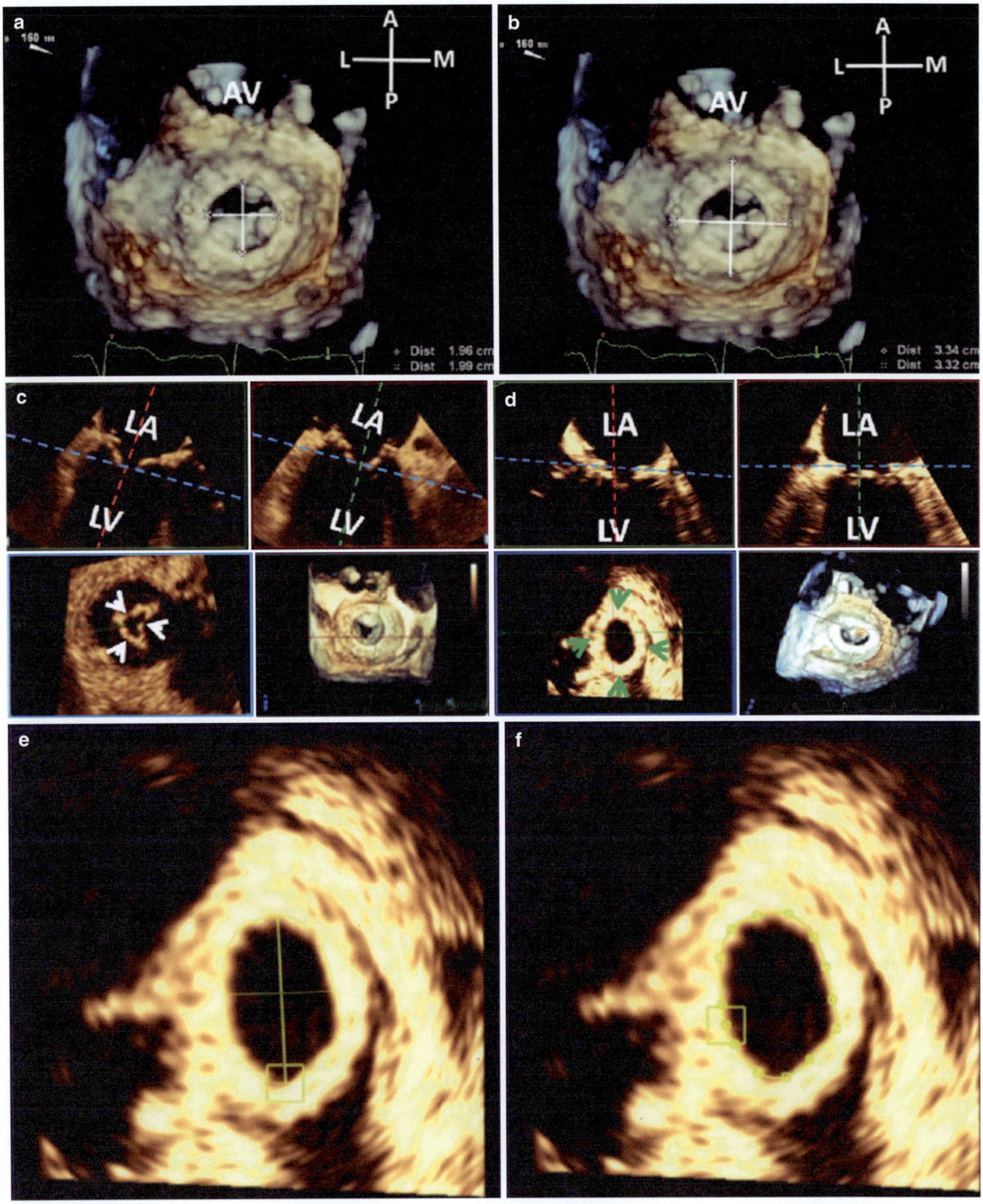

Fig. 31.1 **Top panel:** Internal (**a**) and external (**b**) SR diameters (white lines) of a mitral bioprosthesis using on line calipers. **Middle panel**: MPRs of mitral bioprosthesis stenosis (**c**) and complete annulopasty ring in a patient with failed mitral valve repair (**d**). Alignment of the transverse plane (blue line) and an orthogoanl sagittal plane (red line) at ROI in the coronal plane (green rectangle), and similar alignment of the transverse plane (blue line) with coronal plane (green line) in the sagittal plane (red rectangle) in both MPRs generates the measurement ready ROI (**c**: white arrows, and **d**: green arrows) in the transverse plane (blue rectangle). **Bottom panel:** Complete annuloplasty SR internal diameters (**e**) and circumeference/area (**f**) on MPR. Used with permission of Mayo Foundation for Medical Education and Research. All rights reserved. A, anterior; AV, aortic valve; L, lateral; LA, left atrium; LV, left ventricle; M, medial, MPR, multiplanar reconstruction; P, posterior; ROI, region of interest; SR, sewing ring

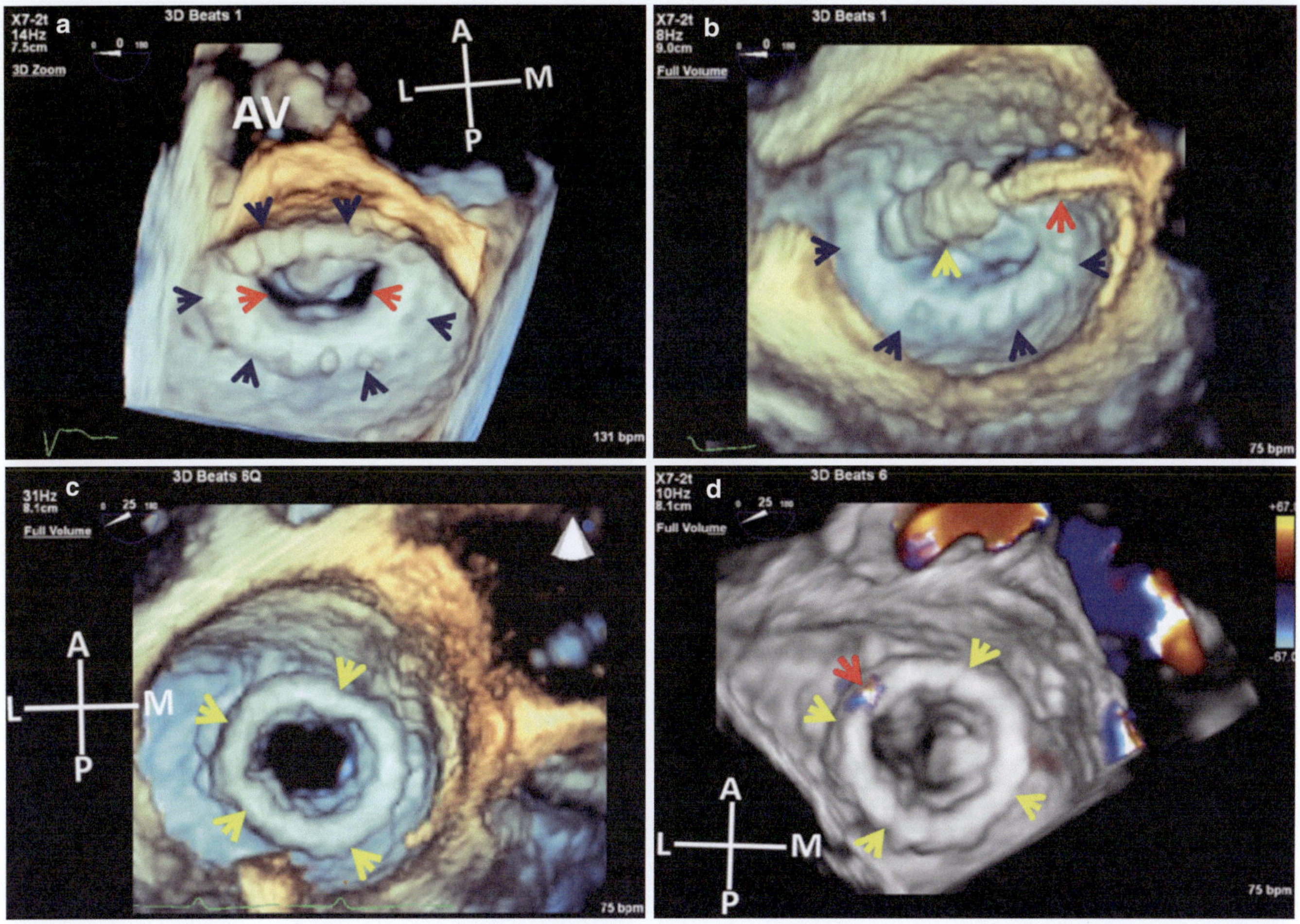

Fig. 31.2 3D TEE enface LA views during valve-in-ring implantation of an Edwards SAPIEN valve. **Top panel:** Real time intraprocedural imaging. (**a**): 3D zoom of complete annuloplasty ring (dark blue arrows) showing severe narrowing of MV orifice (red arrows). (**b**): FV of crimped THV (yellow arrow) on balloon delivery catheter (red arrow) with the complete annuloplasty ring (dark blue arrows) below it. **Bottom panel** (**c** and **d**): Multibeat FV 3D TEE enface LA views of the fully deployed Edwards SAPIEN valve (yellow arrows) with trivial paravalvular regurgitation (red arrow). Used with permission of Mayo Foundation for Medical Education and Research. All rights reserved. A, anterior; AV, aortic valve; FV, Full Volume; L, lateral; LA, left atrium; M, medial; MV, mitral valve; P, posterior; THV, transcatheter heart valve

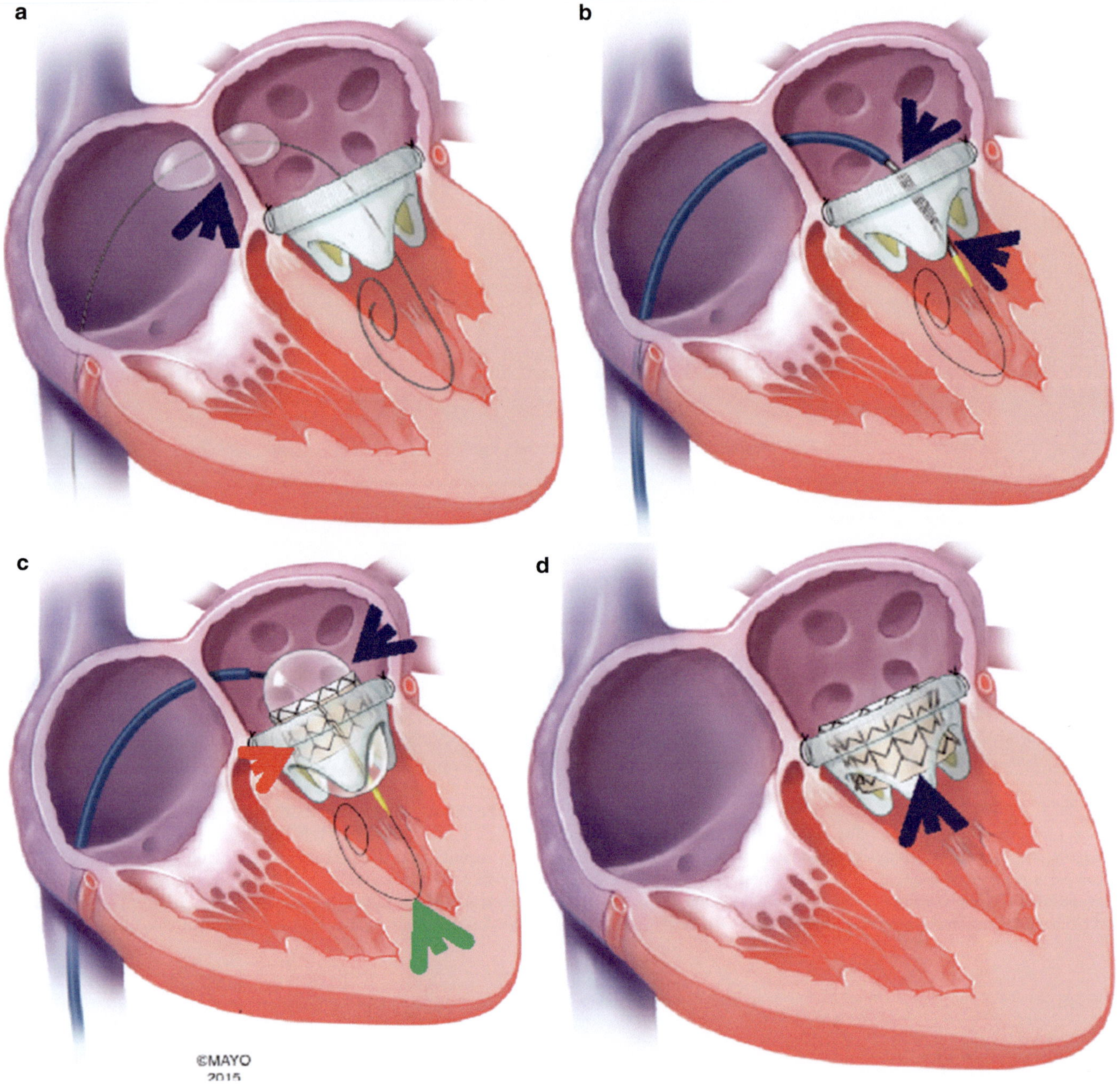

Fig. 31.3 Schematic of the various steps in mitral valve-in-valve (degenerated mitral prosthesis) implantation of a SAPIEN valve via a transeptal technique. (**a**): Balloon atrial septum dilation (arrow); (**b**): Coaxial positioning of the crimped THV (arrows) inside the bioprosthesis; (**c**): Balloon inflation of the transcatheter Edwards SAPIEN valve (dark blue arrow). Red arrow points to the THV and green arrow points to guide wire in LV. (**d**): Fully deployed Edwards SAPIEN valve (arrow) inside the degenrated mitral bioprosthesis. Used with permission of Mayo Foundation for Medical Education and Research. All rights reserved

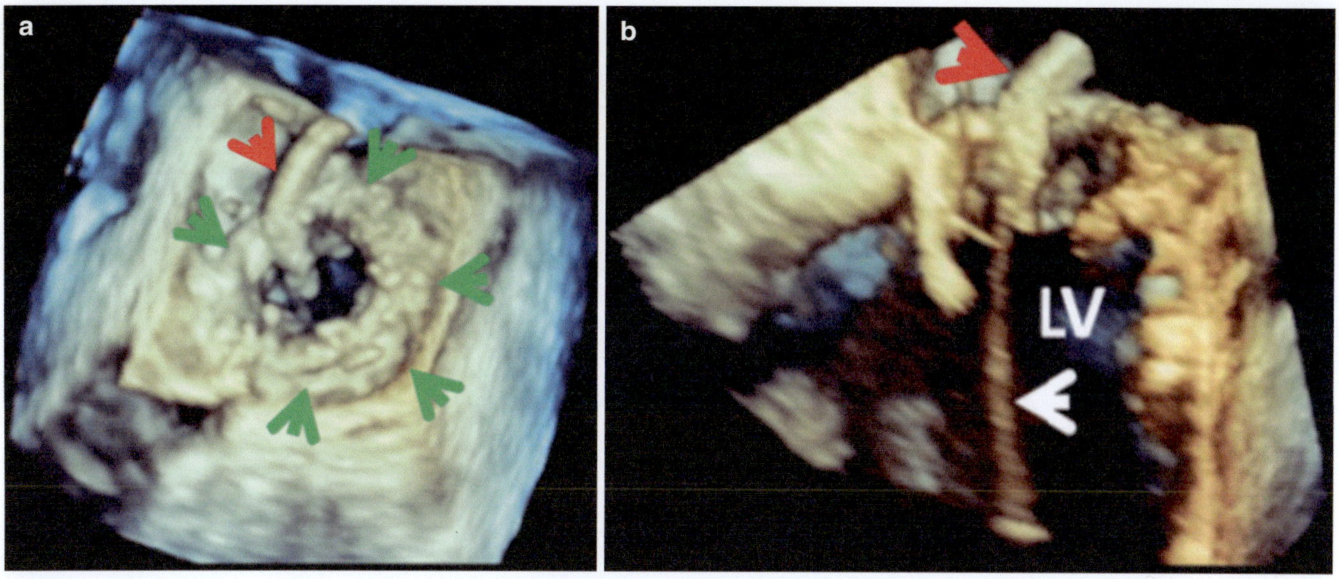

Fig. 31.4 Live 3D TEE of valve in degenerated mitral bioprosthesis implantation of a Melody valve via a transapical rail. (**a**): Following transeptal puncture, coaxial positioning of the delivery sheath (red arrow) within the orifice of the degenrated bioprosthesis; green arrows point to prosthesis SR. (**b**): Delivery sheath (red arrow) in the LA and Glidewire (white arrow) that was advanced through the sheath into the LV, and exteriorized through an LV apical puncture. The resulting arterio- venous rail was used to advance the Melody THV into position within the degenerated bioprosthesis. Used with permission of Mayo Foundation for Medical Education and Research. All rights reserved. LA, left atrium; LV, left ventricle; SR, sewing ring; THV, transcatheter heart valve

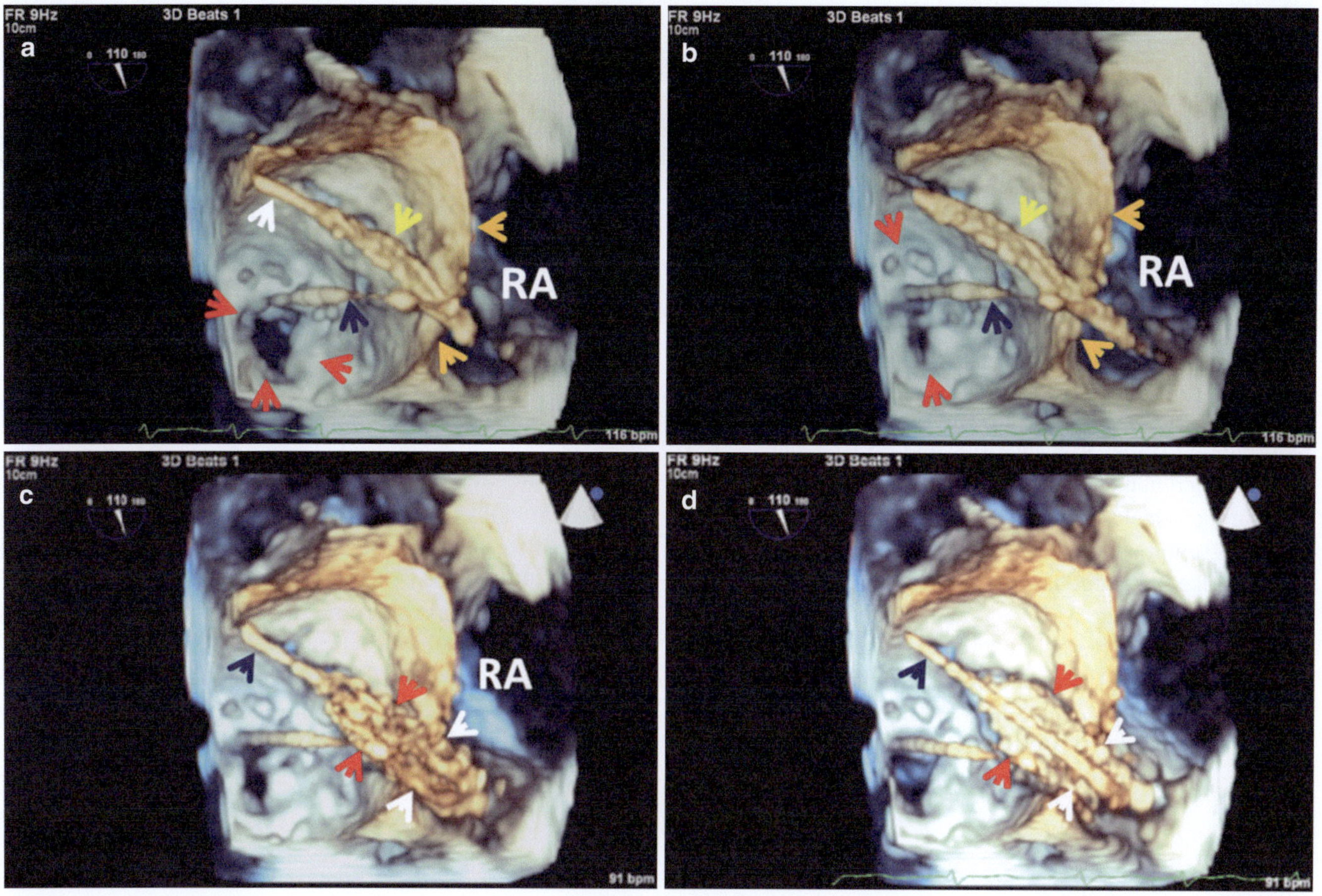

Fig. 31.5 (**a**): Inoue dilator (yellow arrow) on guide wire (white arrow). (**b**): The Inoue dilator is advanced over the wire. Dark blue arrow points to a second stiff wire in the LA. Orange arrows point to atrial septum and red arrows point to the mitral bioprosthesis. (**c** and **d**): Two frames of balloon (red arrows) septal dilation. White arrows point to region of the septum being dilated and dark blue arrow points to the guide wire. Used with permission of Mayo Foundation for Medical Education and Research. All rights reserved. LA, left atrium; RA, right atrium

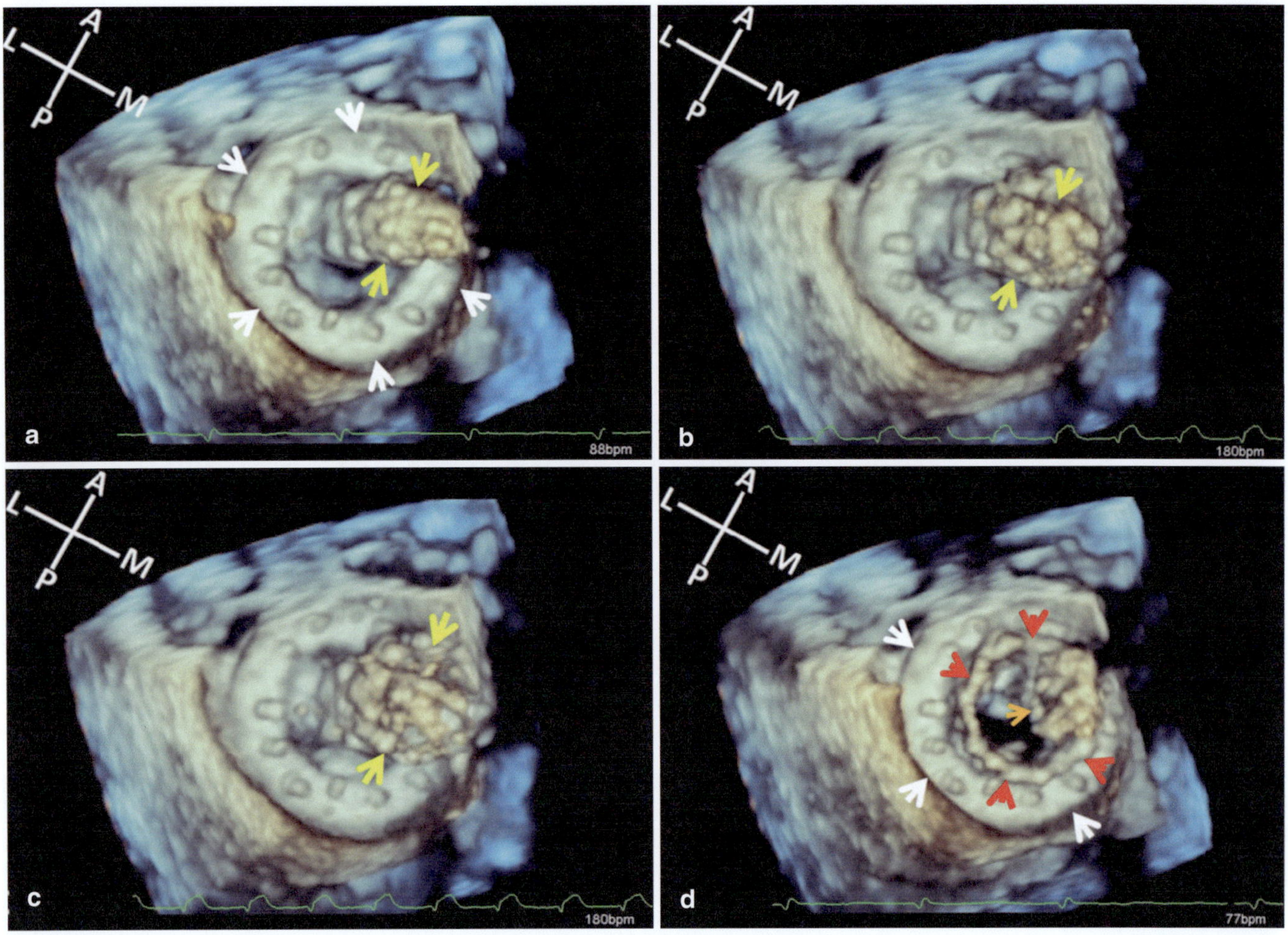

Fig. 31.6 (**a–d**) Live 3D TEE enface LA views of transcatheter Melody valve-in- degenerated mitral bioprosthesis implantation showing a catheter mounted balloon inflatable Melody valve (yellow arrows) at various stages of deployment during rapid ventricular pacing (**b** and **c**). White arrows point to the degenerated mitral bioprosthesis SR and red arrows point to the Melody valve stent frame. Note the excellent seal with the bioprosthesis SR. Threre was no PPL. Orange arrow points to the THV delivery catheter. Used with permission of Mayo Foundation for Medical Education and Research. All rights reserved. A, anterior; L, lateral; LA, left atrium; M, medial; P, posterior; PPL, periprosthetic leak; SR, sewing ring; THV, transcatheter heart valve

prosthesis and severity of any prosthetic or periprosthetic regurgitation (Figs. 30.7 and 30.8, and 30.10, Chap. 30). As with any percutaneous procedure that involves a transseptal puncture, particularly those involving use of large catheters, the atrial septum should be carefully scanned post procedure for evidence of a large iatrogenic ASD that may need transcatheter closure (Fig. 31.9).

For tricuspid valve-in-valve or complete tricuspid sewing ring implants [4, 5], the transcatheter valve is delivered via the right internal jugular vein. Bicaval view of the tricuspid prosthesis inflow (110–130 degrees) offers the optimal imaging window for guiding the procedure (Fig. 31.10).

Valve-in-MAC

Transcatheter valve in native mitral valve implantation is also feasible for patients with severe mitral inflow stenosis caused by heavy mitral annular calcification [3] (Fig. 31.11). Accurate sizing of the mitral annulus is critical for successful outcome because undersizing risks embolization or late migration of the THV as well as paravalvular regurgitation [6] (see Fig. 30.10 Chap. 30). The presence of circumferential annular calcification, needed for optimal device anchoring of balloon-expandable prostheses, is confirmed with reformatted CT images which are

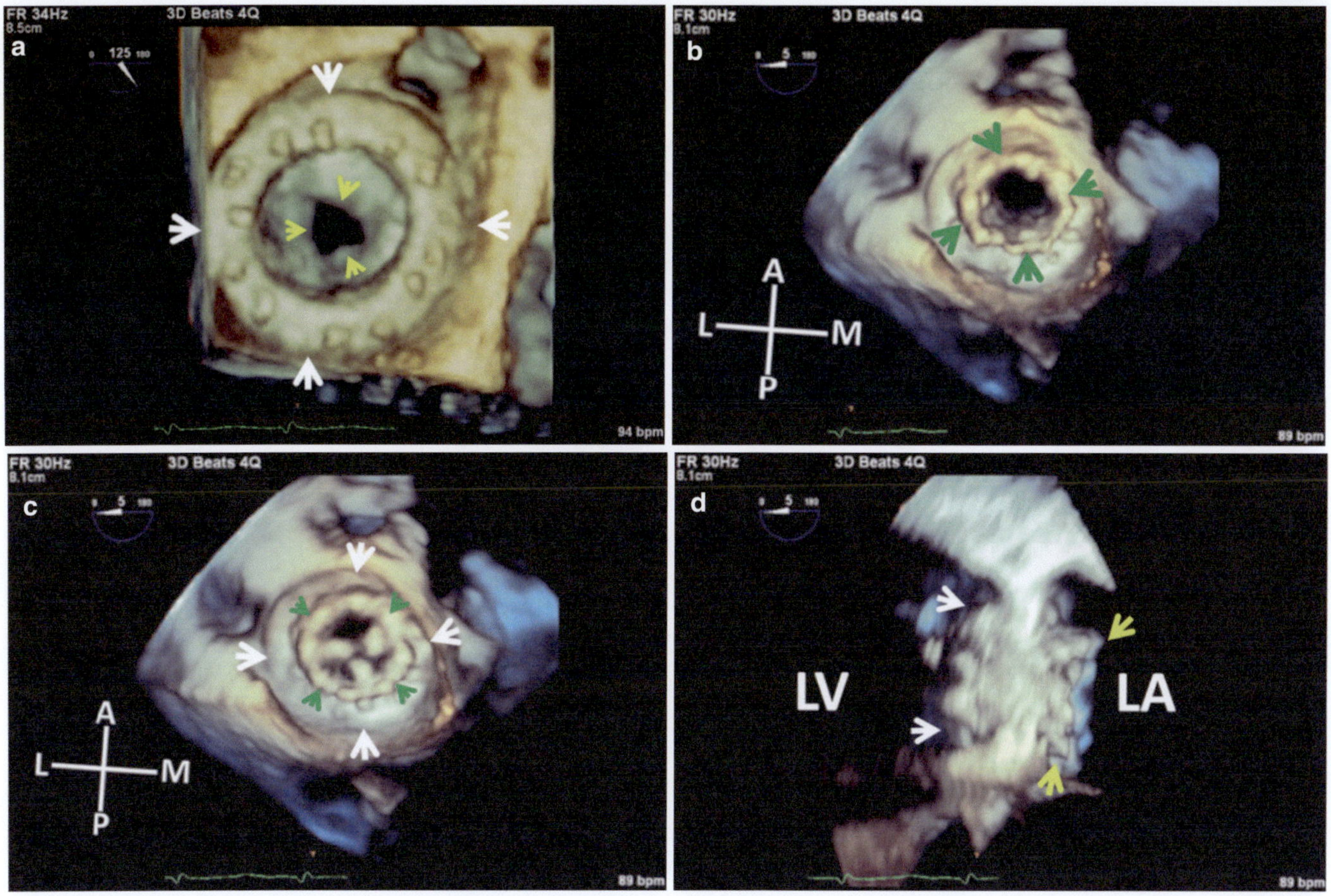

Fig. 31.7 From patient in Fig. 31.6. **Top panel**. 3D TEE enface LA views. (**a**): Pre procedure severe bioprosthesis stenosis (yellow arrows); white arrows point to bioprosthesis SR. (**b**): Fully deployed Melody valve in diastole. **Bottom panel**. (**c**): Same Melody valve in systole. Green arrows point to Melody valve stent . White arrows point to bioprosthesis SR. (**d**): Sideway view of the atrial (yellow arrows) and ventricular (white arrows) surfaces of the Melody valve stent. Used with permission of Mayo Foundation for Medical Education and Research. All rights reserved. A, anterior; L, lateral; LA, left atrium; LV, left ventricle; M, medial; P posterior; SR, sewing ring

also used to obtain the mitral annular dimensions for transcatheter heart valve sizing [3]. Mitral annular measurements are also feasible on 3D TEE multiplanar reconstruction of the volumetric 3D data set (Fig. 31.12), and the extent of circumferential annular calcification including irregularity of calcium distribution (see Chap. 7 Fig. 7.9a and b) can also be assessed on 3D TEE. A major concern with transcatheter mitral valve replacement (TMVR) for valve in MAC or annuloplasty ring, is left ventricular outflow obstruction (LVOT) caused by displacement of the anterior mitral valve leaflet into the left ventricle particularly when there is basal septal hypertrophy or the left ventricular cavity is small [3]. CT scan provides measurements of the projected neo LVOT area [3] which may also be feasible on 3D TEE (Fig. 31.13), and 3D printing (see Chap. 36) derived from 3D TEE has recently become possible [6]. If the risk of LVOT obstruction after TMVR is high, patients can undergo alcohol septal ablation or intentional percutaneous laceration of the anterior mitral leaflet [10] (LAMPOON procedure [10], Figs. 31.14, 31.15, 31.16 and 31.17) or both to reduce the risk of LVOT obstruction before TMVR. Other concerns following transcatheter valve deployment are the same as for valve in degenerated mitral prosthesis implantation.

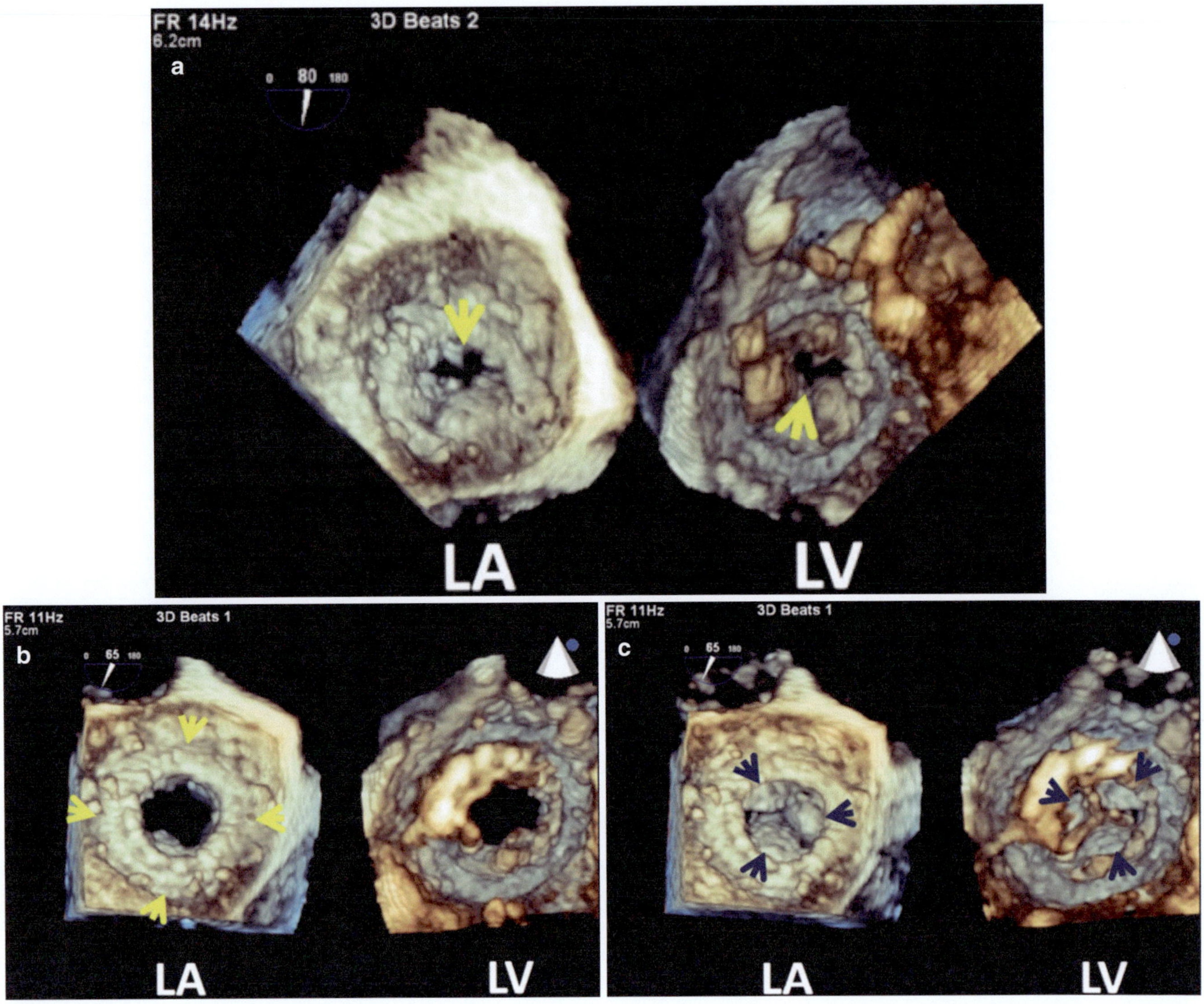

Fig. 31.8 3DTEE enface dual layout LA and LV views of transcatheter Edwards SAPIEN valve-in-degenerated mitral bioprosthesis implantation. (**a**): Degenerated bioprosthesis with severe stenosis (arrows). (**b** and **c**): Diastolic (**b**) and systolic (**c**) frames of the deployed SAPIEN valve. Yellow arrows point to degenrated bioprosthis SR, and dark blue arrows point to the THV cusps. Used with permission of Mayo Foundation for Medical Education and Research. All rights reserved. LA, left atrium; LV, left ventricle; SR, sewing ring; THV, transcatheter heart valve

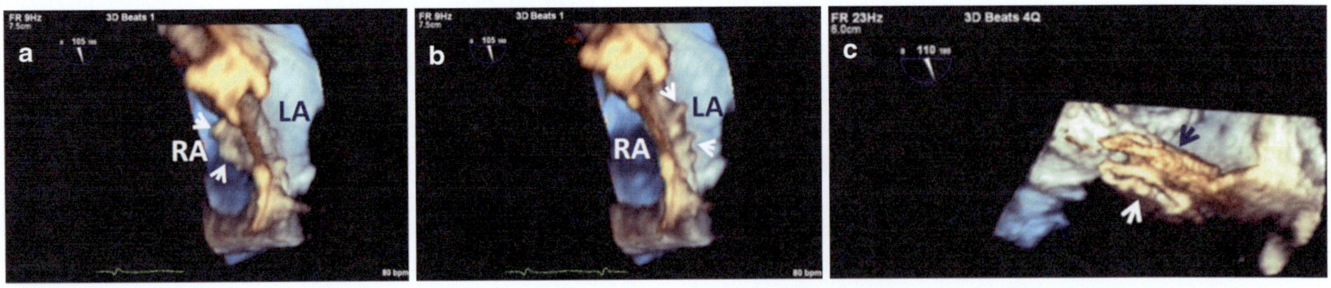

Fig. 31.9 (**a** and **b**): 3D TEE RA and LA views of iatrogenic ASD in diastole (**a**) and systole (**b**) following Melody valve-in- degenerated mitral valve prosthesis implantation. Note the irregular edges of the iatrogenic ASD (arrows). (**c**): left atrial (dark blue arrow) and right atrial (white arrow) surfaces of the Amplatzer ASD occluder device that was deployed percutaneously. Used with permission of Mayo Foundation for Medical Education and Research. All rights reserved. ASD, atrial septal defect; LA, left atrium; RA, right atrium

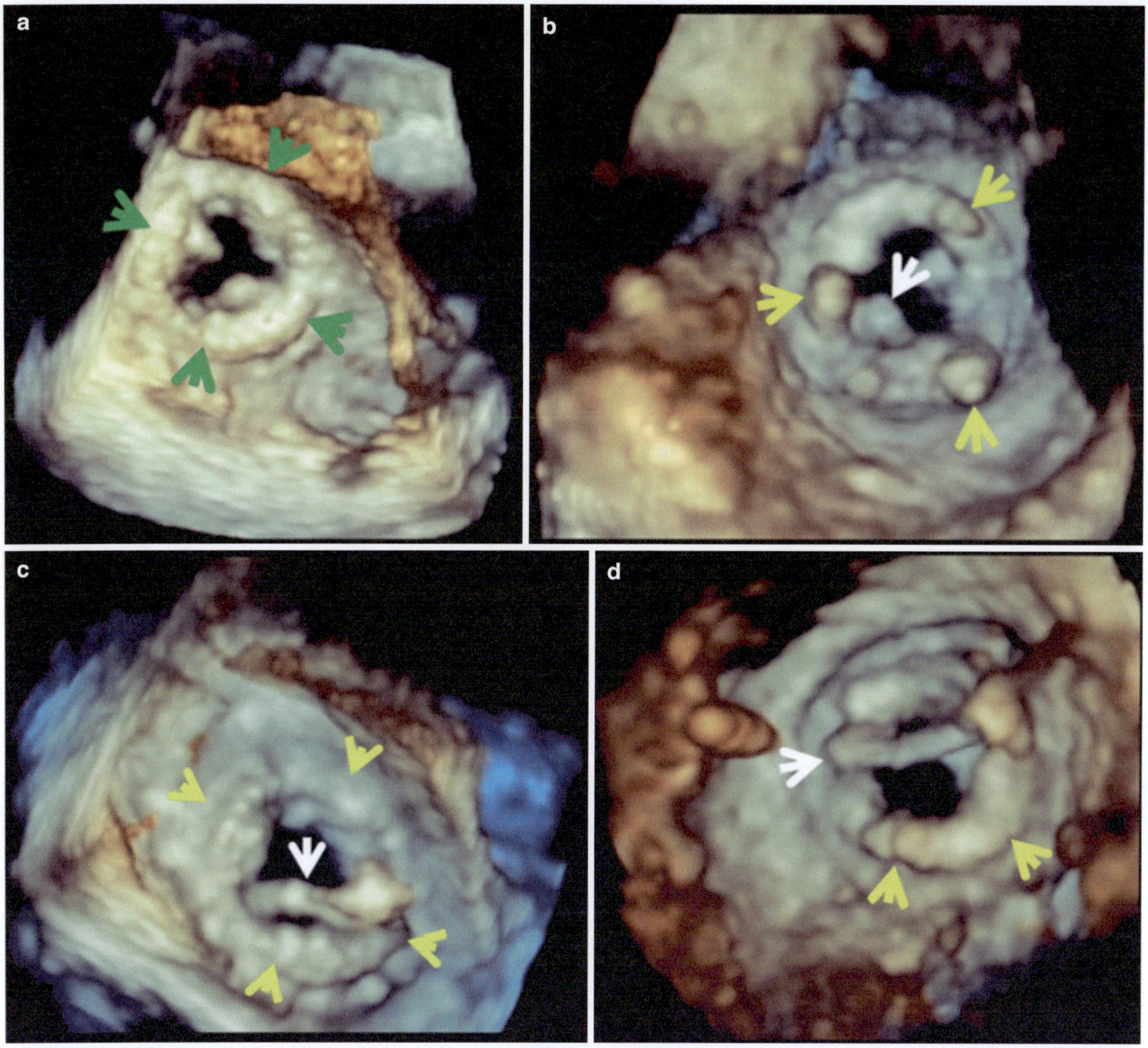

Fig. 31.10 3D TEE enface RA and RVviews of transcatheter Melody valve-in- degenerated tricuspid bioprosthesis implantation. **Top panel:** RA (**a**) and RV (**b**) views of the degenerated bioprosthesis. Green arrows point to bioprosthesis SR and yellow arrows point to the bioprosthesis struts. White arrow points to a catheter in bioprosthesis lumen. **Middle panel:** RA (**c**) and RV (**d**) views of a stiff guide wire (white arrow) inside lumen of degenerated bioprosthesis (yellow arrows). **Bottom panel:** Enface RA (**e**) and RV (**f**) views of the fully deployed transcatheter Melody valve. Green and white arrows point to the degenerated bioprosthesis SR and struts respectively, and yellow arrows point to the three Melody valve cusps. Note the perfect seal between the stented Melody valve and degenerated bioprosthesis SR. RA, right atrium; RV, right ventricle; SR, sewing ring

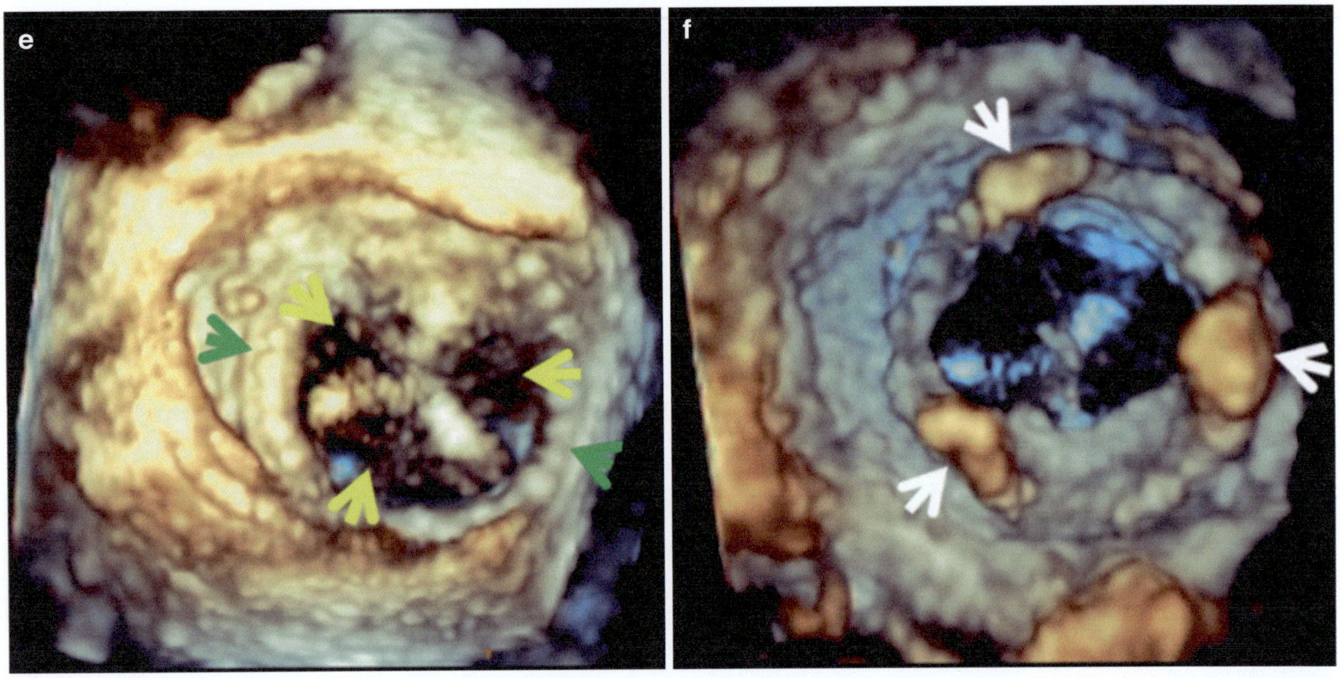

Fig. 31.10 (continued)

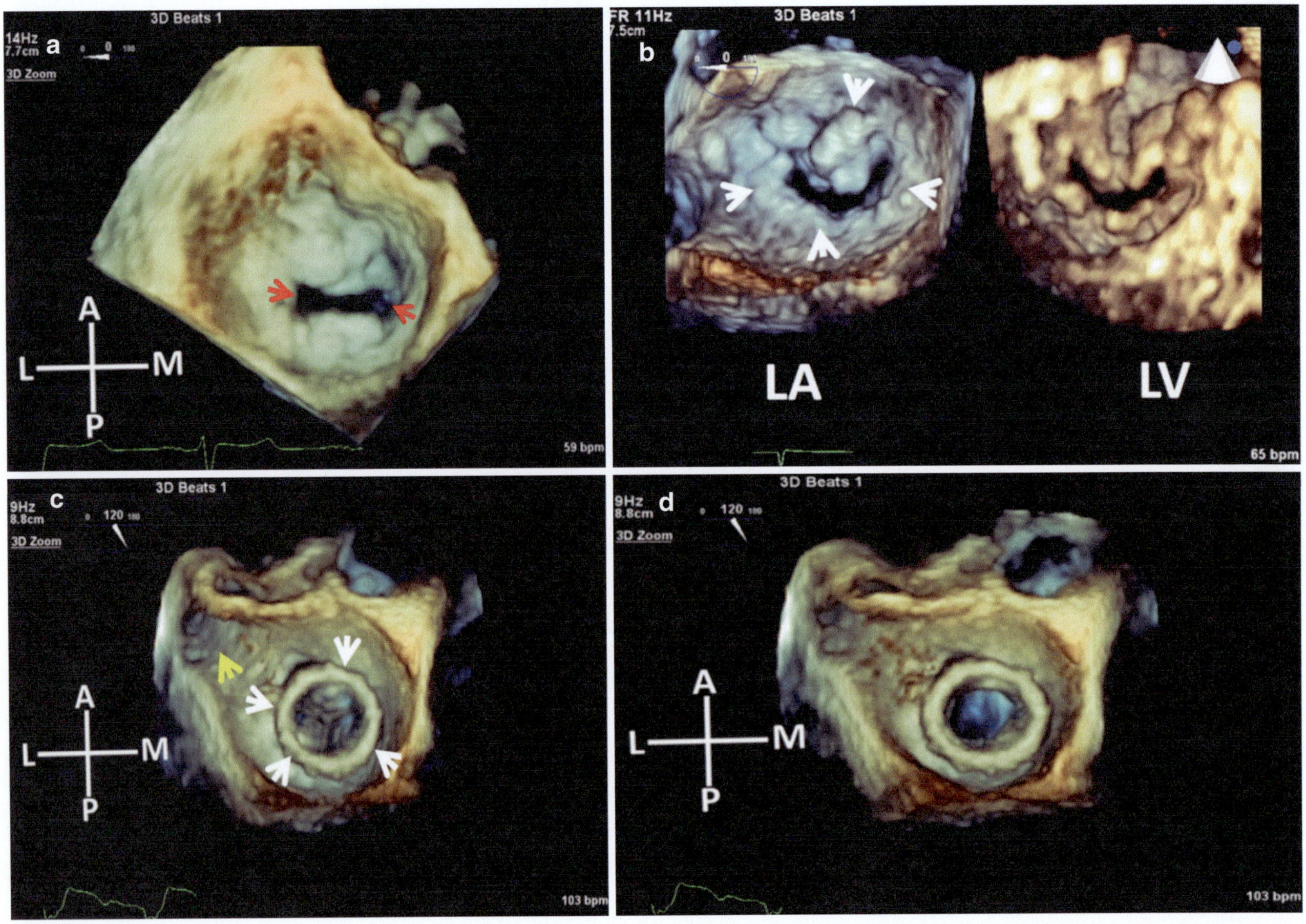

Fig. 31.11 RT 3D TEE Zoom of transcatheter implantation of SAPIEN THV in- native mitral valve with severe stenosis secondary to heavy annular calcification. **Top panel:** LA view of severe mitral stenosis (red arrows) due to MAC (**a**) and dual layout in another patient showing severe MAC (white arrows) with markedly narrowed MV orifice (**b**). **Bottom panel**: from patient in **a**. Enface LA views of fully deployed SAPIEN THV (white arrows) in both systole (**c**) and diastole (**d**). Yellow arrow points to LAA. Used with permission of Mayo Foundation for Medical Education and Research. All rights reserved. A, anterior; L, lateral; LA, left atrium; LAA, left atrial appendage; LV, left ventricle; M, medial; MAC, mitral annular calcification; MV, mitral valve; P, posterior; RT, real time; THV, transcatheter heart valve

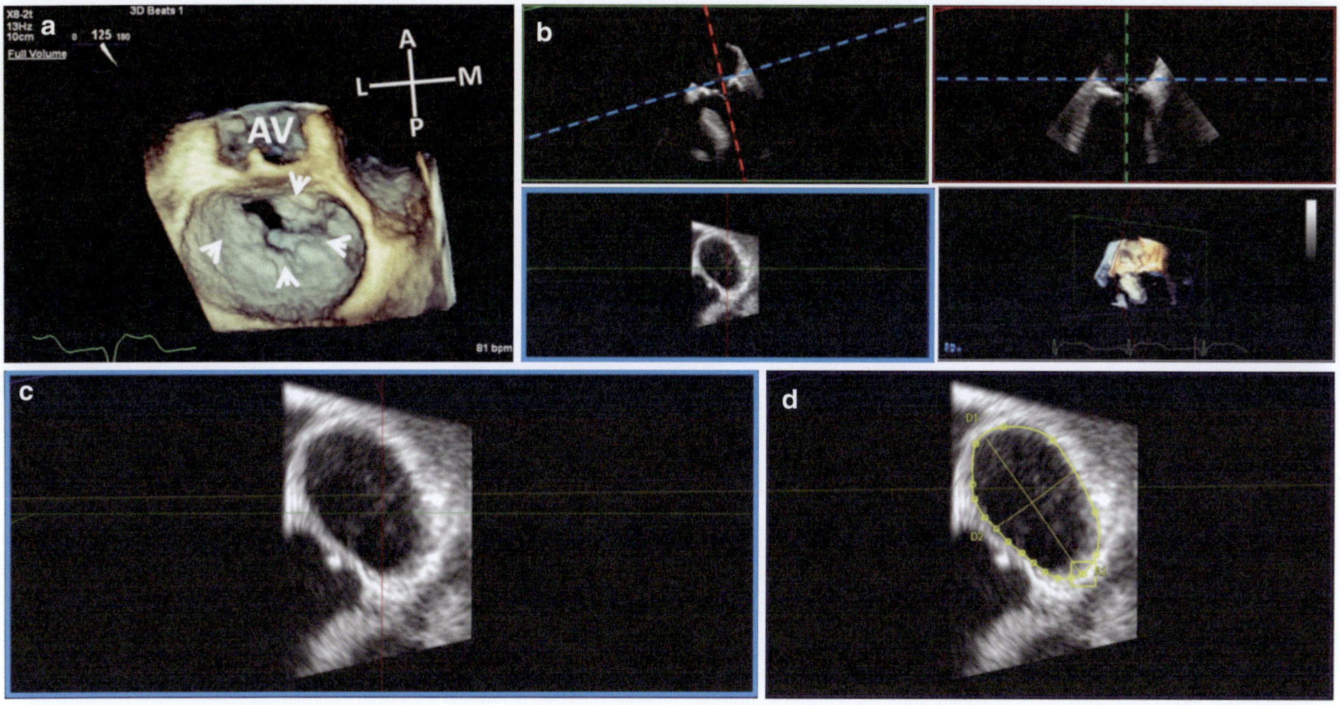

Fig. 31.12 3D TEE mitral annular measuremetns in a patient with severe MS due to MAC prior to TMVR. **Top panel:** FV of MV (**a**) showing severe MAC (white arrows) and the corresponding MPR (**b**). Alignment of the transverse plane (dashed blue lines) with both the orthogonal sagittal (dashed red line) and coronal (dashed green line) planes at mitral annulus in the coronal (green rectangle) and sagittal (red rectangle) 2D tomographic space produces a measurement ready image of the mitral annulus in the transverse plane (blue rectangle). **Bottom panel:** Enlarged images of MPR derived transverse plane showing mitral annulus (**c**) and corresponding area and dimension measurements (**d**). Used with permission of Mayo Foundation for Medical Education and Research. All rights reserved. A, anterior; AV, aortic valve; FV, Full Volume; L, lateral; LA, left atrium; LV, left ventricle; M, medial; MAC, mitral annular calcification; MPR, multiplanar reconstruction; MS, mitral stenosis; MV, mitral valve; P, posterior; TMVR, transcatheter mitral valve replacement

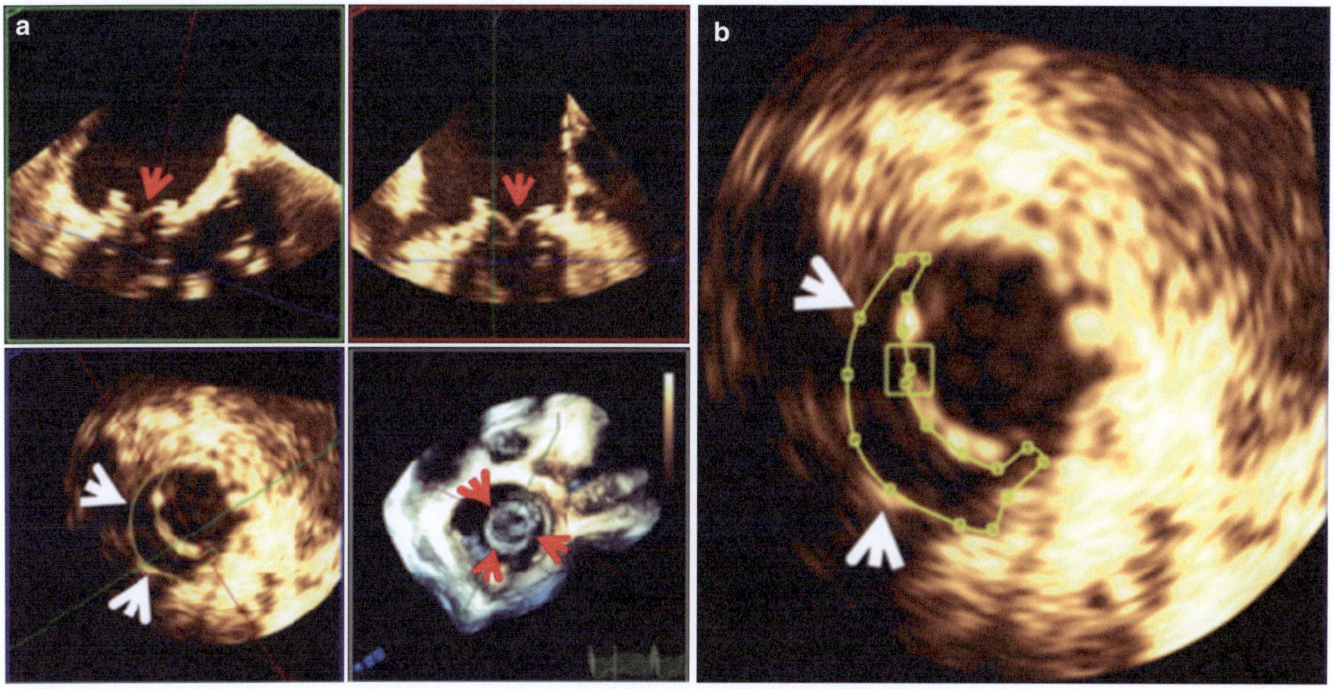

Fig. 31.13 MPR (**a**) following valve-in-ring implantation of a SAPIEN THV(red arrows). The neo LVOT area (**a** and **b**; white arrows) is clearly delineated and can be measured. Used with permission of Mayo Foundation for Medical Education and Research. All rights reserved. LVOT, left ventricular outflow tract; MPR, multiplanar reconstruction; THV, transcathether heart valve

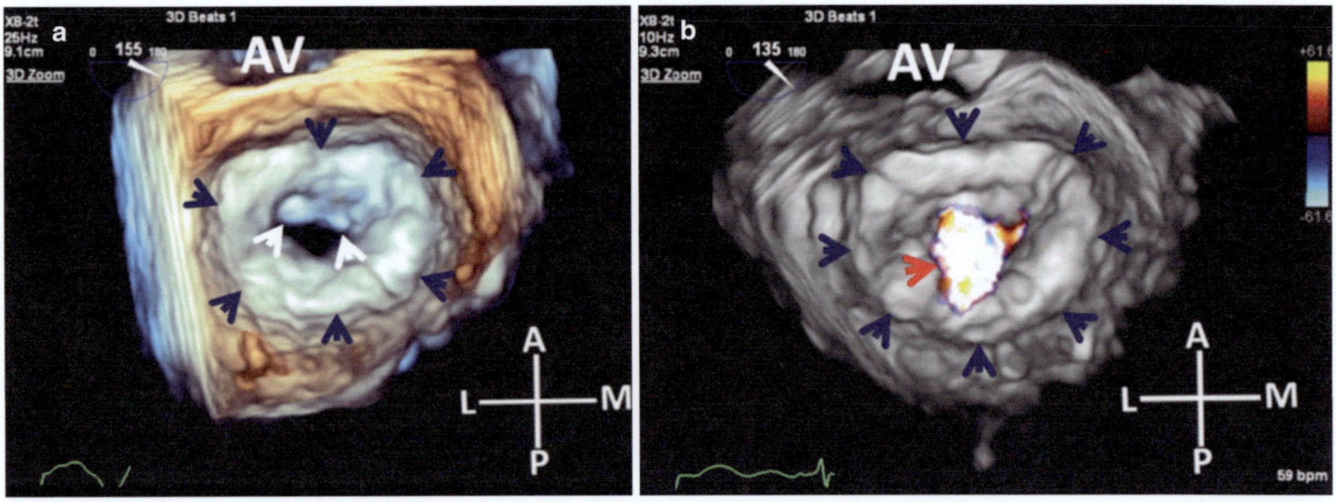

Fig. 31.14 (**a** and **b**): Baseline RT 3D zoom enface LA views of MV prior to LAMPOON procedure and TMVR in a patient with extensive circuferential MAC (dark blue arrows) with the calcification extending into the AML (**a**, white arrows) restricting leaflet motion. The primary pathology was severe MS mainly due to MAC but there was also moderate MR (**b**, red arrow). Patient had a thick septum and small LV cavity with narrow LVOT and underwent alcohol septal ablation without significant improvement in neo-LVOT. Images courtesy of Dr. Sari Padang. Used with permission of Mayo Foundation for Medical Education and Research. All rights reserved. A, anterior; AML, anterior mitral leaflet; AV, aortic valve; L, lateral; LA, left atrium; LV, left ventricle; LVOT, left ventricular outflow tract; M, medial; MAC, mitral annular calcification; MR, mitral regurgitation; MS, mitral stenosis; MV, mitral valve; P, posterior; RT, real time; TMVR, transcatheter mitral valve replacement

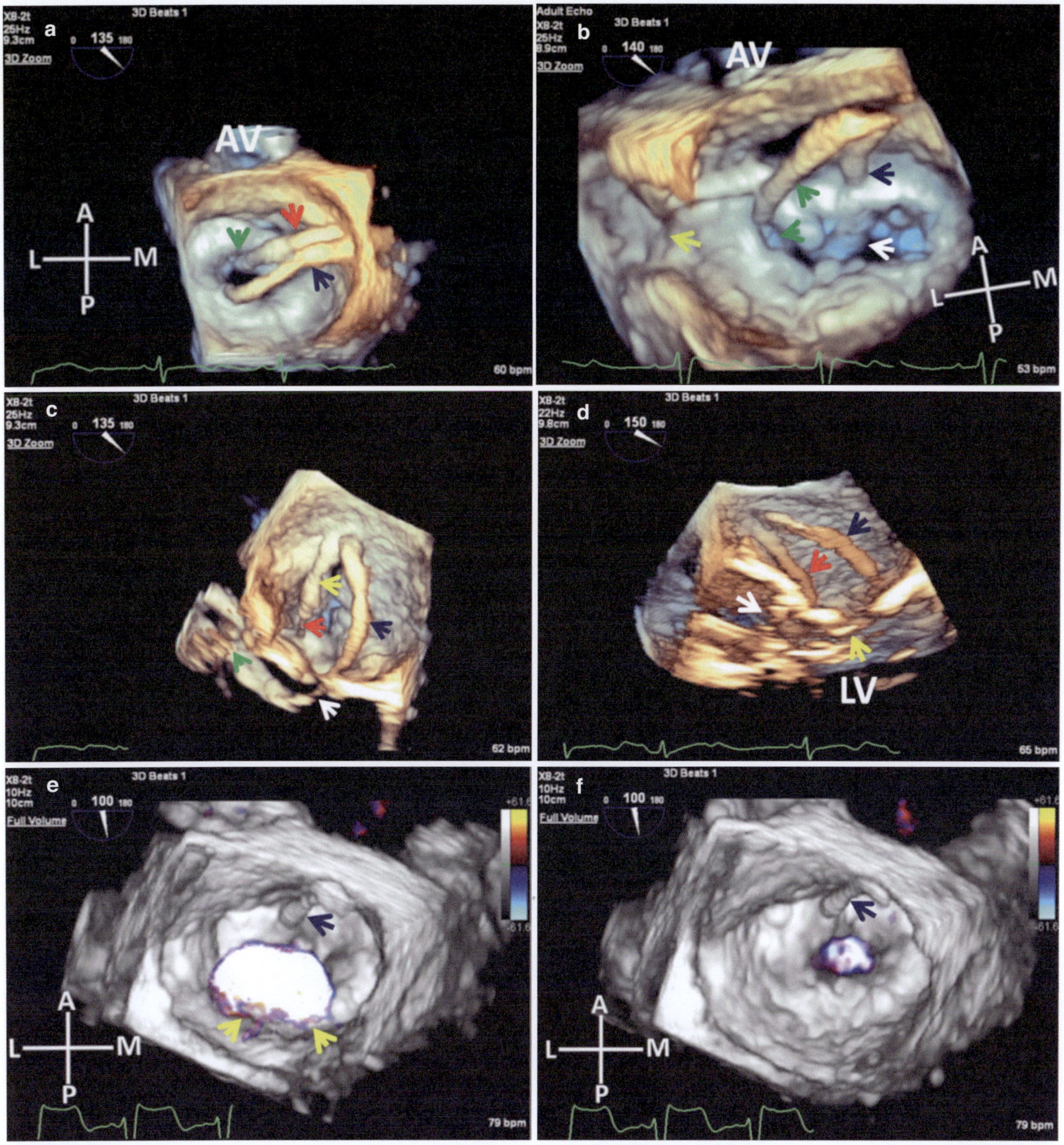

Fig. 31.15 Percutaneous antegrade LAMPOON procedure in preparation for TMVR in patient from Fig. 31.14. **Top panel**. (**a**): Two guide catheters in LA via transseptal approach. One catheter (red arrow) is positioned above the A2 segment of the AML (green arrow) while the other catheter (dark blue arrow) is directed through the MV orifice into the LVOT. (**b**): A catheter (green arrows) is advanced through the MV orifice into the LV and through that catheter a snare is extruded. An Astato wire connected to a Bovie is advanced through the other catheter to perforate the base of the AML (dark blue arrow) and is then advanced into the LV (white arrow) to be be passed into the snare in preparation for laceration of the AML. Note that differentiating catheters from wires can be difficult on 3DE because of blooming artifacts. **Middle panel.** Enface views of giude catheters and wires from both LA and LV perspectives. (**c**): AML directed catheter (yellow arrow) and wire (red arrow) at base of AML. The other guide catheter can be seen in both LA (dark blue arrow) and LVOT (white arrow). Green arrow points to AV. (**d**): Snaring (yellow arrow) of the Astato wire (red arrow) in LVOT**.** White arow points to AV**. Bottom panel**. (**e**): Significant increase in MR (yellow arrows) following laceration of the AMLwith the color filter at the highest setting. (**f**): Diastolic frame. Dark blue arrows in both images point to site of AML Astato wire perforation. Images courtesy of Dr. Sari Padang. Used with permission of Mayo Foundation for Medical Education and Research. A, anterior; AML, anterior mitral leaflet; AV, aortic valve; L, lateral; LA, left atrium; LV, left ventricle; LVOT, left ventricular outflow tract; M, medial; MR, mitral regurgitation; MV, mitral valve; P, posterior, TMVR transcatheter mitral valve replacement

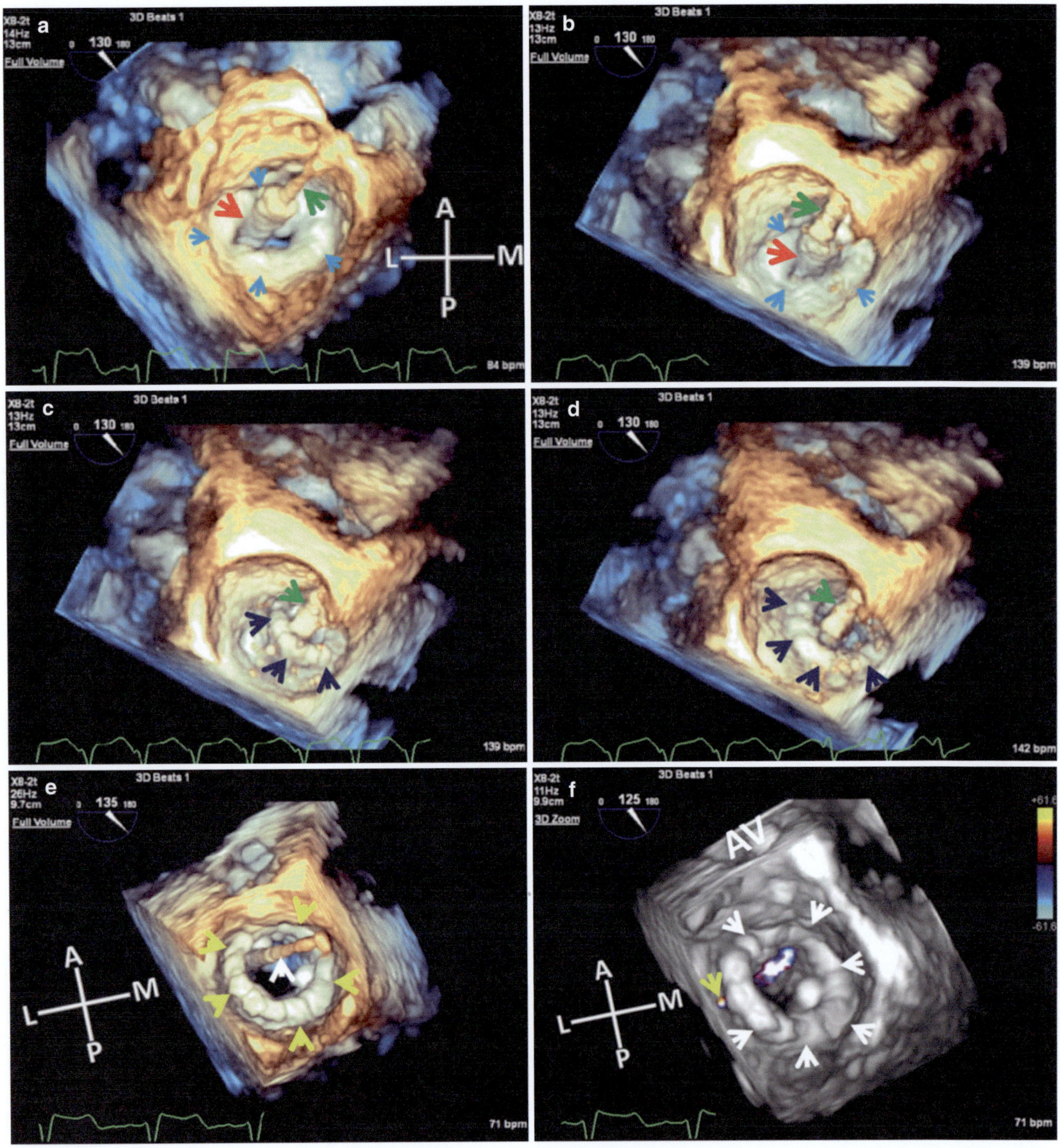

Fig. 31.16 Live 3D TEE enface LA views of TMVR following LAMPOON procedure. (**a**): Positioning of delivery catheter (green arrow) with crimped balloon expandable SAPIEN 3 THV (red arrow) within the MV orifice. (**b**): Initiation of rapid ventricular pacing. Light blue arrows point to circumferential MAC. (**c** and **d**): Two stages of balloon inflation and SAPIEN 3 deployment (dark blue arrows) during rapid ventricular pacing. Green arrow points to delivery catheter. (**e**): Fully deployed SAPIEN 3 THV (yellow arrows) with wire in lumen (white arrow). (**f**): Live 3D Zoom CFD of same THV (white arrows) showing trivial PPL (yellow arrow). Images courtesy of Dr. Sari Padang. Used with permission of Mayo Foundation for Medical Education and Research. All rights reserved. A, anterior; AV, aortic valve; CFD, color flow Doppler; L, lateral; LA, left atrium; M, medial; MAC, mitral annular calcification; MV, mitral valve; P, posterior; PPL, periprosthetic leak; THV, transcatheter heart valve; TMVR, transcatheter mitral valve replacement

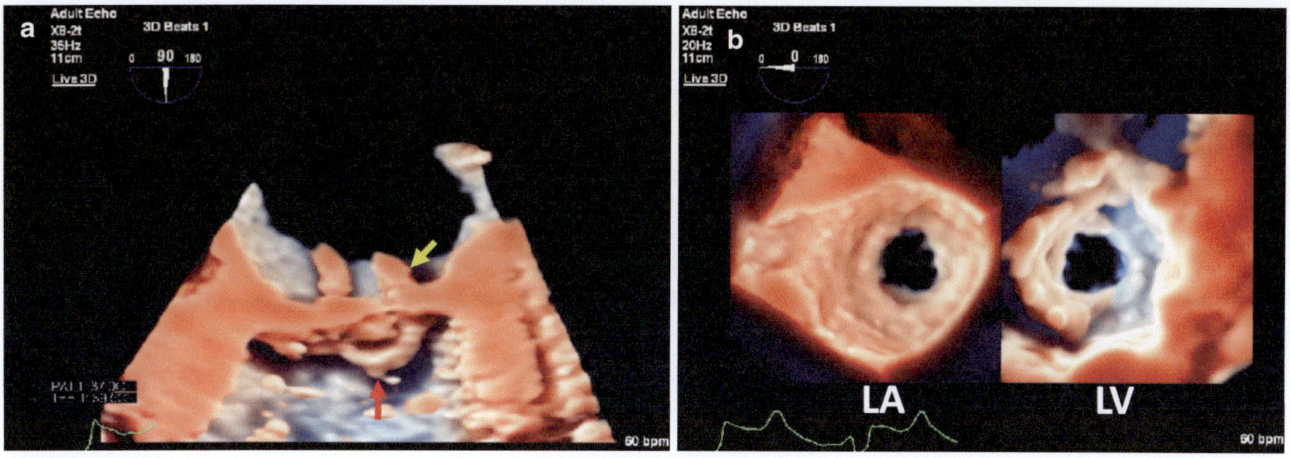

Fig. 31.17 3D TrueVue (Philips Healthcare) of another LAMPOON procedure. (**a**) snaring of AML directed wire (yellow arrow) in LVOT (red arrow). (**b**) Dual layout diastolic frame of MV post deployment of SAPIEN 3 valve. Images courtesy of Dr. Sari Padang. Used with permission of Mayo Foundation for Medical Education and Research. All rights reserved. AML, anterior mitral leaflet; LA, left atrium; LV, left ventricle; LVOT, left ventricular outflow tract; MV, mitral valve

References

1. Rodés-Cabau J, Kalavrouziotis D. Transcatheter mitral valve-in-valve replacement: the new gold standard for treating mitral bioprosthesis failure? JACC Cardiovasc Interv. 2018 June;11(12):1139–41.
2. Coylewright M, Cabalka AK, Malouf JF, Geske JB, Pollak PM, Suri RM, Rihal CS. Percutaneous mitral valve replacement using a transvenous, transseptal approach: transvenous mitral valve replacement. JACC Cardiovasc Interv. 2015 May;8(6):850–7.
3. Guerrero M, Salinger M, Pursnani A, Pearson P, Lampert M, Levisay J, Russell H, Feldman T. Transseptal transcatheter mitral valve-in-valve: a step by step guide from preprocedural planning to postprocedural care. Catheter Cardiovasc Interv. 2018 Sep 1;92(3):E185–96.
4. Sanon S, Cabalka AK, Babaliaros V, Rihal C, Gafoor S, Webb J, Latib A. Transcatheter tricuspid valve-in-valve and valve-in-ring implantation for degenerated surgical prosthesis. JACC Cardiovasc Interv. 2019 August;12(15):1403–12.
5. Aboulhosn J, Cabalka AK, Levi DS, Himbert D, Testa L, Latib A, Makkar RR, Boudjemline Y, Kim DW, Kefer J, Bleiziffer S, Kerst G, Dvir D, McElhinney DB. Transcatheter valve-in-ring implantation for the treatment of residual or recurrent tricuspid valve dysfunction after prior surgical repair. JACC Cardiovasc Interv. 2017 January;10(1):53–63.
6. Burkhard Mackensen G, Lee JC, Wang DD, Pearson PJ, Blanke P, Dvir D, Kirkpatrick JN. Role of echocardiography in transcatheter mitral valve replacement in native mitral valves and mitral rings. JASE. 2018;31(4):475–49.
7. Wunderlich NC, Beigel R, Ho SY, Nietlispach F, Cheng R, Agricola E, Siegel RJ. Imaging for mitral interventions: methods and efficacy. JACC Cardiovasc Imaging. 2018 June;11(6):872–901.
8. Loghin C, Loghin A. Role of imaging in novel mitral technologies—echocardiography and computed tomography. Ann Cardiothorac Surg. 2018 Nov;7(6):799–811.
9. Wilbring M, Kappert U, Matschke K. Transapical transcatheter valve-in-ring implantation for failed mitral valve repair in the absence of radiopaque markers. JTCVS. 2015 June;149(6):e92–4.
10. Babaliaros VC, Greenbaum AB, Khan JM, Rogers T, Wang DD, Eng MH, O'Neill WW, Paone G, Thourani VH, Lerakis S, Kim DW, Chen MY, Lederman RJ. Intentional percutaneous laceration of the anterior mitral leaflet to prevent outflow obstruction during transcatheter mitral valve replacement: first-in-human experience. JACC Cardiovasc Interv. 2017 Apr 24;10(8):798–809.

Part VII

Role of 3DE in Catheter-Based Electrophysiologic Procedures

The Role of Imaging Techniques in Electrophysiologic Procedures

32

Francesco F. Faletra, Francois Regoli, Laura A. Leo, Vera L. Paiocchi, Susanne A. Schlossbauer, and Samuel J. Asirvatham

Introduction

Over the past 25 years, the field of EP has greatly expanded. Sophisticated three-dimensional electro-anatomical mapping systems, novel implantable devices (capable of simultaneously recording electrical signal and intracardiac pressures, or "resynchronizing" ventricular contraction), implantable cardioverter-defibrillators and catheter-based ablation of a wide range of arrhythmias, have become the "armamentarium" of electrophysiologists (EPs). The same time frame has witnessed impressive technological advances in non-invasive imaging techniques. Currently, cardiac magnetic resonance (CMR), computed tomography (CT) and three-dimensional transesophageal echocardiography (3D TEE), are able to provide exquisite anatomical details of cardiac structures, both in two and in three-dimensional format making them an indispensable support for the diagnosis and management of patients with all forms of cardiovascular diseases including EP. The aforementioned non-invasive cardiac imaging techniques, have their own strengths and weaknesses and inevitably there is overlap between techniques. The choice of a single imaging modality may therefore, vary between institutions depending on several factors. Thus, a well thought of approach is required in order to avoid duplication of information and costs.

The use of advanced ultrasound imaging techniques (i.e. 2D/3D TEE) is no longer confined to the echocardiography laboratory, but has immensely expanded in the domain of image-guided structural heart disease interventions. Unfortunately, this trend does not comprise transcatheter-based treatment of atrial and ventricular arrhythmias. Indeed, most imaging cardiologists or radiologists have little exposure to EP procedures. There is also concern that image-guided EP procedures may have a significant impact on the workflow and may increase procedural costs. None-the-less, "potential" advantages of imaging during EP interventions include easier navigation, greater precision in targeting the "terrain" of interest, better catheter stability, avoidance of collateral damage, and reduction of radiation exposure.

In this chapter we review the role of non-invasive imaging techniques in EP. In particular we will focus our attention on 2D/3D TEE pre-procedural assessment and procedural guidance of cavo-tricuspid isthmus radiofrequency (RF) ablation and pulmonary vein isolation using either cryo- or radiofrequency energy.

CVTI Radiofrequency Ablation

Anatomy

The cavo-tricuspid isthmus (CVTI) can be envisioned as a quadrilateral region on the inferior-posterior wall of the right atrium, being delimited anteriorly by the tricuspid hinge line and posteriorly by the Eustachian valve (EV) (Fig. 32.1). The medial and lateral borders however, are less distinct, roughly corresponding to the coronary sinus ostium and to the terminal ramifications of the crista terminalis respec-

F. F. Faletra (✉)
Director of Cardiac Imaging Lab, Cardiocentro Ticino Institute, Lugano, Switzerland
e-mail: Francesco.Faletra@cardiocentro.org

F. Regoli
Division of Arrhythmology and Electrophysiology, Cardiocentro Ticino Institute, Lugano, Switzerland
e-mail: francois.regoli@cardiocentro.org

L. A. Leo · V. L. Paiocchi · S. A. Schlossbauer
Cardiac Imaging Lab, Cardiocentro Ticino Institute, Lugano, Switzerland
e-mail: lauraanna.leo@cardiocentro.org; vera.paiocchi@cardiocentro.org; susanne.schlossbauer@cardiocentro.org

S. J. Asirvatham
James M. and Lee S. Vann Professorship in Cardiovascular Diseases; Consultant, Department of Cardiovascular Medicine; Division of Pediatric Cardiology, Department of Anatomy & Department of Physiology and Biomedical Engineering; Professor of Medicine and Pediatrics; Mayo Clinic College of Medicine; Vice Chair, Innovation in the Midwest; Program Director, EP Fellowship Program; Medical Director, Electrophysiology Laboratory, Mayo Clinic, Rochester, MN, USA
e-mail: Asirvatham.Samuel@mayo.edu

J. F. Maalouf et al. (eds.), *Practical 3D Echocardiography*, https://doi.org/10.1007/978-3-030-72941-7_32

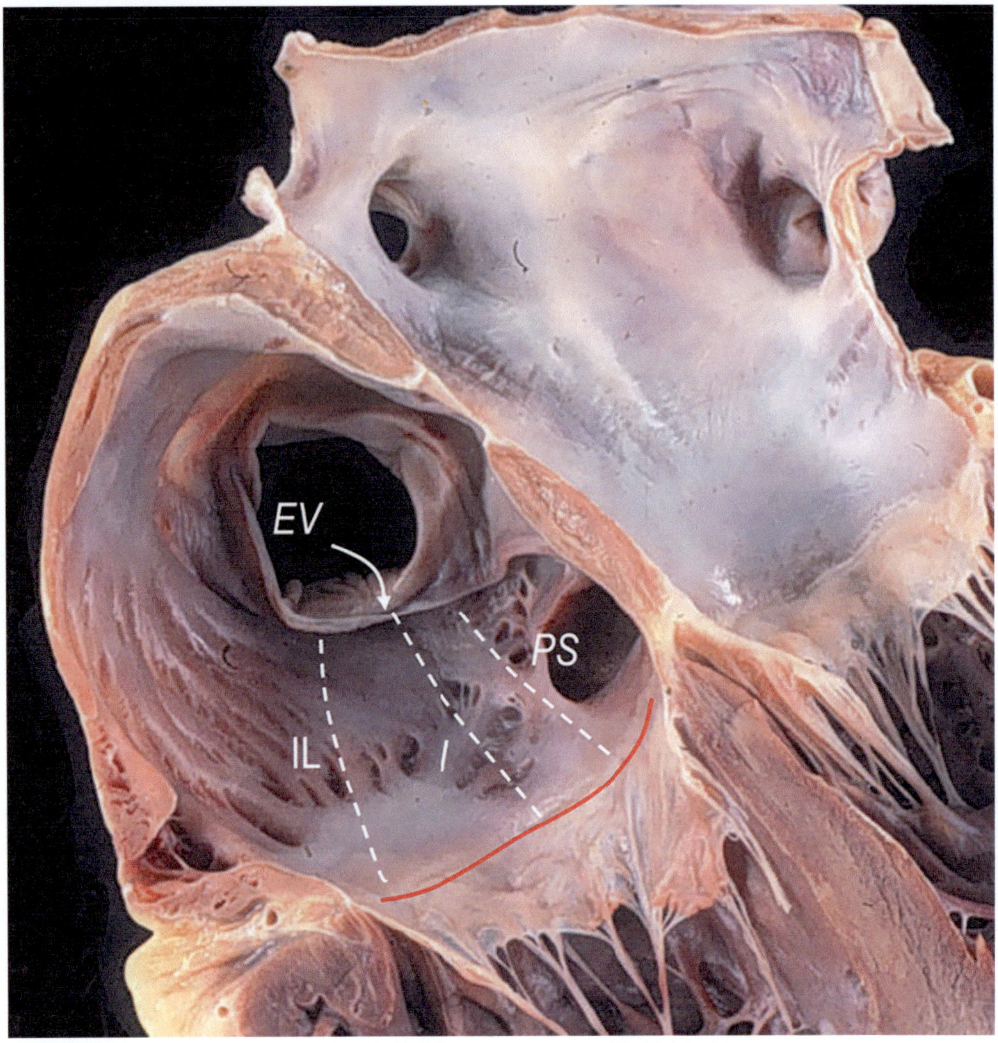

Fig. 32.1 Anatomic specimen showing the cavo-tricuspid isthmus (CVTI). The dotted lines mark the borders of the three sectors within the CVTI: inferolateral (IL), Inferior (I) and para-septal (PS) where the ablation may take place. The red line marks the hinge line of the tricuspid valve. EV, Eustachian valve

tively. The CVTI is the target of linear ablation (i.e. an ablation line which starts at the orifice of the inferior vena cava and ends at the hinge line of the tricuspid valve), which has been shown to be effective in interrupting the macro-reentrant circuit of typical atrial flutter. For this purpose, three sectors within the quadrilateral CVTI have been defined: para-septal, inferior and inferolateral (Fig. 32.1).

The preferred site of linear ablation is the inferior isthmus in the central sector for several reason: (a) the distance between the tricuspid valve hinge line and the orifice of the inferior vena cava is shorter in the inferior isthmus than in the inferolateral isthmus; (b) the ablation line is further away from the atrioventricular node; (c) the atrial wall in this sector is relatively thin and includes small areas of fatty-fibrous tissue which are electrically inert. These characteristics facilitate a completely transmural ablation line.

Anatomical variants of the CVTI may make the ablation difficult by lengthening the duration of the procedure and ablation time [1]. Among these anatomical variants it is worth mentioning the following: (1) a sub-Eustachian pouch-like recess, present in the inferior isthmus in approximately 10% of patients, may cause difficulties in achieving transmural lesions. The catheter tip may, in fact, not reach the deepest area of the recess, resulting in an incomplete ablation line. In such cases, the longer inferolateral isthmus may be preferable; (2) a long isthmus or an angulation between the inferior vena cava and CVTI close to 90° as well as a very prominent and rigid Eustachian valve may render catheter manipulations difficult; (3) pectinate muscles may occasionally extend across the lateral CVTI thus encroaching to some extent on the central CVTI. Their presence may also create gaps in the ablation line, which increases the risk of recurrence of the arrhythmia. Thus, "a priori" knowledge of the detailed anatomy of this region may significantly improve the safety and success rate of the ablation procedure.

Imaging Techniques

Several imaging techniques are able to illustrate "a priori" the anatomy of the CVTI and its anatomical variants:

Right atrial angiography just before the onset of the procedure may define the contour of the CVTI. Historically, angiographic studies first demonstrated that CVTI length and the presence of pouch-like recesses significantly increase the time of the procedure, x-ray exposure, and the number of radiofrequency applications [2].

CT and CMR performed before the onset of the procedure, are valuable non-invasive imaging techniques for assessing anatomy and anatomical variants.

CT has the highest spatial resolution (its isotropic voxel is 0.6 mm) and therefore may be better at defining the anatomical features and providing quantitative assessment of the CVTI. Indeed, CT provides extensive information regarding length, width, depth, thickness, angle with inferior vena cava, length and rigidity of EV, shape (flat, concave) and presence of a sub-Eustachian recess [3]. Additionally, CT provides fine images of the right coronary artery (RCA). Pre-procedural knowledge of the course of the RCA and its branches (including the nodal arteries) may be extremely useful. In particular, at the level of the lateral isthmus, the distance between the RCA and atrial endocardium may be less than 5 mm (which roughly corresponds to the depth that an effective trans-mural lesion should achieve) with potential risk for RCA injury [4]. Thus, a CT study may alert the electrophysiologist, as to whether the course of the RCA is too close to the potential ablation line. Although, CT is probably the most complete imaging technique in assessing CVTI anatomy, there are some limitations. First, a dedicated protocol must be used to obtain contrast images of the right atrium with image acquisition occurring when the first pass contrast is in the right atrial cavity. In order to avoid blooming artefacts due to the large amount of contrast flowing into the right atrium, which may obscure the CVTI border, the contrast must be adequately diluted by a second injection of physiological solution. Of note, this protocol is different from that used for CT coronary angiography which if needed, will impact quality of RA imaging. Second, obtaining clear and dynamic images of the CVTI requires multiphase retrospective acquisition with no dose modulation. With this protocol, even when the acquisition is performed with the new generation of CT machines, the x-ray exposure is no less than 10 mSv.

CMR appears to be a reliable imaging modality to illustrate the anatomy of the CVTI and to predict difficulty of the CVTI ablation. There is no radiation exposure associated with CMR and it is excellent at illustrating the dynamic nature of the CVTI, which shortens and lengthens during the cardiac cycle. However, CMR has its own limitations. First, delineating the EV or hinge line of the tricuspid valve is not always optimal. Second, to cover the entire surface of the CVTI, imaging with CMR relies on acquisition of multiple dedicated cross sections. And, as with CT, CMR visualizes the internal aspect of the CVTI in a two-dimensional plane, making it difficult to distinguish the para-septal, inferior and inferolateral isthmus. Third, in contrast to CT, CMR is unable to reliably determine the thickness of the CVTI, a potential marker of ablation difficulty. Finally, we should not forget the fact that CMR has limited availability in many institutions.

3D TEE provides excellent quality 3D images of the endocardial surface of the right atrium (RA). Indeed, the proximity of the transducer to the atrial cavities allows the use of high frequency crystals (5–7 MHz) with an axial spatial resolution ≤1 mm. Moreover, the high difference in acoustic impedance between blood and the internal surface of the atrial wall, makes possible achieving full visibility of right atrial structures. Finally,the capability of displaying right atrial structures from different perspectives, permits defining anatomic details which approximate the anatomic specimens (Fig. 32.2). In the following paragraphs we focus on this latter technique and its role before and during CVTI ablation.

The Use of 3D TEE Before and During CVTI Ablation

Before CVTI ablation, a pre-procedural 2D/3D TEE study is performed to rule-out thrombus. TEE may also provide the electrophysiologist with useful information regarding important anatomic variants that could require modifying the procedure. For instance, the use of a long transvenous sheath may offer adequate support and stability of the ablation catheter in the presence of a prominent and rigid EV and a long CVTI. A medial ablation line, closer to the coronary sinus ostium, could be more adequate in the presence of abundant pectinate muscles; conversely, a more lateral line may circumvent anatomical obstacles such as a deep sub-Eustachian pouch [1](Fig. 32.3 and Table 32.1).

Although routine use of 3DTEE for the anatomic characterization of the CVTI before RF ablation would be desirable (since these patients should undergo TEE to rule out LAA thrombus), there are limited studies in support of such use. Regoli et al. [5] using 3D TEE, studied patients with typical atrial flutter undergoing CVTI ablation and found that these patients often present with an anatomically complex CVTI. In fact, in this study more than 30% of the patients, had a deep sub-Eustachian septal recess or pouch, one in

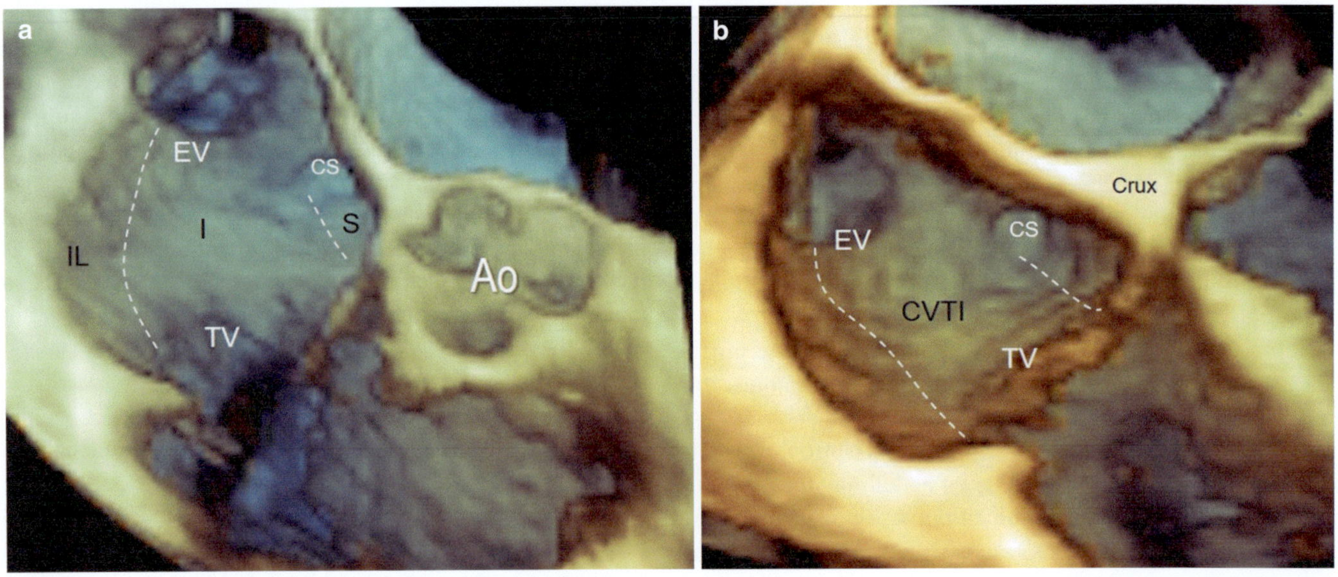

Fig. 32.2 (**a**, **b**) 3D TEE image of the cavo-tricuspid isthmus (CVTI) modified with the permission of Faletra et al. in Real-time 3D interventional echocardiography page 171. Springer-Verlag London 2014. The dotted lines mark the three regions of the CVTI: the inferolateral (IL), the inferior (I) and the para-septal (S). In the image in panel **a** the aortic root (Ao), partially covers the para-septal region. A more posterior plane **b** reveals the entire CVTI. CS, coronary sinus; EV, Eustachean valve; TV, tricuspid valve

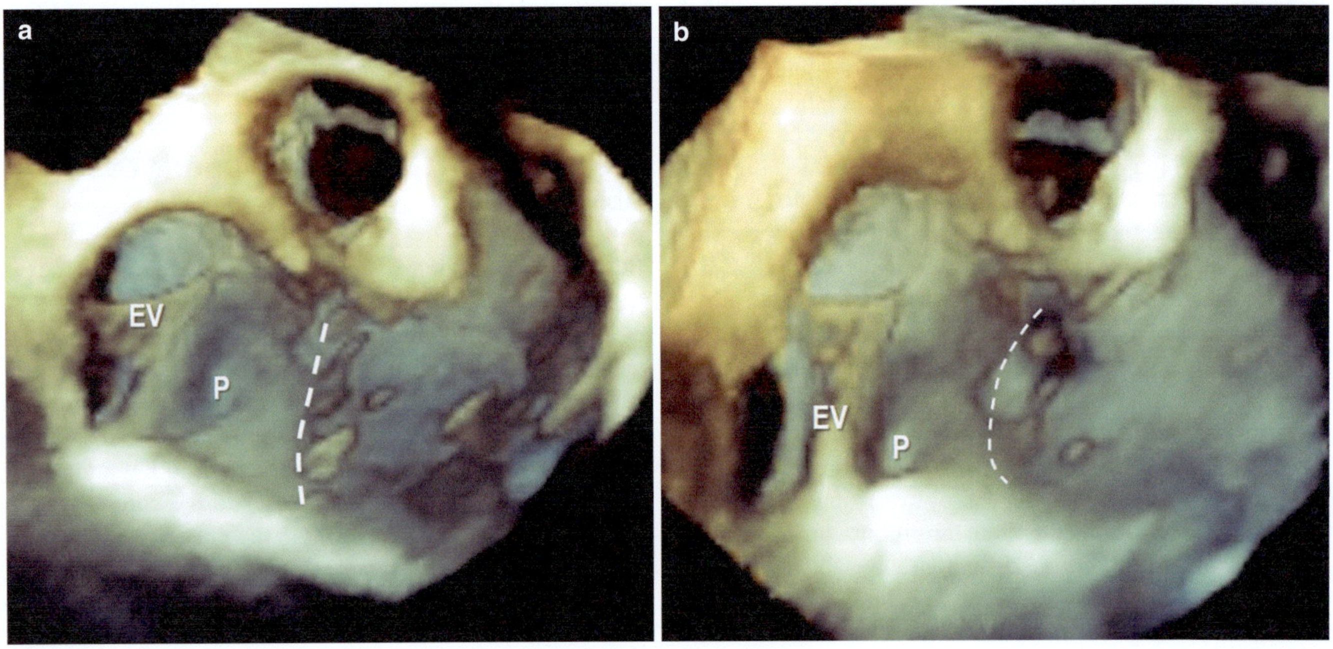

Fig. 32.3 (**a** and **b**): 3D TEE of right atrium in two slightly different perspectives of the right atrium showing Eustachian valve (EV), sub-Eustachian pouch (P) and the hinge line of tricuspid valve (dotted line)

every four patients had a long isthmus, a prominent Eustachian valve and/ or ridge, and/or pectinate muscle encroachment on the central sector of the CVTI. The presence of a deep septal pouch (most often combined with another prominent feature) represented the most important anatomical variant that rendered achievement of a bidirectional isthmus block challenging. However, it must be said that this was a single centre study with a limited number of patients, and randomized, prospectively designed studies are lacking.

In a proof-of-concept study, Regoli et al. [6], also assessed the feasibility and effectiveness of performing an anatomic-driven approach for CVTI ablation based on the intra-procedural use of 3D-TEE during the CVTI ablation

Table 32.1 Key Anatomic and Imaging Features of the CVTI for the Electrophysiologist

Feature	Impact
Prominent pectinates across the CVTI	Create a line more medially or increase power delivery
Prominent sub-Eustachian pouch	Create a line more laterally, use of irrigation
Prominent Eustachian ridge	Pre-formed sheaths, consider a lateral line
Prosthetic tricuspid valve	Find site where the valve has been sutured most ventricular to allow complete ablation

procedure. Procedural data using a real-time 3D TEE-guided approach, were compared with a retrospective patient cohort treated according to the standard fluoroscopy-guided approach. This study showed that (a) guiding the ablation catheter along the isthmus with 3D TEE is feasible, (b) a 3D TEE guided approach was associated with a four-fold reduction in fluoroscopy time; (c) total procedure duration was reduced by a mean of 40 min, and the number of applications needed to achieve bi-directional block were almost halved. It should be mentioned that as remarkable as these results may appear, they were nevertheless influenced by a learning curve effect: only in the last half of the study population, electrophysiologists completely relied on echocardiographic guidance without fluoroscopic guidance.

While the intra-procedural use of 3D TEE appears promising, it has some drawbacks. First, this approach needs general anaesthesia and the presence of a skilled echocardiographer for continuous monitoring during the procedure. This requires the allocation of many resources, making integration of this approach in routine clinical workflow rather difficult. Indeed, today CVTI ablation is an easy and straightforward procedure that does not need to be guided by 3D TEE. A 3D TEE-guided intraprocedural approach may be contemplated in particularly challenging patients who present recurrences despite previous RF ablation (roughly 5% of cases), or in those in whom avoiding x-ray exposure may be desirable.

Pulmonary Veins Isolation

Introduction

The pulmonary veins (PVs) play a relevant role in triggering and sustaining atrial fibrillation (AF). This is due to extension of an electrically active layer of atrial myocardium that discontinuously covers the PVs beyond the atrio-venous junction. This irregular myocardial distribution along the PVs may result in an abnormal electrical activity such as ectopic beats, local re-entry, or sustained focal activity, which may eventually cause AF. Today, the most common interventional treatment strategy for symptomatic, drug-resistant, AF is the electrical isolation of PVs. The procedure consists of radiofrequency or cryoablation delivered around the PVs with or without additional ablation within the LA. A pre-procedural definition of PV anatomy (i.e. number, size and shape) is therefore relevant for accurate targeting during the procedure and for the follow-up in case of PV stenosis. Key anatomic and imaging features of PV isolation are listed in Table 32.2.

Table 32.2 Key anatomic and imaging features of PV isolation for the electrophysiologist

Features	Impact
Aberrant location of pulmonary veins	Include in wide area circle around one side or both superior veins
Prominent vein of Marshall within the endocardial ridge	Consider cannulation and internal ablation
Pseudo diverticula on the left atrial vestibule	May not benefit fully from appendage isolation, potential perforation risk during linear ablation
Visualization of sinus node artery from left circumflex	Avoid lateral transverse linear ablation
Disjunction of mitral valve apparatus	Ablation may be required under the mitral valve to complete ablation of lateral isthmus line

Anatomy

The PVs enter the posterior part of the left atrium (LA). In around 70% of the population, PV entrance consists of two veins for each lung. The right upper PV drains oxygenated blood from the right superior and middle lobes, whereas the left upper PV from the left superior lobe and lingula [7]. The lower right and left PVs receive oxygenated blood from the right and left inferior lobes respectively. Anatomical variants from the usual pattern of four PVs are rather common. In around 15% of the population the upper and lower PVs merge in a common trunk. The most frequent anatomic variant of the right PVs consists of an additional vein entering the LA independently [7]. The pulmonary vein orifices are rather oval with the maximum diameter around 16 to 20 mm. However, quite often PVs enter the atrial cavity with a "funnel-shaped" configuration, making precise delineation of the venous-atrial junction difficult. The region in between two separate ipsilateral veins is referred to as an inter-venous ridge (Figs. 32.4 and 32.5c).

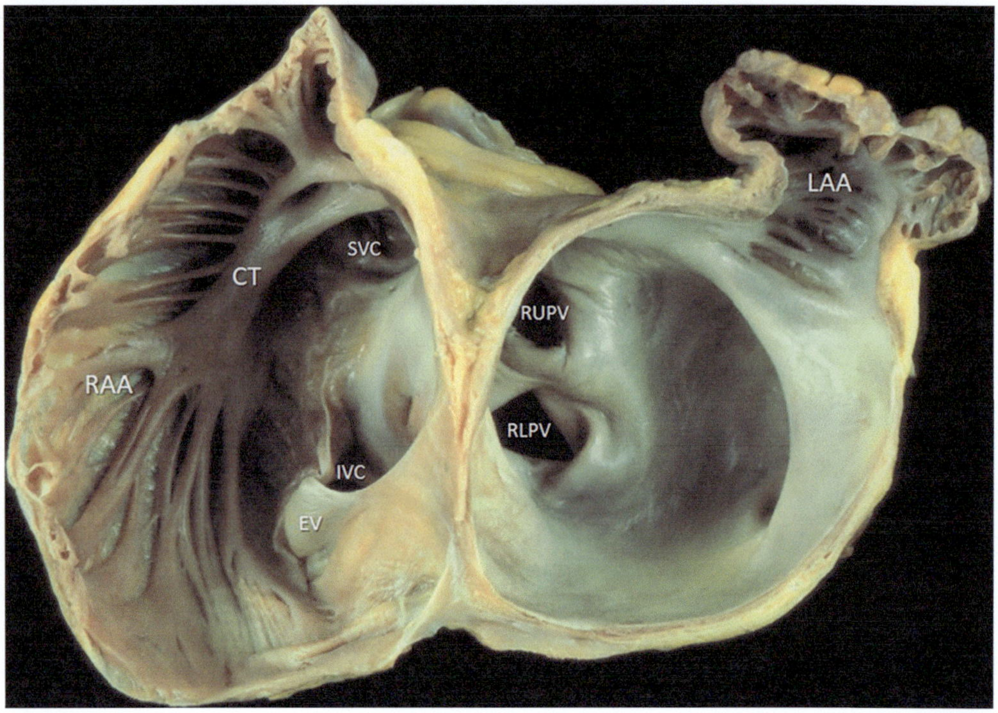

Fig. 32.4 anatomic specimen showing the four pulmonary veins (see text). CT, crista terminalis; EV, Eustachian valve; IVC, inferior vena cava; LAA, left atrial appendage; LLPV, left lower pulmonary vein; LUPV, left upper pulmonary vein; RAA, right atrial appendage; RUPV, right upper pulmonary vein; RLPV, right lower pulmonary vein; SVC, superior vena cava. With permission from McGraw-Hill, Hurst's The Heart, 2017, Maalouf et al., Chap. 4 Functional Anatomy of the Heart

Imaging Techniques

CT and CMR are the non-invasive imaging modalities commonly used for visualizing PV anatomy either in planar or in volume rendering format. Both techniques provide information regarding the size, number, location and anatomic variants of the pulmonary veins. CMR has the unique ability to precisely define the location and extent of myocardial fibrosis. Briefly, in presence of fibrosis, gadolinium accumulates in the interstitial space and its clearance is reduced compared with normal myocardium. Late gadolinium enhancement (LGE) on CMR allows precise delinitation of the fibrotic areas and correlates with amount of fibrosis. LGE is used routinely to detect fibrosis in ventricular myocardium, but it may be adapted to detect atrial or PV fibrosis [8]. It has been speculated that the extension of pre-procedural fibrosis along the atrial wall may predict recurrence of AF and therefore better determine in which patient ablation may be beneficial. However, it must be said that detecting LGE in the atrial myocardium is less obvious than in the thicker ventricular myocardium and is subject to significant interobserver variability. Moreover, patients with atrial fibrillation have an irregular heart rate making it difficult to acquire clear images of atrial LGE.

CT is the second imaging modality used to asses PV anatomy [7]. CT undoubtedly has the highest isotropic spatial resolution (0.6 × 0.6 × 0.6 mm) and produces images of excellent quality both in 2D cross section and in 3D volume rendering. Moreover, a modality called "virtual endoscopy" available using particular CT algorithms, makes the contrast transparent and the cavities opaque allowing for the entire roof of the LA along with the venous-atrial junctions to be visible in a single "panoramic" view. Finally, CT remains the only imaging modality that can provide anatomy of the coronary arteries along with PV anatomy. The main concern remains radiation exposure; however, new CT scanners are able to image the coronary arteries and PVs with an exposure ≤5 mSV.

3D TEE is another modality that allows imaging of the PV orifices [9]. Routinely, patients scheduled for PV ablation must undergo 2D/3D TEE to rule-out LAA or LA thrombus. Thus, theoretically 3D TEE should be the ideal technique for determining the number, size and anatomical variants avoiding more complex and expansive CT or CMR examinations. Unfortunately, while 3D TEE may visualize the CVTI in almost all patients, imaging the four pulmonary veins in individual patients is more challenging. Whereas, the entire contour of the upper right and left PV orifice is visible in almost all cases, visualizing the orifices of the lower PVs may be very difficult. The difficulty in consistently imaging the lower pulmonary veins may be due to the different angulations by which the lower veins drain into the left atrium (Fig. 32.5).

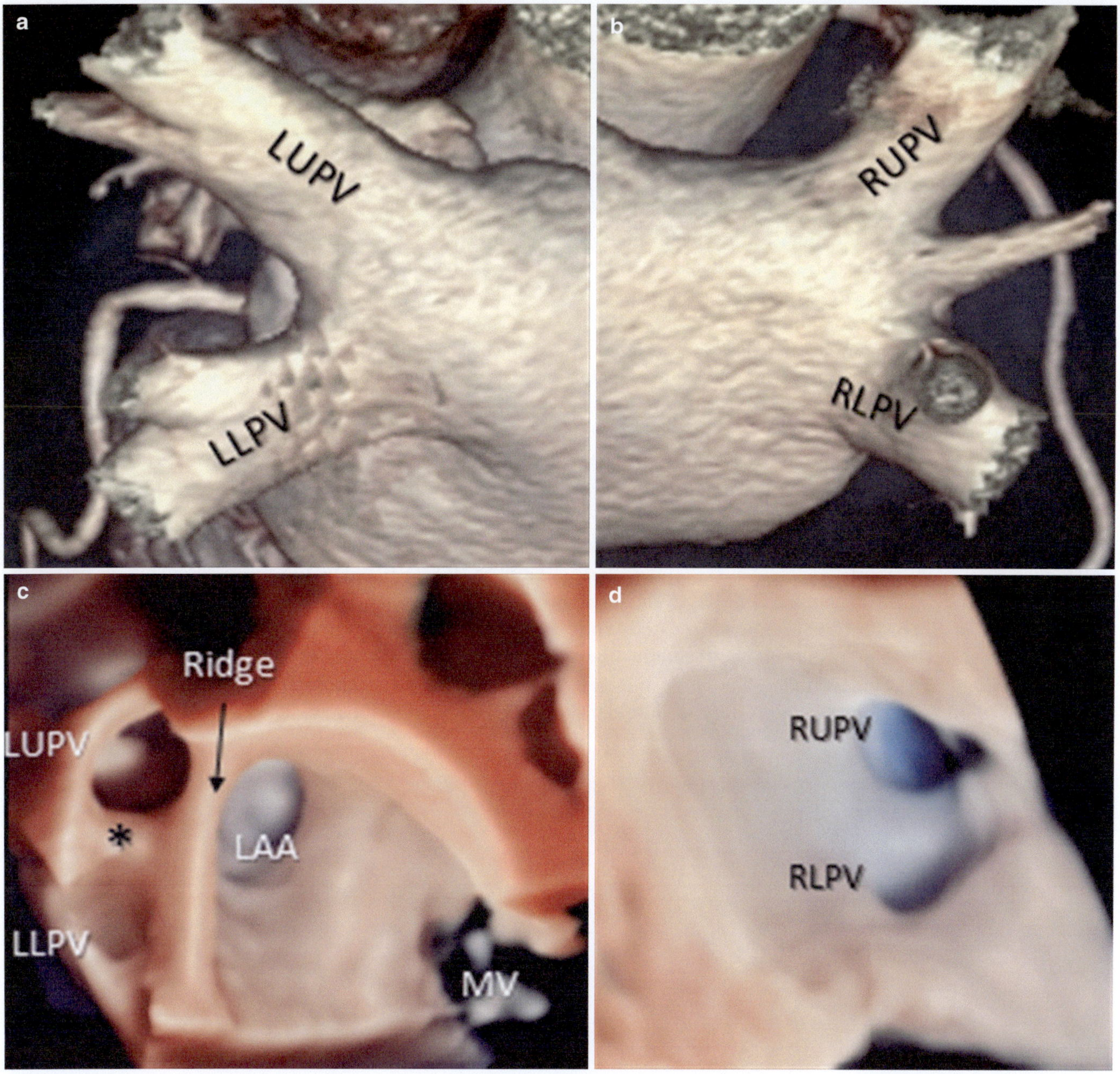

Fig. 32.5 (**a**, **b**) CT scan volume rendering showing the left upper (LUPV) and lower (LLPV) in panel **a** and the right upper (RUPV) and lower (RLPV) in panel **b**. (**c**, **d**): 3D TEE using a new algorithm which allows use of a movable source of light. Panel **c** shows the LUPV and LLPV, the left atrial appendage (LAA) and the left lateral ridge (ridge) and Panel **d** shows the RUPV and RLPV. Asterisk points to the intervenous ridge. MV, mitral valve

3D TEE During PVs Ablation

Despite the aforementioned limitations of 3D TEE, Acena et al. [10]conducted a small study (22 patients), aiming to prospectively evaluate the ability of intra-procedural real time (RT) 3D TEE to visualize the PV orifices and to compare this modality with an electroanatomic mapping system for the localization of the radiofrequency ablation catheter during PV ablation. Visualization of all four PVs was possible in only 18% of cases; 3 veins were visualized in 50% of cases and no veins could be seen in roughly 10% of cases. The "ultrasound pyramidal window" does not allow for imaging structures that are less than 1 cm from the probe, and being supine can produce anteroposterior pressure on the atrium such that the LA posterior wall becomes too close to the TEE probe.

However, these disappointing findings on the intra-procedural use of 3DTEE are in contrast with what was previously reported by Ottaviano and colleagues [11] who used 3DTEE to monitor PVI procedures using cryoablation technology. In 45 patients, real time (RT).

3DTEE, successfully guided the positioning of the cryo-balloon to achieve complete ostium occlusion in all PVs. Moreover, 2DTEE identified peri-ostial leakage in 13% of veins, implicating inadequate cryo-balloon positioning. Therapy without reported complications was effectively delivered in all patients, and freedom from AF recurrence at a median of 9 months was high (82%). In this single-center experience, RT 3D TEE guidance of cryo-balloon ablation was safe and feasible, allowing not only adequate visualization of all PV ostia and neighbouring LA structures, but also effectively guided complete PV occlusion of the cryo-balloon, an essential aspect for effective cryoablation.

A more recent single-center contribution by Sun and colleagues [12] also reports a positive experience with intra-procedural 3DTEE technique on an even larger patient cohort ($n = 80$ patients) in a comparative study considering procedural end-points, namely procedure duration, fluoroscopy time, and volume of contrast injected. While no difference was found in terms of procedure duration and number of cryo-applications to achieve PV isolation, fluoroscopy time was reduced in the 3D TEE group by over 60% (mean fluoroscopy time of less than 7 min) and mean contrast dye volume injected in this group was only 3 ml.

Taken together, based on current evidence that continues to be limited to the experience of single centers, the utility of 3DTEE appears highly dependent on the technique used to perform PV ablation. The RF technique is a lengthy procedure, delivering point-by-point lesions circumferentially around the PV ostia. This implies a lengthy, continuous, and precise monitoring of the ablation catheter position. Imaging with 3DTEE can be distorted by ablation catheter artefact, physiological movement (breathing, movement of the esophagus), and the spatial orientation of the lower PVs, thus rendering continuous monitoring very challenging even for the most experienced echocardiographers. The cryo-balloon technique, in contrast, is a quicker and more straightforward procedure requiring only the assessment of the correct alignment between the balloon and the PV ostia. Switching regularly to 2D TEE mode for the assessment of peri-ostial leakage using color Doppler guides realignment of the balloon by simply applying fine torque/ counter-torque maneuvers to the balloon catheter (Fig. 32.6).

Additional areas where 3D imaging is beneficial beyond CVTI and PV isolation are listed in Table 32.3.

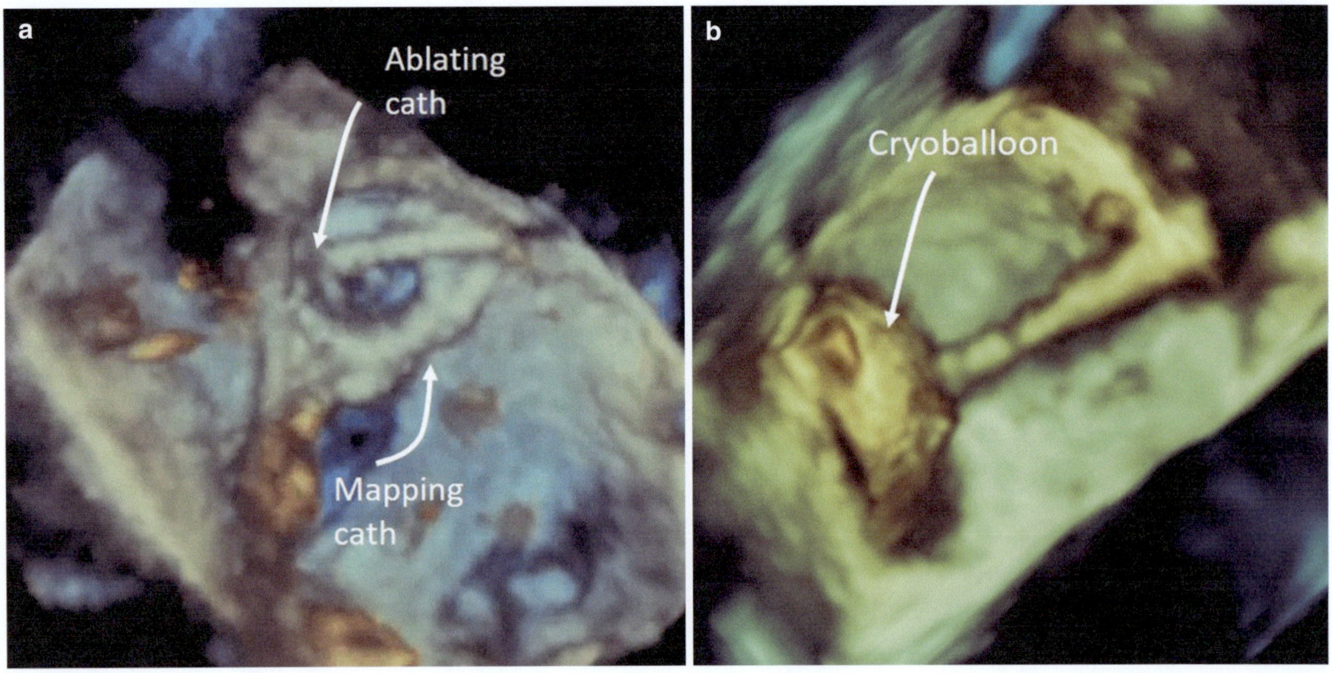

Fig. 32.6 (**a**) 3D TEE of PV ablation with radiofrequency waves; (**b**) 3D TEE of PV ablation with a cryoballoon

Table 32.3 Areas of real-time 3D visualization value beyond CVTI and PV isolation

Features	Impact
Outflow tract relationship [15]	• Appreciate where myocardium exists on either side of the complex outflow septum when ablating. • Avoid injury to distal left main or proximal LAD with direct visualization. • Appreciate the existence of supravalvar extensions of myocardium into the semi-lunar valves
Endocavitary structure ablation [16]	• Appreciate the intraconnectivity and 3D anatomy of the papillary muscles. • Visualize insertion point of neo-chords post-surgery. • Identify and map along the moderator band. • Identify the conus papillary muscle to completely map and ablate as needed [17]
Common congenital heart disease ablation	• Assess catheter contact in neo-let atrium after classic Fontan procedure. • Baffle attachment points visualization. • Atrial septal patch visualization for transseptal access including visualizing fenestrations. • Accessory pathway ablation, identify forme fruste of Ebstein's anomaly. • Identify coronary sinus diverticula.

Conclusions

Although the aforementioned data appear promising, the main limitation is the lack of high-impact, well designed trials that support the routine use of 3D TEE for the treatment of AF. Moreover, it is difficult to conceive how 3DTEE may be integrated in the routine workflow for monitoring PV ablation. These procedures are lengthy and complex. And, although limited available intra-procedural data have reported no complications related to the prolonged use of the TEE probe, the possibility that prolonged TEE monitoring may cause oesophageal heat injury cannot be excluded. This aspect is especially of concern when RF is delivered on the left atrial posterior wall. Heating of the TEE probe coupled with RF delivery heating in this area may act synergistically and cause oesophageal injury.

Lastly, it must be stated that EP procedures in contrast to many other catheter-based structural interventions do not rely on 3D TEE for intra-procedural guidance. Indeed, in recent years, the diffusion of electro-anatomical mapping systems (EAMS) with high-density mapping has considerably improved the overall workflow of RF ablation procedures of complex arrhythmias. This improved technology allows for the simultaneous acquisition of 3D anatomic geometry that integrates both electrical (arrythmia activation/ propagation) as well as ultra-structural (endocardial voltage map) information with a high degree of spatial resolution [13]. Furthermore, all available EAMS are equipped with dedicated algorithms that monitor RF lesion extension and depth [14].

References

1. Asirvatham SJ. Correlative anatomy and electrophysiology for the interventional electrophysiologist: right atrial flutter. J Cardiovasc Electrophysiol. 2009;20:113–22.
2. Hisazaki K, Kaseno K, Miyazaki S, Amaya N, Hasegawa K, Shiomi Y, Tama N, Ikeda H, Fukuoka Y, Morishita T, Ishida K, Uzui H, Tada H. Intra-procedural evaluation of the cavo-tricuspid isthmus anatomy with different techniques: comparison of angiography and intracardiac echocardiography. Heart Vessel. 2019 Oct;34(10):1703–9.
3. Kajihara K, Nakano Y, Hirai Y, Ogi H, Oda N, Suenari K, Makita Y, Sairaku A, Tokuyama T, Motoda C, Fujiwara M, Watanabe Y, Kiguchi M, Kihara Y. Variable procedural strategies adapted to anatomical characteristics in catheter ablation of the cavotricuspid isthmus using a preoperative multidetector computed tomography analysis. J Cardiovasc Electrophysiol. 2013 Dec;24(12):1344–51.
4. Al Aloul B, Sigurdsson G, Adabag S, Li JM, Dykoski R, Tholakanahalli VN. Atrial flutter ablation and risk of right coronary artery injury. J Clin Med Res. 2015 Apr;7(4):270–3.
5. Regoli F, Faletra F, Marcon S, et al. Anatomic characterization of cavotricuspid isthmus by 3D transesophageal echocardiography in patients undergoing radiofrequency ablation of typical atrial flutter. Eur Heart J Cardiovasc Imaging. 2018;19:84–91.
6. Regoli F, Faletra FF, Nucifora G, et al. Feasibility and acute efficacy of radiofrequency ablation of cavotricuspid isthmus-dependent atrial flutter guided by real-time 3D TEE. JACC Cardiovasc Imaging. 2011;4(7):716–26.
7. Hassani C, Saremi F. Comprehensive cross-sectional imaging of the pulmonary veins. Radiographics. 2017 Nov–Dec;37(7):1928–54.
8. Higuchi K, Cates J, Gardner G, Morris A, Burgon NS, Akoum N, Marrouche NF. The spatial distribution of late gadolinium enhancement of left atrial magnetic resonance imaging in patients with atrial fibrillation. JACC Clin Electrophysiol. 2018 Jan;4(1):49–58.
9. Faletra FF, Nucifora G, Regoli F, Ho SY, Moccetti T, Auricchio A. Anatomy of pulmonary veins by real-time 3D TEE: implications for catheter-based pulmonary vein ablation. JACC Cardiovasc Imaging. 2012 Apr;5(4):456–62.
10. Acena M, Regoli F, Faletra FF, et al. 3D real-time TEE during pulmonary vein isolation in atrial fibrillation. JACC Cardiovasc Imaging. 2014;7:737–8.
11. Ottaviano L, Chierchia GB, Bregasi A, et al. Cryoballoon ablation for atrial fibrillation guided by real-time three-dimensional transoesophageal echocardiography: a feasibility study. Europace. 2013;15:944–50.
12. Sun YJ, Yin XM, Cong T, et al. Comparison of cryoballoon ablation for atrial fibrillation guided by real-time three-dimensional transesophageal echocardiography vs. contrast agent injection. Chin Med J (Engl). 2019;132:285–93.
13. Herczeg S, Walsh K, Keaney JJ, et al. Quantitative assessment of left atrial scar using high-density voltage mapping and a novel automated voltage analysis tool. [published online ahead of print, 2019 Jun 5]. J Interv Card Electrophysiol. 2020;59(1):5–12.

14. Holmes D, Fish JM, Byrd IA, et al. Contact sensing provides a highly accurate means to titrate radiofrequency ablation lesion depth. J Cardiovasc Electrophysiol. 2011;22(6):684–90.
15. Gard J, et al. Outflow tract ventricular tachycardia. Texas Heart Inst J. 2012;39(4):526–8.
16. Abouezzeddine O, Suleiman M, Buescher T, Kapa S, Friedman PA, Jahangir A, Mears JA, Ladewig DJ, Munger TM, Hammill SC, Packer DL, Asirvatham SJ. Relevance of endocavitary structures in ablation procedures for ventricular tachycardia. J Cardiovasc Electrophysiol 2010 Mar;21(3):245–254.
17. Hai JJ, Desimone CV, Vaidya VR, Asirvatham SJ. Endocavitary structures in the outflow tract: anatomy and electrophysiology of the conus papillary muscles. J Cardiovasc Electrophysiol. 2014;25(1):94–8.

The Role of CT and MRI in Electrophysiologic Procedures

33

Kathleen A. Young, Jared G. Bird, Thomas A. Foley, and Nandan S. Anavekar

Multimodality imaging utilizing cardiac computed tomography (CT) and/or magnetic resonance imaging (MRI) is commonly employed in the procedural planning for electrophysiology procedures, from ablation to device implantation [1]. Both cardiac CT and MRI can provide additional information regarding the anatomy of surrounding structures and tissue characterization that is not able to be assessed fully by echocardiography.

Cardiac CT in particular has been integrated into procedural planning for atrial fibrillation ablation procedures as it provides information regarding anatomy of pulmonary veins and atria; as well as evaluation for thrombus [2–4]. The left atrial appendage is the most common place for left atrial thrombus, particularly in atrial fibrillation [2]. Transesophageal echocardiography remains the gold standard for detection of left atrial appendage thrombus; however, cardiac CT has also been shown to have high diagnostic accuracy for detection of thrombus (Fig. 33.1, [2]).

For ventricular tachycardia ablation, evaluation for intracardiac thrombus prior to the procedure is also important. While this can be assessed by echocardiography, both cardiac CT and MRI are emerging as superior imaging modalities to fully detail the character of the thrombi if present (Fig. 33.2, [5]). In addition, cardiac MRI is commonly utilized for substrate identification and lesion evaluation, such as scar, prior to and following ventricular tachycardia ablation (Fig. 33.3, [5, 6]). Cardiac CT is a reasonable alternative if there are contraindications to MRI or concern of artifact from a cardiac device (Fig. 33.4, [5]).

Lastly, these advanced imaging modalities are also used to evaluate for post-procedure complications, such as pulmonary vein stenosis, which can be a complication of atrial fibrillation ablation procedures (Figs. 33.5 and 33.6, [2, 7]).

K. A. Young
Instructor in Medicine, Mayo Clinic College of Medicine; Resident, Department of Cardiovascular Medicine, Mayo Clinic, Rochester, MN, USA
e-mail: young.kathleen1@mayo.edu

J. G. Bird
Instructor in Medicine, Mayo Clinic College of Medicine, Senior Associate Consultant, Department of Cardiovascular Medicine, Mayo Clinic, Rochester, MN, USA
e-mail: bird.jared@mayo.edu

T. A. Foley
Assistant Professor of Radiology, Mayo Clinic College of Medicine; Consultant, Division of Cardiovascular Radiology, Department of Radiology, Mayo Clinic, Rochester, MN, USA
e-mail: foley.thomas@mayo.edu

N. S. Anavekar (✉)
Professor of Medicine, Mayo Clinic College of Medicine; Consultant, Department of Cardiovascular Medicine, Mayo Clinic, Rochester, MN, USA
e-mail: anavekar.nandan@mayo.edu

J. F. Maalouf et al. (eds.), *Practical 3D Echocardiography*, https://doi.org/10.1007/978-3-030-72941-7_33

Fig. 33.1 Left Atrial Appendage Thrombus: 80 year old female who underwent contrast CT scan to assess pulmonary veins prior to atrial fibrillation ablation. Top image demonstrates incomplete opacification (arrow) of the left atrial appendage during initial imaging due to slow filling of the atrial appendage with contrast. Bottom image is repeat delayed imaging 25 seconds later which shows opacification of the left atrial appendage with a persistent filling defect (arrow) consistent with left atrial appendage thrombus. Used with permission of Mayo Foundation for Medical Education and Research. All rights reserved

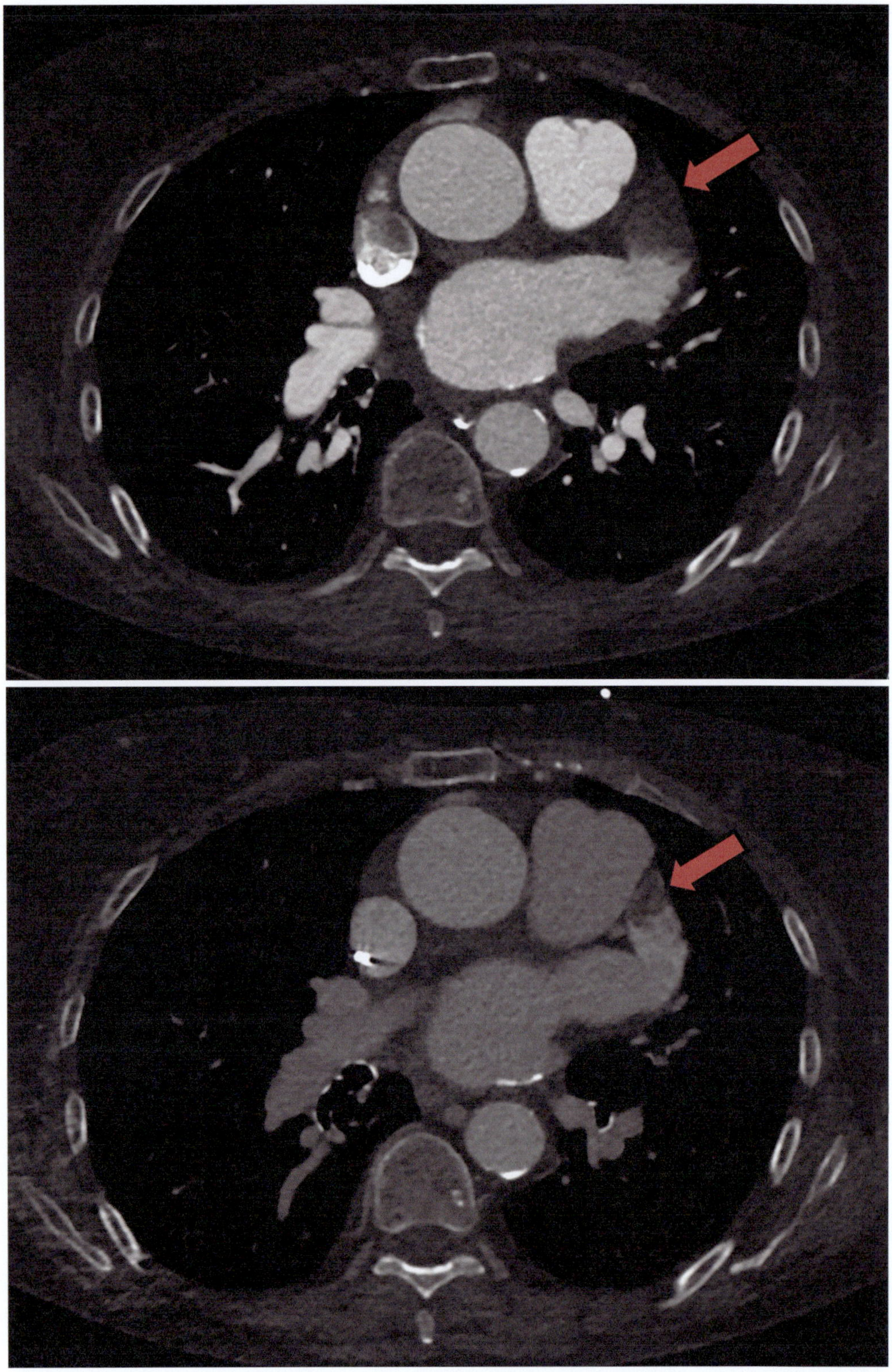

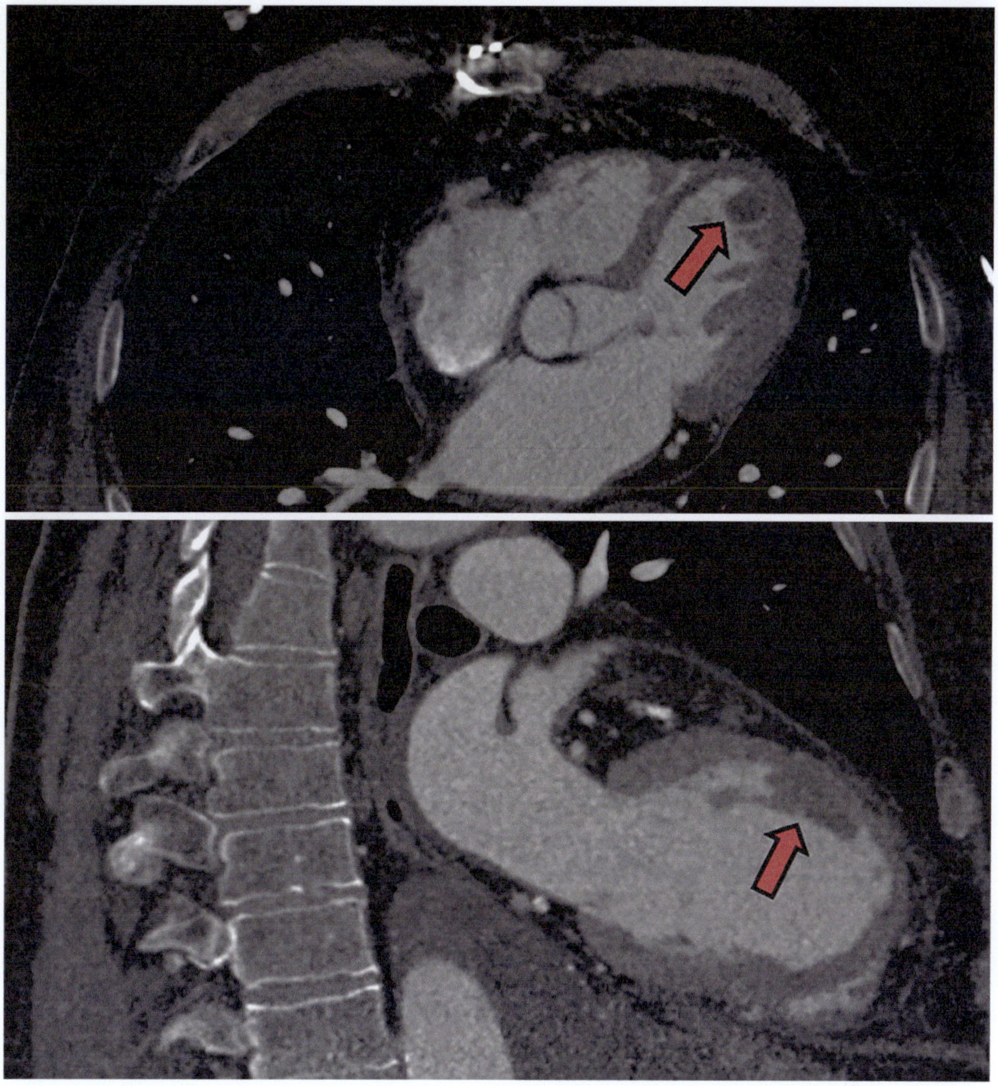

Fig. 33.2 Computed Tomography (CT) Evaluation for Thrombus: Contrast cardiac CT demonstrating laminated apical and anterior wall thrombus (red arrows) in a 72 year old male. He presented with chest pain and was found to have an acute Type A dissection. He underwent surgical repair and post-operative CT scan demonstrated the left ventricular thrombus. Used with permission of Mayo Foundation for Medical Education and Research.

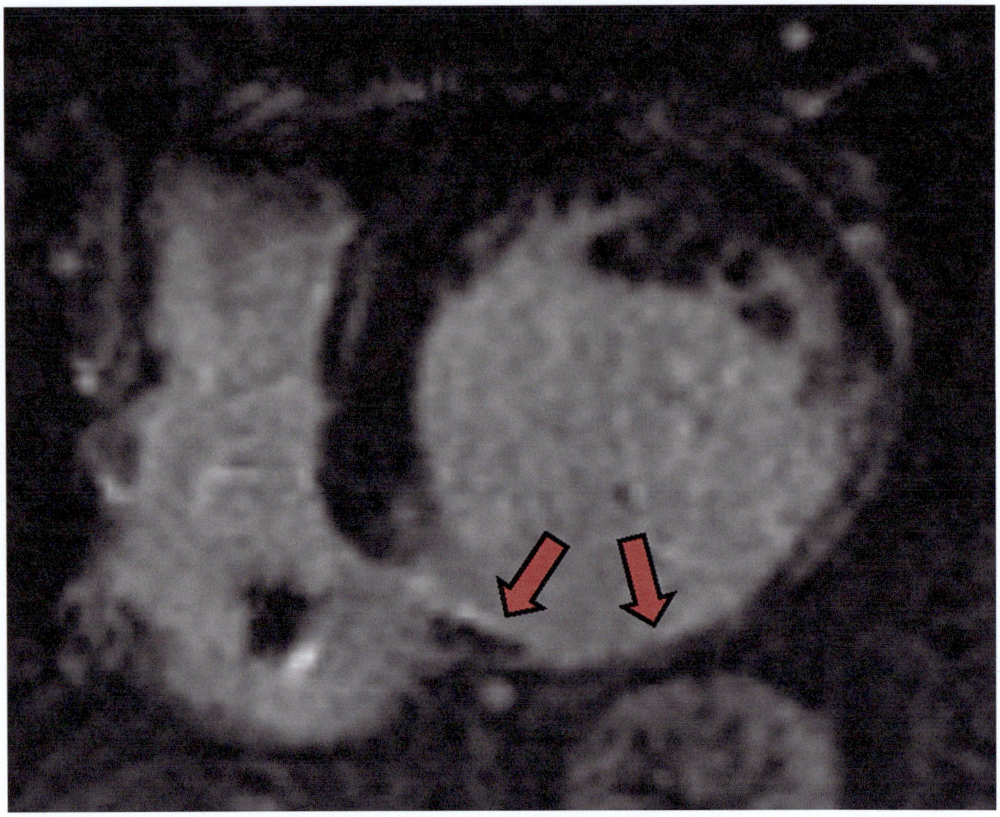

Fig. 33.3 Magnetic Resonance Imaging (MRI) for Evaluation of Scar Prior to Ventricular Tachycardia Ablation: 74 year old male who presented with ventricular tachycardia unresponsive to medical therapy. Cardiac MRI was performed to assess for scarring prior to VT ablation. There is full thickness delayed enhancement of the inferior, inferolateral, and inferoseptal walls consistent with transmural infarction (arrows). The patient underwent successful inferior/inferolateral VT ablation. Used with permission of Mayo Foundation for Medical Education and Research. All rights reserved

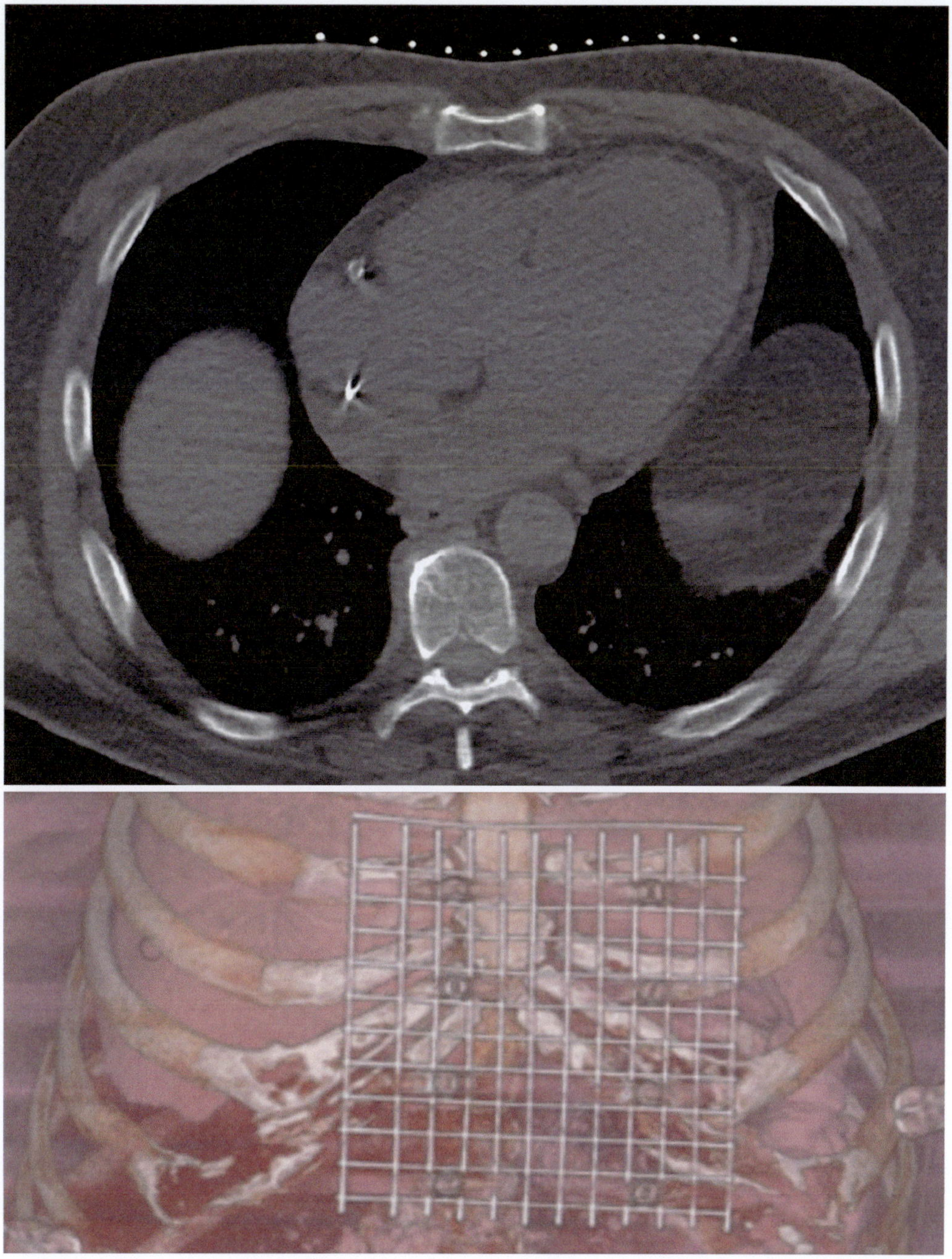

Fig. 33.4 Epicardial Grid Using Computed Tomography (CT): Non-contrast chest CT performed for epicardial grid planning in a 69 year old male prior to pericardial access for epicardial VT ablation. The upper image demonstrates an axial non-contrast CT slice with radiopaque markers on the chest (white circles) for mapping of the internal structures prior to pericardial access. The bottom image is a 3D reconstruction of the chest with the epicardial grid superimposed. Images are taken in both inspiration and expiration for procedural planning. Used with permission of Mayo Foundation for Medical Education and Research. All rights reserved

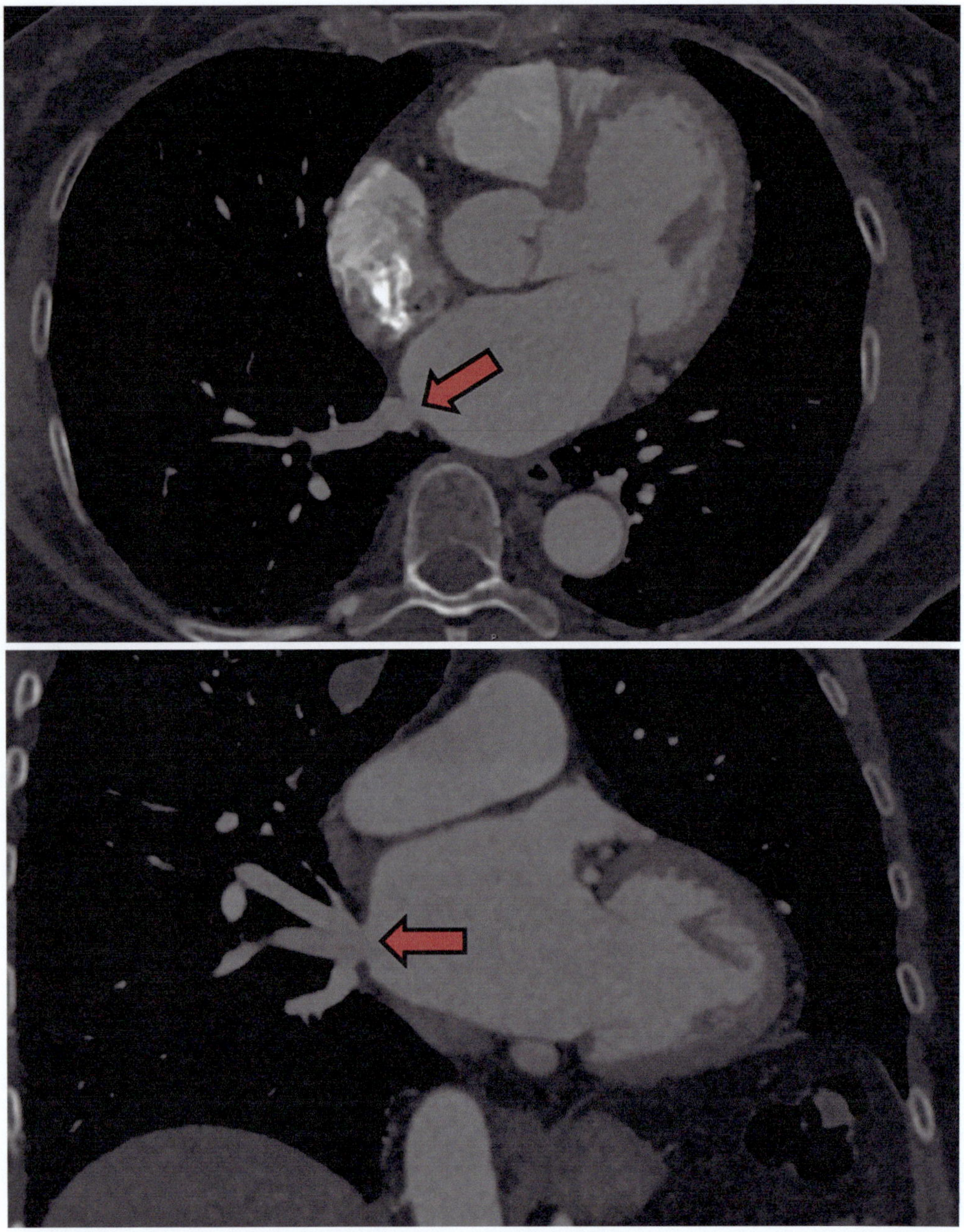

Fig. 33.5 Pulmonary Vein Stenosis on Cardiac Computed Tomography (CT): Cardiac CT demonstrating stenosis of the right inferior pulmonary vein after pulmonary vein isolation in a 73 year old female. Note the ostial stenosis demonstrated by the red arrow in both the axial (top image) and coronal (bottom image) planes. Used with permission of Mayo Foundation for Medical Education and Research. All rights reserved

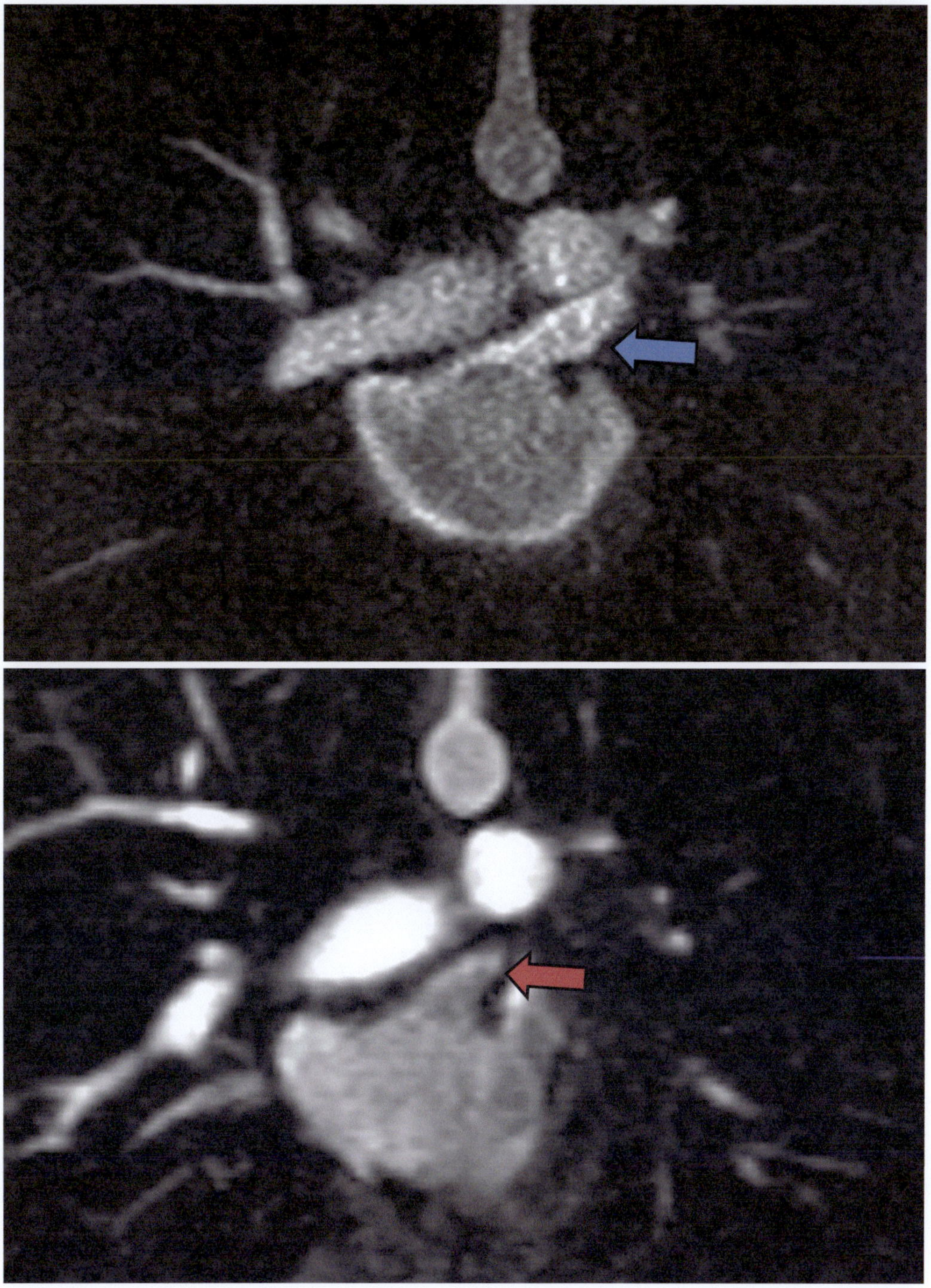

Fig. 33.6 Pulmonary Vein Stenosis on Magnetic Resonance Imaging (MRI). Cardiac MRI demonstrating interval left superior pulmonary vein occlusion after pulmonary vein isolation in a 49 year old male. Pre-procedure imaging demonstrated patent left superior pulmonary vein (blue arrow). Post-procedure imaging 6 months later demonstrated proximal occlusion of the left superior pulmonary vein (red arrow). Used with permission of Mayo Foundation for Medical Education and Research. All rights reserved

References

1. Pison L, et al. Imaging techniques in electrophysiology and implantable device procedures: results of the European heart rhythm association survey. Europace. 2013;15(9):1333–6.
2. Donal E, et al. EACVI/EHRA expert consensus document on the role of multi-modality imaging for the evaluation of patients with atrial fibrillation. Eur Heart J Cardiovasc Imaging. 2016;17(4):355–83.
3. Robinson MR, Hutchinson MD. Use of imaging techniques to guide catheter ablation procedures. Curr Cardiol Rep. 2010;12(5):374–81.
4. Joshi SB, et al. CT applications in electrophysiology. Cardiol Clin. 2009;27(4):619–31.
5. Mahida S, et al. Cardiac imaging in patients with ventricular tachycardia. Circulation. 2017;136(25):2491–507.
6. Chubb H, et al. Cardiac electrophysiology under MRI guidance: an emerging technology. Arrhythm Electrophysiol Rev. 2017;6(2):85–93.
7. Calkins H, et al. 2017 HRS/EHRA/ECAS/APHRS/SOLAECE expert consensus statement on catheter and surgical ablation of atrial fibrillation: executive summary. J Arrhythm. 2017;33(5):369–409.

Part VIII

New Trends for 3DE in Catheter-Based Interventions

34 Novel Percutaneous Techniques for Mitral and Tricuspid Valve Repair

Joseph F. Maalouf, Sushil Allen Luis, and Jeremy J. Thaden

Mitral Regurgitation

There are currently several transcatheter devices undergoing evaluation for percutaneous mitral valve repair or replacement in select patients with severe mitral regurgitation (MR) and the list continues to grow [1–6]. A comprehensive review, therefore, is beyond the scope of this chapter. Deployment of these novel percutaneous valve therapies is heavily dependent on 2D and 3D TEE guidance. One such device is the Edwards-SAPIEN M3 transcatheter heart valve (THV) [2, 3], a modified SAPIEN 3 valve (Edwards Lifesciences, Irvine-California) that is implanted via a transseptal approach using a nitinol dock delivery system that is designed to encircle and capture the native mitral leaflets and provide an anchor location for the M3 THV (Fig. 34.1). The dock is made up of an encirling turn, functional turns, and an atrial turn. The transcatheter docking system is advanced through the medial mitral valve commissure into the left ventricle to encircle the mitral chordae (Fig. 34.1), and thus acts as a secure anchor for the M3 valve that is then deployed into the dock using a standard valve-in-valve implantation technique. The atrial turn is released upon withdrawing the dock delivery steerable catheter into the left atrium creating the equivalent of a surgical ring. 3D TEE plays a pivotal role in guiding the steerable catheter towards the mitral valve medial commissure.

Another THV that underwent early feasibility study is the Caisson transcatheter mitral valve replacement system (Caisson Interventional LivaNova Maple Grove, Minnesota) [1, 2]. This THV system is composed of a self-expanding nitinol docking anchor frame and a trileaflet porcine pericardial valve that is housed within the docking anchor (Fig. 34.2). En face 3D TEE LA views are critical to align the advancing anchor frame feet to the mitral valve apparatus and commissures (Fig. 34.2). 3D TEE is also very useful to monitor the THV descent towards the anchor, and to assess anchor alignment with the mitral valve after the atrial holding frames are lowered. 3D color flow Doppler post implantation is used to confirm stability of the newly implanted transcatheter valve and to exclude significant regurgitation.

Transcatheter edge-to-edge mitral valve repair is also evolving. The Edwards PASCAL transcatheter valve repair system (Edwards Lifesciences Corp, Irvine, CA) is currently being evaluated for treatment of functional and degenerative mitral regurgitation [6]. It consists of a central spacer to fill the regurgitant orifice area, two broad paddles and two clasps that allow for independent leaflet capture between the paddles and spacer (Fig. 34.3). As with transcatheter edge-to-edge mitral valve repair using the MitraClip device, 3D TEE plays a pivotal role in guiding deployment of the PASCAL device (Fig. 34.4).

Tricuspid Regurgitation

Until recently, trans-catheter interventions for tricuspid valve (TV) disease were restricted primarily to patients with a degenerating bioprosthesis (see Chap. 31). The realization that severe tricuspid regurgitation (TR), left untreated, has

Supplementary Information The online version of this chapter (https://doi.org/10.1007/978-3-030-72941-7_34) contains supplementary material, which is available to authorized users.

J. F. Maalouf (✉)
Professor of Medicine, Mayo Clinic College of Medicine; Director, Interventional Echocardiography; Consultant, Department of Cardiovascular Medicine, Mayo Clinic, Rochester, MN, USA
e-mail: maalouf.joseph@mayo.edu

S. A. Luis
Associate Professor of Medicine, Mayo Clinic College of Medicine; Consultant, Rochester, MN, USA
e-mail: Luis.S@mayo.edu

J. J. Thaden
Assistant Professor of Medicine, Mayo Clinic College of Medicine; Co-Chair for Clinical Practice and Quality, Division of Cardiovascular Ultrasound; Consultant, Department of Cardiovascular Medicine, Mayo Clinic, Rochester, MN, USA
e-mail: thaden.jeremy@mayo.edu

J. F. Maalouf et al. (eds.), *Practical 3D Echocardiography*, https://doi.org/10.1007/978-3-030-72941-7_34

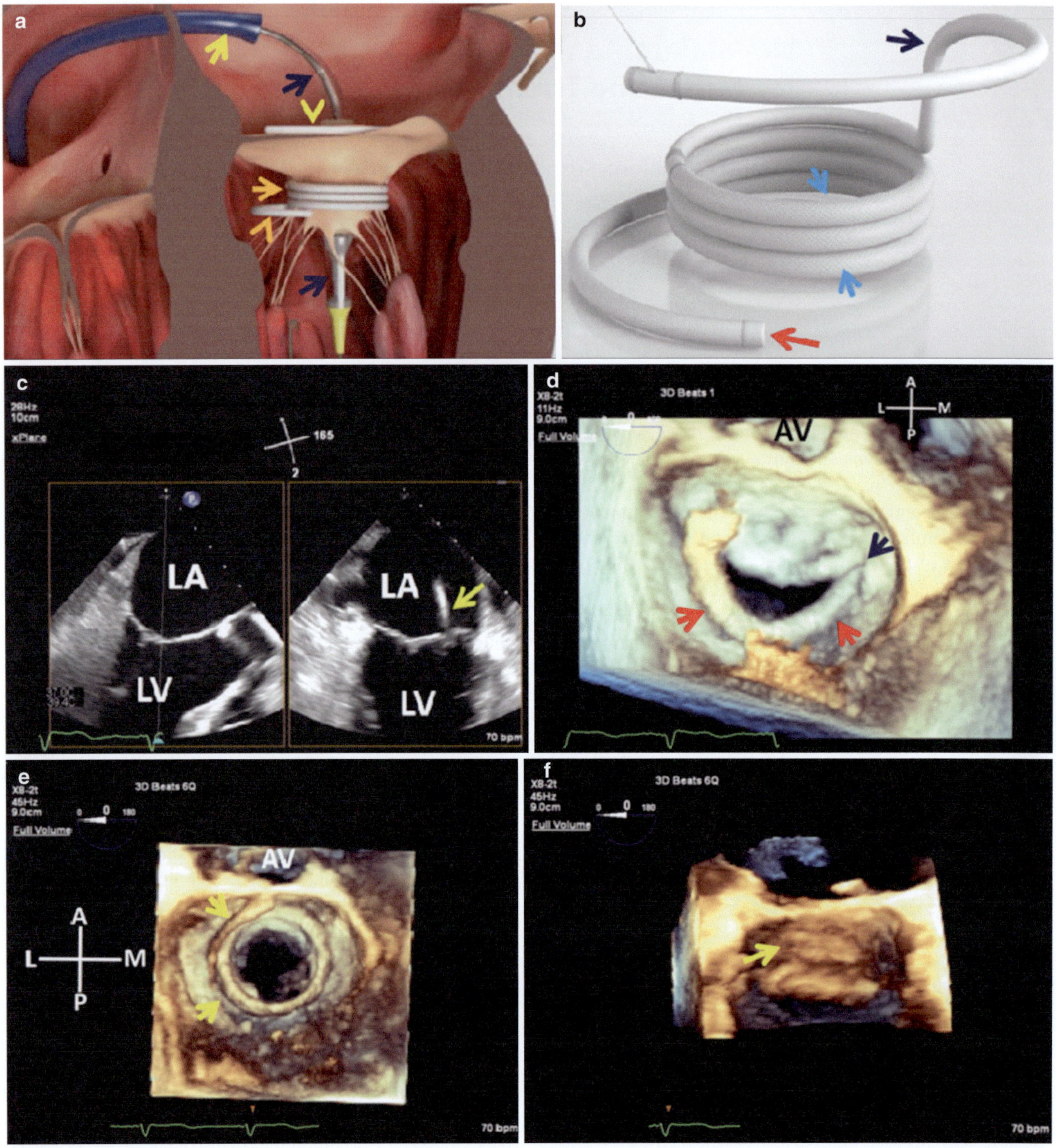

Fig. 34.1 **Top panel**. (**a**): Edwards -SAPIEN M3 system showing the steerable catheter delivery sheath (yellow arrow), steerable catheter (blue arrows), SAPIEN M3 dock functional turns encircling the native mitral leaflets and chordae (orange arrow), encircling turn (orange arrowhead), and atrial turn (yellow arrowhead) (**b**): SAPIEN M3 dock showing the encircling turn (red arrow) that guides the dock implant in capturing the native mitral chordae, the functional series of turns that provide a rigid landing zone and anchor for the SAPIEN M3 valve (light blue arrows), and the atrial turn that suspends the device against the mitral annulus by anchoring it in the LA (dark blue arrow). Images **a** and **b** courtesy of Edwards Lifesciences LLC. **Middle panel**. (**c**): x-Plane showing the steerable catheter (yellow arrow) in the LA. (**d**): 3D TEE enface LA view showing the steerable dock delivery catheter (red arrows) being directed towards the medial mitral commissure (dark blue arrow). **Bottom panel**: (**e**): 3D TEE enface LA view of the fully deployed Edwards-SAPIEN M3 valve showing the atrial turn (arrows). (**f**): 3D TEE ventricular view of the depolyed THV showing the functional series of turns (arrow). Images **c-f** used with permission of Mayo Foundation for Medical Education and Research. All rights reserved. A, anterior; AV, aortic valve; L, lateral; LA, left atrium; LV, left ventricle; M, medial; P, posterior; THV, transcatheter heart valve

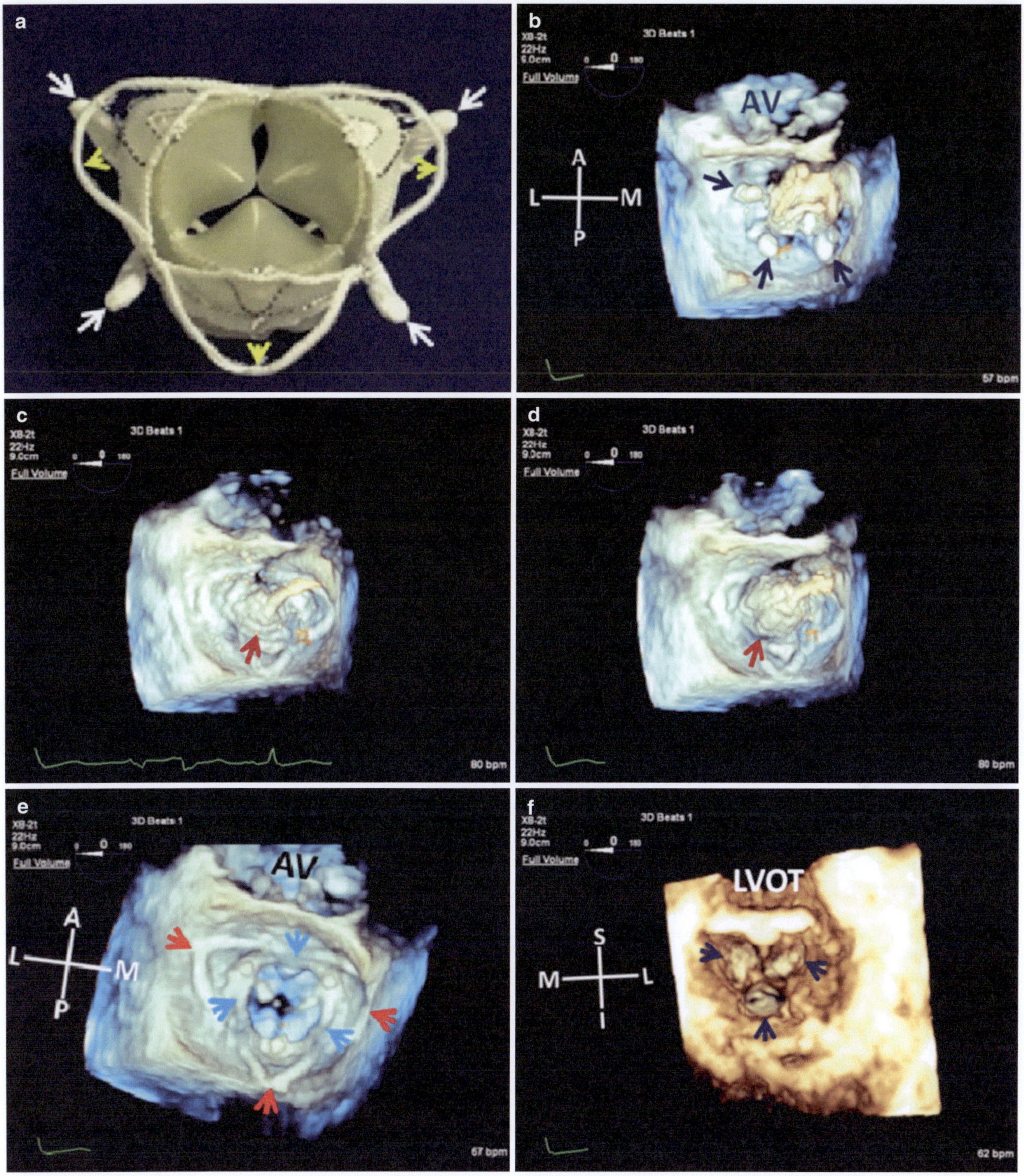

Fig. 34.2 **Top panel** (**a**): Caisson TMVR system showing anchor frame and valve. Note the four anchor feet (white arrows) and lowered semicircular atrial holding frames (yellow arrowheads). Image courtsey of Dr. Saric (**b**): Enface 3D TEE LA view of three of the four feet (arrows) of the anchor frame above the MV.**Second panel** (**c** and **d**): Two stages of the Caisson THV (arrows) descent towards the anchor frame in the LA as viewed on 3D TEE. **Third panel** (**e**): 3D TEE enface LA view of the fully deployed Caisson THV (light blue arrows) and lowered atrial holding frames (red arrows). (**f**): 3D TEE enface LV view of the fully deployed Caisson THV showing the three bioprosthesis cusps (dark blue arrows). **Bottom panel:** 3D TEE CFD enface LA views of the fully deployed Caisson THV in diastole (**g**) and systole (**h**). Note the trivial prosthesis regurgitation (arrow). Used with permission of Mayo Foundation for Medical Education and Research. All rights reserved. A, anterior; AV, aortic valve; CFD, color flow Doppler; I, inferior; L, lateral; LA, left atrium; LV, left ventricle; LVOT, left ventricular outflow tract; M, medial; P, posterior; S, superior; TMVR, transcatheter mitral valve replacement; THV, transcatheter heart valve

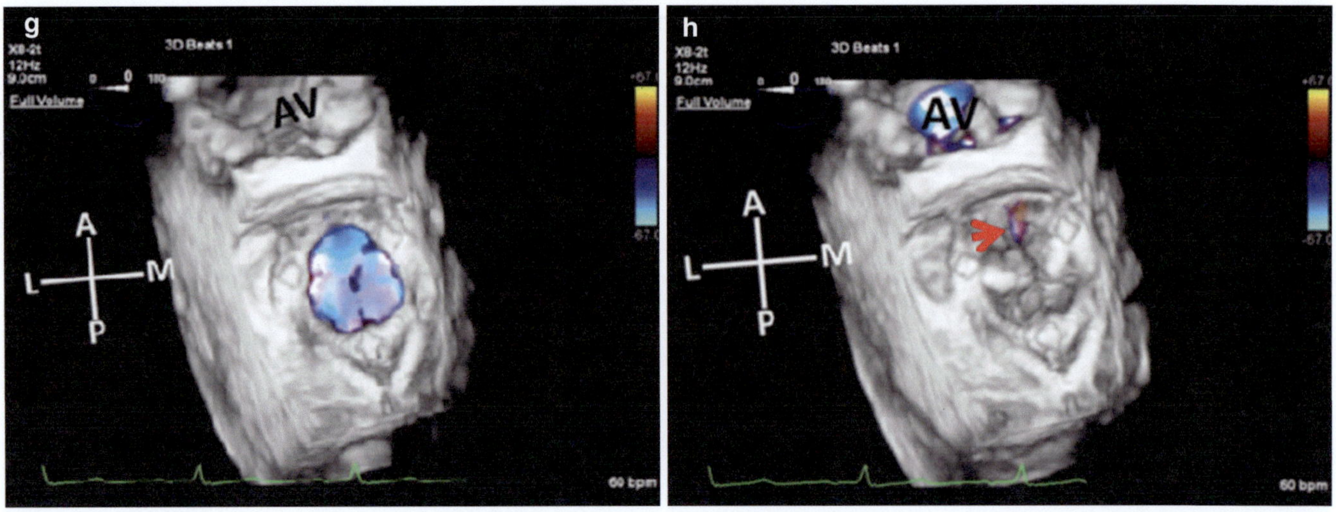

Fig. 34.2 (continued)

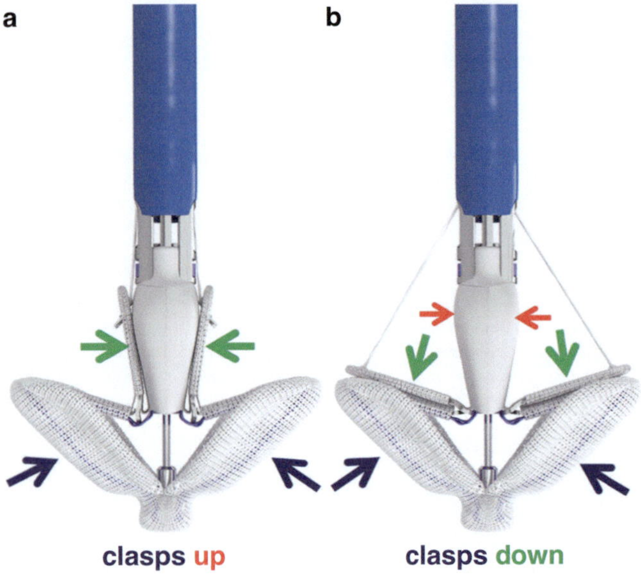

Fig. 34.3 PASCAL transcatheter edge-to-edge repair device. (**a**): capture ready with clasps (green arrows) up. (**b**): in capture mode with clasps (green arrows) down. Dark blue arrows point to the paddles and red arrows point to spacer. Image courtesy of Edwards Lifesciences LLC

adverse prognostic implications prompted interest in corrective percutaneous therapies in patients considered to be high surgical risk [7–15]. The majority of severe TR cases are functional, arising from the complex interplay of the tricuspid valve annulus (TVA) and right ventricle (RV) and not due to intrinsic anatomic TV abnormalities [16, 17]. Progressive dilatation of the RV and TVA leads to malcoaptation of the TV leaflets which with time become tethered [16, 17]. Because RV dilatation mainly affects the free wall, the posterior and in particular the larger anterior TV leaflets that are anchored to the free wall are pulled away from the septal leaflet resulting in TV leaflet malcoaptation [16, 17]. Because of the varying and complex etiology of severe TR, percutaneous devices undergoing evaluation have sought to address the problem by either treating annular dilatation or leaflet malcoaptation, or by replacing the TV [7–15], and the list of transcatheter tricuspid devices being tested or in development, analogous to mitral valve interventions, continues to grow [7–15]. Determination of the mechanism(s) of TR including site(s) of leaflet malcoaptation is therefore, critical prior to any intervention. With 3D transthoracic and transesophageal echocardiography, enface views of the ventricular and atrial surfaces of the tricuspid valve can be obtained from a single imaging window analogous to imaging of the mitral valve (Figs. 34.5, 34.6, and 34.7) [7], TR severity and tricuspid annular dimensions can also be assessed on mutiplanar reconstruction of the 3D volumetric data sets (Fig. 34.7).

The FORMA device (Edwards Lifesciences, Irvine, California) is a valve spacer that occupies the regurgitant orifice of the tricuspid valve, producing a platform for leaflet coaptation to reduce TR [12, 13] (Fig. 34.8). A steerable delivery catheter is advanced into the RV to deliver an anchor and rail to the RV wall perpendicular to the annulus [12, 13] (Fig. 34.8). Under 2D and 3D TEE guidance, the valve spacer is advanced to the regurgitant orifice and positioned for maximal reduction in TR (Fig. 34.8). As with any transcatheter intervention, a clear understanding of all steps involved is a prerequisite for guiding the procedure.

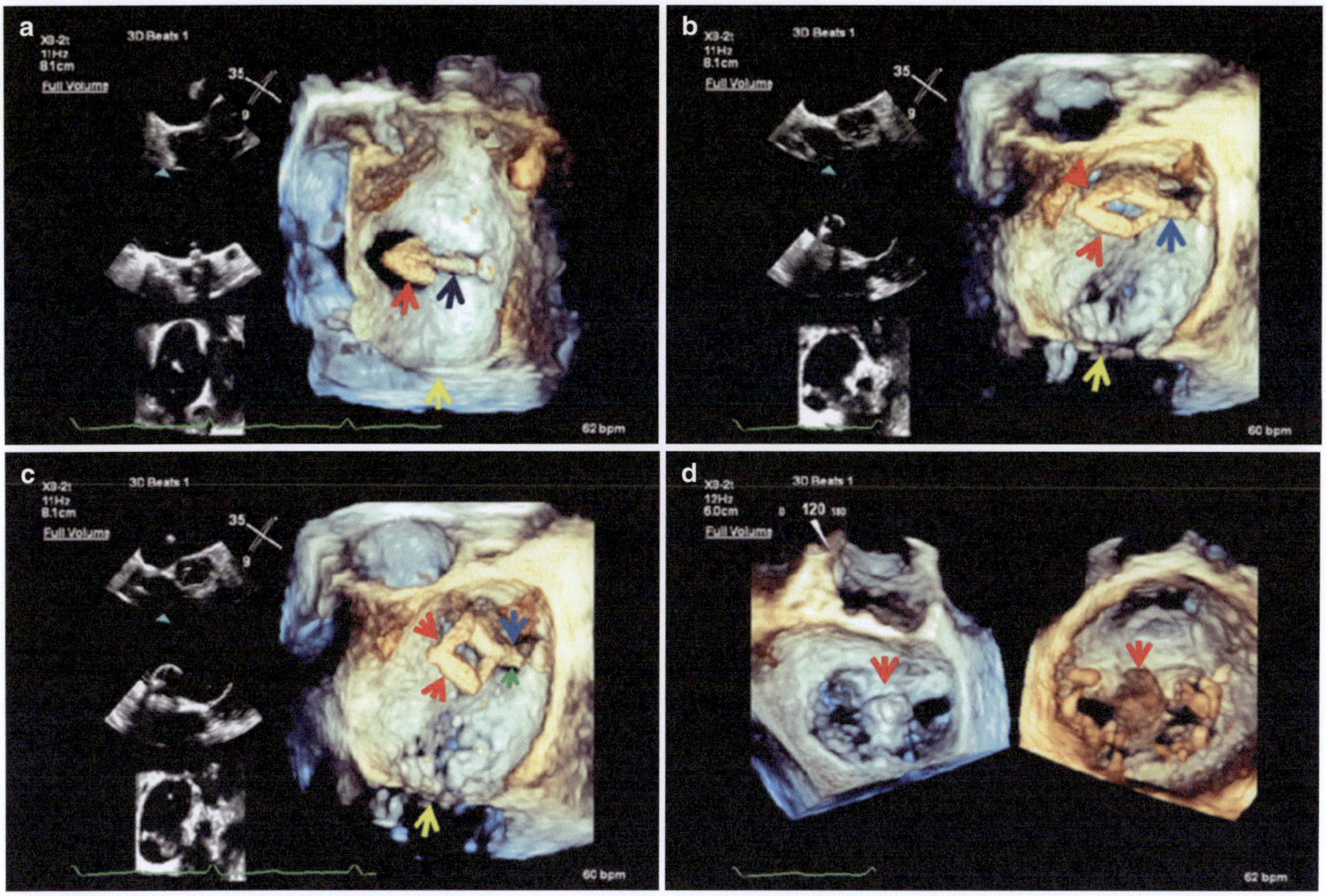

Fig. 34.4 **Top panel**. (**a**): The crimped PASCAL device (red arrow) at tip of implant catheter (dark blue arrow). (**b**): Partially open paddles (red arrows) and spacer (light blue arrow). **Bottom panel**. (**c**): capture ready PASCAL device with open paddle arms (red arrows) and spacer (light blue arrow). One clasp (green arrow) can be seen pulled up along side of the spacer. Yellow arrow in all images points to MV. (**d**): Live3D FV dual LA and LV layout of MV showing the fully deployed PASCAL device (red arrows). Used with permission of Mayo Foundation for Medical Education and Research. All rights reserved. FV, Full Volume; LA, left atrium; LV, left ventricle; MV, mitral valve

Annular perimeter and area are also important measurements for sizing and positioning of annular devices (Trialign, Cardioband, and TriCinch) [8, 9, 14, 15]. The Trialign system (Mitralign, Inc.) attempts to replicate the Kay bicusipdation procedure by plication of the posterior TV leaflet annulus thus improving coaptation of the anterior and septal leaflet and reduction in functional TR [14]. Implantion of the Trialign device relies primarily on TEE. 3D TEE in combination with biplane imaging is used to visualize the guide delivery system and to confirm positioning of the two transannular wires and pledgets necessary for annular plication on the posterior annulus, including distance between pledgets [14]. Cinching of the two pledget sutures and plication of the annulus can be monitored using Live 3D TEE [14]. Tricuspid annular reduction can also be achieved using the Cardioband system [9, 14, 15] (Edwards Lifesciences Fig. 34.9).

Edge-to-Edge TV Repair

For patients with severe TR, TEE guided edge-to-edge TV repair using the MitraClip device (Abbott Vascular, Santa Clara, California) is being increasingly performed either in conjunction with MV repair or as a stand-alone procedure [7]. The PASCAL transcatheter valve repair system (Edwards Lifesciences, Irvine-California), is another edge-to-edge TV repair device that is undergoing clinical evaluation [10, 11]. Compared with the MV, anatomy of the TV is more complex however, and imaging by TEE is challenging because the TV is in the far field of the ultrasound beam, thus vulnerable to shadowing by the mitral and aortic valves especially when calcified or in presence of prosthetic valves [16]. Moreover, because the TV leaflets are thin when the etiology of TR is functional, the most common indication for edge-to-edge repair, imaging using 3D TEE may be suboptimal due to

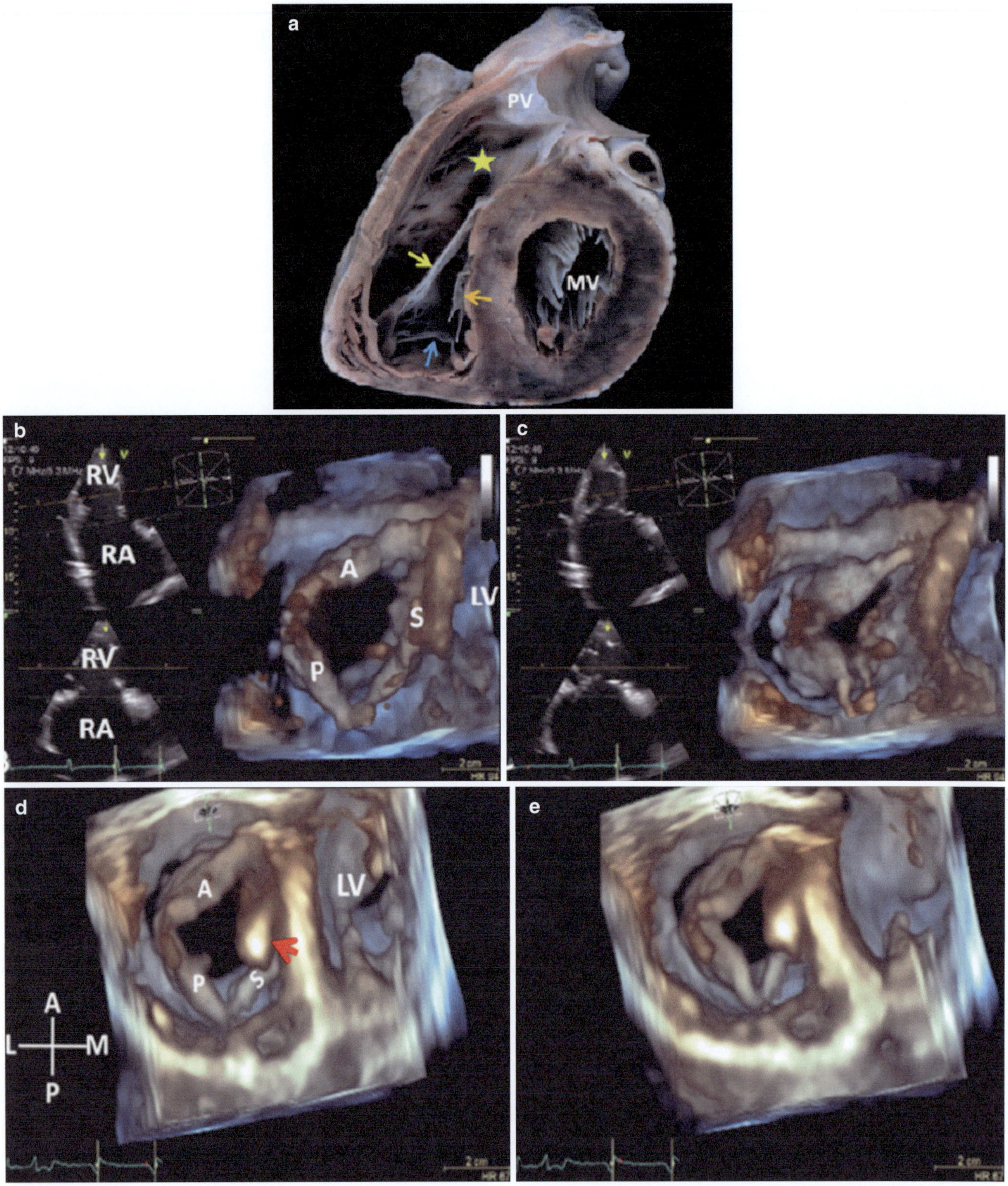

Fig. 34.5 (**a**): Anatomic view of the triangular-shaped tricuspid orifice at mid-leaflet level. This view corresponds to the echocardiographic short-axis view. The anterior tricuspid leaflet (yellow arrow), septal leaflet (orange arrow), posterior leaflet (blue arrow) and right ventricular outflow tract (star) can be appreciated. Permission for image **a** from McGraw-Hill, Hurst's The Heart, 2017, Maalouf et al., Chap. 4 Functional Anatomy of the Heart. (**b–e**): 3D TTE RV short-axis views of the TV from two patients showing mechanism of TR (**b**): end diastolic frame showing all three leaflets. (**c**): systolic frame showing central malcoaptation due to annular dilatation. (**d** and **e**): Pacemaker (red arrow) induced TR due to tethering of septal leaflet. (**d**): end diastolic frame; (**e**): early systolic frame. Used with permission of Mayo Foundation for Medical Education and Research. All rights reserved. A, anterior; L, lateral; LV, left ventricle; M, medial; MV, mitral valve; P, posterior; PV, pulmonary valve; RA, right atrium; RV, right ventricle; S, septal; TR, tricuspid regurgitation; TV, tricuspid valve

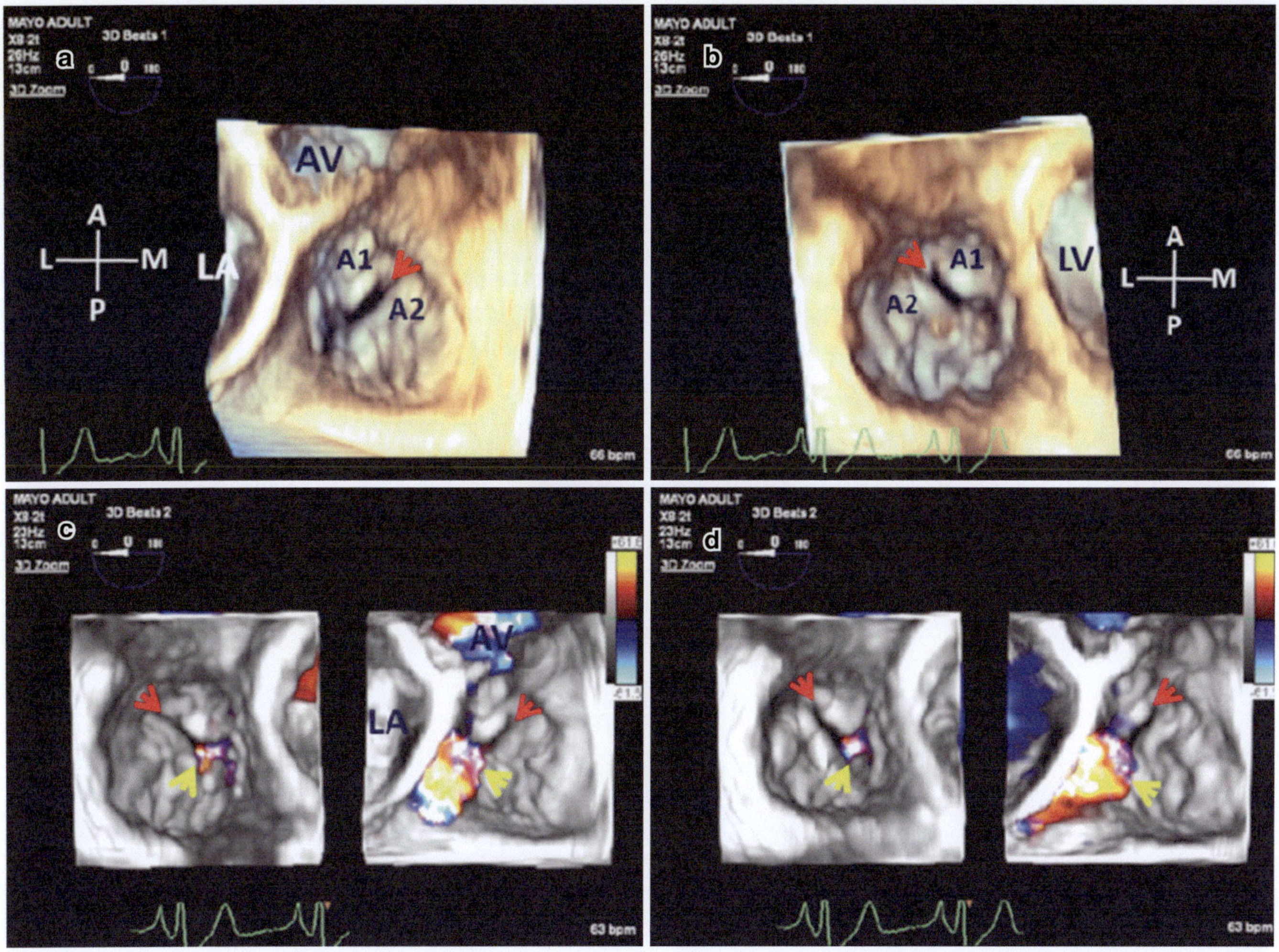

Fig. 34.6 Mechanism of TR: 3D Zoom TEE of TV from midesophageal window. **Top panel:** Real time enface RA (**a**) and RV (**b**) views of the TV showing two anterior leaflet scallops (A1 and A2) separated by a cleft like indentation (red arrows). **Bottom panel:** Dual layout multibeat CFD in mid (**c**) and late (**d**) systole showing site of TR (yellow arrows). Note that there is no regurgitation through the cleft like indentation (red arrows) separating the two anterior leaflet scallops. Used with permission of Mayo Foundation for Medical Education and Research. All rights reserved. A, anterior; AV, aortic valve; CFD, color flow Doppler; L, lateral; LA, left atrium; M, medial; P, posterior; RA, right atrium; RV, right ventricle; TR, tricuspid regurgitation; TV, tricuspid valve

drop out artifacts. *In patients with a pacemaker or ICD lead, edge-to-edge TV repair may be feasible if the TR is not device lead induced.* These limitations notwithstanding, 3D TEE complements 2D TEE in pre procedure assessment and intraprocedural guidance. Whereas with 2D TEE, identifying the individual TV leaflets requires careful probe manipulation (midesophageal horizontal 4-chamber view for septal leaflet, short-axis aortic valve view for anterior and posterior leaflets, and transgastric short-axis view to image all three leaflets simultaneously), the entire TV (annulus and leaflets) can be imaged in real time from any midesophagel window using single beat Full Volume/Large volume 3D or 3D zoom (generated from the two orthogonal midesophageal views of the TV that include all three leaflets) [16] (Fig. 34.10). This in turn allows for clear delineation of the mechanism(s) of TR including site(s) of tricuspid leaflet malcoaptation (Figs. 34.5, 34.6, and 34.10). And analogous to 3D imaging of the MV, it is important to include fixed anatomy (aortic or mitral valve, atrial or ventricular septum, and right ventricular outflow tract) that can provide the necessary intraprocedural spatial coordinates (Figs. 34.7, 34.10, 34.11, and 34.12).

A critical role for TEE during transcatheter tricuspid valve edge-to- edge repair (TTVR) is to ensure correct MitraClip or PASCAL device trajectory with the open arms/paddles clearly seen as they approach the TV and to ensure that this trajectory is maintained as the MitraClip arms or PASCAL device paddles are advanced into the right ventricle. Toward these ends, 3D MultiVue (Philips Healthcare) multiplanar reconstruction (MPR) can be a very useful tool for rapid real time imaging of the TV (Figs. 34.13, 34.14,

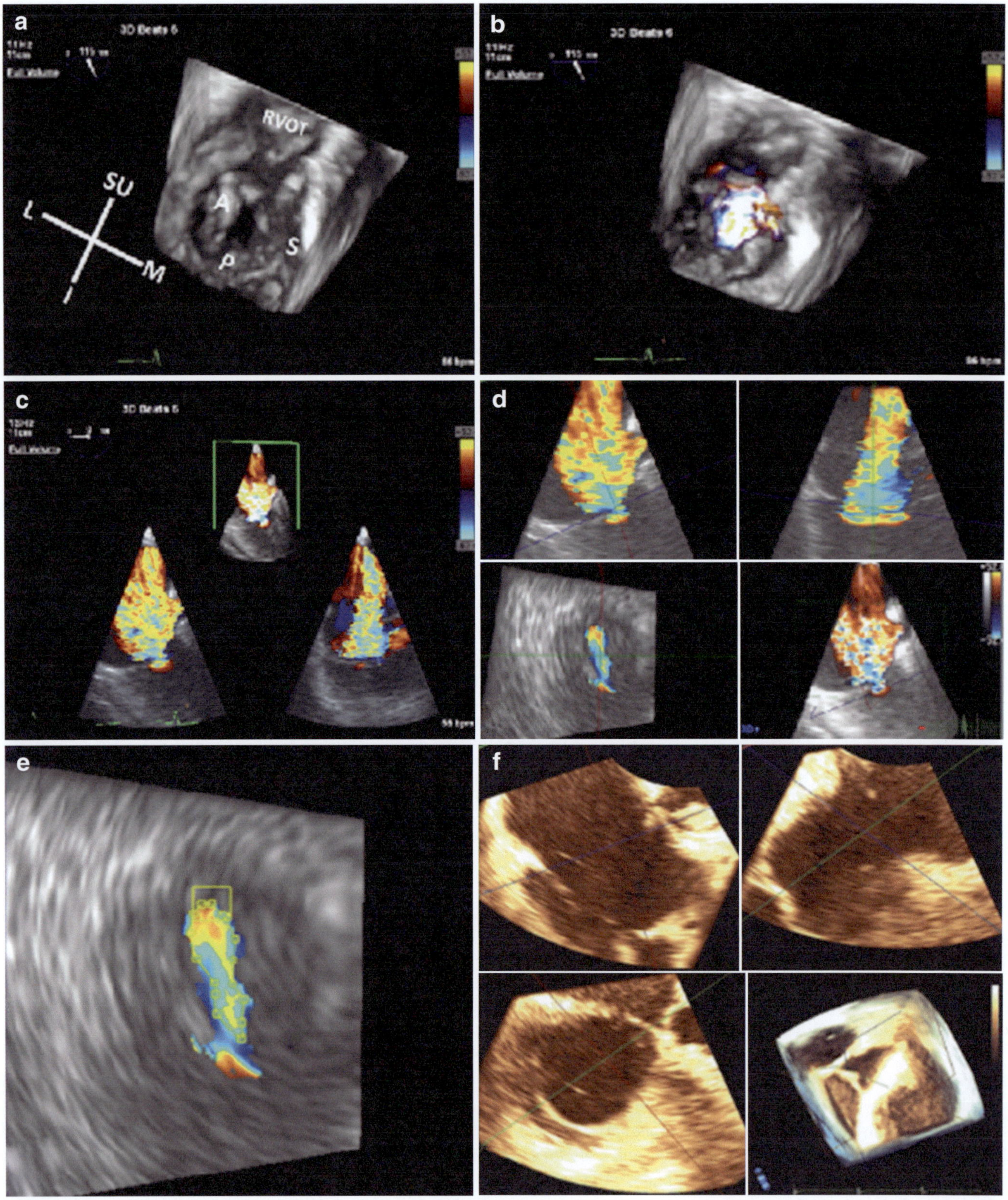

Fig. 34.7 Pre FORMA TV device intervention 3D TEE assessment of mechanism and severity of TR. **Top panel**: 3D TEE enface RV TV views showing central malcoaptation of the TV leaflets (**a**) with secondary central regurgitation (**b**). **Middle panel**: Multibeat FV 3D CFD of TR (**c**) and MPR of the 3D CFD volumetric data set to quantify severity of TR (**d**). VC can be seen in transverse plane (blue box, lower left). **Bottom panel**: Measurement of TR vena contracta area (**e**) and TV annular measurement using MPR (**f**). Images courtesy Dr. Sorin Pislaru, used with permission of Mayo Foundation for Medical Education and Research. All rights reserved. A, anterior tricuspid leaflet; CFD, color flow Doppler; FV, Full Volume; I, inferior; L, lateral; M, medial; MPR, multiplanar reconstruction; P, posterior tricuspid leaflet; R, right; RV, right ventricle; RVOT, right ventricular outflow tract; S, septal tricuspid leaflet; SU, superior; TR, tricuspid regurgitation; TV, tricuspid valve; VC, vena contracta

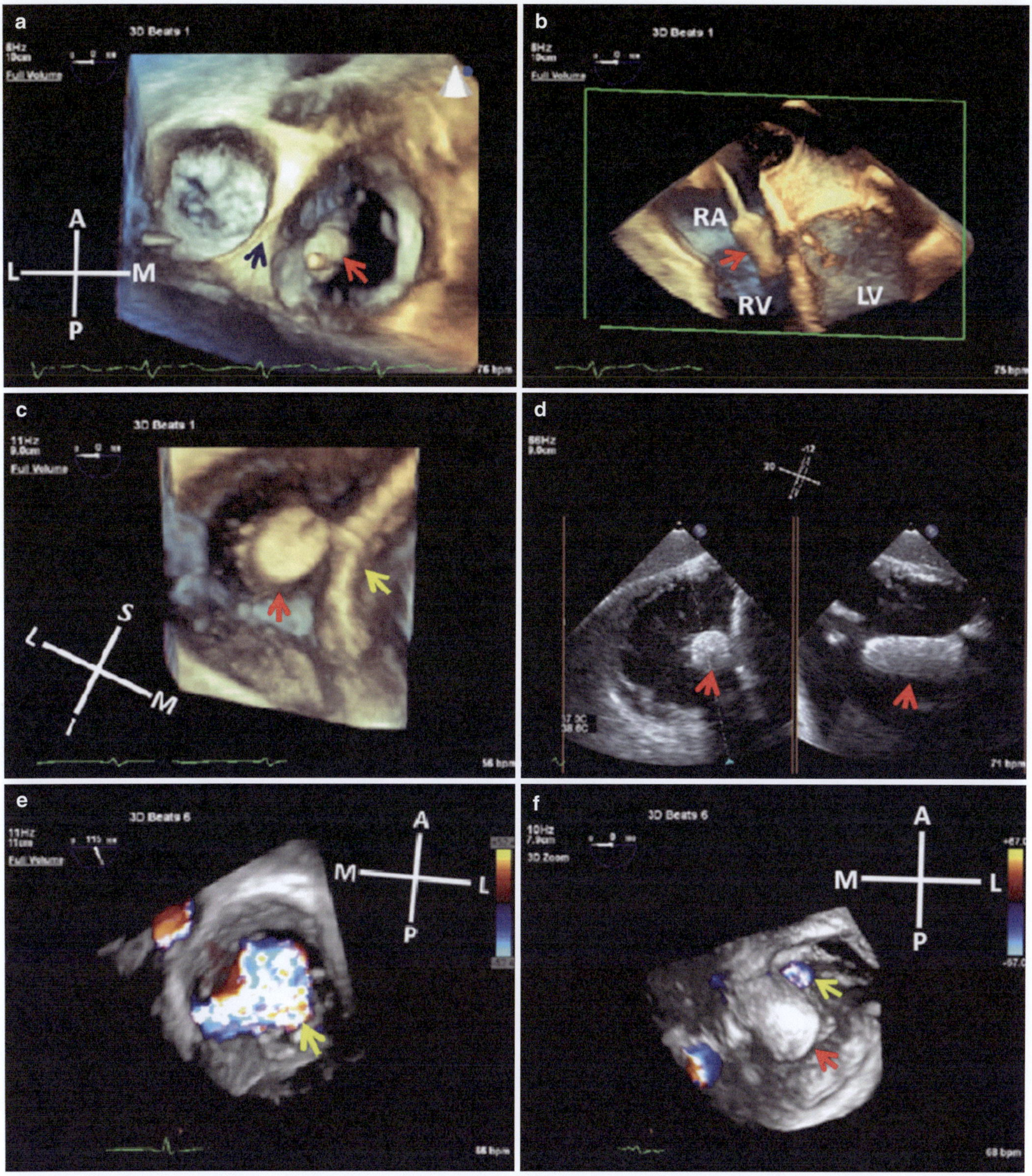

Fig. 34.8 Intraprocedural imaging during deployment of FORMA TV device. **Top panel**. (**a**): 3D TEE enface RA view of TV showing FORMA device within TV orifice(red arrow; dark blue arrow points to atrial septum). (**b**): autocropped FV of the FORMA device (red arrow) as it crosses the TV orifice into the RV. **Second panel**. (**c**): 3D TEE enface RV view of the FORMA device (red arrow) and (**d**): xPlane of the device within the RV (red arrows). Yellow arrow points to ventricular septum**. Third panel** 3D CFD (**e**): pre procedure TR (arrow). (**f**): residual TR (yellow arrow) post deployment of FORMA device (red arrow). **Bottom panel**: TG xPlane CFD of TR (arrows) prior to (**g**) and following deployment of FORMA device (**h**). Both 3D and xPlane CFD panels show significant reduction in TR severity. Used with permission of Mayo Foundation for Medical Education and Research. All rights reserved. A, anterior; CFD, color flow Doppler; FV, Full Volume; I, inferior; L, lateral; LV, left ventricle; M, medial; MPR, multiplane reconstruction; P, posterior; R, right; RA, right atrium; RV, right ventricle; RVOT, right ventricular outflow tract; S, superior; TG, transgastric; TR, tricuspid regurgitation; TV, tricuspid valve

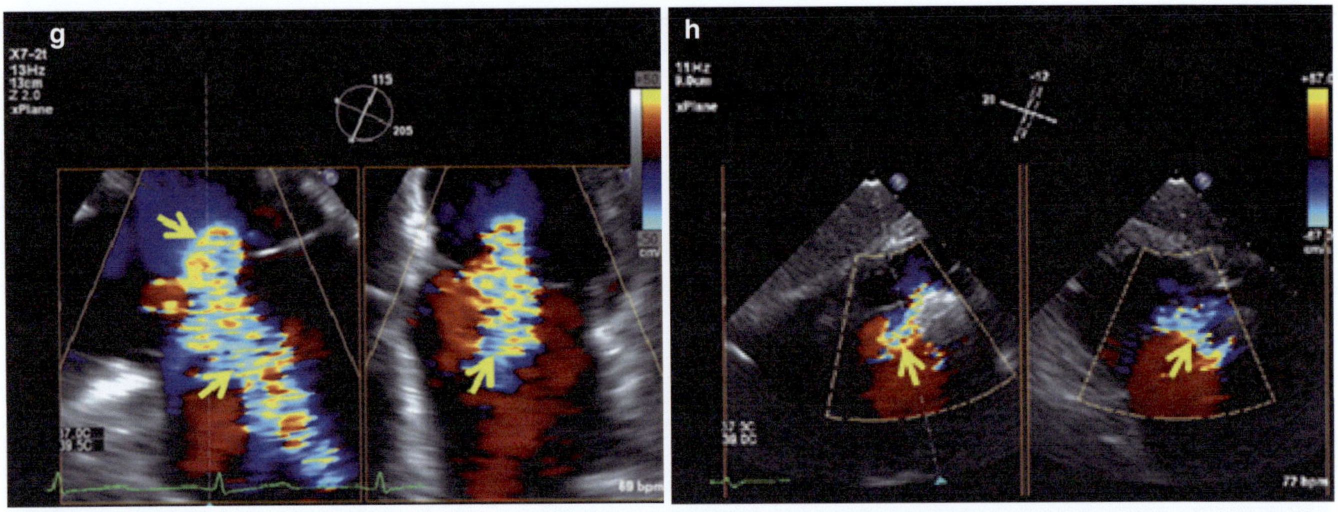

Fig. 34.8 (continued)

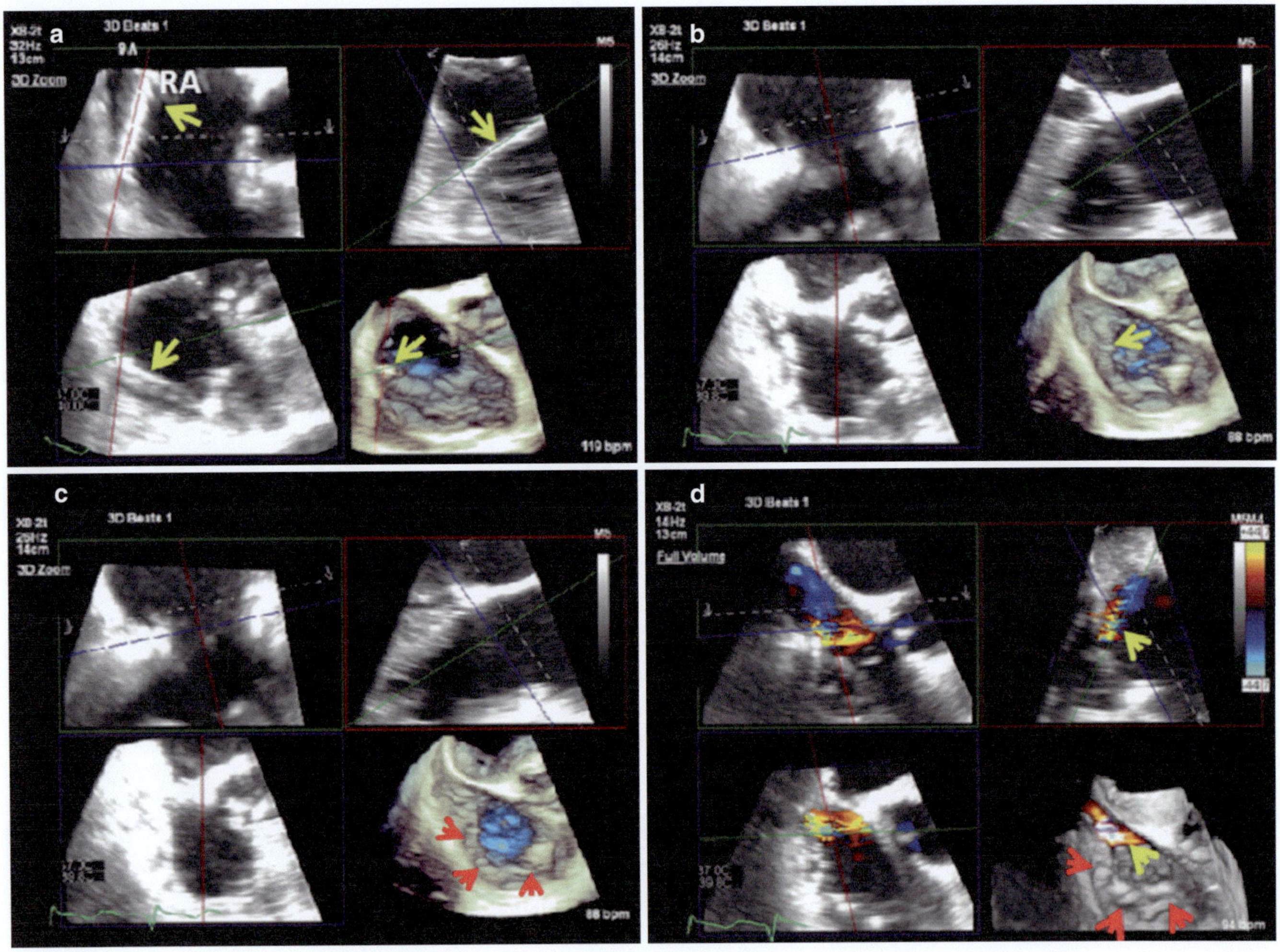

Fig. 34.9 **Top panel** (**a** and **b**): Live 3D zoom MultiVue guidance of Cardioband system (arrows). **Middle panel** (**c** and **d**): Live 3D zoom MultiVue of fully deployed Cardioband (red arrows) and residual TR on CFD (yellow arrow). **Bottom panel:** MPR TV annular measurements before (**e**) and after deployment of Cardioband (**f**) showing reduction in annular area. Used with permission of Mayo Foundation for Medical Education and Research. All rights reserved. CFD, color flow Doppler; MPR, multiplane reconstruction; RA, right atrium; TR, tricuspid regurgitation; TV, tricuspid valve

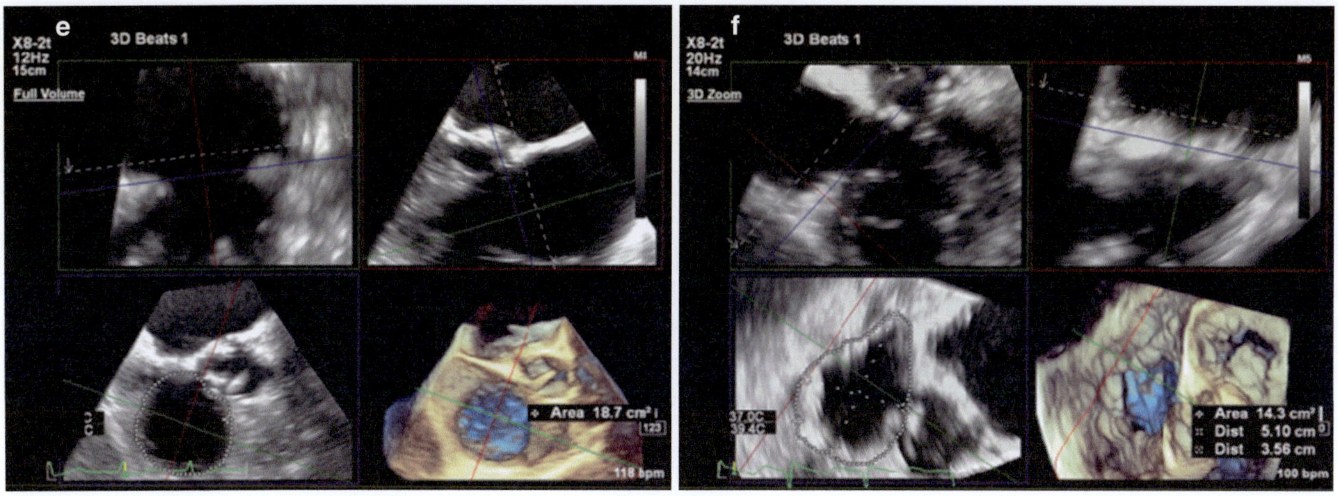

Fig. 34.9 (continued)

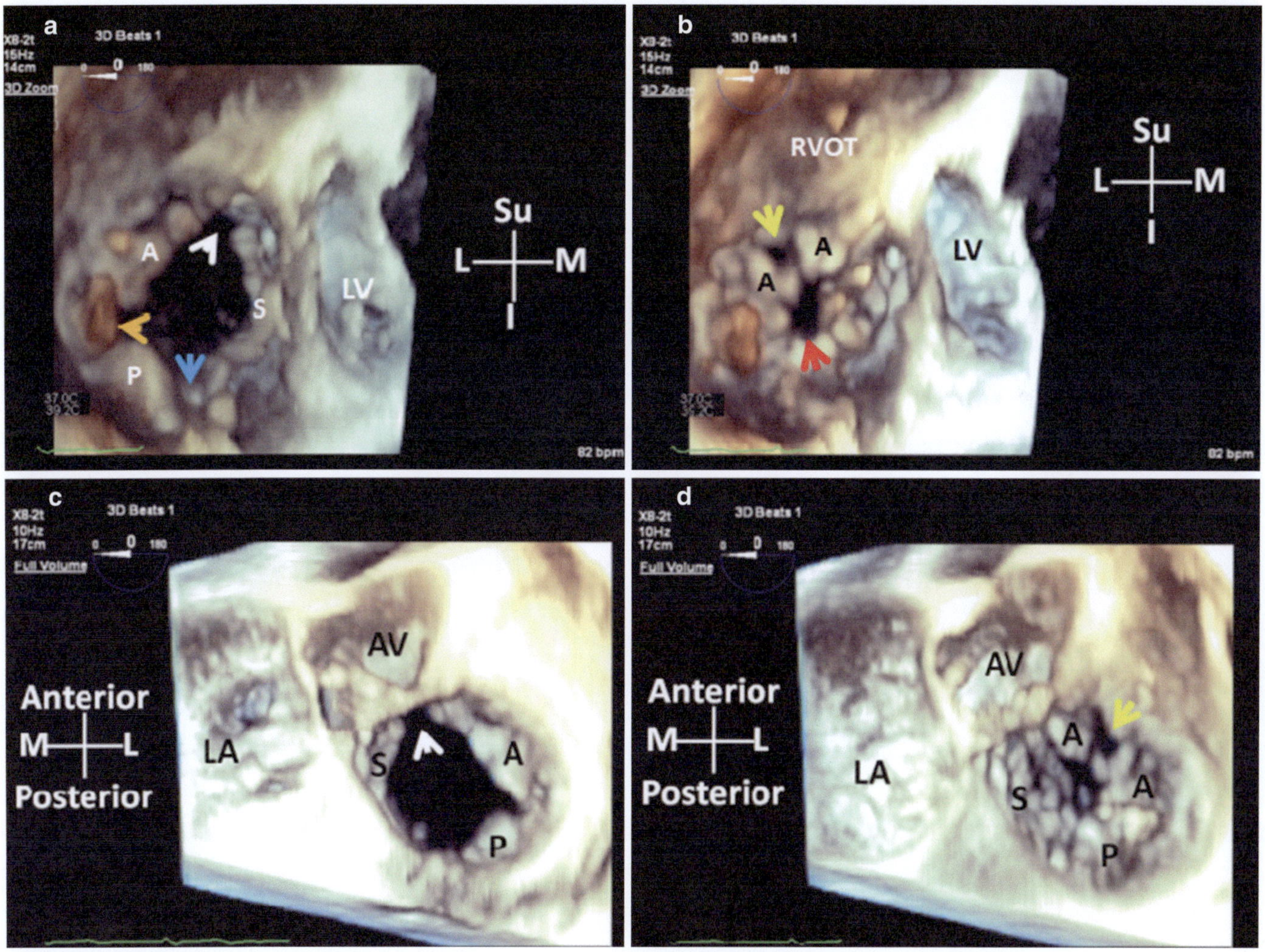

Fig. 34.10 3D TEE views of TV with leaflet malcoaptation. **Top panel** (**a** and **b**): Enface RV views in diastole (**a**) and systole (**b**) showing central leaflet malcoaptation (red arrow) and a cleft like space (yellow arrow) between two scallops of the anterior TV leaflet (A). Note the antero-septal commissure (white arrow), postero-septal commissure (blue arrow) and papillary muscle (orange arrow). **Bottom panel** (**c** and **d**): Same views from an enface RA perspective showing the anterior leaflet inter-scallop cleft (yellow arrow) and central TV leaflets malcoaptation in systole (**d**). White arrow points to antero-septal commissure in diastole (**c**). Used with permission of Mayo Foundation for Medical Education and Research. All rights reserved. A, anterior leaflet; AV, aortic valve; I, inferior; LA, left atrium; LV, left ventricle; M, medial; L, lateral; P, posterior leaflet; RA, right atrium; RV, right ventricle; RVOT, right ventricular outflow tract; S, septal leaflet; Su, superior; TV, tricuspid valve

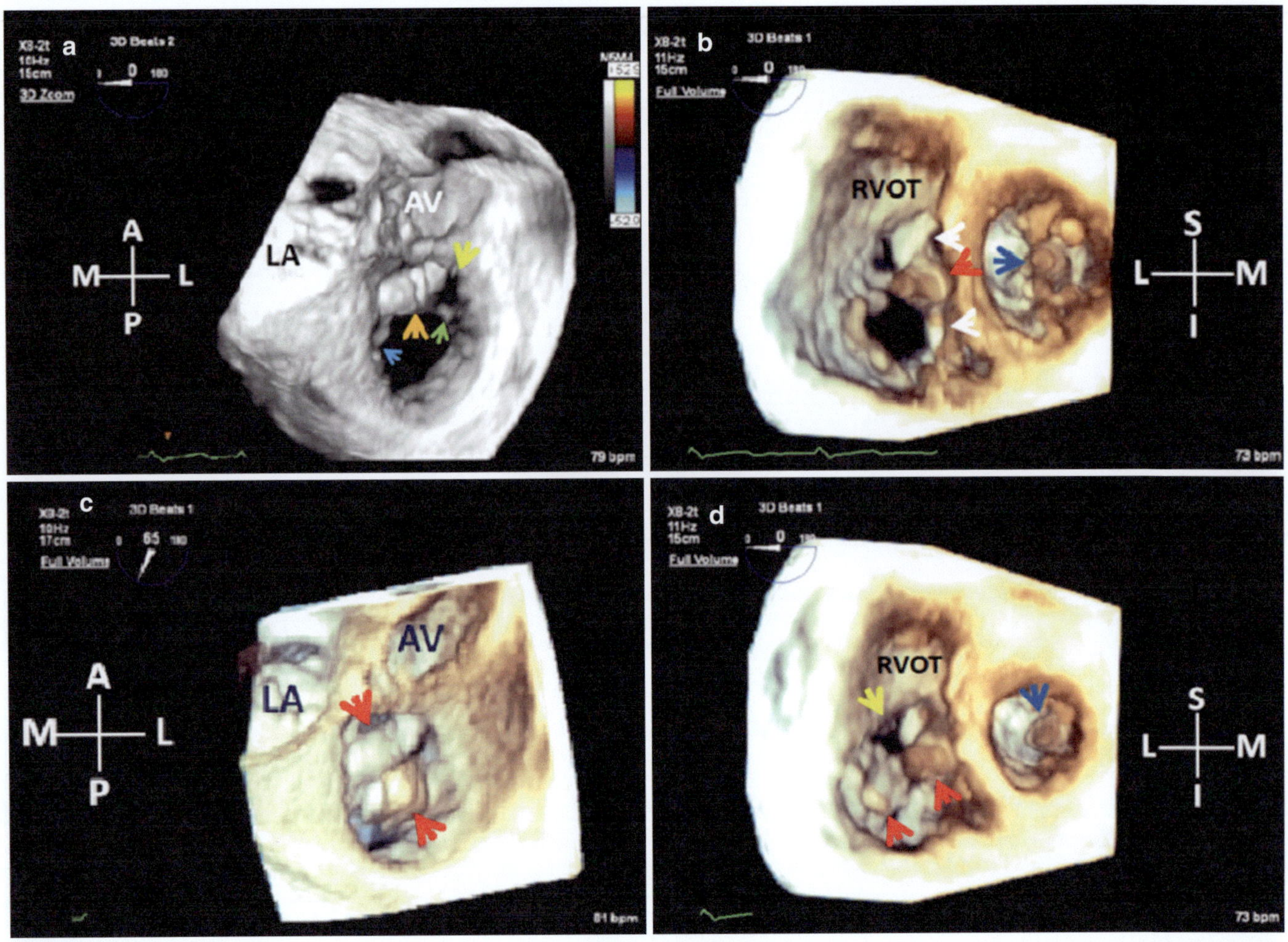

Fig. 34.11 Same patient as in Fig. 34.10. 3D TEE enface views of the TV post deployment of two PASCAL devices. **Top panel:** First PASCAL device. (**a**): Enface RA view shows grasping of the anterior (green arrow) and septal (blue arrow) leaflets by the PASCAL device (orange arrow) close to the anteroseptal commissure. Note the anterior leaflet cleft (yellow arrow). (**b**): Enface RV view of the PASCAL device (red arrow) showing the fully deployed device paddles (white arrows) in relation to the anterior and septal leaflets. Blue arrow points to a MitraClip following edge-to-edge MV repair. **Bottom panel:** Post deployment of a second PASCAL device. Red arrows show the two PASCAL devices from RA (**c**) and RV (**d**) perspectives. Yellow arrow shows persistence of the anterior leaflet interscallop cleft, and blue arrow points to the MitraClip. Used with permission of Mayo Foundation for Medical Education and Research. All rights reserved. A, anterior; AV, aortic valve; I, inferior; L, lateral; LA, left atrium; M, medial; MV, mitral valve; P, posterior; RA, right atrium; RV, right ventricle; RVOT, right ventricular outflow tract; S, superior; TV, tricuspid valve

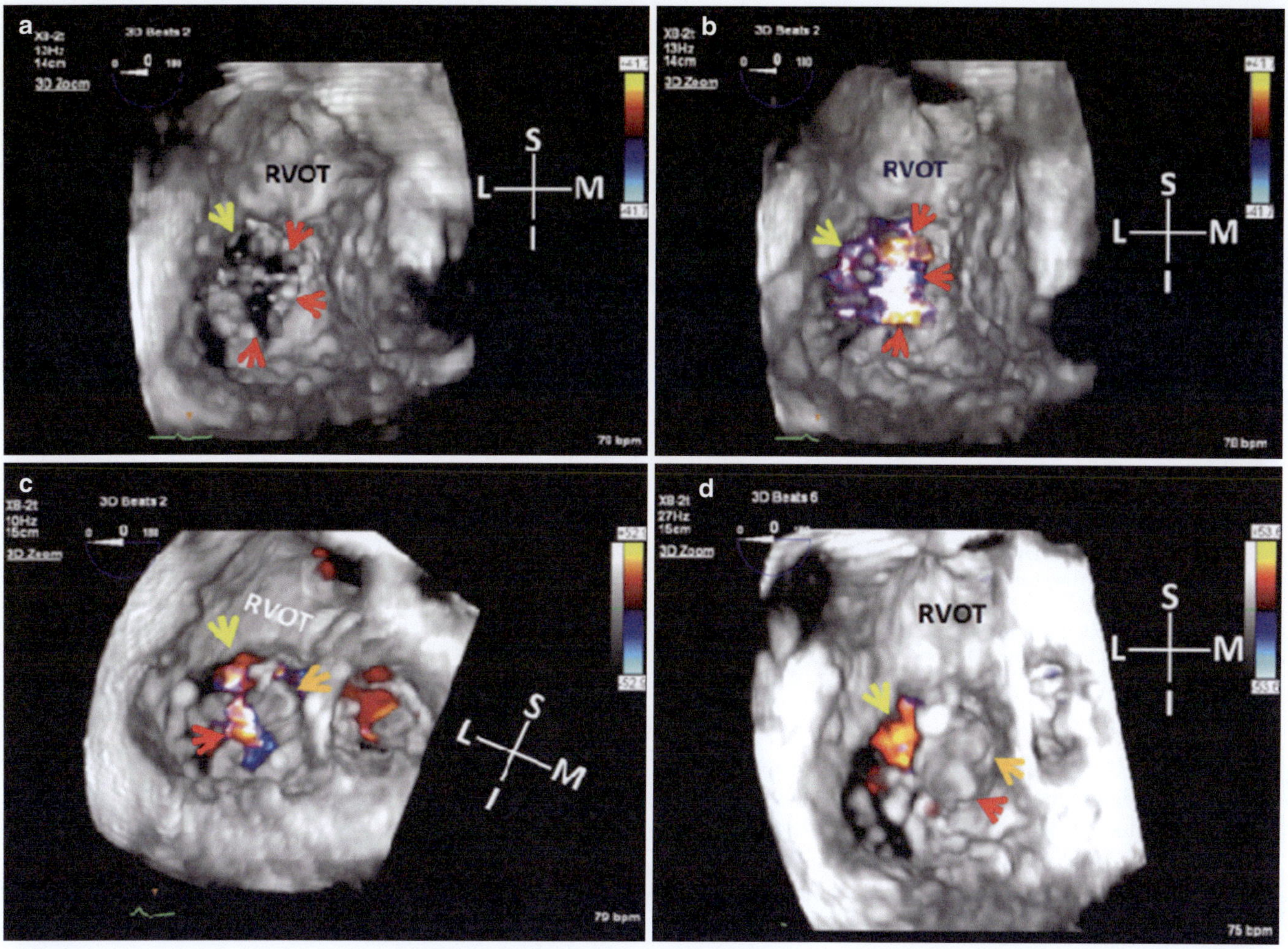

Fig. 34.12 3D TEE CFD enface RV views of TV from same patient in Fig. 34.11. **Top panel**: Baseline pre procedure images showing central malcoaptation (red arrows) and anterior leaflet interscallop cleft (yellow arrow) with CFD off (**a**) and on (**b**). Note that in addition to regurgitation through the central leaflet malcoaptation, there is also regurgitation through the cleft. **Bottom panel**. (**c**): persistent central regurgitation (red arrow) and regurgitation through the anterior leaflet cleft (yellow arrow) following deployment of first PASCAL device (orange arrow). (**d**): Resolution of central regurgitation following deployment of a second PASCAL device (red arrow), but persistence of regurgitation through the anterior leaflet interscallop cleft (yellow arrow). Used with permission of Mayo Foundation for Medical Education and Research. All rights reserved. A, anterior; CFD, color flow Doppler; I, inferior; L, lateral; M, medial; RV, right ventricle; RVOT, right ventricular outflow tract; S, superior; TV, tricuspid valve

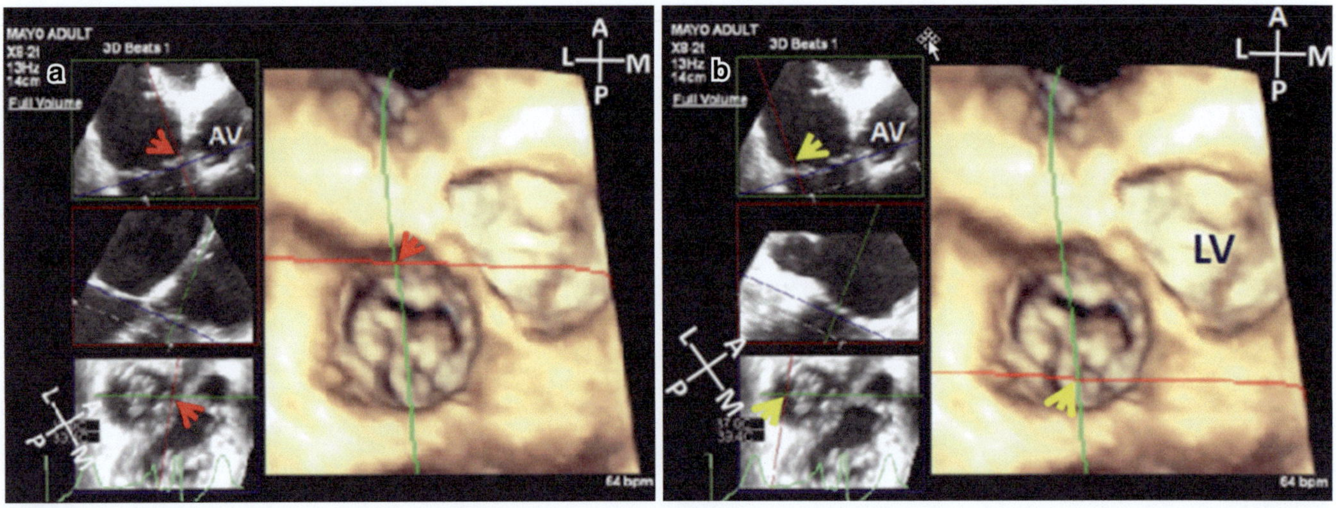

Fig. 34.13 Live single beat 3D FV MPR of TV obtained from mid-esophageal short-axis AV view to illustrate how the ATL (**a**, red arrows) and PTL (**b**, yellow arrows) are identified. Note that the leaflet adjacent to the AV is the ATL (**a**; red arrow top left) and the leaflet away from the AV is the PTL (**b**, yellow arrow top left). Also note that the intersection of the red and green lines in the 2D short-axis tomographic space (bottom left **a** and **b**) and in the corresponding 3D space points to the tricuspid leaflet being viewed. Used with permission of Mayo Foundation for Medical Education and Research. All rights reserved. A, anterior; AV, aortic valve; ATL, anterior tricuspid leaflet; FV, Full Volume; L, lateral; LV, left ventricle; M, medial; MPR, muliplanar reconstruction; P, posterior; PTL, posterior tricuspid leaflet; TV, tricuspid valve

34.15, and 34.16), and for guiding device advancement into the RV and alignment of MitraClip arms/PASCAL paddles with the targeted TV leaflets (Figs. 34.17, 34.18, and 34.19). 3D MultiVue is usually generated from the horizontal or short axis midesophageal views in any 3D modality, but most commonly Full Volume or 3D zoom (Figs. 34.14, 34.15, and 34.16).

Although the MultiVue function can be used to guide grasping of the targeted TV leaflets (usually anterior and septal with additional anterior and posterior if need be), image resolution for this purpose is usually suboptimal. We therefore, prefer the x-Plane (biplane) RV views of the TV from the transgastric window when feasible to guide this stage of the procedure (Fig. 34.20). We also prefer the transgastric short-axis window to ascertain adequate tissue bridging post clip deployment.

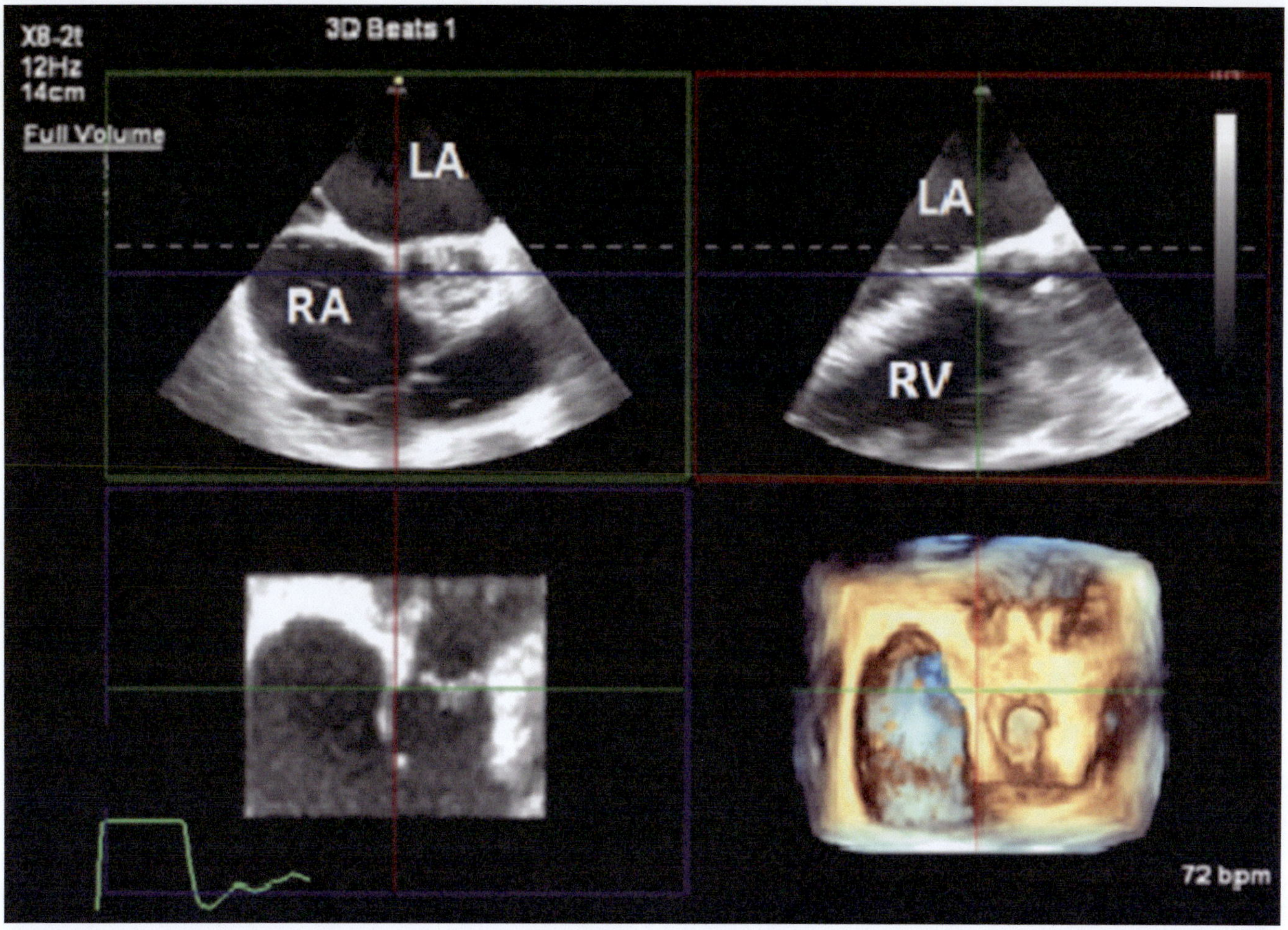

Fig. 34.14 3D FV MultiVue of the TV from mid esophageal window in three orthogonal planes color coded green, red, and blue rectangles or lines. Alignment of one plane in the form of a color coded line with a structure of interest will display that structure in the other two orthogonal planes in the form of color coded rectangles. The orientation of the dashed white line (see Fig. 34.15) determines the TV perspective being viewed (i.e. atrial or ventricular). Used with permission of Mayo Foundation for Medical Education and Research. All rights reserved. FV, Full Volume; LA, left atrium; RA, right atrium; RV, right ventricle; TV, tricuspid valve

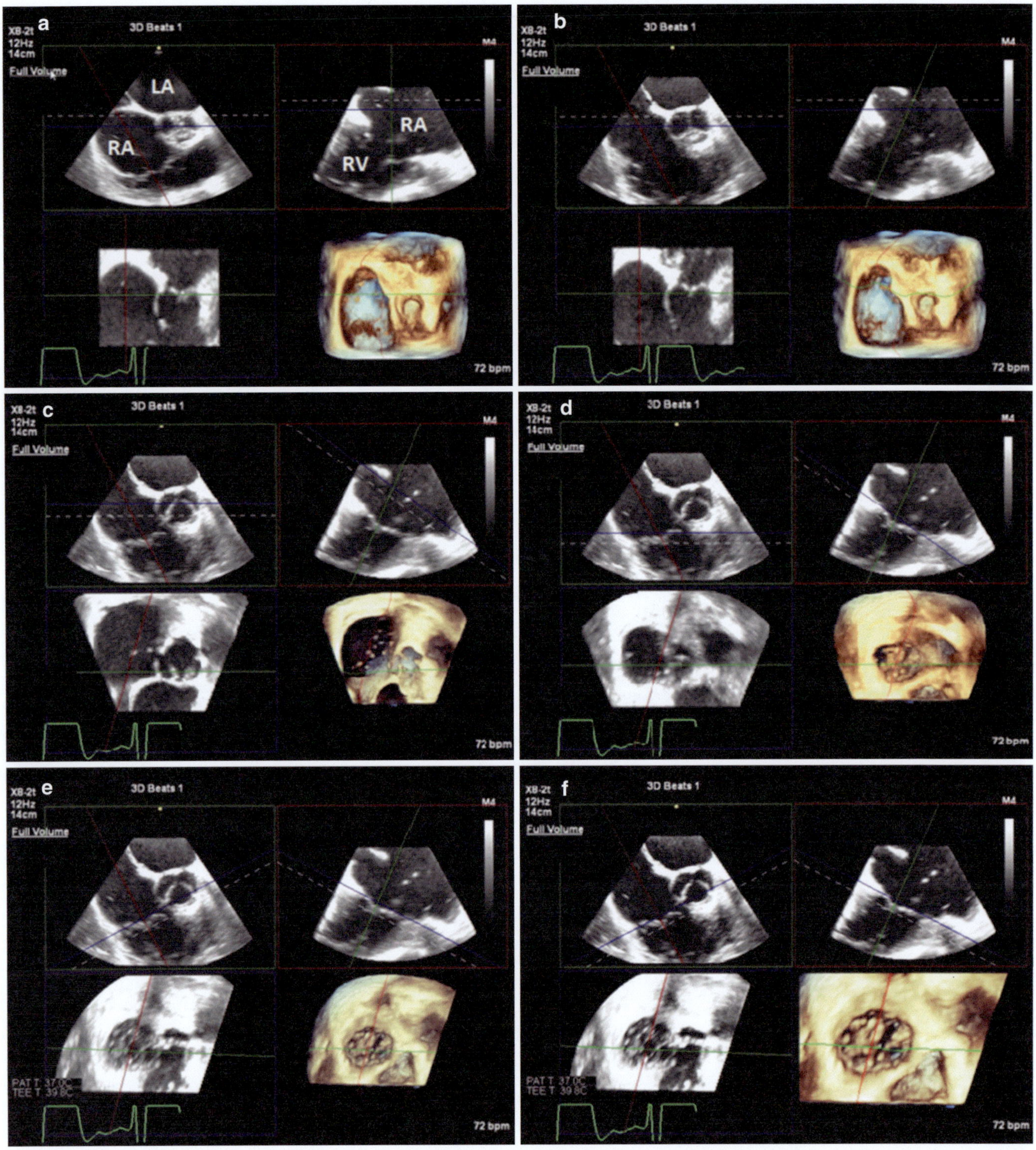

Fig. 34.15 Step by step approach to MultiVue imaging of the TV shown in Fig. 34.14 to guide TTVR: Baseline pre procedure images. (**a**): Alignment of the redline (top left, green rectangle) parallel to TV inflow. (**b**): Alignment of the green line (top right, red rectangle) parallel to TV inflow. (**c** and **d**): Rotation of the dashed white line together with the blue line in both green and red rectangles so as to view the TV from its ventricular surface. (**e**): Alignment of the dashed white line with tips of the TV leaflets so as to view all three leaflets in the short-axis 2D tomographic space (bottom left), and adjacent 3D space. (**f**): same views with 3D image magnified. Used with permission of Mayo Foundation for Medical Education and Research. All rights reserved. LA, left atrium; RA, right atrium; RV, right ventricle; TTVR, transcatheter tricuspid valve repair; TV, tricuspid valve

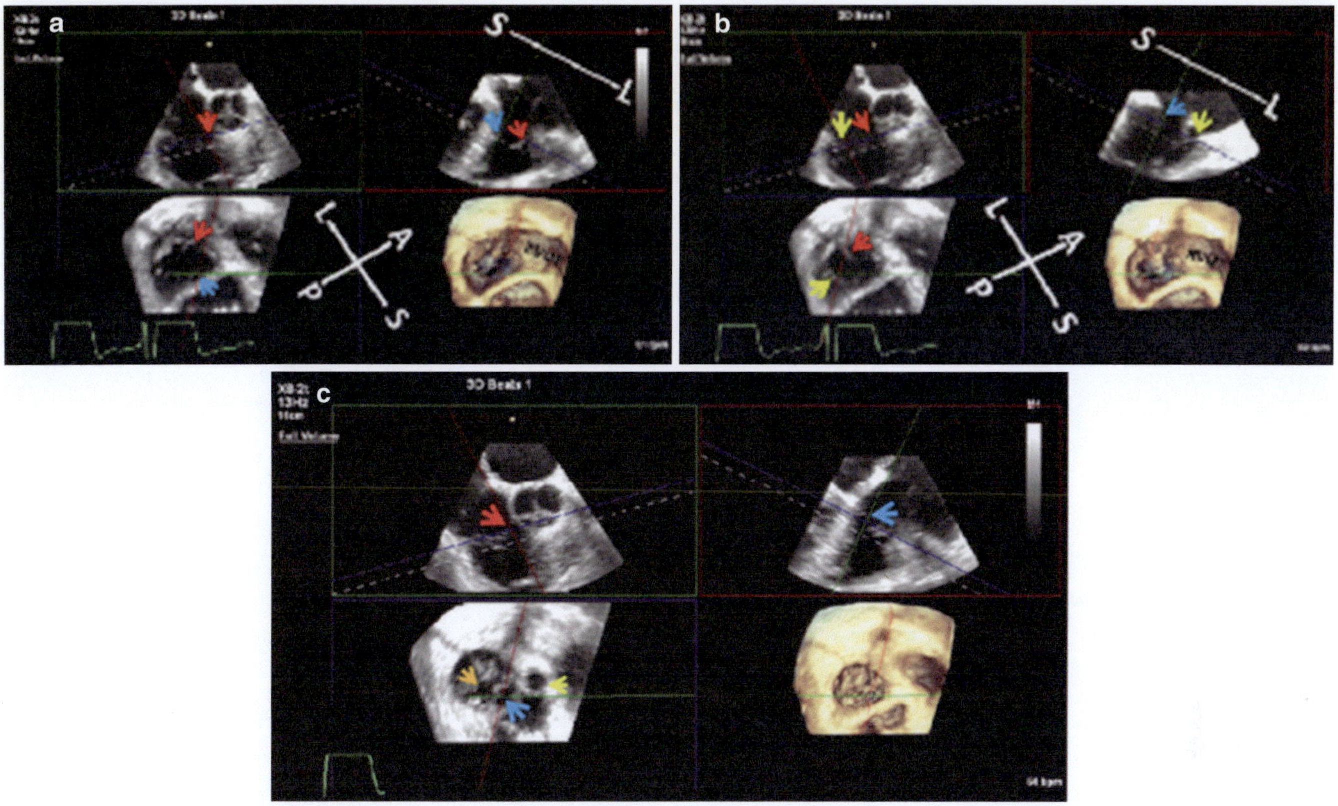

Fig. 34.16 Identifying individual TV leaflets. 3D MultiVue obtained from a single beat FV data set of the TV from the aortic valve short-axis midesophageal window. (**a** and **b**): Diastolic frames of TV. (**a**): Red line positioned at the anterior TV leaflet (red arrow). The septal leaflet (blue arrow) can also be seen at intersection of the green line with the TV in the adjacent red plane (red rectangle, top right). The lateral leaflet (red arrow) in this plane corresponds to the anterior leaflet because the red plane (red line) does not cross the posterior leaflet in the 2D short-axis tomographic space (blue rectangle bottom left) or adjacent 3D space. Note the intersection of the red and green lines at the septal leaflet in the 2D short-axis and 3D space. (**b**): The red line (top left, green rectangle) is now positioned at the posterior leaflet (yellow arrow).The lateral leaflet (yellow arrow) in the adjacent red plane (top right, red rectangle) corresponds to the posterior leaflet. The septal leaflet (blue arrow) is also seen. Note the intersection of the red and green lines at the posterior leaflet (yellow arrow) in the 2D short-axis (blue rectangle bottom left) tomographic space and adjacent 3D space; red arrows point to anterior leaflet. (**c**): Systolic frame showing the anterior tricuspid leaflet (red arrow), septal tricuspid leaflet (blue arrow) and central leaflet malcoaptation (orange arrow). Yellow arrow points to AV. Used with permission of Mayo Foundation for Medical Education and Research. A, anterior; AV, aortic valve; CFD, color flow Doppler; FV, Full Volume; L, lateral; P, posterior; RVOT, right ventricular outflow tract; S, ventricular septal; TR, tricuspid regurgitation; TV, tricuspid valve

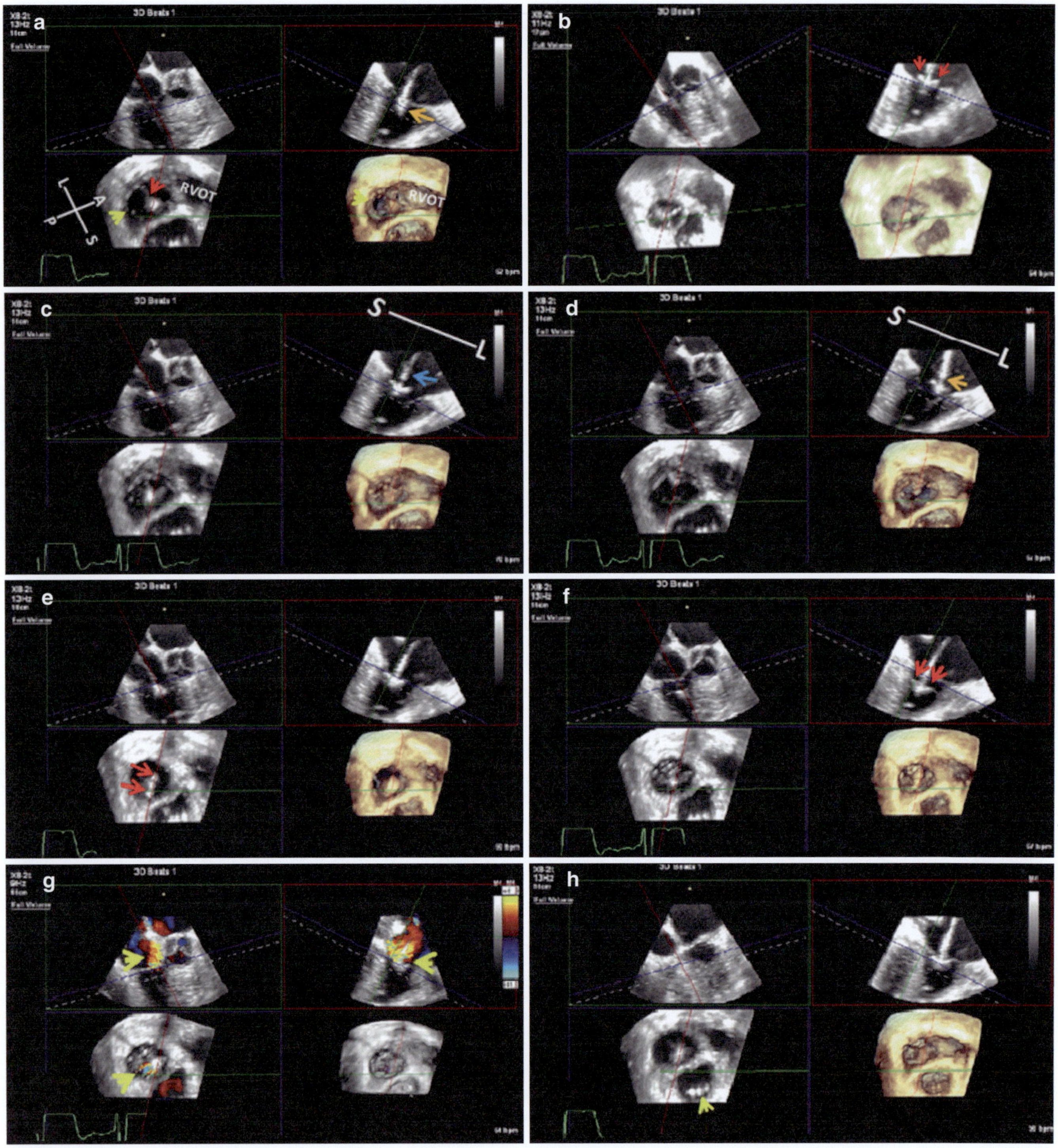

Fig. 34.17 Real time 3D guidance of TTVR with MitraClip using FV MultiVue MPR. (**a**): MitraClip (orange arrow) in the red plane (top right, red rectangle) but the clip arms are not seen. The anterior (red arrow) and posterior (yellow arrow) tricuspid leaflets are seen in the short-axis tomographic space at bottom left. (**b**): MitraClip arms (red arrows) are now clearly seen in the red plane. (**c** and **d**): MitraClip arms are too septal (**c**, blue arrow) or too lateral (**d**, orange arrow). (**e**): MitraClip arms are in correct trajectory with the open clip arms perpendicular to septal and anterior leaflets (red arrows) in the short-axis tomographic space at bottom left of image. (**f**): correct clip arm(red arrows) trajectory is maintained as the MitraClip is advanced into the RV. (**g**): Splitting of the TR jet (yellow arrow) by MitraClip in the red plane (top right). (**h**): leaflet capture (red plane, top right). Yellow arrow points to MitraClip deployed on the MV. Used with permission of Mayo Foundation for Medical Education and Research. All rights reserved. A, anterior; FV, Full Volume; L, lateral; MPR, multiplanar reconstruction; MV, mitral valve; P, posterior; RV, right ventricle; RVOT, right ventricular outflow tract; S, ventricular septal; TR, tricuspid regurgitation; TTVR, transcatheter tricuspid valve repair; TV, tricuspid valve

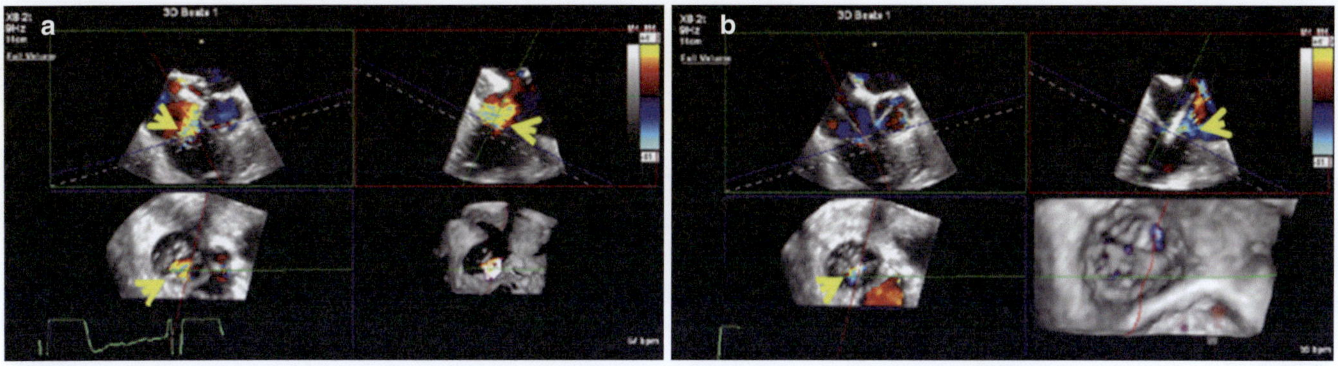

Fig. 34.18 Real time 3D FV MultiVue CFD TEE enface views of the TV from the RV showing TR (arrows) before (**a**) and after MitraClip deployment (**b**). Note the reduction in TR following MitraClip. Used with permission of Mayo Foundation for Medical Education and Research. All rights reserved. CFD, color flow Doppler; FV, Full Volume; RV, right ventricle; TR, tricuspid regurgitation

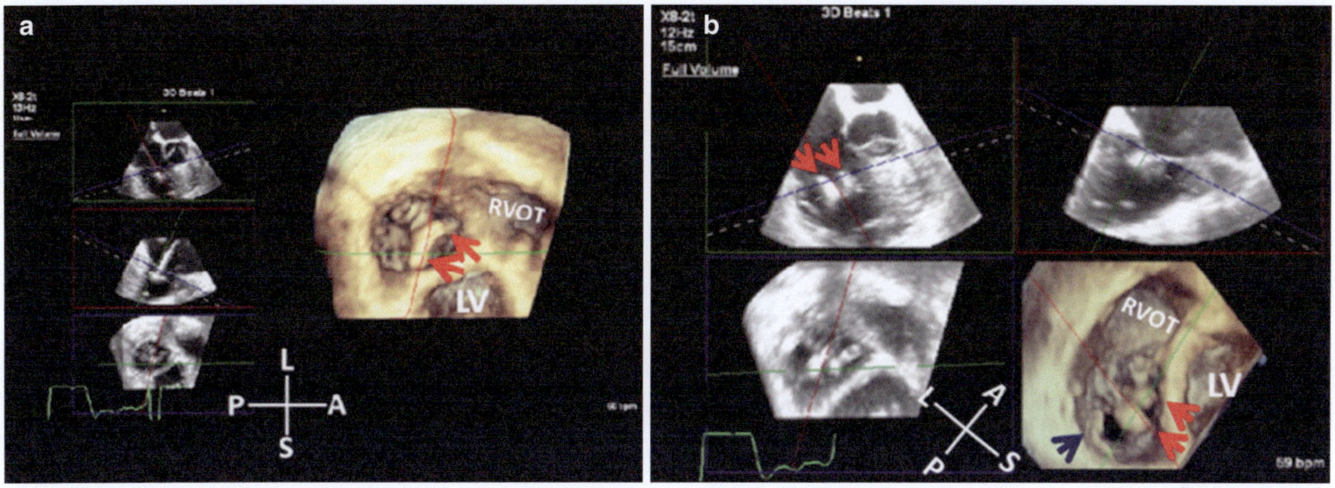

Fig. 34.19 Real time 3D FV TEE enface RV views of the TV following deployment of one MitraClip device (**a**, systole) showing the open clip arms (red, arrows), and after deployment of two MitraClip devices in diastole (**b**, red arrows). Blue arrow points to the posterior TV leaflet. Used with permission of Mayo Foundation for Medical Education and Research. All rights reserved. A, anterior; FV, Full Volume; L, lateral; LV, left ventricle; P, posterior; RV, right ventricle; RVOT, right ventricular outflow tract; S, septal; TV, tricuspid valve

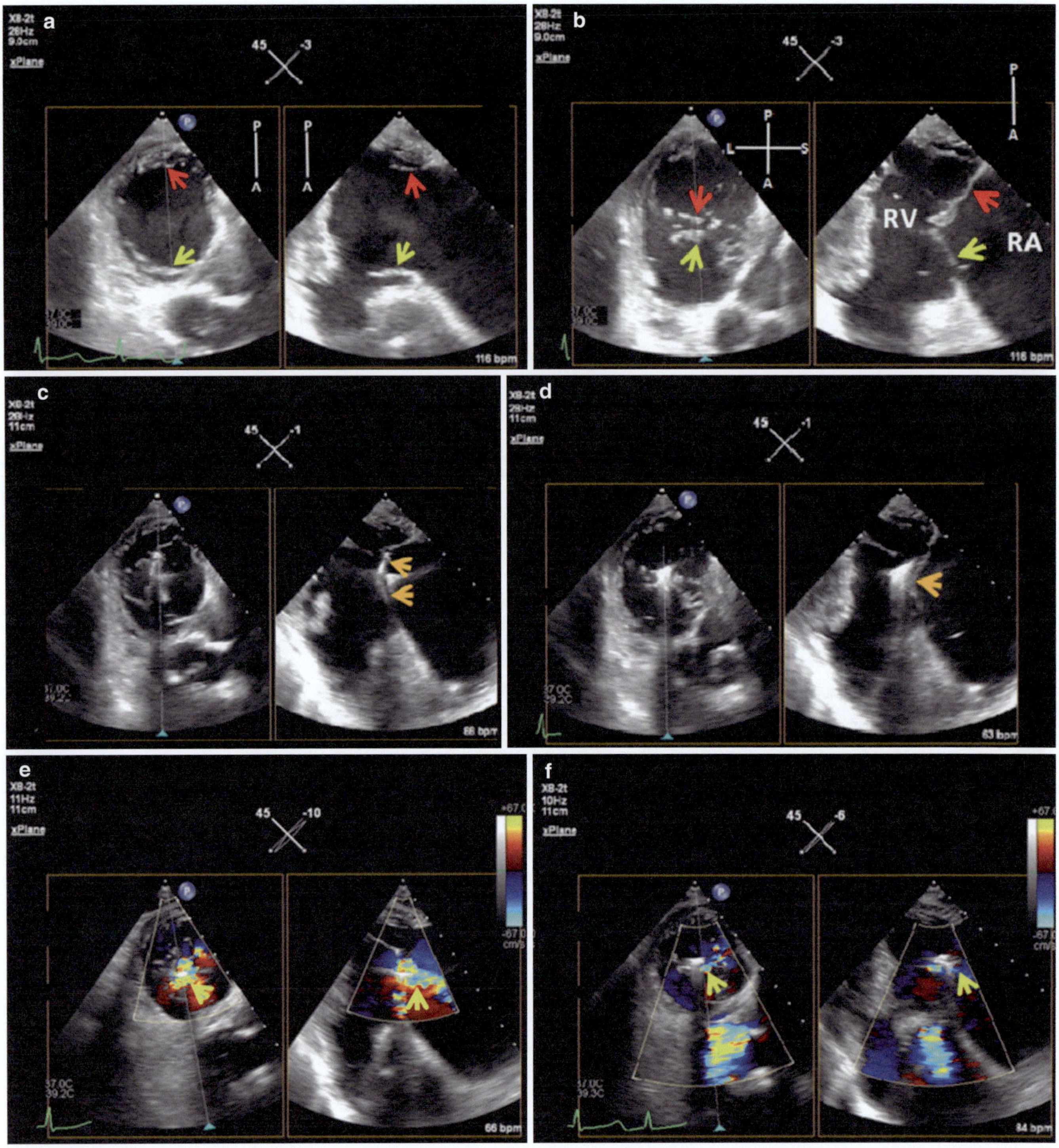

Fig. 34.20 Guiding transcatheter edge-to-edge TV repair using x-Plane. **Top panel:** TG views of TV in diastole (**a**) and systole (**b**) showing the posterior (red arrows) and anterior (yellow arrows) tricuspid leaflets in short axis and corresponding orthogonal long-axis views. **Middle panel:** Advancing the MitraClip arms to capture the anterior and posterior leaflets. (**c**): open MitraClip arms (arrows) on ventricular surface of the targeted TV leaflets ready to be grasped. (**d**): Post deployment of MitraClip (arrow). **Bottom panel:** TR (arrows) before (**e**) and after MitraClip deployment (**f**). Note marked reduction in TR severity. A, anterior; L, lateral; P, posterior; RA, right atrium; RV, right ventricle; S, septal; TG, transgastric; TR, tricuspid regurgitation; TV, tricuspid valve

References

1. Prendegast BD, Baumgartner H, Delgado V, Bax JJ. Transcatheter heart valve interventions: where are we? Where are we going? Eur Heart J. 2019 February 01;40(5):422–40.
2. Del Val D, Ferreira-Neto AN, Wintzer-Wehekind J, et al. Early experience with transcatheter mitral valve replacement: a systematic review. J Am Heart Assoc. 2019 September;8(17):e013332.
3. Webb JG, Murdoch DJ, Boone RH, Moss R, Attinger-Toller A, Blanke P, Cheung A, Hensey M, Leipsic J, Ong K, Sathananthan J, Wood DA, Ye J, Tartara P. Percutaneous transcatheter mitral valve replacement first-in-human experience with a new transseptal system. J Am Coll Cardiol. 2019;73(11):1239–46.
4. Regueiro A, Granada JF, Dagenais F. Rodes-Cabau. J: Transcatheter mitral valve replacement: Insights from early clinical experience and future challenges Journal of the American College of Cardiology volume. 2017;69:2175–92.
5. Testa L, Latib A, Montone RA, Bedogni F. Transcatheter mitral valve regurgitation treatment: state of the art and a glimpse to the future. J Thorac Cardiovasc Surg. 2016 August;152(2):319–27.
6. Grasso C, Rubbio AP. The PASCAL transcatheter mitral valve repair system for the treatment of mitral regurgitation: another piece to the puzzle of edge-to-edge technique. Lancet. 2017;390:773–80.
7. Nickenig G, Kowalski M, Hausleiter J, et al. Transcatheter treatment of severe tricuspid regurgitation with the edge-to-edge MitraClip technique. Circulation. 2017;135:1802–14.
8. Taramasso M, Hahn RT, Alessandrini H, et al. The international multicenter TriValve registry: which patients are undergoing transcatheter tricuspid repair? J Am Coll Cardiol Intv. 2017;10:1982–90.
9. Curio J, Demir OM, Pagnesi M, Mangieri A, Giannini F, Weisz G, Azeem LA. Update on the current landscape of Transcatheter options for tricuspid regurgitation treatment. Interv Cardiol. 2019 May;14(2):54–61.
10. Fam NP, Braun D, von Bardeleben RS, Nabauer M, Ruf T, Connelly KA, Ho E, Thiele H, Lurz P, Weber M, Nickenig G, Narang A, Davidson CJ, Hausleiter J. Compassionate use of the PASCAL transcatheter valve repair system for severe tricuspid regurgitation: a multicenter, observational, first-in-human experience. JACC: Cardiovasc Interv. 2019 December;12(24):2488–95.
11. Fam NP, Ho EC, Zahrani M, Samargandy S, Connelly KA. Transcatheter tricuspid valve repair with the PASCAL system. JACC: Cardiovasc Interv. 2018 February;11(4):407–8.
12. Perlman GY, Dvir D. Treatment of tricuspid regurgitation with the FORMA repair system. Front Cardiovasc Med. 2018;5:140.
13. Muntané-Carol G, Del Val D, Bédard E, Philippon F, Rodés-Cabau J. Transcatheter innovations in tricuspid regurgitation: FORMA device. Prog Cardiovasc Dis. 2019 Nov–Dec;62(6):496–9.
14. Hahn RT, Nabauer M, Zuber M, Nazif TM, Hausleiter J, Taramasso M, Pozzoli A, George I, Kodali S, Bapat V, Maisano F. Intraprocedural imaging of transcatheter tricuspid valve interventions. JACC Cardiovasc Imag. 2019 March;12(3):532.
15. Kalra A, Uberoi AS, Latib A, Khera S, Little SH, Bhatt DL, Reardon MJ, Kleiman NS, Barker CM. Emerging Transcatheter options for tricuspid regurgitation. Methodist Debakey Cardiovasc J. 2017 Jul–Sep;13(3):120–5.
16. Muraru D, Hahn RT, Soliman OI, Faletra FF, Basso C, Badano LP. 3-dimensional echocardiography in imaging the tricuspid valve. JACC Cardiovasc Imaging. 2019 March;12(3):500–15.
17. Dreyfus GD, Corbi PJ, Chan J, Bahrami T. Secondary tricuspid regurgitation or dilatation: which should be the criteria for surgical repair? Ann Thoracic Surg. 2005;79:127–32.

Echo-Navigation

35

Jeremy J. Thaden and Joseph F. Maalouf

Introduction

Traditionally, guidance of structural heart interventions has been performed using a combination of fluoroscopy and echocardiography. Fluoroscopy affords a wide field of view with excellent visualization of catheters and devices, but only limited soft tissue visualization. By contrast, echocardiography affords excellent visualization of cardiac soft tissue anatomy but has a limited field of view and complete visualization of catheters and devices can be challenging. Additionally, fluoroscopy and TEE are typically displayed in different orientations, making it more challenging to mentally integrate the data obtained from the two modalities.

Systems are now clinically available that provide real-time, automated TEE-fluoroscopic fusion imaging for procedural guidance (Fig. 35.1) [1]. Currently available systems allow the imager to transpose a point or location from the echocardiographic image to the fluoroscopic image, thus serving as a reference point on the fluoroscopic image, and also to overlay live 2D or 3D echocardiographic data on top of the fluoroscopic image [1, 2]. And, with any movement of the C arm of fluoroscopy, the TEE image and reference points are automatically relocated in accordance with the new x-ray projection [1]. Moreover, with 3D TEE, the echocardiographer can crop, rotate, or change the transparency of the 3D image relative to fluoroscopy in order to highlight the soft tissues most relevant to the procedure and to best visualize catheters and devices [1, 3]. The potential benefits include common TEE and fluoroscopic image orientation and the ability to simultaneously view catheters and devices (seen well by fluoroscopy) and cardiac soft tissue anatomy (seen well by TEE) to enhance communication and procedural guidance. In this chapter we will review the use of TEE-fluoroscopic fusion imaging for guidance of several commonly performed structural heart procedures.

Transseptal Puncture

Transseptal puncture (TSP) is a common first step for a growing list of transseptal procedures. Precise localization of the TSP location is often critical to safely and effectively complete the procedure. TEE is the predominant imaging modality used to identify the location of TSP in current clinical practice, but fusion imaging may facilitate a more precise septal puncture location and may decrease the time required for TSP [3, 4]. With TEE-fluoroscopic fusion imaging, the optimal TSP location can be identified by TEE and a fiducial marker can be transposed onto the fluoscopic image thus serving as a reference point when manipulating the catheter. Live 2D and 3D TEE images can also be superimposed on the fluoroscopic image, allowing good visualization of the catheter by fluoroscopy and the interatrial septum and adjacent soft tissue anatomy by TEE (Fig. 35.2). Following successful TSP, the fiducial marker placed at the site of TSP can also be helpful to confirm guide catheter position relative to the atrial septum (e.g. to ensure a guide catheter in the left atrium has not slipped back to the right atrium).

Supplementary Information The online version of this chapter (https://doi.org/10.1007/978-3-030-72941-7_35) contains supplementary material, which is available to authorized users.

J. J. Thaden (✉)
Assistant Professor of Medicine, Mayo Clinic College of Medicine; Co-Chair for Clinical Practice and Quality, Division of Cardiovascular Ultrasound; Consultant, Department of Cardiovascular Medicine, Mayo Clinic, Rochester, MN, USA
e-mail: thaden.jeremy@mayo.edu

J. F. Maalouf
Professor of Medicine, Mayo Clinic College of Medicine; Director, Interventional Echocardiography; Consultant, Department of Cardiovascular Medicine, Mayo Clinic, Rochester, MN, USA
e-mail: maalouf.joseph@mayo.edu

J. F. Maalouf et al. (eds.), *Practical 3D Echocardiography*, https://doi.org/10.1007/978-3-030-72941-7_35

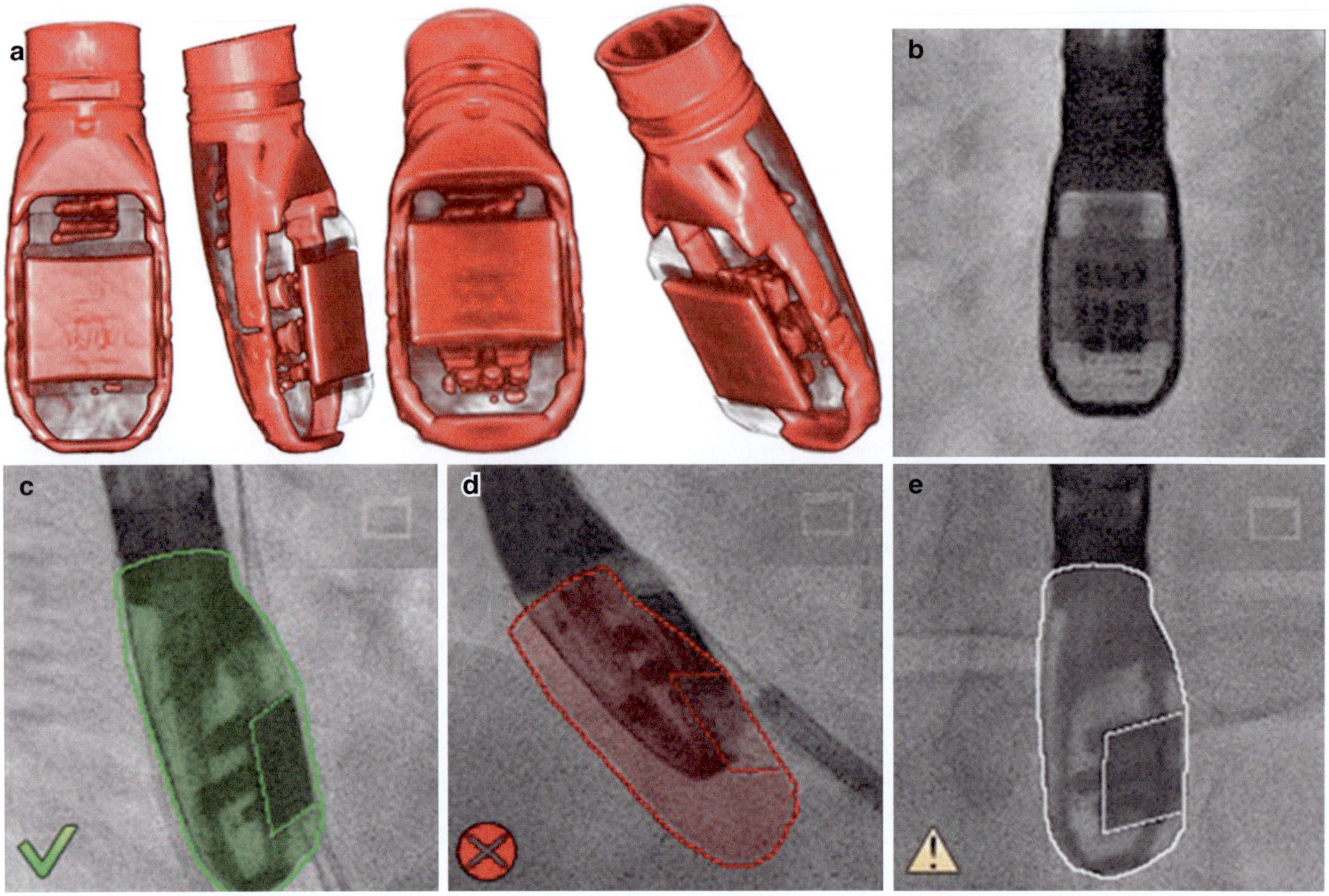

Fig. 35.1 Automated TEE probe registration for live TEE-fluoroscopic fusion imaging. Automated image registration relies on a high-resolution 3D reconstruction of the TEE probe (**a**). The 3D datasest is used as a template and matched with the observed fluoroscopic signature seen on live fluoroscopy to achieve a dynamic, automated and near-real time registration (**b**). The probe registration status is denoted using a color overlay, with green denoting successful registration (**c**), red denoting unsuccessful registration (D), and a transparent overlay relaying indeterminate registration (**e**). By permission- Thaden et al. *JASE* 2016 [1]

Left Atrial Appendage Occlusion

TEE-fluoroscopic fusion imaging holds promise in guiding left atrial appendage occlusion. 3D TEE image overlay on the fluoroscopic image provides better appreciation of the guide catheter and device position relative to the soft tissue anatomy and has the potential to facilitate more efficient and safe cannulation of the left atrial appendage (Fig. 35.3). We frequently also mark the ostium of the left atrial appendage with a fiducial marker, transposed on the fluoroscopic image, and additional markers can be useful to better visualize the circumflex coronary artery and the most proximal lobe of the left atrial appendage, if relevant. There is potential to improve safety and reduce radiation exposure although supporting data are currently lacking.

Transcatheter Edge-to-Edge Mitral Valve Repair

There is early data validating the safety of TEE-fluoroscopic fusion for guidance of transcatheter mitral valve repair [5]. In our experience, we have used fiducial markers to mark the site of TSP and the left upper pulmonary vein (see Chap. 29) on the fluoroscopic image. Live 2D and 3D TEE imaging with or without color Doppler imaging is also helpful to guide clip trajectory (Figs. 35.4 and 35.5). More data are needed on the impact of TEE-fluoroscopic imaging on safety and procedural outcomes.

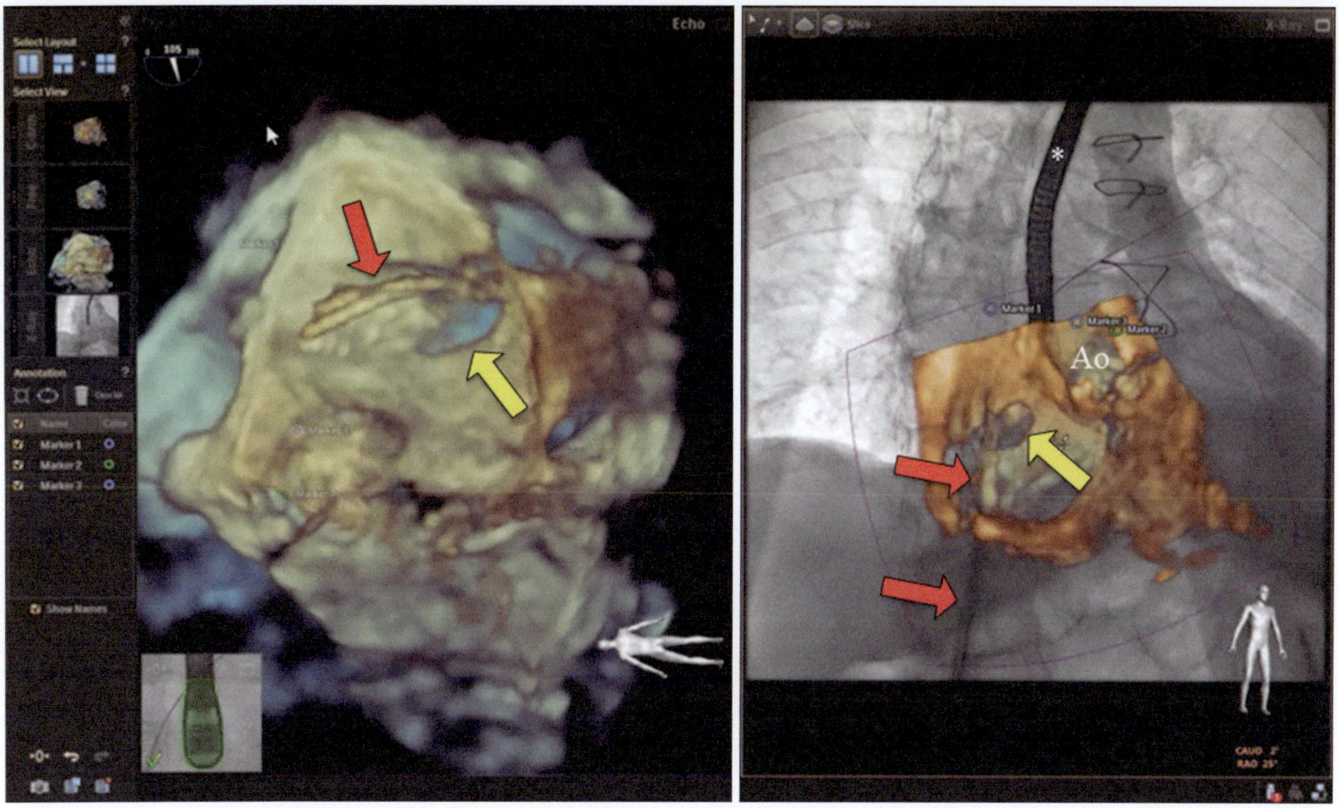

Fig. 35.2 Live 3D TEE-fluoroscopic fusion imaging for transseptal puncture. The image in the left panel shows a view of the atrial septum from the perspective of the left atrium. The 3D TEE image shows a guide catheter (red arrow) crossing the fossa ovalis (yellow arrow). The panel on the right shows the fluoroscopic view with live 3D TEE images re-oriented to the fluoroscopic perspective. The guide catheter (red arrows) is seen traversing the inferior vena cava on the fluoroscopic image and the 3D TEE shows the catheter crossing at the level of the fossa ovalis (yellow arrow). Used with permission of Mayo Foundation for Medical Education and Research. All rights reserved. *, TEE probe; Ao, aortic root

Percutaneous Paravalvular Regurgitation Closure

In our practice, aortic paravalvular regurgitation is typically closed from a retrograde (aortic) approach and mitral paravalvular regurgitation is closed from an antegrade (left atrial approach). For aortic closure, annotation markers placed at the site of the defect or live echocardiographic fusion can be helpful to guide cannulation. Additional annotation markers at adjacent structures of interest such as the left main coronary artery can also be helpful to avoid iatrogenic trauma from devices and catheters. Similarly, live fusion imaging can be helpful to guide cannulation of mitral paravalvular regurgitation defects. Fiducial markers can also be used to guide cannulation (Fig. 35.6), but one limitation of fiducial markers is that they are static markers which is less useful when the mitral and aortic annuli are dynamic.

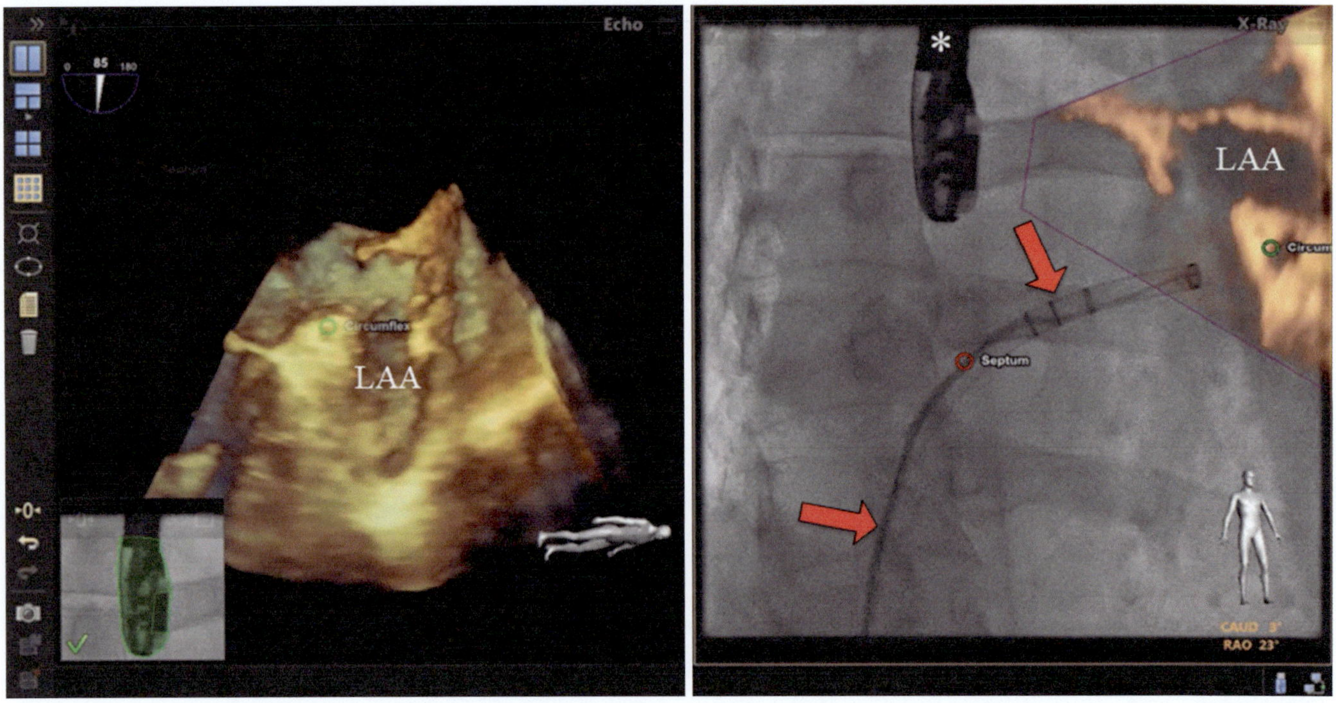

Fig. 35.3 Live 3D TEE-fluoroscopic fusion imaging for left atrial appendage occlusion. The image in the left panel shows a 3D TEE view of the left atrial appendage (LAA). The circumflex coronary artery was marked with an annotation marker (green marker) and the guide catheter is not well seen in the dedicated 3D TEE image. The panel on the right shows the fluoroscopic view with live 3D TEE images re-oriented to the fluoroscopic perspective. The guide catheter (red arrows) is seen traversing the atrial septum by fluoroscopy with the tip of the catheter inferior to the ostium of the LAA seen on the fused 3D TEE image. In this case the transseptal puncture site was marked (red circle) at the start of the case and serves as a reference annotation marker on the fluoroscopic view for the puncture site. Used with permission of Mayo Foundation for Medical Education and Research. All rights reserved. *, TEE, transducer; LAA, left atrial appendage

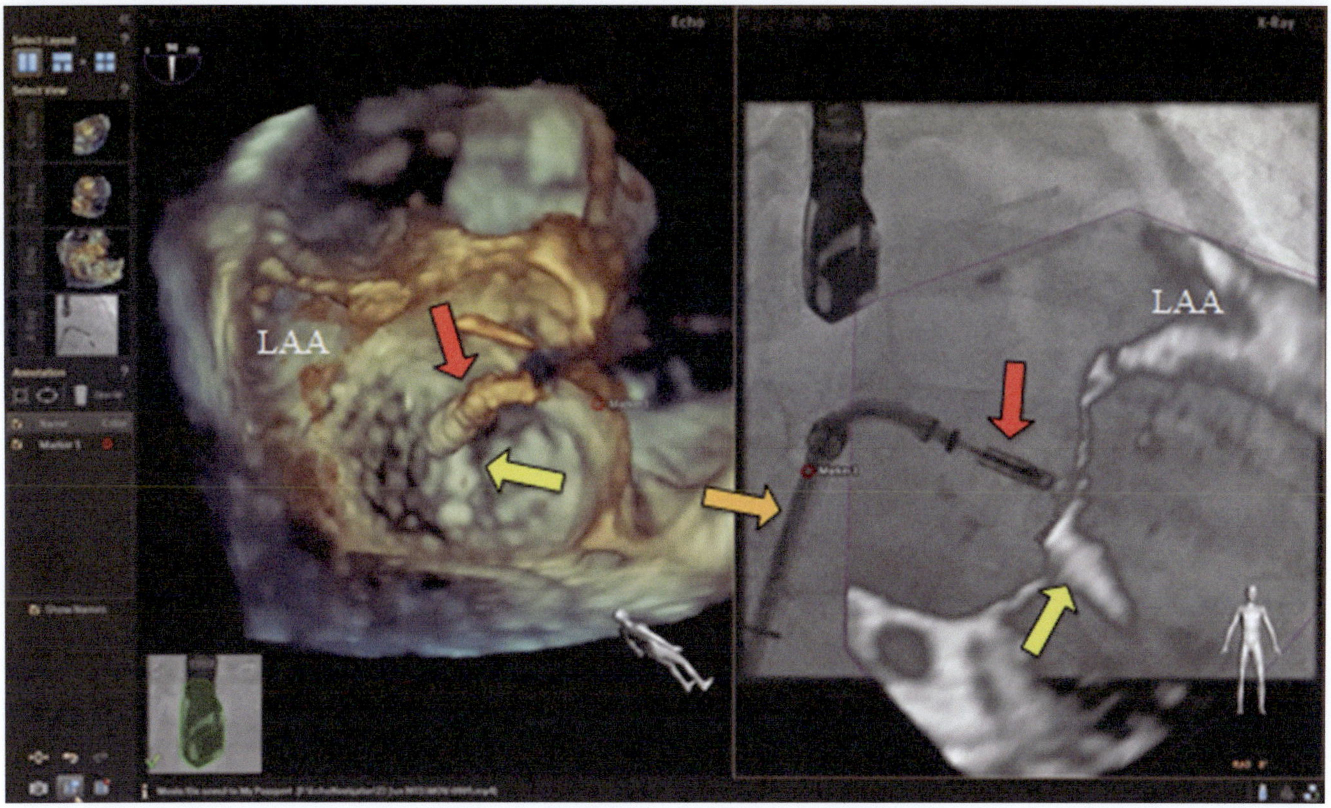

Fig. 35.4 Live 3D TEE-fluoroscopic fusion imaging for transcatheter edge-to-edge mitral valve repair. The image in the left panel shows a 3D TEE view of the mitral valve and MitraClip (Abbott Vascular, Abbott Park, IL). In the left atrial view, a previously deployed clip with tissue bridge (yellow arrow) is seen alongside a delivery system and second clip (red arrow). The TEE-fluoroscopic fusion image on the right more clearly shows the position of the steerable guide catheter (orange arrow) and MitraClip (red arrow) delivery system trajectory in relation to the mitral valve leaflets and the first clip (yellow arrow). The optimal trans-septal puncture site was marked at the beginning of the case and can be seen as an annotation marker on the fluoroscopic image on the right (red circle). LAA, left atrial appendage

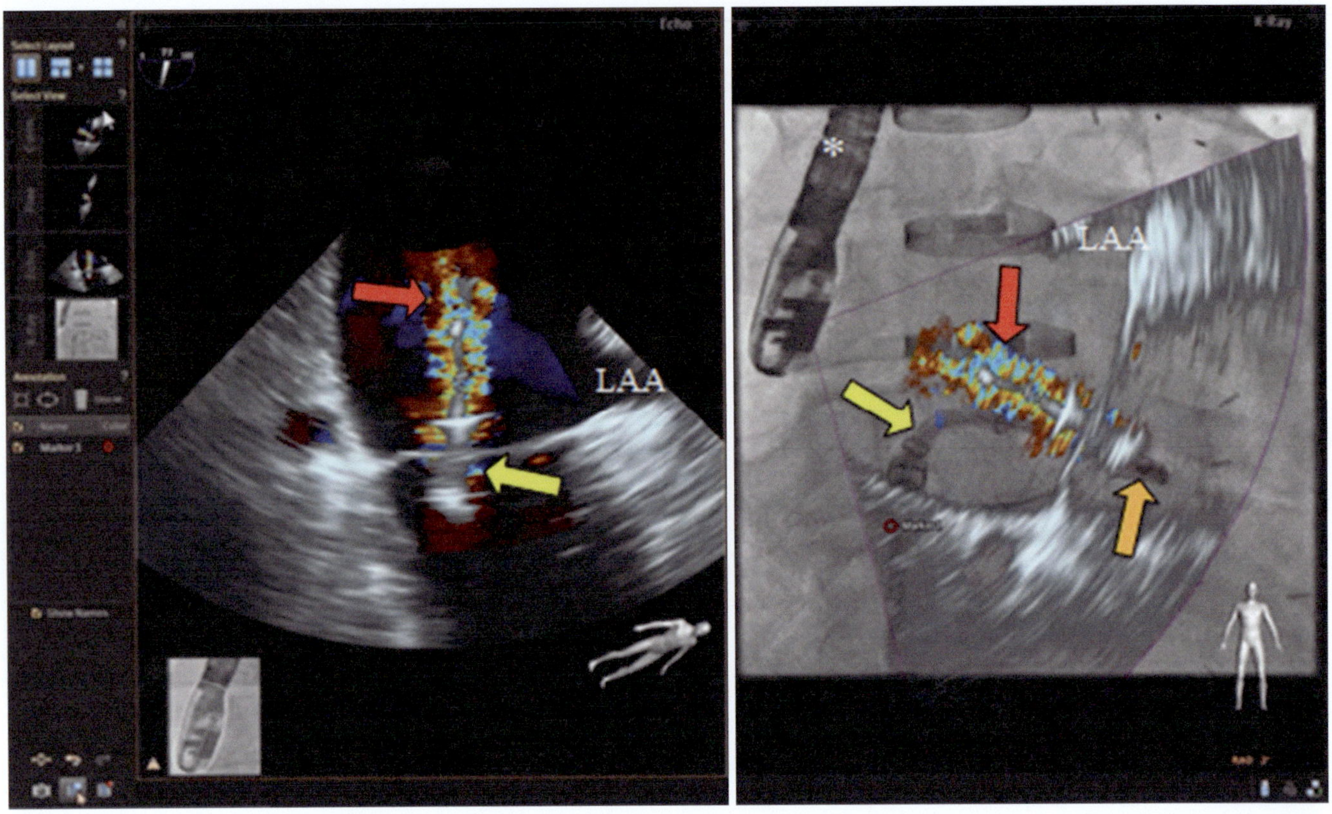

Fig. 35.5 Live 2D TEE with color Doppler and fluoroscopic fusion imaging for transcatheter edge-to-edge mitral valve repair. The image in the left panel shows a 2D TEE view of the mitral valve and MitraClip (yellow arrow; Abbott Vascular, Abbott Park, IL) directed at a central jet of mitral regurgitation (red arrow). The TEE-fluoroscopic fusion image on the right shows the 2D and color Doppler data re-oriented and superimposed on the fluoroscopic image. The position of the guide catheter (yellow arrow) and MitraClip delivery system (orange arrow) is better appreciated in relation to the mitral valve leaflets and mitral regurgitant jet (red arrow) on the fusion image. Used with permission of Mayo Foundation for Medical Education and Research. All rights reserved. *, TEE, transducer; LAA, left atrial appendage

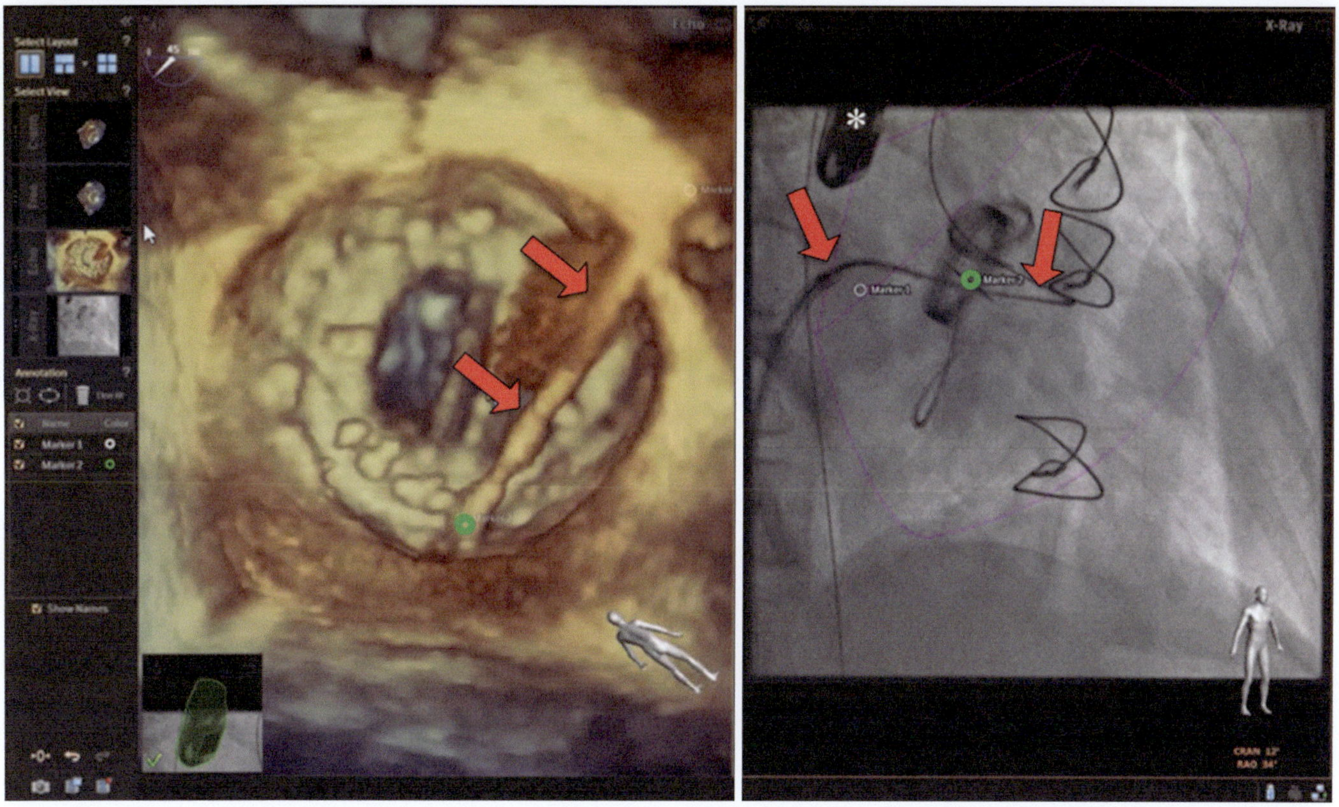

Fig. 35.6 Live 3D TEE-fluoroscopic fusion imaging for mitral paravalvular regurgitation closure in a patient with a mitral prosthesis. The image in the left panel shows a 3D TEE view of a mitral valve prosthesis and a transseptal catheter (red arrows) for cannulation of a posterior paravalvular regurgitation defect. In this case the site of the defect was marked using a green annotation marker (green circle). The site of the regurgitant jet was marked using the echocardiographic image and the corresponding location is shown by the annotation marker on the fluoroscopic view on the right (green circle). The position of the transseptal catheter is better seen in the fluoroscopic view on the right (red arrows), which shows the catheter traversing the atrial septum, the mitral paravalvular defect, followed by the ascending aorta. Used with permission of Mayo Foundation for Medical Education and Research. All rights reserved. *, TEE, transducer

Conclusions and Limitations

TEE-fluoroscopic fusion imaging is an emerging tool which shows promise for guiding complex transcatheter structural heart interventions. Currently available systems provide automated, near-real time registration of TEE and fluoroscopic views for procedural guidance. Features include transposing markers of interest (e.g. TSP puncture site, paravalvular regurgitant jet location, etc) from the echocardiographic space to the fluoroscopic space and the capability to superimpose live 2D, 3D, and color Doppler echocardiographic images on the live fluoroscopic views. Potential advantages include enhanced communication and anatomical understanding amongst the various team members. Particularly as we see an increase in the complexity of transcatheter procedures there is also potential to improve the efficiency of these procedures and to improve outcomes, but additional studies are needed on how best to apply this novel technology and precisely what advantages it can provide. Limitations of 3D TEE-fluoroscopic fusion imaging are suboptimal 3D spatial resolution and inability to always display desired enface perspectives. Another limitation of fusion imaging is inability to keep track of fiducial markers with respiratory movements or during cardiac contraction which may result in location annotation errors [3].

References

1. Thaden JJ, Sanon S, Geske JB, Eleid MF, Nijhof N, Malouf JF, et al. Echocardiographic and fluoroscopic fusion imaging for procedural guidance: an overview and early clinical experience. J Am Soc Echocardiogr. 2016;29:503–12.
2. Faletra FF, Pedrazzini G, Pasotti E, Murzilli R, Leo LA, Moccetti T. Echocardiography-X-ray image fusion. JACC Cardiovasc Imaging. 2016;9:1114–7.
3. Faletra FF, Biasco L, Pedrazzini G, Moccetti M, Pasotti E, Leo LA, et al. Echocardiographic-fluoroscopic fusion imaging in Transseptal puncture: a new Technology for an old Procedure. J Am Soc Echocardiogr. 2017;30:885–95.
4. Afzal S, Veulemans V, Balzer J, Rassaf T, Hellhammer K, Polzin A, et al. Safety and efficacy of transseptal puncture guided by real-time fusion of echocardiography and fluoroscopy. Neth Heart J. 2017;25:131–6.
5. Sundermann SH, Biaggi P, Grunenfelder J, Gessat M, Felix C, Bettex D, et al. Safety and feasibility of novel technology fusing echocardiography and fluoroscopy images during MitraClip interventions. EuroIntervention. 2014;9:1210–6.

Evolving Role of 3D Printing in Guiding Interventional Procedures

36

Thomas A. Foley and Nandan S. Anavekar

Imaging has been central to the evolution of contemporary cardiovascular practice which has entered the frontier of therapies for complex structural heart and vascular disease. Underpinning the ability to successfully manage these complex situations is a detailed understanding of the complex spatial relationships in the heart and vascular system that is required by cardiac surgeons, cardiologists, cardiac radiologists, and the cardiovascular device industry. In reality the three-dimensional (3D) relationships of cardiovascular structures vary greatly from patient to patient and is often not immediately intuitive from two dimensional (2D) images.

Despite advanced 3D imaging and display, whether from echocardiography, CT, or MRI, the understanding of spatial relationships remains limited when the images are viewed on a two dimensional screen (Fig. 36.1). Also, as image size can be scaled, it is difficult to get an accurate sense of size relationships when viewing 3D images on a 2D screen (Fig. 36.2a and b). These limitations can be addressed by creating a physical model of patient specific anatomy using 3D printing [1]. 3D printing is the process of creating a physical 3D model from volumetric tomographic images. 3D printed physical models allow more intuitive understanding of 3D spatial relationships and can be printed at 1:1 size ratio to the imaged structure so that life size models are created (Fig. 36.2c).

The process of creating a physical 3D model is composed of four basic steps. The first is acquisition of volumetric imaging data of the anatomy of interest. For cardiac imaging, this can be from 3D echocardiography (3DE), volumetric MRI, or CT. The second step is the identification and segmentation of the anatomy of interest to be displayed in the model. There are multiple software packages available, many FDA approved, for segmentation of medical images. The third step is the preparation of the segmented data for 3D printing. This often requires the use of computer aided design (CAD) software to process the digital data. The processing can involve removing artifact from the data, combining parts in the model, adding support structure, creating openings in the model to improve visualization of internal structures, labelling anatomy, etc. The fourth step is printing the model. There are multiple types of 3D printers which use different technology to create a physical model. The printers vary in cost, speed, physical properties of material, build volume size, and ease of use. Depending on the printer and material used, the models can be full color, transparent, hard, soft, or flexible; however, most printers are not able to do all of these in one model.

The 3D printed models can be used for planning/simulation of procedures and surgeries. 3D printed models can be used for a variety of indications for guiding interventional procedures. The models can be used to aid in visualization of anatomy or location of pathology prior to a procedure to determine procedure feasibility or to assess for likelihood of potential complications (Fig. 36.3). Models which provide patient specific anatomy have been used to aid in sizing of devices such as percutaneously placed valves or atrial appendage closure devices (Figs. 36.4 and 36.5). Models can also been used for simulation of patient specific procedures and can be connected to flow pumps to simulate physiologic conditions. These models have been used to teach practitioners new procedures, rehearse complex procedures, and to aid in the learning of procedures which trainees may not be able to perform on live patients.

Most 3D printed models currently come from CT imaging due to high spatial resolution, easy availability, large image field of view, and frequent use of CT prior to procedures for

T. A. Foley (✉)
Assistant Professor of Radiology, Mayo Clinic College of Medicine; Consultant, Division of Cardiovascular Radiology, Department of Radiology, Mayo Clinic, Rochester, MN, USA
e-mail: foley.thomas@mayo.edu

N. S. Anavekar
Professor of Medicine, Mayo Clinic College of Medicine; Consultant, Department of Cardiovascular Medicine, Mayo Clinic, Rochester, MN, USA
e-mail: anavekar.nandan@mayo.edu

J. F. Maalouf et al. (eds.), *Practical 3D Echocardiography*, https://doi.org/10.1007/978-3-030-72941-7_36

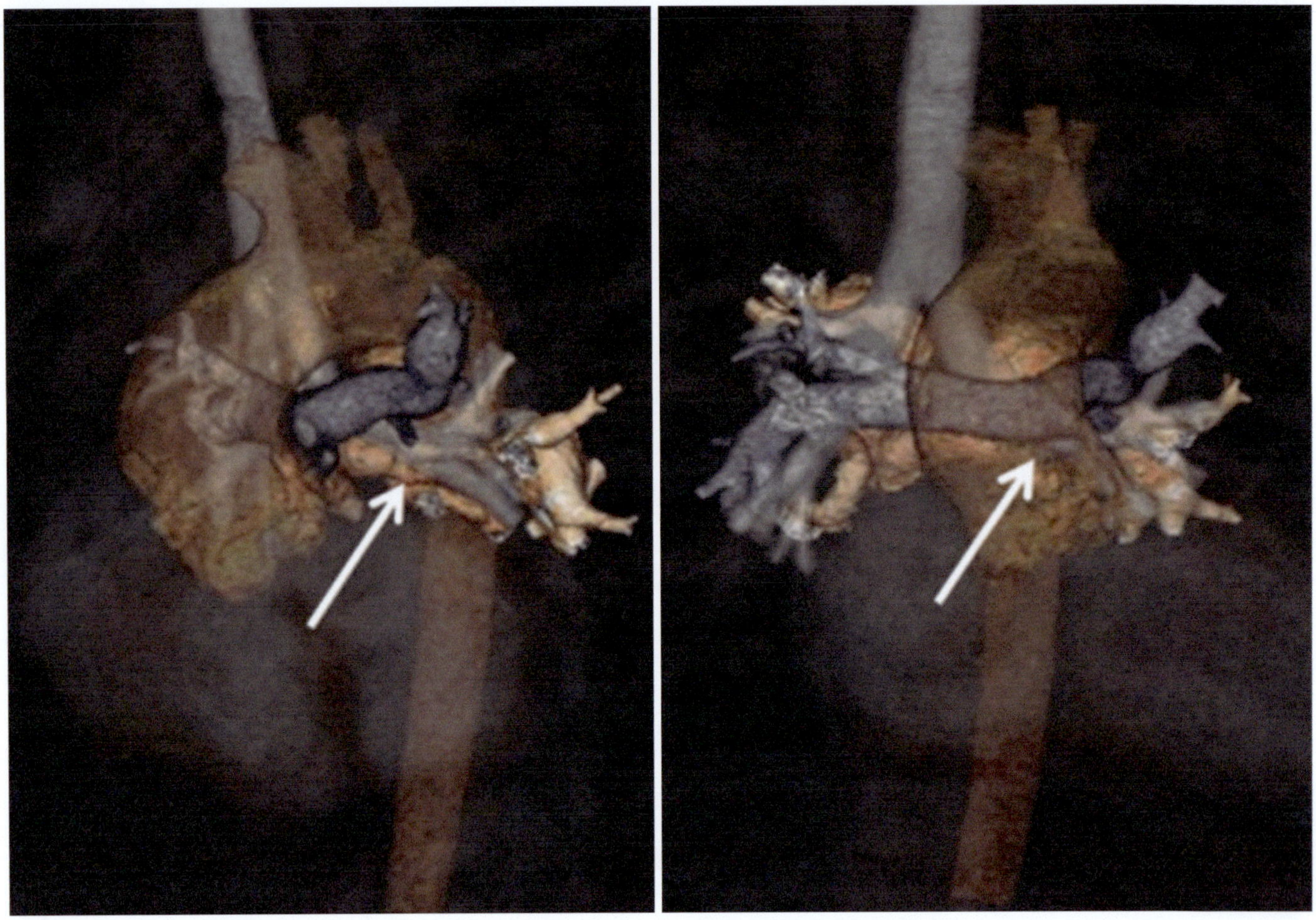

Fig. 36.1 3D volume rendered images from a CT angiogram in a 6 year old male with pulmonary atresia and ventricular septal defect. The aorta, pulmonary arteries, and trachea are displayed. Aorto-pulmonary collateral vessels are also displayed (arrows); however, relationship of the collaterals with adjacent structures such as the trachea was limited and difficult to fully understand from these images. Used with permission of Mayo Foundation for Medical Education and Research.

planning and/or coronary artery assessment. Cardiac MRI is also frequently used; however, a special imaging sequence with high spatial resolution in all three planes needs to be obtained at the time of image acquisition to allow for a high quality model to be made. 3DE images can also be used to create a model (Fig. 36.6); however, 3DE images are limited by smaller field of view and image noise. Currently most reported models for 3DE have been focused models of the cardiac valves or septal defects.

Moreover, the use of 3D printed models can be used to tailor education to different learners. 3D printed models are being used to effectively teach complex cardiac anatomy to cardiology and cardiovascular surgery fellows. Training procedural techniques has been traditionally time consuming and has the potential to be implicated in procedural complications. Simulation using 3D models is emerging as a fundamental resource for teaching procedural techniques for trainees acquiring advanced skill sets in the field and may evolve to represent a new standard of care. Finally, we have found that 3D printed models are also effective tools for communication within healthcare teams and with patients. Within the practice, specific 3D models used to explain disease processes and planned procedures enhanced patient understanding and facilitated shared decision making and informed consent, which ultimately improves patient satisfaction.

Current limitations for 3D printing are availability of 3D printers. Segmentation and processing can require significant amounts of time to create the model. While 3D printers have seen reduction in prices, there remains a cost to purchase, maintain, and buy 3D printing material. There are also limited studies demonstrating the effectiveness of 3D printing in reducing costs, complications, or time of procedures.

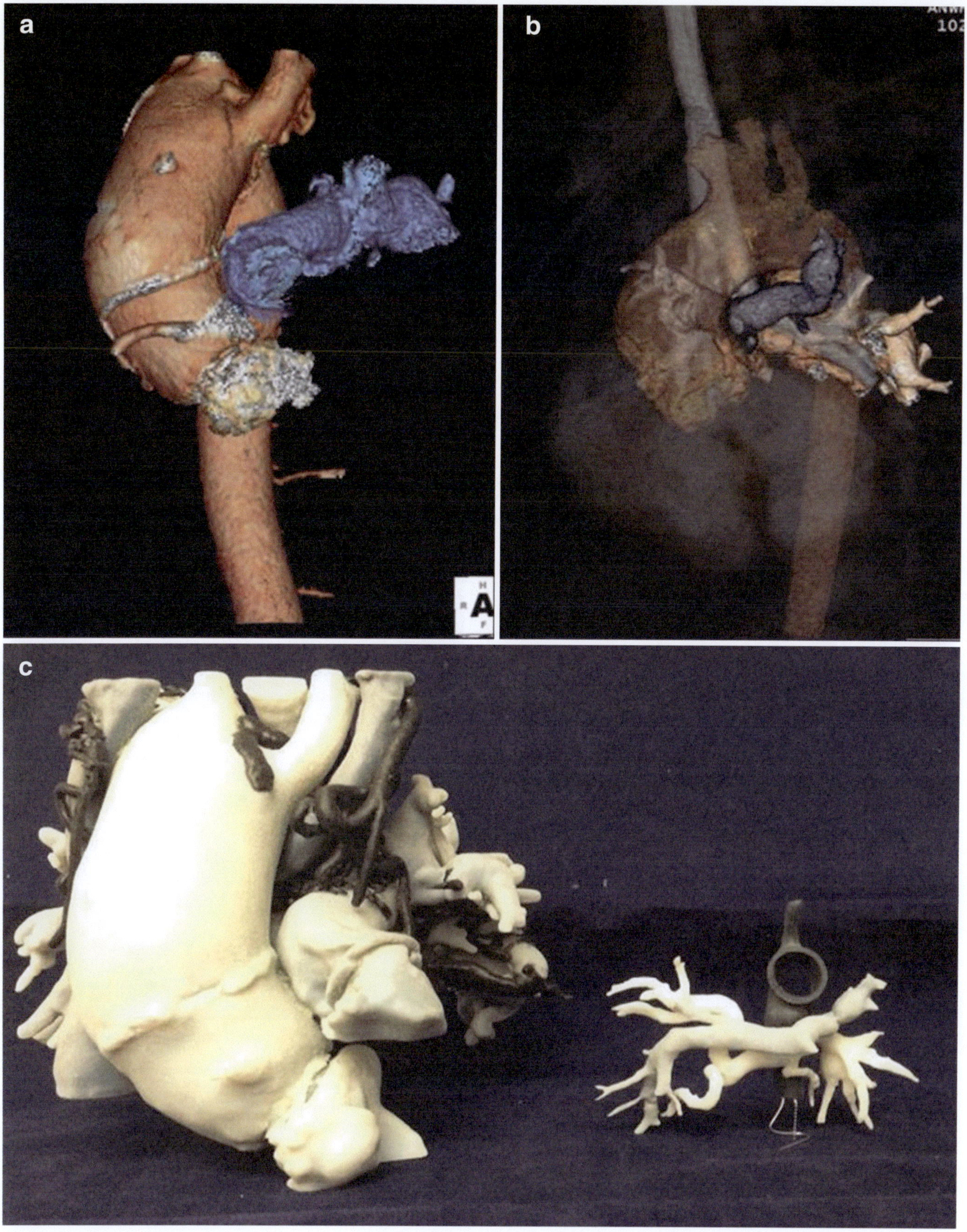

Fig. 36.2 3D volume rendered image showing the aorta and pulmonary arteries created from a CT angiogram of a 60 year old man with a 6 cm ascending aortic aneurysm (**a**) and 3D volume rendered image showing the aorta, pulmonary arteries, trachea and collateral arteries in the 6 year old with pulmonary atresia and VSD from Fig. 36.1(b). Because of scaling of the images, the size of the aorta looks similar in both cases. (**c**). Life size 3D printed models show the actual size of the aorta in patient from Fig. 36.2a and the relationship of the collaterals to the trachea in patient from Fig. 36.1 and 36.2b. Used with permission of Mayo Foundation for Medical Education and Research.

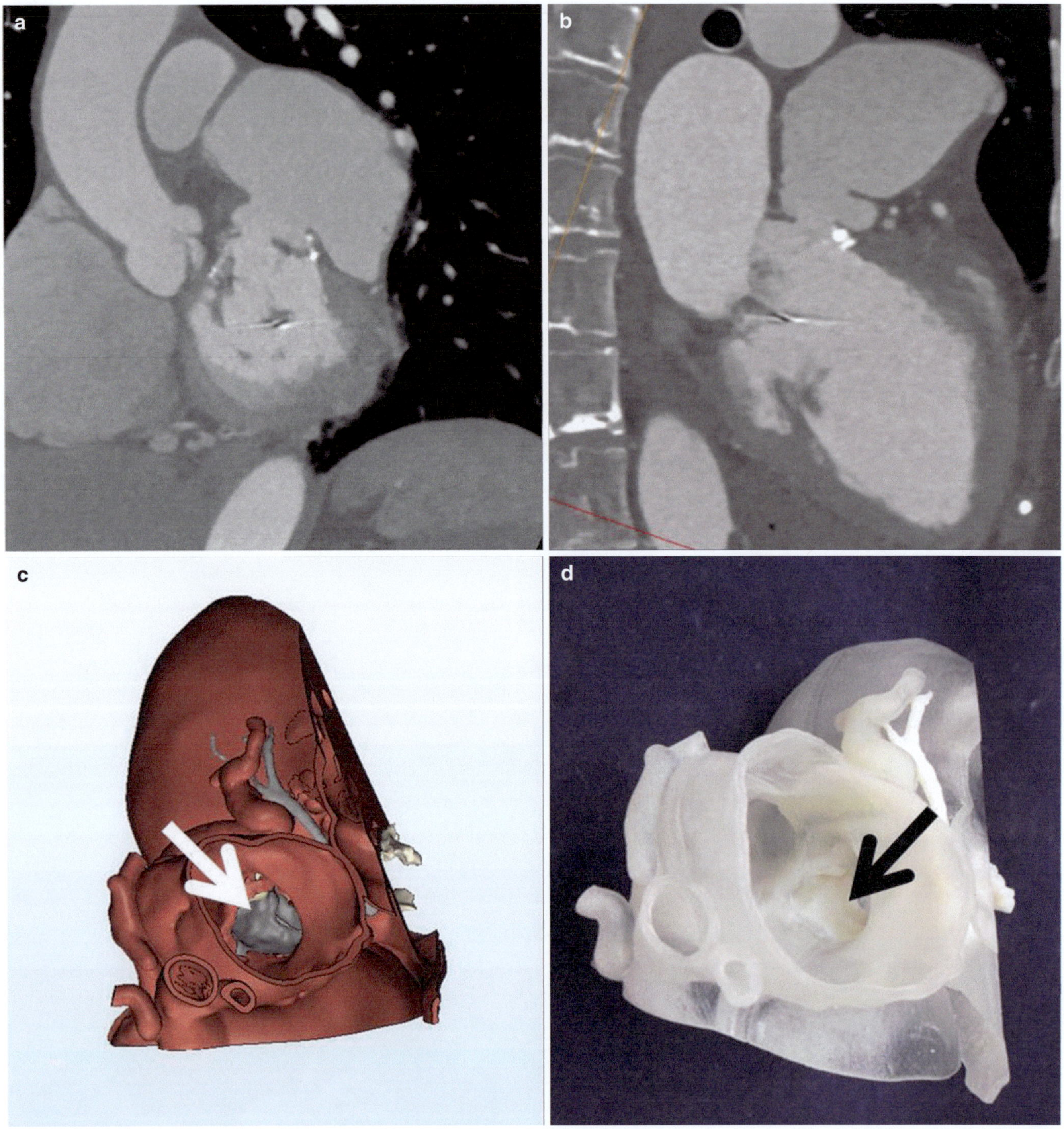

Fig. 36.3 Short axis (**a**) and long axis (**b**) reformmated CT angiogram images from a patient with a mitral valve prosthesis and left ventricle to left atrial appendage fistula. Virtual 3D model (**c**) created from the CT images viewing the fistulous connection through the dilated left atrial appendage (arrow). The prosthetic mitral valve is seen through the fistula opening (gray structure, white arrow). 3D printed model (**d**) showing the location of the fistulous connection and the prosthetic valve (black arrow). The 3D printed model showed that the opening of the fistula was too close to the prosthetic valve to allow for a percutaneous closure. Used with permission of Mayo Foundation for Medical Education and Research.

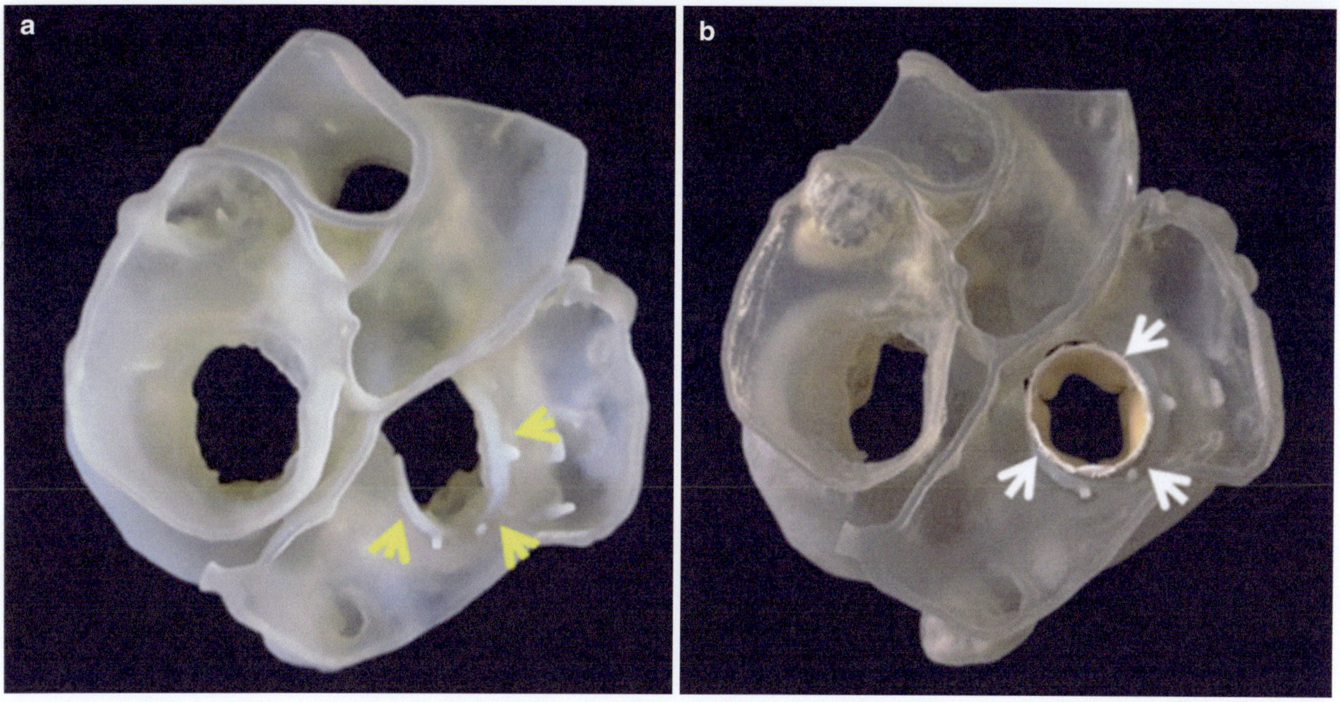

Fig. 36.4 3D printed models from a patient with a prior tricuspid annuloplasty and severe tricupsid valve regurgitation used to size a percutaneous tricuspid valve placement (**a**). Model before showing site of tricuspid annuloplasty, yellow arrows). Used with permission of Mayo Foundation for Medical Education and Research. All rights reserved. (**b**). Model after off label placement of a percutaneous prosthetic valve (white arrows) [2] (By permission- Cabasa et al. *JACC 2015*)

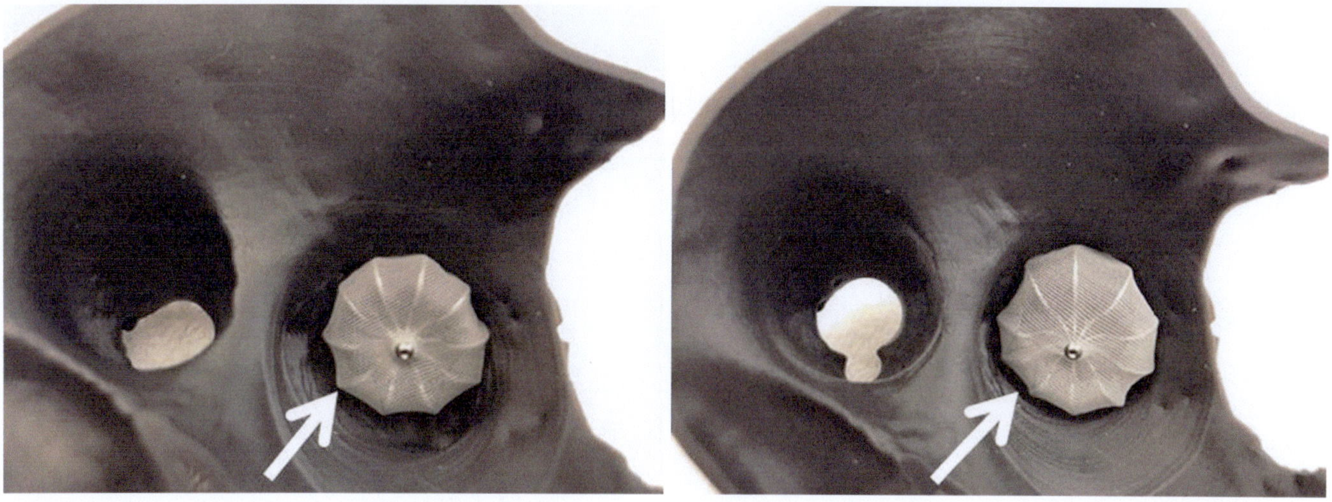

Fig. 36.5 3D printed models from CT data used to test various sizes of left atrial appendage occluder devices (white arrows) for prediction of leak around the device. Used with permission of Mayo Foundation for Medical Education and Research. All rights reserved

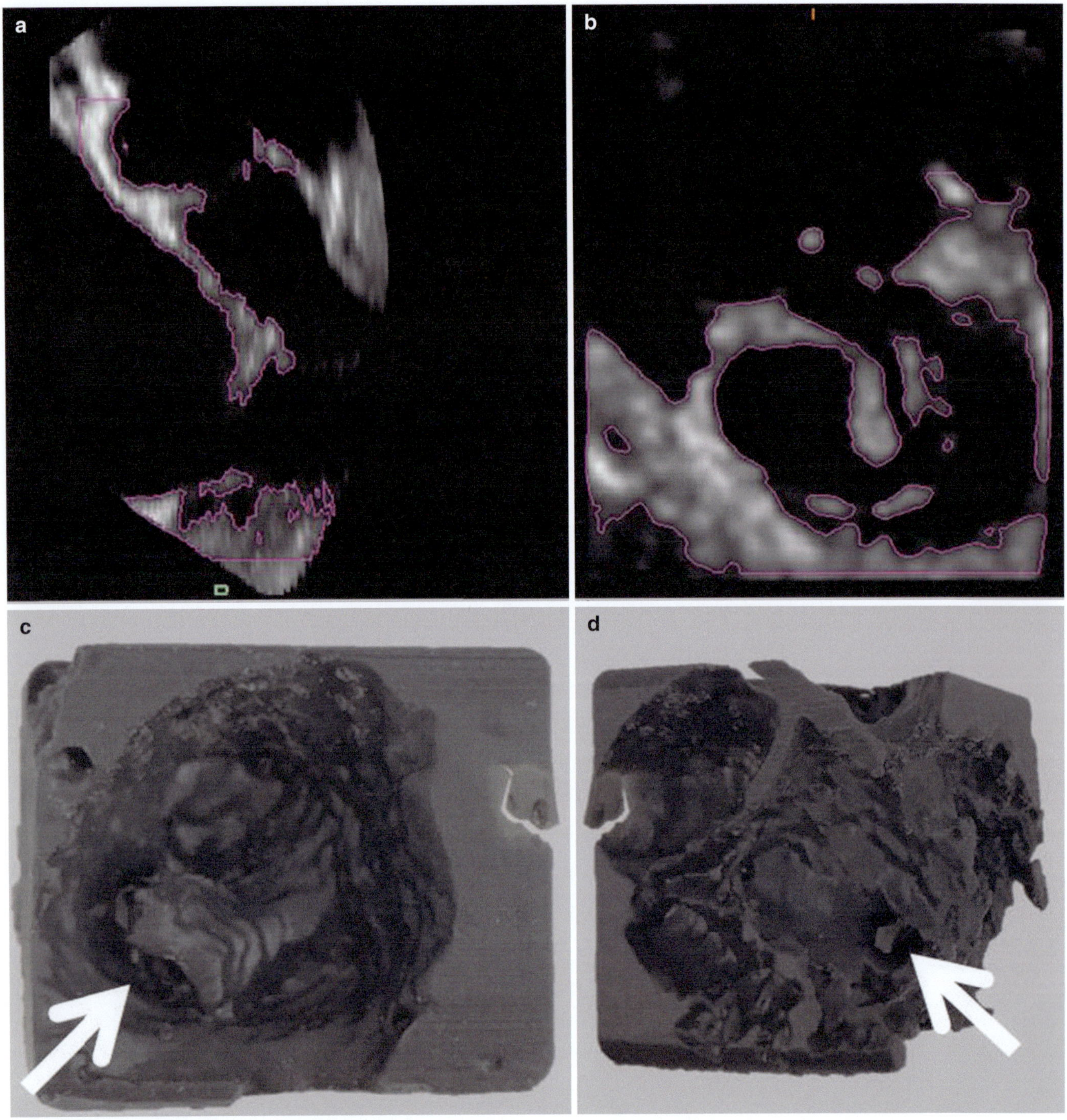

Fig. 36.6 Reformated images from a 3D transesophageal echocardiogram (**a** and **b**) showing valve anatomy segmented for printing (purple outline) in a patient with a history of endocarditis complicated by perforation and windsock deformity. 3D printed models from the same patient shown from the atrial (**c**) and ventricular (**d**) perpective showing the windsock deformity and perforation (white arrows). Used with permission of Mayo Foundation for Medical Education and Research. All rights reserved

References

1. Vukicevic M, Mosadegh B, Min JK, Little SH. Cardiac 3D printing and its future directions. JACC Cardiovasc Imaging. 2017;10(2):171–84.
2. Cabasa AS, Eleid MF, Rihal CS, Villaraga HR, Foley TA, Suri RM. Tricuspid valve replacement: a percutaneous transfemoral Valve-in-Ring approach. JACC Cardiovasc interv. 2015;8(8):1126–8.

MIX
Papier aus verantwortungsvollen Quellen
Paper from responsible sources
FSC® C105338

If you have any concerns about our products,
you can contact us on
ProductSafety@springernature.com

In case Publisher is established outside the EU,
the EU authorized representative is:
Springer Nature Customer Service Center GmbH
Europaplatz 3, 69115 Heidelberg, Germany

Printed by Libri Plureos GmbH
in Hamburg, Germany